OTHER PMIC TITLES OF INTEREST

CODING AND REIMBURSEMENT TITLES

Collections Made Easy!
CPT & HCPCS Coding Made Easy!
CPT Coding Guides by Medical Specialty
CPT Plus! Coders Choice®
DRG Plus!
E/M Coding Made Easy!
Getting Paid for What You Do
HCPCS Coders Choice®,
Health Insurance Carrier Directory
HIPAA Compliance Manual
ICD-9-CM, Coders Choice®,
ICD-9-CM Coding for Physicians' Offices
ICD-9-CM Coding Made Easy!
ICD-9-CM, Home Health Edition
Medical Fees in the United States
Medicare Compliance Manual
Medicare Rules & Regulations
Physicians Fee Guide
Reimbursement Manual for the Medical Office

PRACTICE MANAGEMENT TITLES

Accounts Receivable Management for the Medical Practice
Achieving Profitability With a Medical Office System
Encyclopedia of Practice and Financial Management
Managed Care Organizations
Managing Medical Office Personnel
Marketing Strategies for Physicians
Medical Marketing Handbook
Medical Office Policy Manual
Medical Practice Forms
Medical Practice Handbook
Medical Staff Privileges
Negotiating Managed Care Contracts
Patient Satisfaction
Performance Standards for the Laboratory
Professional and Practice Development
Promoting Your Medical Practice
Starting in Medical Practice
Working With Insurance and Managed Care Plans

OTHER PMIC TITLES OF INTEREST

RISK MANAGEMENT TITLES

Malpractice Depositions
Medical Risk Management
Preparing for Your Deposition
Preventing Emergency Malpractice
Testifying in Court

FINANCIAL MANAGEMENT TITLES

A Physician's Guide to Financial Independence
Business Ventures for Physicians
Financial Valuation of Your Practice
Personal Money Management for Physicians
Personal Pension Plan Strategies for Physicians
Securing Your Assets

DICTIONARIES AND OTHER REFERENCE TITLES

Dictionary of Coding & Billing Terminology
Drugs of Abuse
Health and Medicine on the Internet
Medical Acronyms and Abbreviations
Medical Phrase Index
Medical Word Building
Medico Mnemonica
Medico-Legal Glossary
Spanish/English Handbook for Medical Professionals

MEDICAL REFERENCE AND CLINICAL TITLES

Advance Medical Directives
Clinical Research Opportunities
Gastroenterology: Problems in Primary Care
Manual of IV Therapy
Medical Care of the Adolescent Athlete
Medical Procedures for Referral
Neurology: Problems in Primary Care
Orthopaedics: Problems in Primary Care
Patient Care Emergency Handbook
Patient Care Flowchart Manual
Patient Care Procedures for Your Practice
Physician's Office Laboratory
Pulmonary Medicine: Problems in Primary Care
Questions and Answers on AIDS

H•C•P•C•S

Health Care
Procedure Coding System

National Level II
Medicare Codes

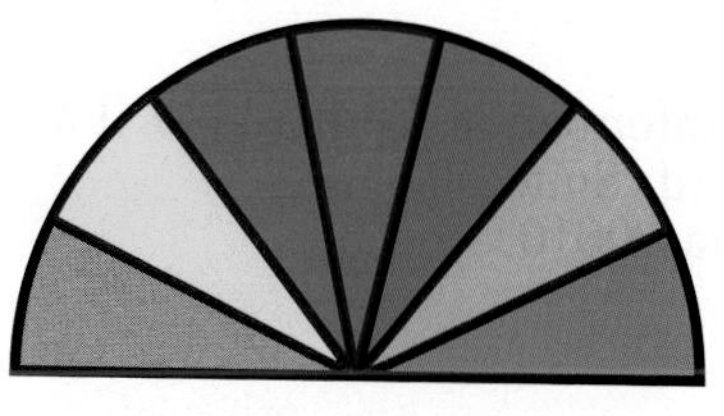

Color Coded

2014

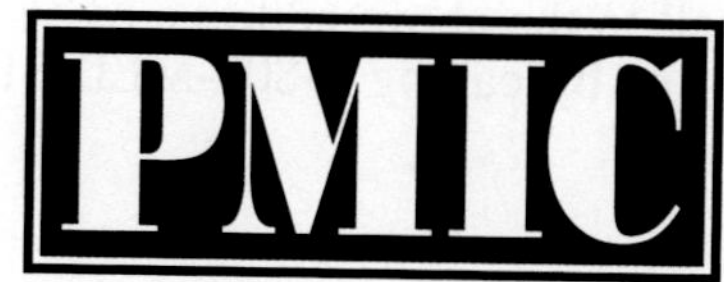

ISBN 978-1-936977-91-8 (Coder's Choice®)
ISBN 978-1-936977-89-5 (Spiral Bound)
ISBN 978-1-936977-92-5 (e-book)

Practice Management Information Corporation (PMIC)
4727 Wilshire Boulevard, Suite 300
Los Angeles, California 90010
1-800-MED-SHOP

http://pmiconline.com

Printed in China

Additional copies of this book may be purchased from any medical book store, from PMIC by mail to the above address, by visiting our web site at http://pmiconline.com or by calling 1-800-MED-SHOP.

FOREWORD

The Health Care Procedure Coding System (HCPCS), National Level II, is a listing of codes and descriptive terminology used for reporting the provision of supplies, materials, injections and certain services and procedures to Medicare. HCPCS 2014 is the most recent revision of the HCPCS National Level II codes. The changes that appear in this revision have been prepared by our editorial staff using the HCPCS revisions released by the Center for Medicare and Medicaid Services (CMS), which is overseen by the Department of Health and Human Services (DHHS). HCPCS National Level II codes are now effective January 1st of each year.

Even though HCPCS National Level II codes have been in use since 1983, there is still some confusion among health care professionals regarding when and how to use these codes instead of the more familiar CPT codes. In addition, due to what is known as "carrier discretion," the use, interpretation, and reimbursement policies for HCPCS National Level II codes, which should be uniform nationwide, vary from carrier to carrier.

One of our goals as a publisher is to educate our customers about the business of medicine. One of our most successful methods of accomplishing this goal is to create publications about new or unfamiliar concepts, such as HCPCS, that are similar in format and content to related publications, such as CPT. This provides our customers with an opportunity to learn and implement new concepts of vital importance to their medical practice using formats, conventions and terminology that they already use and understand.

James B. Davis, President

DISCLAIMER

This publication is designed to offer basic information regarding coding and billing of medical services, supplies and procedures using the HCPCS coding system. The information presented is based upon material obtained from the Center for Medicare and Medicaid Services (CMS), and the experience and interpretations of the editors and publisher. Though all of the information has been carefully researched and checked for accuracy and completeness, the publisher accepts no responsibility or liability with regard to errors, omissions, misuse or misinterpretation.

CONTENTS

INTRODUCTION

HCPCS is an acronym for Health Care Procedure Coding System. This coding system was developed in 1983 by the Health Care Financing Administration (HCFA) for the purpose of standardizing the coding systems used to process Medicare claims. In 2001, HCFA changed its name to the Center for Medicare and Medicaid Services (CMS) to reflect its increased emphasis on improving Medicare and Medicaid beneficiary services and information.

The HCPCS coding system is primarily used to bill Medicare for supplies, materials and injections. It is also used to bill for certain services and procedures which are not defined in CPT. HCPCS codes must be used when billing Medicare carriers, and in some states, Medicaid carriers. Some private insurance carriers also allow or mandate the use of HCPCS codes, mostly those that are processing Medicare claims.

STRUCTURE OF HCPCS

HCPCS is a systematic method for coding supplies, materials, injections and services performed by health care professionals. Each supply, material, injection or service is identified with a five digit alphanumeric code. With the HCPCS coding system, the supplies, materials and injections can be accurately identified and properly reimbursed. There are three levels of codes within the HCPCS coding system.

LEVEL I CPT CODES

The major portion of the HCPCS coding system, referred to as Level I, is CPT. Most of the procedures and services you perform, even for Medicare patients, are billed using CPT codes. However, one of the major deficiencies of CPT is that it has limited code selections to describe supplies, materials and injections.

LEVEL II NATIONAL CODES

HCPCS National Level II codes are alphanumeric codes which start with a letter followed by four numbers. The range of HCPCS National Level II codes is from A0000 through V0000. There are also HCPCS National Level II modifiers. HCPCS National Level II codes are uniform in description throughout the United States. However, due to what is known as “carrier discretion” the processing and reimbursement of HCPCS National Level II codes is not necessarily uniform.

There are over 2,400 HCPCS National Level II codes covering supplies, materials, injections and services. A fundamental understanding of when and how to use HCPCS National Level II or Local Level III codes can have a significant impact on your Medicare reimbursement. The majority of health care professionals use codes from the Medical and Surgical Supplies section and Drugs Administered by Other Than Oral Method, commonly referred to as "A" codes and "J" codes.

HCPCS CODE OVERLAP

As may be expected, there is some overlap among the three HCPCS code levels. On occasion you may have a coding situation where a specific code exists at all three levels for the same service or material. When faced with this situation, the general rule is that Local Level II codes have the highest priority, followed by CPT codes. You should consult your local Medicare carrier if you have any questions regarding HCPCS code overlap.

SECTIONS

The main body of HCPCS National Level II codes is divided into 22 sections. The supplies, materials, injections and services are presented in alphanumeric order within each section. The sections of HCPCS National Level II are:

Transportation Services	A0000-A0999
Medical And Surgical Supplies	A4000-A7509
Miscellaneous And Experimental	A9000-A9999
Enteral And Parenteral Therapy	B0000-B9999
Temporary Hospital Outpatient PPS	C0000-C9999
Durable Medical Equipment (DME)	E0000-E9999
Temporary Procedures & Professional Services	G0000-G9999
Rehabilitative Services	H0000-H9999
Drugs Administered Other Than Oral Method	J0000-J8999
Chemotherapy Drugs	J9000-J9999
Temporary Codes For DMERCS	K0000-K9999
Orthotic Procedures	L0000-L4999
Prosthetic Procedures	L5000-L9999
Medical Services	M0000-M9999
Pathology And Laboratory	P0000-P9999
Temporary Codes	Q0000-Q9999
Diagnostic Radiology Services	R0000-R9999
Private Payer Codes	S0000-S9999

State Medicaid Agency Codes	T0000-T9999
Vision Services	V0000-V2999
Hearing Services	V5000-V5999

INSTRUCTIONS FOR USE OF HCPCS NATIONAL LEVEL II CODES

A health care professional using the HCPCS National Level II codes selects the name of the material, supply, injection, service or procedure that most accurately identifies the service performed or supply delivered. Most often, HCPCS National Level II codes will be used instead of, or in addition to, CPT codes for visits, evaluation and management services, or other procedures performed at the same time or during the same visit. All services, procedures, supplies, materials and injections should be properly documented in the medical record.

The listing of a supply, material, injection or service and its code number in a specific section of HCPCS does not usually restrict its use to a specific profession or specialty group. However, there are some HCPCS National Level II codes that are by definition, profession or specialty specific.

FORMAT OF THE TERMINOLOGY

HCPCS National Level II terminology has been developed as stand-alone descriptions of supplies, materials, injections, services and procedures. However, some of the procedures in HCPCS National Level II are not printed in their entirety but refer back to a common portion of the procedure listed in a preceding entry. This is evident when an entry is followed by one or more indentations. For example:

L1610 Hip orthosis (HO), abduction control of hip joints; flexible, (Frejka cover only), prefabricated, includes fitting and adjustment

L1640 static, pelvic band or spreader bar, thigh cuffs, custom fabricated

Note that the common part of code L1610 (the part before the semicolon) should be considered part of code L1640. Therefore the full procedure description represented by code L1640 would read:

L1640 Hip orthosis (HO), abduction control of hip joints; static, pelvic band or spreader bar, thight cuffs, custom fabricated

GUIDELINES

Specific GUIDELINES are presented at the beginning of most of the sections. These GUIDELINES define items that are necessary to appropriately interpret and report the supplies, materials, injections, services and procedures listed in that section.

HCPCS MODIFIERS

A modifier provides the means by which the health care professional can indicate that a service or procedure that has been performed has been altered by some specific circumstance but not changed in its definition or code. HCPCS modifiers may be used to indicate the following:

- A service was supervised by an anesthesiologist
- A service was performed by a specific health care professional, for example, a clinical psychologist, clinical social worker, nurse practitioner, or physician assistant.
- A service was provided as part of a specific government program
- A service was provided to a specific side of the body
- Equipment was purchased or rented
- Single or multiple patients were seen during nursing home visits

It is important to note that HCPCS National Level II modifiers can be combined with CPT codes when reporting services to Medicare.

An example of the use of HCPCS National Level II modifiers is:

E1280-NR Heavy duty wheelchair; detachable arms (desk or full length) elevating leg rests - new when rented

A listing of modifiers pertinent to each section of HCPCS National Level II are located in the GUIDELINES of each section. A complete listing of HCPCS National Level II modifiers is found in APPENDIX A.

UNLISTED PROCEDURE OR SERVICE

A service or procedure may be provided that is not listed in this edition of HCPCS National Level II. When reporting such a service, the appropriate "unlisted procedure" code may be used to indicate the service, identifying it by "special report" as defined below. HCPCS National Level II terminology is inconsistent in defining unlisted procedures. The procedure definition may include the term(s) "unlisted," "not otherwise classified," "unspecified," "unclassified," "other" and "miscellaneous." Prior to using these codes, try to determine if a Local Level III or CPT code is available. When an unlisted procedure code is used, the supply, material, injection, service or procedure must be described. Each of these unlisted procedure codes relates to a specific section of HCPCS National Level II and is presented in the GUIDELINES of that section.

SPECIAL REPORT

A supply, material, injection, service or procedure that is rarely provided, unusual, variable or new may require a special report for reimbursement purposes. Pertinent information should include an adequate definition or description of the nature, extent, and need for the supply, material, injection, service or procedure.

HCPCS CODE CHANGES

Each year numerous codes are added, changed or deleted. A summary of revisions to HCPCS 2014 is found in APPENDIX B. The following symbols, identical to those used in CPT, are used to indicate additions, changes and deletions in HCPCS National Level II.

ADDITIONS TO HCPCS

New HCPCS National Level II codes are identified with a small black circle placed to the left of the code number. An example of a new code in HCPCS 2014 is:

● **C1841** Retinal prosthesis, includes all internal and external components

CHANGES TO HCPCS

Changes in HCPCS National Level II code definitions are identified with a small black triangle placed to the left of the code number. An example of a changed code in HCPCS 2014 is:

▲ **L3710** Elbow orthosis, elastic with metal joints, prefabricated, off-the-shelf

DELETIONS FROM HCPCS

Deleted HCPCS National Level II codes are enclosed within parentheses, along with an italicized reference to replacement codes when available. Examples of codes deleted from HCPCS 2014 are:

(C1204) Code deleted December 31, 2013. Use A9520

and

(Q0090) Code deleted December 31, 2013. Use J7301

PHYSICIAN QUALITY REVIEW SYSTEM (PQRS) INDICATOR

Ⓟ Indicates a code included in one or more PQRS measures. The specific measures may be found in Appendix E.

SPECIAL COVERAGE SYMBOLS

NOT VALID FOR MEDICARE

There are codes listed in HCPCS which are not valid for Medicare. These codes are identified by a red bar over the HCPCS code. These codes should not be used to report services to Medicare.

NON-COVERED BY MEDICARE

There are numerous supplies, materials, injections, services and procedures which are not covered by Medicare, either by program definition or by legislative statute. Examples of non-covered services include routine services and appliances, foot care and supportive devices for feet, custodial care, personal comfort items, and cosmetic surgery. These codes are identified by an orange bar over the HCPCS code. These codes should not be used to report services to Medicare; however, in most cases, you may bill the patient directly for non-covered services.

SPECIAL COVERAGE INSTRUCTIONS

Your local Medicare carrier has specific coverage instructions for processing certain HCPCS codes. These codes are identified by a yellow bar over the HCPCS code. While these codes are covered by the Medicare program, the use of these codes does not guarantee payment. If you have a question about a specific code in this category, review your Medicare provider manual or consult with your local Medicare carrier.

CARRIER DISCRETION

Processing and payment for these codes is done at the discretion of each insurance carrier. These codes are identified by a blue bar over the HCPCS code. For codes in this category, you should check with your Medicare carrier for proper billing instructions prior to filing an insurance claim.

DURABLE MEDICAL EQUIPMENT MEDICARE ADMINISTRATIVE CONTRACTORS (DME-MACs)

All Medicare claims for durable medical equipment (DME), prosthetics, orthotics and supplies go to one of four durable medical equipment Medicare administrative contractors, or DME-MACs (formerly known as DMERCs).

MEDICARE SUPPLIER NUMBER

Before submitting claims to DME-MACs, you must apply for a supplier number. You must use this number when submitting claims to all four carriers. To find out more information, go to the Medicare website at http://www.cms.gov.

REGIONALIZATION OF CLAIM PROCESSING

Listed below are the contracted carriers and the states that they serve. The residence of the beneficiary is what determines which regional carrier processes the claim.

Region A: CT, DE, DC, MA, MD, ME, NH, NJ, NY, PA, RI, VT

National Heritage Insurance Co
PO Box 9146
Hingham, MA 02043-9146
(866) 419-9458
(800) 633-4227
http://www.medicarenhic.com

Region B: IL, IN, KY, MI, MN, OH, WI

National Government Services
8115 Knue Road
PO Box 6036
Indianapolis, IN 46206
(877) 299-7900
http://www.ngsmedicare.com

Region C: AL, AR, CO, FL, GA, LA, MS, NM, NC, OK, PR, SC, TN, TX, VA, WV

Cigna Government Services
PO Box 20010
Nashville, TN 37202
(866) 270-4909
(866) 238-9650
http://www.cignagovernmentservices.com/jc

Region D: AK, AZ, CA, Guam, HI, IA, ID, KS, MO, MT, ND, NE, NV, OR, SD, UT, WA, WY

Noridian Mutual Insurance Co
901 40th St. South, Suite 1
Fargo, ND 58103
(866) 243-7272
http://www.noridianmedicare.com

CHANGE OF CLAIM JURISDICTION

Prior to October 1, 1993, Medicare carriers processed durable medical equipment (DME), prosthetics, and orthotics claims based on where the transaction for the sale or rental took place. This is called the point of sale. Beginning October 1, 1993 and according to the state by state transfer schedule, regional processing of supplier claims began using beneficiary residence to determine which regional carrier had claim jurisdiction.

ELECTRONIC CLAIM FILING

The Center for Medicare and Medicaid Services is strongly encouraging electronic claims submission to DME-MACs. Suppliers submitting claims electronic must use the designated National Standard Format which meets all Medicare billing requirements and is accepted by other third-party insurance carriers. The regional carriers will assist you in converting to electronic claims submission. You can contact the Electronic Media Coordinater (EMC) at the DME-MACs listed above.

APPENDICES

APPENDIX A: Modifiers: Lists all National Level II modifiers, ambulance service, and PET scan modifiers.

APPENDIX B: Summary of Changes: Includes a summary of official additions, changes, and deletions to the current edition of HCPCS.

APPENDIX C: Table of Drugs: Includes drug names, cross references along with selected dosage, administration route, and HCPCS codes from the official HCPCS Table of Drugs.

APPENDIX D: Medicare References: Includes the complete text from all Medicare Coverage Instruction Manual (CIM) and Medicare Carriers Manual (MCM) citations in the body of the HCPCS book.

APPENDIX E: Physician Quality Review System (PQRS) measures. Includes all PQRS measures that reference HCPCS codes.

HCPCS 2014 ON DISK

HCPCS codes are available on CD-ROM. The HCPCS short description datafile includes all official HCPCS codes with descriptions of 35 characters or fewer. The datafile can be uploaded to your PC for inclusion in billing programs. For more information regarding HCPCS codes on CD-ROM, call PMIC at 1-800-MED-SHOP or visit http://pmiconline.com.

TRANSPORTATION SERVICES

Guidelines

In addition to the information presented in the INTRODUCTION, several other items unique to this section are defined or identified here:

1. VEHICLE AND CREW REQUIREMENTS: The ambulance must be designed and equipped for transporting the sick or injured and include patient care equipment, such as a stretcher, clean linens, first aid supplies, oxygen equipment and other safety and lifesaving equipment required by state or local authorities. The ambulance crew must have two members, one of which has medical training equivalent to the standard and advanced Red Cross training. The vehicle and personnel supplier must provide a statement that describes the first-aid, safety and other patient-care items in the vehicle, the extent of first-aid training of the personnel and the supplier's agreement to notify Medicare of any changes that could affect coverage.

2. AIR AMBULANCE SERVICE: Air ambulance services are covered when the point of pick-up is inaccessible by land vehicle; distances or other obstacles are involved in getting the patient to the nearest hospital with appropriate facilities; and, all other conditions of coverage are met.

3. AMBULANCE SERVICE CLAIMS: Reimbursement may be made for expenses incurred for ambulance services when specific conditions have been met and the appropriate medical documentation is provided.

4. MATERIALS SUPPLIED BY AMBULANCE SERVICE: Reusable devices, such as back boards, neck boards and inflatable leg and arm splints, are considered part of general ambulance services and included in the charge for the trip. A separate reasonable charge may be recognized for non-reusable items and disposable supplies, such as oxygen, gauze and dressings, that are required for patient care during the trip.

5. UNLISTED SERVICE OR PROCEDURE: A service or procedure may be provided that is not listed in this edition of HCPCS. When reporting such a service, the appropriate "unlisted procedure" code may be used to indicate the service, identifying it by "special report" as defined below. HCPCS terminology is inconsistent in defining

unlisted procedures. The procedure definition may include the term(s) "unlisted", "not otherwise classified", "unspecified", "unclassified", "other" and "miscellaneous". Prior to using these codes, try to determine if a Local Level III code or CPT code is available. The "unlisted procedures" and accompanying codes for TRANSPORTATION SERVICES are as follows:

A0999 Unlisted ambulance service

6. SPECIAL REPORT: A service, material or supply that is rarely provided, unusual, variable or new may require a special report in determining medical appropriateness for reimbursement purposes. Pertinent information should include an adequate definition or description of the nature, extent, and need for the service, material or supply.

7. MODIFIERS: Listed services may be modified under certain circumstances. When appropriate, the modifying circumstance is identified by adding a modifier to the basic procedure code. CPT and HCPCS National Level II modifiers may be used with CPT and HCPCS National Level II procedure codes. One digit codes are to be used in combination. The first digit should indicate the origin; the second digit should indicate the destination.

   The Level II modifiers commonly used with TRANSPORTATION codes are as follows:

   -GM Multiple patients on one ambulance trip

   -QM Ambulance service provided under arrangement by a provider of services

   -QN Ambulance services furnished directly by a provider of services

   AMBULANCE SERVICE MODIFIERS

   For ambulance service, one-digit modifiers are combined to form a two-digit modifier that identifies the ambulance's place of origin with the first digit, and ambulance's destination with the second digit. They are used in items 12 and 13 on the CMS Form 1491.

   One digit ambulance modifiers:

-D Diagnostic or therapeutic site other than -P or -H when these are used as origin codes

-E Residential, domiciliary, custodial facility (other than an 1819 facility)

-G Hospital-based dialysis facility (hospital or hospital related)

-H Hospital

-I Site of transfer (for example, airport or helicopter pad) between types of ambulance

-J Non-hospital-based dialysis facility

-N Skilled nursing facility (SNF) (1819 facility)

-P Physician's office (includes HMO non-hospital facility, clinic, etc.)

-R Residence

-S Scene of accident or acute event

-X (Destination code only) Intermediate stop at physician's office on the way to the hospital (includes HMO non-hospital facility, clinic, etc.)

8. CPT CODE CROSS-REFERENCE: Unless specified otherwise, there is no equivalent CPT code for listings in this section.

Transportation Services Including Ambulance

A0021 Ambulance service; outside state per mile, transport (Medicaid only)

Ambulance Waiting Time Table

Units	Time (Hrs)	Units	Time (Hrs)
1	1/2 to 1	6	3 to 3 1/2
2	1 to 1 1/2	7	3 1/2 to 4
3	1 1/2 to 2	8	4 to 4 1/2
4	2 to 2 1/2	9	4 1/2 to 5
5	2 to 3	10	5 to 5 1/2

A0080 Non-emergency transportation, per mile—vehicle provided by volunteer (individual or organization), with no vested interest

A0090 Non-emergency transportation, per mile—vehicle provided by individual (family member, self, neighbor) with vested interest

A0100 Non-emergency transportation; taxi

A0110 Non-emergency transportation and bus, intra or inter state carrier

A0120 Non-emergency transportation: mini-bus, mountain area transports, or other transportation systems

A0130 Non-emergency transportation: wheel-chair van

A0140 Non-emergency transportation and air travel (private or commercial) intra or inter state

A0160 Non-emergency transportation: per mile—case worker or social worker

A0170 Transportation ancillary: parking fees, tolls, other

A0180 Non-emergency transportation; ancillary: lodging-recipient

A0190 ancillary: meals-recipient

A0200 ancillary: lodging-escort

A0210 ancillary: meals-escort

A0225 Ambulance service; neonatal transport, base rate, emergency transport, one way

A0380 BLS mileage (per mile); Medicare use A0425

A0382 BLS routine disposable supplies

A0384 BLS specialized service disposable supplies, defibrillation (used by ALS ambulances and BLS ambulances in jurisdictions where defibrillation is permitted in BLS ambulances)

A0390 ALS mileage (per mile); Medicare use A0425

A0392 ALS specialized service disposable supplies; defibrillation (to be used only in jurisdictions where defibrillation cannot be performed in BLS ambulances)

A0394 ALS specialized service disposable supplies; IV drug therapy

A0396 ALS specialized service disposable supplies; esophageal intubation

A0398 ALS routine disposable supplies

A0420 Ambulance waiting time (ALS or BLS), one-half (1/2) hour increments

A0422 Ambulance (ALS or BLS) oxygen and oxygen supplies, life sustaining situation

A0424 Extra ambulance attendant, ground (ALS or BLS) or air (fixed or rotary winged); (requires medical review)

A0425 Ground mileage, per statue mile

A0426 Ambulance service, advanced life support, non-emergency transport, level 1 (ALS1)

A0427 Ambulance service, advanced life support, emergency transport, level 1 (ALS1-emergency)

A0428 Ambulance service, basic life support, non-emergency transport (BLS)

A0429 Ambulance service, basic life support, emergency transport (BLS-emergency)

A0430 Ambulance service, conventional air services, transport, one way (fixed wing)

A0431 Ambulance service, conventional air services, transport, one way (rotary wing)

A0432 Paramedic intercept (PI), rural area, transport furnished by a volunteer ambulance company which is prohibited by state law from billing third party payers

A0433 Advanced life support, level 2 (ALS2)

A0434 Specialty care transport (SCT)

A0435 Fixed wing air mileage, per statute mile

A0436 Rotary wing air mileage, per statute mile

A0888 Noncovered ambulance mileage, per mile (e.g., for miles traveled beyond closest appropriate facility)
MCM: 2125

A0998 Ambulance response and treatment, no transport

A0999 Unlisted ambulance service
MCM: 2120.1, 2125

MEDICAL AND SURGICAL SUPPLIES

Guidelines

In addition to the information presented in the INTRODUCTION, several other items unique to this section are defined or identified here:

1. SUBSECTION INFORMATION: Some of the listed subheadings or subsections have special needs or instructions unique to that section. Where these are indicated, special "notes" will be presented preceding or following the listings. Those subsections within the MEDICAL AND SURGICAL SUPPLIES section that have "notes" are as follows:

Subsection	Code Numbers
External urinary supplies	A4356-A4358
Tracheostomy supplies	A4622-A4626
Supplies for ESRD	A4650-A4927

2. UNLISTED SERVICE OR PROCEDURE: A service or procedure may be provided that is not listed in this edition of HCPCS. When reporting such a service, the appropriate "unlisted procedure" code may be used to indicate the service, identifying it by "special report" as defined below. HCPCS terminology is inconsistent in defining unlisted procedures. The procedure definition may include the term(s) "unlisted", "not otherwise classified", "unspecified", "unclassified", "other" and "miscellaneous". Prior to using these codes, try to determine if a Local Level III code or CPT code is available. The "unlisted procedures" and accompanying codes for MEDICAL AND SURGICAL SUPPLIES are as follows:

A4335	Incontinence supply; miscellaneous
A4421	Ostomy supply; miscellaneous
A4649	Surgical supply; miscellaneous
A4913	Miscellaneous dialysis supplies, not otherwise specified
A6261	Wound filler, gel/paste, per fluid ounce, not elsewhere classified
A6262	Wound filler, dry foam, per gram, not elsewhere classified

3. SPECIAL REPORT: A service, material or supply that is rarely provided, unusual, variable or new may require a special report in determining medical appropriateness for reimbursement purposes.

Pertinent information should include an adequate definition or description of the nature, extent, and need for the service, material or supply.

4. MODIFIERS: Listed services may be modified under certain circumstances. When appropriate, the modifying circumstance is identified by adding a modifier to the basic procedure code. CPT and HCPCS National Level II modifiers may be used with CPT and HCPCS National Level II procedure codes. Modifiers commonly used with MEDICAL AND SURGICAL SUPPLIES are as follows:

   -CC Procedure code change (use "CC" when the procedure code submitted was changed either for administrative reasons or because an incorrect code was filed)

   -LT Left side (used to identify procedures performed on the left side of the body)

   -RT Right side (used to identify procedures performed on the right side of the body)

5. CPT CODE CROSS-REFERENCE: Unless specified otherwise, the equivalent CPT code for all listings in this section is 99070.

6. DURABLE MEDICAL EQUIPMENT REGIONAL CARRIERS (DMERCS): Effective October 1, 1993 claims for supplies must be billed to one of four regional carriers depending upon the residence of the beneficiary. The transition dates for DMERC claims is from November 1, 1993 to March 1, 1994, also depending upon the state you practice in. See the Introduction for a complete discussion of DMERCs.

Medical and Surgical Supplies

A4206 Syringe with needle; sterile 1cc or less, each

A4207 sterile 2cc, each

A4208 sterile 3cc, each

A4209 sterile 5cc or greater, each

A4210 Needle-free injection device, each
CIM: 60-9

A4211 Supplies for self-administered injections
MCM: 2049

A4212 Non-coring needle or stylet with or without catheter

A4213 Syringe, sterile, 20cc or greater, each

A4215 Needle, sterile, any size, each

A4216 Sterile water, saline and/or dextrose (diluent/flush), 10 ml
MCM: 2049

A4217 Sterile water/saline, 500 ml
MCM: 2049

A4218 Sterile saline or water, metered dose dispenser, 10 ml

A4220 Refill kit for implantable infusion pump
CIM: 60-14

A4221 Supplies for maintenance of drug infusion catheter, per week (list drug separately)

A4222 Infusion supplies for external drug infusion pump, per cassette or bag (list drugs separately)

A4223 Infusion supplies not used with external infusion pump, per cassette or bag (list drugs separately)

A4230 Infusion set for external insulin pump, non needle cannula type
CIM: 60-14

A4231 Infusion set for external insulin pump, needle type
CIM: 60-14

A4232 Syringe with needle for external insulin pump, sterile, 3cc
CIM: 60-14

A4233 Replacement battery, alkaline (other than j cell), for use with medically necessary home blood glucose monitor owned by patient, each

A4234 Replacement battery, alkaline, j cell, for use with medically necessary home blood glucose monitor owned by patient, each

A4235 Replacement battery, lithium, for use with medically necessary home blood glucose monitor owned by patient, each

A4236 Replacement battery, silver oxide, for use with medically necessary home blood glucose monitor owned by patient, each

A4244 Alcohol or peroxide, per pint

A4245 Alcohol wipes, per box

A4246 Betadine or phisohex solution, per pint

A4247 Betadine or iodine swabs/wipes, per box

A4248 Chlorhexidine containing antiseptic, 1 ml

A4250 Urine test or reagent strips or tablets (100 tablets or strips)
MCM: 2100

A4252 Blood ketone test or reagent strip, each

A4253 Blood glucose test or reagent strips for home blood glucose monitor, per 50 strips
CIM: 60-11

A4255 Platforms for home blood glucose monitor, 50 per box
CIM: 60-11

A4256 Normal, low and high calibrator solution/chips
CIM: 60-11

A4257 Replacement lens shield cartridge for use with laser skin piercing device, each

A4258 Spring-powered device for lancet, each
CIM: 60-11

A4259 Lancets, per box of 100
CIM: 60-11

A4261 Cervical cap for contraceptive use

A4262 Temporary, absorbable lacrimal duct implant, each

A4263 Permanent, long term, non-dissolvable lacrimal duct implant, each
MCM: 15030

A4264 Permanent implantable contraceptive intratubal occlusion device(s) and delivery system

A4265 Paraffin, per pound
CIM: 60-9

A4266 Diaphragm for contraceptive use

A4267 Contraceptive supply, condom, male, each

A4268 Contraceptive supply, condom, female, each

A4269 Contraceptive supply, spermicide (e.g., Foam, gel), each

A4270 Disposable endoscope sheath, each

A4280 Adhesive skin support attachment for use with external breast prosthesis, each

A4281 Tubing for breast pump, replacement

A4282 Adapter for breast pump, replacement

A4283 Cap for breast pump bottle, replacement

A4284 Breast shield and splash protector for use with breast pump, replacement

A4285 Polycarbonate bottle for use with breast pump, replacement

A4286 Locking ring for breast pump, replacement

A4290 Sacral nerve stimulation test lead, each

VASCULAR CATHETERS

A4300 Implantable access catheter, (eg, venous, arterial, epidural subarachnoid, or peritoneal, etc) External access
MCM: 2130

A4301 Implantable access total catheter, port/reservoir (eg, venous, arterial, epidural, subarachnoid, peritoneal, etc.)

A4305 Disposable drug delivery system, flow rate of 50 ml or greater per hour

A4306 Disposable drug delivery system, flow rate of less than 50 ml per hour

Not valid for Medicare | Non-covered by Medicare | Special coverage instructions | Carrier discretion

INCONTINENCE APPLIANCES AND CARE SUPPLIES

A4310 Insertion tray without drainage bag; and without catheter (accessories only)
MCM: 2130

A4311 Insertion tray without drainage bag; with indwelling catheter, foley type, two-way latex with coating (teflon, silicone, silicone elastomer or hydrophilic, etc.)
MCM: 2130

A4312 with indwelling catheter, foley type, two-way, all silicone
MCM: 2130

A4313 with indwelling catheter, foley type, three-way, for continuous irrigation
MCM: 2130

A4314 Insertion tray with drainage bag; with indwelling catheter, foley type, two-way latex with coating (teflon, silicone, silicone elastomer or hydrophilic, etc.)
MCM: 2130

A4315 with indwelling catheter, foley type, two-way, all silicone
MCM: 2130

A4316 with indwelling catheter, foley type, three-way, for continuous irrigation
MCM: 2130

A4320 Irrigation tray with bulb or piston syringe, any purpose
MCM: 2130

A4321 Therapeutic agent for urinary catheter irrigation
MCM: 2130

A4322 Irrigation syringe, bulb or piston, each
MCM: 2130

A4326 Male external catheter specialty type with integral collection chamber, any type, each
MCM: 2130

A4327 Female external urinary collection device; meatal cup, each
MCM: 2130

A4328 pouch, each
MCM: 2130

A4330 Perianal fecal collection pouch with adhesive, each
MCM: 2130

A4331 Extension drainage tubing, any type, any length, with connector/adaptor, for use with urinary leg bag or urostomy pouch, each
MCM: 2130

A4332 Lubricant, individual sterile packet, each
MCM: 2130

A4333 Urinary catheter anchoring device, adhesive skin attachment, each
MCM: 2130

A4334 Urinary catheter anchoring device, leg strap, each
MCM: 2130

A4335 Incontinence supply; miscellaneous
MCM: 2130

A4336 Incontinence supply, urethral insert, any type, each

A4338 Indwelling catheter; foley type, two-way latex with coating (teflon, silicone, silicone elastomer, or hydrophilic, etc.), each
MCM: 2130

A4340 Indwelling catheter; specialty type, (e.g.; coude, mushroom, wing, etc.), each
MCM: 2130

A4344 Indwelling catheter, foley type; two-way all silicone, each
MCM: 2130

A4346 three-way for continuous irrigation, each
MCM: 2130

A4349 Male external catheter, with or without adhesive, disposable, each
MCM: 2130

A4351 Intermittent urinary catheter; straight tip, with or without coating (teflon, silicone, silicone elastomer, or hydrophilic, etc), each
MCM: 2130

A4352 Intermittent urinary catheter; coude (curved) tip, with or without coating (teflon, silicone, silicone elastomer, or hydrophilic, etc), each
MCM: 2130

A4353 Intermittent urinary catheter, with insertion supplies
MCM: 2130

A4354 Insertion tray with drainage bag, but without catheter
MCM: 2130

A4355 Irrigation tubing set for continuous bladder irrigation through a three-way indwelling foley catheter, each
MCM: 2130

EXTERNAL URINARY SUPPLIES

A4356 External urethral clamp or compression device (not to be used for catheter clamp), each
MCM: 2130

A4357 Bedside drainage bag, day or night with or without anti-reflux device, with or without tube, each
MCM: 2130

A4358 Urinary drainage bag, leg or abdomen, vinyl, with or without tube, with straps, each
MCM: 2130

NOTE: See DME section for male or female urinals

OSTOMY SUPPLIES

A4360 Disposable external urethral clamp or compression device, with pad and/or pouch, each

A4361 Ostomy faceplate, each
MCM: 2130

A4362 Skin barrier; solid, 4 x 4 or equivalent; each
MCM: 2130

A4363 Ostomy clamp, any type, replacement only, each

A4364 Adhesive, liquid or equal, any type, per ounce
MCM: 2130

A4366 Ostomy vent, any type, each

A4367 Ostomy belt, each
MCM: 2130.A

A4368 Ostomy filter, any type, each

A4369 Ostomy skin barrier, liquid (spray, brush, etc.), per oz.
MCM: 2130

A4371 Ostomy skin barrier, powder, per oz.
MCM: 2130

A4372 Ostomy skin barrier, solid 4x4 or equivalent, standard wear, with built-in convexity, each
MCM: 2130

A4373 Ostomy skin barrier, with flange (solid, flexible or accordion), with built-in convexity, any size, each
MCM: 2130

A4375 Ostomy pouch, drainable, with faceplate attached, plastic, each
MCM: 2130

A4376 Ostomy pouch, drainable, with faceplate attached, rubber each
MCM: 2130

A4377 Ostomy pouch, drainable, for use on faceplate, plastic, each
MCM: 2130

A4378 Ostomy pouch, drainable, for use on faceplate, rubber, each
MCM: 2130

A4379 Ostomy pouch, urinary, with faceplate attached, plastic, each
MCM: 2130

A4380 Ostomy pouch, urinary, with faceplate attached, rubber, each
MCM: 2130

A4381 Ostomy pouch, urinary, for use on faceplate, plastic, each
MCM: 2130

A4382 Ostomy pouch, urinary, for use on faceplate, heavy plastic, each
MCM: 2130

A4383 Ostomy pouch, urinary, for use on faceplate, rubber, each
MCM: 2130

A4384 Ostomy faceplate equivalent, silicone ring, each
MCM: 2130

A4385 Ostomy skin barrier, solid 4x4 or equivalent, extended wear, without built-in convexity, each
MCM: 2130

A4387 Ostomy pouch, closed, with barrier attached, with built-in convexity (1 piece), each
MCM: 2130

A4388 Ostomy pouch, drainable, with extended wear barrier attached, (1 piece), each
MCM: 2130

A4389 Ostomy pouch, drainable, with barrier attached, with built-in convexity (1 piece), each
MCM: 2130

A4390 Ostomy pouch, drainable, with extended wear barrier attached, with built-in convexity (1 piece), each
MCM: 2130

A4391 Ostomy pouch, urinary, with extended wear barrier attached, (1 piece), each
MCM: 2130

A4392 Ostomy pouch, urinary, with standard wear barrier attached, with built-in convexity (1 piece), each
MCM: 2130

A4393 Ostomy pouch, urinary, with extended wear barrier attached, with built-in convexity (1 piece), each
MCM: 2130

A4394 Ostomy deodorant, with or without lubricant, for use in ostomy pouch, per fluid ounce
MCM: 2130

A4395 Ostomy deodorant for use in ostomy pouch, solid, per tablet
MCM: 2130

A4396 Ostomy belt with peristomal hernia support
MCM: 2130

A4397 Irrigation supply; sleeve, each
MCM: 2130

A4398 Ostomy irrigation supply; bag, each
MCM: 2130

A4399 cone/catheter, with or without brush
MCM: 2130

A4400 Ostomy irrigation set
MCM: 2130

A4402 Lubricant, per ounce
MCM: 2130

A4404 Ostomy ring, each
MCM: 2130

A4405 Ostomy skin barrier, non-pectin based, paste, per ounce
MCM: 2130

A4406 Ostomy skin barrier, pectin-based, paste, per ounce
MCM: 2130

A4407 Ostomy skin barrier, with flange (solid, flexible, or accordion), extended wear, with built-in convexity, 4 x 4 inches or smaller, each
MCM: 2130

A4408 Ostomy skin barrier, with flange (solid, flexible or accordion), extended wear, with built-in convexity, larger than 4 x 4 inches, each
MCM: 2130

A4409 Ostomy skin barrier, with flange (solid, flexible or accordion), extended wear, without built-in convexity, 4 x 4 inches or smaller, each
MCM: 2130

A4410 Ostomy skin barrier, with flange (solid, flexible or accordion), extended wear, without built-in convexity, larger than 4 x 4 inches, each
MCM: 2130

A4411 Ostomy skin barrier, solid 4x4 or equivalent, extended wear, with built-in convexity, each

A4412 Ostomy pouch, drainable, high output, for use on a barrier with flange (2 piece system), without filter, each
MCM: 2130

A4413 Ostomy pouch, drainable, high output, for use on a barrier with flange (2 piece system), with filter, each
MCM: 2130

A4414 Ostomy skin barrier, with flange (solid, flexible or accordion), without built-in convexity, 4 x 4 inches or smaller, each
MCM: 2130

A4415 Ostomy skin barrier, with flange (solid, flexible or accordion), without built-in convexity, larger than 4x4 inches, each
MCM: 2130

A4416 Ostomy pouch, closed, with barrier attached, with filter (1 piece), each

A4417 Ostomy pouch, closed, with barrier attached, with built-in convexity, with filter (1 piece), each

A4418 Ostomy pouch, closed; without barrier attached, with filter (1 piece), each

A4419 Ostomy pouch, closed; for use on barrier with non-locking flange, with filter (2 piece), each

A4420 Ostomy pouch, closed; for use on barrier with locking flange (2 piece), each

A4421 Ostomy supply; miscellaneous

A4422 Ostomy absorbent material (sheet/pad/crystal packet) for use in ostomy pouch to thicken liquid stomal output, each
MCM: 2130

A4423 Ostomy pouch, closed; for use on barrier with locking flange, with filter (2 piece), each

A4424 Ostomy pouch, drainable, with barrier attached, with filter (1 piece), each

A4425 Ostomy pouch, drainable; for use on barrier with non-locking flange, with filter (2 piece system), each

A4426 Ostomy pouch, drainable; for use on barrier with locking flange (2 piece system), each

A4427 Ostomy pouch, drainable; for use on barrier with locking flange, with filter (2 piece system), each

A4428 Ostomy pouch, urinary, with extended wear barrier attached, with faucet-type tap with valve (1 piece), each

A4429 Ostomy pouch, urinary, with barrier attached, with built-in convexity, with faucet-type tap with valve (1 piece), each

A4430 Ostomy pouch, urinary, with extended wear barrier attached, with built-in convexity, with faucet-type tap with valve (1 piece), each

A4431 Ostomy pouch, urinary; with barrier attached, with faucet-type tap with valve (1 piece), each

A4432 Ostomy pouch, urinary; for use on barrier with non-locking flange, with faucet-type tap with valve (2 piece), each

A4433 Ostomy pouch, urinary; for use on barrier with locking flange (2 piece), each

A4434 Ostomy pouch, urinary; for use on barrier with locking flange, with faucet-type tap with valve (2 piece), each

A4435 Ostomy pouch, drainable, high output, with extended wear barrier (one-piece system), with or without filter, each

SUPPLIES

A4450 Tape, non-waterproof, per 18 square inches
MCM: 2130

A4452 Tape, waterproof, per 18 square inches
MCM: 2130

A4455 Adhesive remover or solvent (for tape, cement or other adhesive), per ounce
MCM: 2130

A4456 Adhesive remover, wipes, any type, each
MCM: 2130

A4458 Enema bag with tubing, reusable

A4461 Surgical dressing holder, non-reusable, each

A4463 Surgical dressing holder, reusable, each

A4465 Non-elastic binder for extremity

A4466 Garment, belt, sleeve or other covering, elastic or similar stretchable material, any type, each

A4470 Gravlee jet washer
CIM: 50-4 MCM: 2320

A4480 Vabra aspirator
CIM: 50-10 MCM: 2320

A4481 Tracheostoma filter, any type, any size, each
MCM: 2130

A4483 Moisture exchanger, disposable, for use with invasive mechanical ventilation
MCM: 2130

A4490 Surgical stockings; above knee length, each
CIM: 60-9 MCM: 2079, 2100

A4495 thigh length, each
CIM: 60-9 MCM: 2079, 2100

A4500 below knee length, each
CIM: 60-9 MCM: 2079, 2100

A4510 full length, each
CIM: 60-9 MCM: 2079, 2100

A4520 Incontinence garment, any type (e.g. brief, diaper), each
CIM: 60-9

A4550 Surgical trays
MCM: 15030

A4554 Disposable underpads, all sizes
CIM: 60-9

● **A4555** Electrode/transducer for use with electrical stimulation device used for cancer treatment, replacement only

A4556 Electrodes, (e.g., apnea monitor), per pair

A4557 Lead wires, (e.g., apnea monitor), per pair

A4558 Conductive gel or paste, for use with electrical device (e.g., tens, nmes), per oz.

A4559 Coupling gel or paste, for use with ultrasound device, per oz

A4561 Pessary, rubber, any type

A4562 Pessary, non rubber, any type

A4565 Slings

A4566 Shoulder sling or vest design, abduction restrainer, with or without swathe control, prefabricated, includes fitting and adjustment

A4570 Splint
MCM: 2079

A4575 Topical hyperbaric oxygen chamber, disposable
CIM: 35-10

A4580 Cast supplies (e.g., plaster)
MCM: 2079

A4590 Special casting materials (e.g., fiberglass)
MCM: 2079

A4595 Electrical stimulator supplies, 2 lead, per month, (e.g. TENS, NMES)
CIM: 45-25

SUPPLIES FOR OXYGEN AND RELATED RESPIRATORY EQUIPMENT

A4600 Sleeve for intermittent limb compression device, replacement only, each

A4601 Lithium ion battery for non-prosthetic use, replacement

A4604 Tubing with integrated heating element for use with positive airway pressure device

A4605 Tracheal suction catheter, closed system, each

A4606 Oxygen probe for use with oximeter device, replacement

A4608 Transtracheal oxygen catheter, each

A4611 Battery, heavy duty; replacement for patient-owned ventilator

A4612 Battery cables; replacement for patient-owned ventilator

A4613 Battery charger; replacement for patient-owned ventilator

A4614 Peak expiratory flow rate meter, hand held

A4615 Cannula, nasal
CIM: 60-4 MCM: 3312

A4616 Tubing (oxygen), per foot
CIM: 60-4 MCM: 3312

A4617 Mouth piece
CIM: 60-4 MCM: 3312

A4618 Breathing circuits
CIM: 60-4 MCM: 3312

A4619 Face tent
CIM: 60-4 MCM: 3312

A4620 Variable concentration mask
CIM: 60-4 MCM: 3312

A4623 Tracheostomy, inner cannula
CIM: 65-16 MCM: 2130

A4624 Tracheal suction catheter, any type other than closed system, each

A4625 Tracheostomy care kit for new tracheostomy
MCM: 2130

A4626 Tracheostomy cleaning brush, each
MCM: 2130

NOTE: All of the descriptions for tracheostomy supplies, codes A4622-A4626 are "per item". The correct number of items purchased must be entered in the days or units field (box 24-G) on the CMS1500 claim form. The terms "items" and "units" are used interchangeably.

A4627 Spacer, bag or reservoir, with or without mask, for use with metered dose inhaler
MCM: 2100

A4628 Oropharyngeal suction catheter, each

A4629 Tracheostomy care kit for established tracheostomy
MCM: 2130

SUPPLIES FOR OTHER DURABLE MEDICAL EQUIPMENT

A4630 Replacement batteries, medically necessary, transcutaneous electrical stimulator, owned by patient
CIM: 65-8

A4633 Replacement bulb/lamp for ultraviolet light therapy system, each

A4634 Replacement bulb for therapeutic light box, tabletop model

A4635 Underarm pad, crutch, replacement, each
CIM: 60-9

A4636 Replacement, handgrip, cane, crutch, or walker, each
CIM: 60-9

A4637 Replacement, tip, cane, crutch, walker, each
CIM: 60-9

A4638 Replacement battery for patient-owned ear pulse generator, each

A4639 Replacement pad for infrared heating pad system, each

A4640 Replacement pad for use with medically necessary alternating pressure pad owned by patient
CIM: 60-9 MCM: 4107.6

SUPPLIES FOR RADIOLOGICAL PROCEDURES

A4641 Radiopharmaceutical, diagnostic, not otherwise classified

A4642 Indium IN-111 satumomab pendetide, diagnostic, per study dose, up to 6 millicuries

A4648 Tissue marker, implantable, any type, each

A4649 Surgical supply, miscellaneous

SUPPLIES FOR ESRD

NOTE: For DME items for ESRD see procedure codes D1500-E1699. For dialysis Procedures, see M0900-M0999.

A4650 Implantable radiation dosimeter, each

A4651 Calibrated microcapillary tube, each
MCM: 4270

A4652 Microcapillary tube sealant
MCM: 4270

A4653 Peritoneal dialysis catheter anchoring device, belt, each

A4657 Syringe, with or without needle, each
MCM: 4270

A4660 Sphygmomanometer/blood pressure apparatus with cuff and stethoscope
MCM: 4270

A4663 Blood pressure cuff only
MCM: 4270

A4670 Automatic blood pressure monitor
CIM: 50-42 MCM: 4270

A4671 Disposable cycler set used with cycler dialysis machine, each
MCM: 4270

A4672 Drainage extension line, sterile, for dialysis, each
MCM: 4270

A4673 Extension line with easy lock connectors, used with dialysis
MCM: 4270

A4674 Chemicals/antiseptics solution used to clean/sterilize dialysis equipment, per 8 oz.
MCM: 4270

A4680 Activated carbon filter for hemodialysis, each
CIM: 55-1 MCM: 4270

A4690 Dialyzer (artificial kidneys), all types, all sizes, for hemodialysis, each
MCM: 4270

A4706 Bicarbonate concentrate, solution, for hemodialysis, per gallon
MCM: 4270

A4707 Bicarbonate concentrate, powder, for hemodialysis, per packet

MCM: 4270

A4708 Acetate concentrate solution, for hemodialysis, per gallon
MCM: 4270

A4709 Acid concentrate solution, for hemodialysis, per gallon
MCM: 4270

A4714 Treated water (deionized, distilled, or reverse osmosis) for peritoneal dialysis, per gallon
CIM: 55-1 MCM: 4270

A4719 Y set tubing for peritoneal dialysis
MCM: 4270

A4720 Dialysate solution, any concentration of dextrose, fluid volume greater than 249cc, but less than or equal to 999cc, for peritoneal dialysis
MCM: 4270

A4721 Dialysate solution, any concentration of dextrose, fluid volume greater than 999cc, but less than or equal to 1999cc, for peritoneal dialysis
MCM: 4270

A4722 Dialysate solution, any concentration of dextrose, fluid volume greater than 1999cc, but less than or equal to 2999cc, for peritoneal dialysis
MCM: 4270

A4723 Dialysate solution, any concentration of dextrose, fluid volume greater than 2999cc, but less than or equal to 3999cc, for peritoneal dialysis
MCM: 4270

A4724 Dialysate solution, any concentration of dextrose, fluid volume greater than 3999cc, but less than or equal to 4999cc, for peritoneal dialysis
MCM: 4270

A4725 Dialysate solution, any concentration of dextrose, fluid volume greater than 4999cc, but less than or equal to 5999cc, for peritoneal dialysis
MCM: 4270

A4726 Dialysate solution, any concentration of dextrose, fluid volume greater than 5999cc, for peritoneal dialysis
MCM: 4270

A4728 Dialysate solution, non-dextrose containing, 500 ml

Not valid for Medicare | Non-covered by Medicare | Special coverage instructions | Carrier discretion

A4730 Fistula cannulation set for hemodialysis, each
MCM: 4270

A4736 Topical anesthetic, for dialysis, per gram
MCM: 4270

A4737 Injectable anesthetic, for dialysis, per 10 ml
MCM: 4270

A4740 Shunt accessory, for hemodialysis, any type, each
MCM: 4270

A4750 Blood tubing, arterial or venous, for hemodialysis, each
MCM: 4270

A4755 Blood tubing, arterial and venous combined, for hemodialysis, each
MCM: 4270

A4760 Dialysate solution test kit, for peritoneal dialysis, any type, each
MCM: 4270

A4765 Dialysate concentrate, powder, additive for peritoneal dialysis, per packet
MCM: 4270

A4766 Dialysate concentrate, solution, additive for peritoneal dialysis, per 10 ml
MCM: 4270

A4770 Blood collection tube, vacuum, for dialysis, per 50
MCM: 4270

A4771 Serum clotting time tube, for dialysis, per 50
MCM: 4270

A4772 Blood glucose test strips, for dialysis, per 50
MCM: 4270

A4773 Occult blood test strips, for dialysis, per 50
MCM: 4270

A4774 Ammonia test strips, for dialysis, per 50
MCM: 4270

A4802 Protamine sulfate, for hemodialysis, per 50 mg
MCM: 4270

A4860 Disposable catheter tips for peritoneal dialysis, per 10
MCM: 4270

A4870 Plumbing and/or electrical work for home hemodialysis equipment
MCM: 4270

A4890 Contracts, repair and maintenance, for hemodialysis equipment
MCM: 2100.4

NOTE: The above procedure includes the following: scale, scissors, stopwatch, surgical brush, thermometer, tool kit, tourniquet, tube occluding forceps/clamps.

A4911 Drain bag/bottle, for dialysis, each

A4913 Miscellaneous dialysis supplies, not otherwise specified

A4918 Venous pressure clamp, for hemodialysis, each

A4927 Gloves, non-sterile, per 100

A4928 Surgical mask, per 20

A4929 Tourniquet for dialysis, each

A4930 Gloves, sterile, per pair

A4931 Oral thermometer, reusable, any type, each

A4932 Rectal thermometer, reusable, any type, each

ADDITIONAL OSTOMY SUPPLIES

A5051 Ostomy pouch, closed; with barrier attached (1 piece), each
MCM: 2130

A5052 without barrier attached (1 piece), each
MCM: 2130

A5053 for use on faceplate, each
MCM: 2130

A5054 for use on barrier with flange (2 piece), each
MCM: 2130

A5055 Stoma cap
MCM: 2130

A5056 Ostomy pouch, drainable, with extended wear barrier attached, with filter, (1 piece each)
MCM: 2130

A5057 Ostomy pouch, drainable, with extended wear barrier attached, with built in convexity, with filter, (1 piece), each
MCM: 2130

A5061 Ostomy pouch, drainable; with barrier attached (1 piece), each

A5062 without barrier attached (1 piece), each
MCM: 2130

A5063 for use on barrier with flange (2-piece system), each
MCM: 2130

A5071 Ostomy pouch, urinary; with barrier attached (1 piece), each
MCM: 2130

A5072 without barrier attached (1 piece), each
MCM: 2130

A5073 for use on barrier with flange (2 piece), each
MCM: 2130

▲**A5081** Stoma plug or seal, any type
MCM: 2130

A5082 catheter for continent stoma
MCM: 2130

A5083 Continent device, stoma absorptive cover for continent stom

A5093 Ostomy accessory; convex insert
MCM: 2130

ADDITIONAL INCONTINENCE APPLIANCES/SUPPLIES

A5102 Bedside drainage bottle with or without tubing, rigid or expandable, each
MCM: 2130

A5105 Urinary suspensory with leg bag, with or without tube, each
MCM: 2130

A5112 Urinary drainage bag, leg or abdomen, latex, with or without tube, with straps, each
MCM: 2130

A5113 Leg strap; latex, replacement only, per set
MCM: 2130

A5114 foam or fabric, replacement only, per set
MCM: 2130

SUPPLIES FOR EITHER INCONTINENCE OR OSTOMY APPLIANCES

A5120 Skin barrier, wipes or swabs, each
MCM: 2130

A5121 solid, 6 x 6 or equivalent, each
MCM: 2130

A5122 solid, 8 x 8 or equivalent, each
MCM: 2130

A5126 Adhesive or non-adhesive; disk or foam pad
MCM: 2130

A5131 Appliance cleaner, incontinence and ostomy appliances, per 16 oz.
MCM: 2130

A5200 Percutaneous catheter/tube anchoring device, adhesive skin attachment
MCM: 2130

SHOE SUPPLIES FOR DIABETICS

A5500 For diabetics only, fitting (including follow-up), custom preparation and supply of off-the-shelf depth-inlay shoe manufactured to accommodate multi-density insert(s), per shoe
MCM: 2134

A5501 For diabetics only, fitting (including follow-up), custom preparation and supply of shoe molded from cast(s) of patient's foot (custom molded shoe), per shoe
MCM: 2134

A5503 For diabetics only, modification (including fitting) of off-the-shelf depth-inlay shoe or custom-molded shoe with roller or rigid rocker bottom, per shoe
MCM: 2134

A5504 For diabetics only, modification (including fitting) of off-the-shelf depth-inlay shoe or custom-molded shoe with wedge(s), per shoe
MCM: 2134

A5505 For diabetics only, modification (including fitting) of off-the-shelf depth-inlay shoe or custom-molded shoe with metatarsal bar, per shoe
MCM: 2134

A5506 For diabetics only, modification (including fitting) of off-the-shelf depth-inlay shoe or custom-molded shoe with off-set heel(s), per shoe
MCM: 2134

A5507 For diabetics only, not otherwise specified modification (including fitting) of off-the-shelf depth-inlay shoe or custom-molded shoe, per shoe
MCM: 2134

A5508 For diabetics only, deluxe feature of off-the-shelf depth-inlay shoe or custom-molded shoe, per shoe
MCM: 2134

A5510 For diabetics only, direct formed, compression molded to patient's foot without external heat source, multiple-density insert(s), prefabricated, per shoe
MCM: 2134

A5512 For diabetics only, multiple density insert, direct formed, molded to foot after external heat source of 230 degrees fahrenheit or higher, total contact with patient's foot, including arch, base layer minimum of 1/4 inch material of shore a 35 durometer or 3/16 inch material of shore a 40 durometer (or higher), prefabricated, each

A5513 For diabetics only, multiple density insert, custom molded from model of patient's foot, total contact with patient's foot, including arch, base layer minimum of 3/16 inch material of shore a 35 durometer (or higher), includes arch filler and other shaping material, custom fabricated, each

WOUND DRESSINGS

A6000 Non-contact wound warming wound cover for use with the non-contact wound warming device and warming card
MCM: 2303

A6010 Collagen based wound filler, dry form, sterile, per gram of collagen
MCM: 2079

A6011 Collagen based wound filler, gel/paste, per gram of collagen
MCM: 2079

A6021 Collagen dressing, sterile, pad size 16 sq. in. or less, each
MCM: 2079

A6022 Collagen dressing, sterile, pad size more than 16 sq. in. but less than or equal to 48 sq. in., each
MCM: 2079

A6023 Collagen dressing, sterile, pad size more than 48 sq. in., each
MCM: 2079

A6024 Collagen dressing wound filler, sterile, per 6 inches
MCM: 2079

A6025 Gel sheet for dermal or epidermal application, (eg., silicone, hydrogel, other), each

A6154 Wound pouch, each
MCM: 2079

A6196 Alginate or other fiber gelling dressing, wound cover, sterile, pad size 16 sq. in. or less, each dressing
MCM: 2079

A6197 Alginate or other fiber gelling dressing, wound cover, sterile, pad size more than 16 sq. in. but less than or equal to 48 sq. in., each dressing
MCM: 2079

A6198 Alginate or other fiber gelling dressing, wound cover, sterile, pad size more than 48 sq. in., each dressing
MCM: 2079

A6199 Alginate or other fiber gelling dressing, wound filler, sterile, per 6 inches
MCM: 2079

A6203 Composite dressing, sterile, pad size 16 sq. in. or less, with any size adhesive border, each dressing
MCM: 2079

A6204 Composite dressing, sterile, pad size more than 16 sq. in. but less than or equal to 48 sq. in., with any size adhesive border, each dressing
MCM: 2079

A6205 Composite dressing, sterile, pad size more than 48 sq. in., with any size adhesive border, each dressing
MCM: 2079

A6206 Contact layer, sterile, 16 sq. in. or less, each dressing
MCM: 2079

A6207 Contact layer, sterile, more than 16 sq. in. but less than or equal to 48 sq. in., each dressing
MCM: 2079

A6208 Contact layer, sterile, more than 48 sq. in., each dressing
MCM: 2079

A6209 Foam dressing, wound cover, sterile, pad size 16 sq. in. or less, without adhesive border, each dressing
MCM: 2079

A6210 Foam dressing, wound cover, sterile, pad size more than 16 sq. in. but less than or equal to 48 sq. in., without adhesive border, each dressing
MCM: 2079

A6211 Foam dressing, wound cover, sterile, pad size more than 48 sq. in., without adhesive border, each dressing
MCM: 2079

A6212 Foam dressing, wound cover, sterile, pad size 16 sq. in. or less, with any size adhesive border, each dressing
MCM: 2079

A6213 Foam dressing, wound cover, sterile, pad size more than 16 sq. in. but less than or equal to 48 sq. in., with any size adhesive border, each dressing
MCM: 2079

A6214 Foam dressing, wound cover, sterile, pad size more than 48 sq. in., with any size adhesive border, each dressing
MCM: 2079

A6215 Foam dressing, wound filler, sterile, per gram
MCM: 2079

A6216 Gauze, non-impregnated, non-sterile, pad size 16 sq. in. or less, without adhesive border, each dressing
MCM: 2079

A6217 Gauze, non-impregnated, non-sterile, pad size more than 16 sq. in. but less than or equal to 48 sq. in., without adhesive border, each dressing
MCM: 2079

A6218 Gauze, non-impregnated, non-sterile, pad size more than 48 sq. in., without adhesive border, each dressing
MCM: 2079

A6219 Gauze, non-impregnated, sterile, pad size 16 sq. in. or less, with any size adhesive border, each dressing
MCM: 2079

A6220 Gauze, non-impregnated, sterile, pad size more than 16 sq. in. but less than or equal to 48 sq. in., with any size adhesive border, each dressing
MCM: 2079

A6221 Gauze, non-impregnated, sterile, pad size more than 48 sq. in., with any size adhesive border, each dressing
MCM: 2079

A6222 Gauze, impregnated with other than water, normal saline, or hydrogel, sterile, pad size 16 sq. in. or less, without adhesive border, each dressing
MCM: 2079

A6223 Gauze, impregnated with other than water, normal saline, or hydrogel, sterile, pad size more than 16 sq. in. but less than or equal to 48 sq. in., without adhesive border, each dressing
MCM: 2079

A6224 Gauze, impregnated with other than water, normal saline, or hydrogel, sterile, pad size more than 48 sq. in., without adhesive border, each dressing
MCM: 2079

A6228 Gauze, impregnated, water or normal saline, sterile, pad size 16 sq. in. or less, without adhesive border, each dressing
MCM: 2079

A6229 Gauze, impregnated, water or normal saline, sterile, pad size more than 16 sq. in. but less than or equal to 48 sq. in., without adhesive border, each dressing
MCM: 2079

A6230 Gauze, impregnated, water or normal saline, sterile, pad size more than 48 sq. in., without adhesive border, each dressing

MCM: 2079

A6231 Gauze, impregnated, hydrogel, for direct wound contact, sterile, pad size 16 sq. in. or less, each dressing
MCM: 2079

A6232 Gauze, impregnated, hydrogel, for direct wound contact, sterile, pad size greater than 16 sq. in., but less than or equal to 48 sq. in., each dressing
MCM: 2079

A6233 Gauze, impregnated, hydrogel, for direct wound contact, sterile, pad size more than 48 sq. in., each dressing
MCM: 2079

A6234 Hydrocolloid dressing, wound cover, sterile, pad size 16 sq. in. or less, without adhesive border, each dressing
MCM: 2079

A6235 Hydrocolloid dressing, wound cover, sterile, pad size more than 16 sq. in. but less than or equal to 48 sq. in., without adhesive border, each dressing
MCM: 2079

A6236 Hydrocolloid dressing, wound cover, sterile, pad size more than 48 sq. in., without adhesive border, each dressing
MCM: 2079

A6237 Hydrocolloid dressing, wound cover, sterile, pad size 16 sq. in. or less, with any size adhesive border, each dressing
MCM: 2079

A6238 Hydrocolloid dressing, wound cover, sterile, pad size more than 16 sq. in. but less than or equal to 48 sq. in., with any size adhesive border, each dressing
MCM: 2079

A6239 Hydrocolloid dressing, wound cover, sterile, pad size more than 48 sq. in., with any size adhesive border, each dressing
MCM: 2079

A6240 Hydrocolloid dressing, wound filler, paste, sterile, per ounce
MCM: 2079

A6241 Hydrocolloid dressing, wound filler, dry form, sterile, per gram
MCM: 2079

A6242 Hydrogel dressing, wound cover, sterile, pad size 16 sq. in. or less, without adhesive border, each dressing
MCM: 2079

A6243 Hydrogel dressing, wound cover, sterile, pad size more than 16 sq. in. but less than or equal to 48 sq. in., without adhesive border, each dressing
MCM: 2079

A6244 Hydrogel dressing, wound cover, sterile, pad size more than 48 sq. in., without adhesive border, each dressing
MCM: 2079

A6245 Hydrogel dressing, wound cover, sterile, pad size 16 sq. in. or less, with any size adhesive border, each dressing
MCM: 2079

A6246 Hydrogel dressing, wound cover, sterile, pad size more than 16 sq. in. but less than or equal to 48 sq. in., with any size adhesive border, each dressing
MCM: 2079

A6247 Hydrogel dressing, wound cover, sterile, pad size more than 48 sq. in., with any size adhesive border, each dressing
MCM: 2079

A6248 Hydrogel dressing, wound filler, gel, per fluid ounce
MCM: 2079

A6250 Skin sealants, protectants, moisturizers, ointments, any type, any size
MCM: 2079

A6251 Specialty absorptive dressing, wound cover, sterile, pad size 16 sq. in. or less, without adhesive border, each dressing
MCM: 2079

A6252 Specialty absorptive dressing, wound cover, sterile, pad size more than 16 sq. in. but less than or equal to 48 sq. in., without adhesive border, each dressing
MCM: 2079

A6253 Specialty absorptive dressing, wound cover, sterile, pad size more than 48 sq. in., without adhesive border, each dressing
MCM: 2079

A6254 Specialty absorptive dressing, wound cover, sterile, pad size 16 sq. in. or less, with any size adhesive border, each dressing
MCM: 2079

A6255 Specialty absorptive dressing, wound cover, sterile, pad size more than 16 sq. in. but less than or equal to 48 sq. in., with any size adhesive border, each dressing
MCM: 2079

A6256 Specialty absorptive dressing, wound cover, sterile, pad size more than 48 sq. in., with any size adhesive border, each dressing
MCM: 2079

A6257 Transparent film, sterile, 16 sq. in. or less, each dressing
MCM: 2079

A6258 Transparent film, sterile, more than 16 sq. in. but less than or equal to 48 sq. in., each dressing
MCM: 2079

A6259 Transparent film, sterile, more than 48 sq. in., each dressing
MCM: 2079

A6260 Wound cleansers, any type, any size
MCM: 2079

A6261 Wound filler, gel/paste, per fluid ounce, not otherwise specified
MCM: 2079

A6262 Wound filler, dry form, per gram, not otherwise specified
MCM: 2079

A6266 Gauze, impregnated, other than water, normal saline or zinc paste, sterile, any width, per linear yard
MCM: 2079

A6402 Gauze, non-impregnated, sterile, pad size 16 sq. in. or less, without adhesive border, each dressing
MCM: 2079

A6403 Gauze, non-impregnated, sterile, pad size more than 16 sq. in. but less than or equal to 48 sq. in., without adhesive border, each dressing
MCM: 2079

A6404 Gauze, non-impregnated, sterile, pad size more than 48 sq. in., without adhesive border, each dressing

MCM: 2079

A6407 Packing strips, non-impregnated, sterile, up to 2 inches in width, per linear yard

A6410 Eye pad, sterile, each
MCM: 2079

A6411 Eye pad, non-sterile, each
MCM: 2079

A6412 Eye patch, occlusive, each

A6413 Adhesive bandage, first-aid type, any size, each

A6441 Padding bandage, non-elastic, non-woven/non-knitted, width greater than or equal to three inches and less than five inches, per yard

A6442 Conforming bandage, non-elastic, knitted-woven, non-sterile, width less than three inches, per yard

A6443 Conforming bandage, non-elastic, knitted/woven, non-sterile, width greater than or equal to three inches and less than five inches, per yard

A6444 Conforming bandage, non-elastic, knitted/woven, non-sterile, width greater than or equal to 5 inches, per yard

A6445 Conforming bandage, non-elastic, knitted/woven, sterile, width less than three inches, per yard

A6446 Conforming bandage, non-elastic, knitted/woven, sterile, width greater than or equal to three inches and less than five inches, per yard

A6447 Conforming bandage, non-elastic, knitted/woven, sterile, width greater than or equal to five inches, per yard

A6448 Light compression bandage, elastic, knitted/woven, width less than three inches, per yard

A6449 Light compression bandage, elastic, knitted/woven, width greater than or equal to three inches and less than five inches, per yard

A6450 Light compression bandage, elastic, knitted/woven, width greater than or equal to five inches, per yard

A6451 Moderate compression bandage, elastic, knitted/woven, load resistance of 1.25 to 1.34 foot pounds at 50% maximum stretch, width greater than or equal to three inches and less than five inches, per yard

A6452 High compression bandage, elastic, knitted/woven, load resistance greater than or equal to 1.35 foot pounds at 50% maximum stretch, width greater than or equal to three inches and less than five inches, per yard

A6453 Self-adherent bandage, elastic, non-knitted/non-woven, width less than three inches, per yard

A6454 Self-adherent bandage, elastic, non-knitted/non-woven, width greater than or equal to three inches and less than five inches, per yard

A6455 Self-adherent bandage, elastic, non-knitted/non-woven, width greater than or equal to five inches, per yard

A6456 Zinc paste impregnated bandage, non-elastic, knitted/woven, width greater than or equal to three inches and less than five inches, per yard

A6457 Tubular dressing with or without elastic, any width, per linear yard

A6501 Compression burn garment, bodysuit (head to foot), custom fabricated
MCM: 2079

A6502 Compression burn garment, chin strap, custom fabricated
MCM: 2079

A6503 Compression burn garment, facial hood, custom fabricated
MCM: 2079

A6504 Compression burn garment, glove to wrist, custom fabricated
MCM: 2079

A6505 Compression burn garment, glove to elbow, custom fabricated
MCM: 2079

A6506 Compression burn garment, glove to axilla, custom fabricated
MCM: 2079

A6507 Compression burn garment, foot to knee length, custom fabricated
MCM: 2079

A6508 Compression burn garment, foot to thigh length, custom fabricated
MCM: 2079

A6509 Compression burn garment, upper trunk to waist including arm openings (vest), custom fabricated
MCM: 2079

A6510 Compression burn garment, trunk, including arms down to leg openings (leotard), custom fabricated
MCM: 2079

A6511 Compression burn garment, lower trunk including leg openings (panty), custom fabricated
MCM: 2079

A6512 Compression burn garment, not otherwise classified
MCM: 2079

A6513 Compression burn mask, face and/or neck, plastic or equal, custom fabricated

A6530 Gradient compression stocking, below knee, 18-30 mmhg, each
CIM: 60-9

A6531 Gradient compression stocking, below knee, 30-40 mmhg, each
MCM: 2079

A6532 Gradient compression stocking, below knee, 40-50 mmhg, each
MCM: 2079

A6533 Gradient compression stocking, thigh length, 18-30 mmhg, each
CIM: 60-9 MCM: 2133

A6534 Gradient compression stocking, thigh length, 30-40 mmhg, each
CIM: 60-9 MCM: 2133

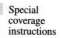

A6535 Gradient compression stocking, thigh length, 40-50 mmhg, each
CIM: 60-9 MCM: 2133

A6536 Gradient compression stocking, full length/chap style, 18-30 mmhg, each
CIM: 60-9 MCM: 2133

A6537 Gradient compression stocking, full length/chap style, 30-40 mmhg, each
CIM: 60-9 MCM: 2133

A6538 Gradient compression stocking, full length/chap style, 40-50 mmhg, each
CIM: 60-9 MCM: 2133

A6539 Gradient compression stocking, waist length, 18-30 mmhg, each
CIM: 60-9 MCM: 2133

A6540 Gradient compression stocking, waist length, 30-40 mmhg, each
CIM: 60-9 MCM: 2133

A6541 Gradient compression stocking, waist length, 40-50 mmhg, each
CIM: 60-9 MCM: 2133

A6544 Gradient compression stocking, garter belt
CIM: 60-9 MCM: 2133

A6545 Gradient compression wrap, non-elastic, below knee, 30-50 mm hg, each
MCM: 2079

A6549 Gradient compression stocking/sleeve, not otherwise specified
CIM: 60-9 MCM: 2133

A6550 Wound care set, for negative pressure wound therapy electrical pump, includes all supplies and accessories

A7000 Canister, disposable, used with suction pump, each

A7001 Canister, non-disposable, used with suction pump, each

A7002 Tubing, used with suction pump, each

A7003 Administration set, with small volume nonfiltered pneumatic nebulizer, disposable

A7004 Small volume nonfiltered pneumatic nebulizer, disposable

A7005 Administration set, with small volume nonfiltered pneumatic nebulizer, non-disposable

A7006 Administration set, with small volume filtered pneumatic nebulizer

A7007 Large volume nebulizer, disposable, unfilled, used with aerosol compressor

A7008 Large volume nebulizer, disposable, prefilled, used with aerosol compressor

A7009 Reservoir bottle, non-disposable, used with large volume ultrasonic nebulizer

A7010 Corrugated tubing, disposable, used with large volume nebulizer, 100 feet

A7011 Corrugated tubing, non-disposable, used with large volume nebulizer, 10 feet

A7012 Water collection device, used with large volume nebulizer

A7013 Filter, disposable, used with aerosol compressor or ultrasonic generator

A7014 Filter, non-disposable, used with aerosol compressor or ultrasonic generator

A7015 Aerosol mask, used with DME nebulizer

A7016 Dome and mouthpiece, used with small volume ultrasonic nebulizer

A7017 Nebulizer, durable, glass or autoclavable plastic, bottle type, not used with oxygen
CIM: 60-9

A7018 Water, distilled, used with large volume nebulizer, 1000 ml

A7020 Interface for cough stimulating device, includes all components, replacement only

A7025 High frequency chest wall oscillation system vest, replacement for use with patient owned equipment, each

A7026 High frequency chest wall oscillation system hose, replacement for use with patient owned equipment, each

A7027 Combination oral/nasal mask, used with continuous positive airway pressure device, each

A7028 Oral cushion for combination oral/nasal mask, replacement only, each

A7029 Nasal pillows for combination oral/nasal mask, replacement only, pair

A7030 Full face mask used with positive airway pressure device, each

A7031 Face mask interface, replacement for full face mask, each

A7032 Cushion for use on nasal mask interface, replacement only, each

A7033 Pillow for use on nasal cannula type interface, replacement only, pair

A7034 Nasal interface (mask or cannula type) used with positive airway pressure device, with or without head strap

A7035 Headgear used with positive airway pressure device

A7036 Chinstrap used with positive airway pressure device

A7037 Tubing used with positive airway pressure device

A7038 Filter, disposable, used with positive airway pressure device

A7039 Filter, non-disposable, used with positive airway pressure device

A7040 One way chest drain valve

A7041 Water seal drainage container and tubing for use with implanted chest tube

A7042 Implanted pleural catheter, each

A7043 Vacuum drainage bottle and tubing for use with implanted catheter

A7044 Oral interface used with positive airway pressure device, each

A7045 Exhalation port with or without swivel used with accessories for positive airway devices, replacement only
CIM: 60-17

A7046 Water chamber for humidifier, used with positive airway pressure device, replacement, each
CIM: 60-17

● **A7047** Oral interface used with respiratory suction pump, each

A7501 Tracheostoma valve, including diaphram, each
MCM: 2130

A7502 Replacement diaphram/faceplate for tracheostoma valve, each
MCM: 2130

A7503 Filter holder or filter cap, reusable, for use in a tracheostoma heat and moisture exchange system, each
MCM: 2130

A7504 Filter for use in a tracheostoma heat and moisture exchange system, each
MCM: 2130

A7505 Housing, reusable without adhesive, for use in a heat and moisture exchange system and/or with a tracheostoma valve, each
MCM: 2130

A7506 Adhesive disc for use in a heat and moisture exchange system and/or with tracheostoma valve, any type, each
MCM: 2130

A7507 Filter holder and integrated filter without adhesive, for use in a tracheostoma heat and moisture exchange system, each
MCM: 2130

A7508 Housing and integrated adhesive, for use in a tracheostoma heat and moisture exchange system and/or with a tracheostoma valve, each
MCM: 2130

A7509 Filter holder and integrated filter housing, and adhesive, for use as a tracheostoma heat and moisture exchange system, each
MCM: 2130

A7520 Tracheostomy/laryngectomy tube, non-cuffed, polyvinylchloride (PVC), silicone or equal, each

A7521 Tracheostomy/laryngectomy tube, cuffed, polyvinylchloride (PVC), silicone or equal, each

A7522 Tracheostomy/laryngectomy tube, stainless steel or equal (sterilizable and reusable), each

A7523 Tracheostomy shower protector, each

A7524 Tracheostoma stent/stud/button, each

A7525 Tracheostomy mask, each

A7526 Tracheostomy tube collar/holder, each

A7527 Tracheostomy/laryngectomy tube plug/stop, each

A8000 Helmet, protective, soft, pre-fabricated, includes all components and accessories

A8001 Helmet, protective, hard, pre-fabricated, includes all components and accessories

A8002 Helmet, protective, soft, custom fabricated, includes all components and accessories

A8003 Helmet, protective, hard, custom fabricated, includes all components and accessories

A8004 Soft interface for helmet, replacement only

ADMINISTRATIVE, MISCELLANEOUS AND INVESTIGATIONAL

NOTE: The following codes do not imply that codes in other sections are necessarily covered.

Guidelines

In addition to the information presented in the INTRODUCTION, several other items unique to this section are defined or identified here:

1. SPECIAL REPORT: A service, material or supply that is rarely provided, unusual, variable or new may require a special report in determining medical appropriateness for reimbursement purposes. Pertinent information should include an adequate definition or description of the nature, extent, and need for the service, material or supply.

2. CPT CODE CROSS-REFERENCE: Unless specified otherwise, there is no equivalent CPT code for listings in this section.

Miscellaneous and Experimental

A9150 Non-prescription drugs
MCM: 2050.5

A9152 Single vitamin/mineral/trace element, oral, per dose, not otherwise specified

A9153 Multiple vitamins, with or without minerals and trace elements, oral, per dose, not otherwise specified

A9155 Artificial saliva, 30 ml

A9180 Pediculosis (lice infestation) treatment, topical, for administration by patient/caretaker

A9270 Non-covered item or service
MCM: 2303

▲**A9272** Wound suction, disposable, includes dressing, all accessories and components, any type, each

A9273 Hot water bottle, ice cap or collar, heat and/or cold wrap, any type

A9274 External ambulatory insulin delivery system, disposable, each, includes all supplies and accessories

A9275 Home glucose disposable monitor, includes test strips

A9276 Sensor; invasive (e.g. subcutaneous), disposable, for use with interstitial continuous glucose monitoring system, one unit = 1 day supply

A9277 Transmitter; external, for use with interstitial continuous glucose monitoring system

A9278 Receiver (monitor); external, for use with interstitial continuous glucose monitoring system

A9279 Monitoring feature/device, stand-alone or integrated, any type, includes all

A9280 Alert or alarm device, not otherwise classified

A9281 Reaching/grabbing device, any type, any length, each

A9282 Wig, any type, each

A9283 Foot pressure off loading/supportive device, any type, each

A9284 Spirometer, non-electronic, includes all accessories

A9300 Exercise equipment
CIM: 60-9 MCM: 2100.1

A9500 Technetium Tc-99m sestamibi, diagnostic, per study dose

A9501 Technetium tc-99m teboroxime, diagnostic, per study dose

A9502 Technetium Tc-99m tetrofosmin, diagnostic, per study dose

A9503 Technetium Tc-99m medronate, diagnostic, per study dose, up to 30 millicuries

A9504 Technetium Tc-99m apcitide, diagnostic, per study dose, up to 20 millicuries

A9505 Thallium Tl-201 thallous chloride, diagnostic, per millicurie

A9507 Indium In-111 capromablue pendetide, diagnostic, per study dose, up to 10 millicuries

A9508 Iodine I-131 ioblueenguane sulfate, diagnostic, per 0.5 millicurie

A9509 Iodine i-123 sodium iodide, diagnostic, per millicurie

A9510 Technetium Tc-99m disofenin, diagnostic, per study dose, up to 15 millicuries

A9512 Technetium Tc-99m pertechnetate, diagnostic, per millicurie

A9516 Iodine I-123 sodium iodide, diagnostic, per 100 microcuries, up to 999 microcuries

A9517 Iodine I-131 sodium iodide capsule(s), therapeutic, per millicurie

● **A9520** Technetium tc-99m, tilmanocept, diagnostic, up to 0.5 millicuries

A9521 Technetium Tc-99m exametazime, diagnostic, per study dose, up to 25 millicuries

A9524 Iodine I-131 iodinated serum alblueumin, diagnostic, per 5 microcuries

A9526 Nitrogen N-13 ammonia, diagnostic, per study dose, up to 40 millicuries

A9527 Iodine I-125, sodium iodide solution, therapeutic, per millicurie

A9528 Iodine I-131 sodium iodide capsule(s), diagnostic, per millicurie

A9529 Iodine I-131 sodium iodide solution, diagnostic, per millicurie

A9530 Iodine I-131 sodium iodide solution, therapeutic, per millicurie

A9531 Iodine I-131 sodium iodide, diagnostic, per microcurie (up to 100 microcuries)

A9532 Iodine I-125 serum alblueumin, diagnostic, per 5 microcuries

A9536 Technetium Tc-99m depreotide, diagnostic, per study dose, up to 35 millicuries

A9537 Technetium Tc-99m mebrofenin, diagnostic, per study dose, up to 15 millicuries

A9538 Technetium Tc-99m pyrophosphate, diagnostic, per study dose, up to 25 millicuries

A9539 Technetium Tc-99m pentetate, diagnostic, per study dose, up to 25 millicuries

A9540 Technetium Tc-99m macroaggregated albumin, diagnostic, per study dose, up to 10 millicuries

A9541 Technetium Tc-99m sulfur colloid, diagnostic, per study dose, up to 20 millicuries

A9542 Indium In-111 ibritumomab tiuxetan, diagnostic, per study dose, up to 5 millicuries

A9543 Yttrium Y-90 ibritumomab tiuxetan, therapeutic, per treatment dose, up to 40 millicuries

A9544 Iodine I-131 tositumomab, diagnostic, per study dose

A9545 Iodine I-131 tositumomab, therapeutic, per treatment dose

A9546 Cobalt Co-57/58, cyanocobalamin, diagnostic, per study dose, up to 1 microcurie

A9547 Indium In-111 oxyquinoline, diagnostic, per 0.5 millicurie

A9548 Indium In-111 pentetate, diagnostic, per 0.5 millicurie

A9550 Technetium Tc-99m sodium gluceptate, diagnostic, per study dose, up to 25 millicuries

A9551 Technetium Tc-99m succimer, diagnostic, per study dose, up to 10 millicuries

A9552 Fluorodeoxyglucose F-18 fdg, diagnostic, per study dose, up to 45 millicuries

A9553 Chromium Cr-51 sodium chromate, diagnostic, per study dose, up to 250 microcuries

A9554 Iodine I-125 sodium iothalamate, diagnostic, per study dose, up to 10 microcuries

A9555 Rubidium Rb-82, diagnostic, per study dose, up to 60 millicuries

A9556 Gallium Ga-67 citrate, diagnostic, per millicurie

A9557 Technetium Tc-99m bicisate, diagnostic, per study dose, up to 25 millicuries

A9558 Xenon Xe-133 gas, diagnostic, per 10 millicuries

A9559 Cobalt Co-57 cyanocobalamin, oral, diagnostic, per study dose, up to 1 microcurie

A9560 Technetium Tc-99m labeled red blood cells, diagnostic, per study dose, up to 30 millicuries

A9561 Technetium Tc-99m oxidronate, diagnostic, per study dose, up to 30 millicuries

A9562 Technetium Tc-99m mertiatide, diagnostic, per study dose, up to 15 millicuries

A9563 Sodium phosphate P-32, therapeutic, per millicurie

A9564 Chromic phosphate P-32 suspension, therapeutic, per millicurie

A9566 Technetium Tc-99m fanolesomab, diagnostic, per study dose, up to 25 millicuries

A9567 Technetium Tc-99m pentetate, diagnostic, aerosol, per study dose, up to 75 millicuries

A9568 Technetium Tc-99m arcitumomab, diagnostic, per study dose, up to 45 millicuries

A9569 Technetium Tc-99m exametazime labeled autologous white blood cells, diagnostic, per study dose

A9570 Indium IN-111 labeled autologous white blood cells, diagnostic, per study dose

A9571 Indium IN-111 labeled autologous platelets, diagnostic, per study dose

A9572 Indium IN-111 pentetreotide, diagnostic, per study dose, up to 6 millicuries

● **A9575** Injection, gadoterate meglumine, 0.1 ml

A9576 Injection, gadoteridol, (prohance multipack), per ml

A9577 Injection, gadobenate dimeglumine (multihance), per ml

A9578 Injection, gadobenate dimeglumine (multihance multipack), per ml

A9579 Injection, gadolinium-based magnetic resonance contrast agent, not otherwise specified (NOS), per ml

A9580 Sodium fluoride f-18, diagnostic, per study dose, up to 30 millicuries

A9581 Injection, gadoxetate disodium, 1 ml

A9582 Iodine I-123 iobenguane, diagnostic, per study dose, up to 15 millicuries

A9583 Injection, gadofosveset trisodium, 1 ml

A9584 Iodine 1-123 ioflupane, diagnostic, per study dose, up to 5 millicuries

A9585 Injection, gadobutrol, 0.1 ml

A9586 Florbetapir F18, diagnostic, per study dose, up to 10 millicuries

● **A9599** Radiopharmaceutical, diagnostic, for beta-amyloid positron emission tomography (PET)

A9600 Strontium Sr-89 chloride, therapeutic, per millicurie

A9604 Samarium SM-153 lexidronam, therapeutic, per treatment dose, up to 150 millicuries

A9698 Non-radioactive contrast imaging material, not otherwise classified, per study
MCM: 15022

A9699 Radiopharmaceutical, therapeutic, not otherwise classified

A9700 Supply of injectable contrast material for use in echocardiography, per study
MCM: 15360

A9900 Miscellaneous DME supply, accessory, and/or service component of another HCPCS code

A9901 DME delivery, set up, and/or dispensing service component of another HCPCS code

A9999 Miscellaneous DME supply or accessory, not otherwise specified

This page intentionally left blank

ENTERAL AND PARENTERAL THERAPY

Guidelines

In addition to the information presented in the INTRODUCTION, several other items unique to this section are defined or identified here:

1. SUBSECTION INFORMATION: Some of the listed subheadings or subsections have special needs or instructions unique to that section. Where these are indicated, special "notes" will be presented preceding or following the listings. Those subsections within the ENTERAL AND PARENTERAL THERAPY section that have "notes" are as follows:

Subsection	Code Numbers
Enteral formulae and enteral medical supplies	B4034-B5200

2. UNLISTED SERVICE OR PROCEDURE: A service or procedure may be provided that is not listed in this edition of HCPCS. When reporting such a service, the appropriate "unlisted procedure" code may be used to indicate the service, identifying it by "special report" as defined below. HCPCS terminology is inconsistent in defining unlisted procedures. The procedure definition may include the term(s) "unlisted", "not otherwise classified", "unspecified", "unclassified", "other" and "miscellaneous". Prior to using these codes, try to determine if a Local Level III code or CPT code is available. The "unlisted procedures" and accompanying codes for ENTERAL AND PARENTERAL THERAPY are as follows:

   B9998 NOC for enteral supplies
   B9999 NOC for parenteral supplies

3. SPECIAL REPORT: A service, material or supply that is rarely provided, unusual, variable or new may require a special report in determining medical appropriateness for reimbursement purposes. Pertinent information should include an adequate definition or description of the nature, extent, and need for the service, material or supply.

4. MODIFIERS: Listed services may be modified under certain circumstances. When appropriate, the modifying circumstance is identified by adding a modifier to the basic procedure code. CPT and HCPCS National Level II modifiers may be used with CPT and

HCPCS National Level II procedure codes. Modifiers commonly used with ENTERAL AND PARENTERAL THERAPY are as follows:

-CC Procedure code change (used when the procedure code submitted was changed either for administrative reasons or because an incorrect code was filed)

5. CPT CODE CROSS-REFERENCE: Unless specified otherwise, the equivalent CPT code for all listings in this section is 99070.

Enteral Formulae and Enteral Medical Supplies

B4034 Enteral feeding supply kit; syringe fed, per day, includes but not limited to feeding/flushing syringe, administration set tubing, dressings, tape
CIM: 65-10 MCM: 2130, 4450

B4035 pump fed, per day, includes but not limited to feeding/flushing syringe, administration set tubing, dressings, tape
CIM: 65-10 MCM: 2130, 4450

B4036 gravity fed, per day, includes but not limited to feeding/flushing syringe, administration set tubing, dressings, tape
CIM: 65-10 MCM: 2130, 4450

B4081 Nasogastric tubing; with stylet
CIM: 65-10 MCM: 2130, 4450

B4082 without stylet
CIM: 65-10 MCM: 2130, 4450

B4083 Stomach tube - levine type
CIM: 65-10 MCM: 2130, 4450

B4087 Gastrostomy/jejunostomy tube, standard, any material, any type, each

B4088 Gastrostomy/jejunostomy tube, low-profile, any material, any type, each

B4100 Food thickener, administered orally, per ounce
CIM: 60-9

B4102 Enteral formula, for adults, used to replace fluids and electrolytes (e.g. clear liquids), 500 ml = 1 unit
CIM: 65-10

B4103 Enteral formula, for pediatrics, used to replace fluids and electrolytes (e.g. clear liquids), 500 ml = 1 unit
CIM: 65-10

B4104 Additive for enteral formula (e.g. fiber)
CIM: 65-10

B4149 Enteral formula, manufactured bluelenderized natural foods with intact nutrients, includes proteins, fats, carblueohydrates, vitamins and minerals, may include fiblueer, administered through an enteral feeding tube, 100 calories = 1 unit
CIM: 65-10 MCM: 2130, 4450

B4150 Enteral formula, nutritionally complete with intact nutrients, includes proteins, fats, carbohydrates, vitamins and minerals, may include fiber, administered through an enteral feeding tube, 100 calories = 1 unit
CIM: 65-10 MCM: 2130, 4450

B4152 Enteral formula, nutritionally complete, calorically dense (equal to or greater than 1.5 Kcal/ml) with intact nutrients, includes proteins, fats, carbohydrates, vitamins and minerals, may include fiber, administered through an enteral feeding tube, 100 calories = 1 unit
CIM: 65-10 MCM: 2130, 4450

B4153 Enteral formula, nutritionally complete, hydrolyzed proteins (amino acids and peptide chain), includes fats, carbohydrates, vitamins and minerals, may include fiber, administered through an enteral feeding tube, 100 calories = 1 unit
CIM: 65-10 MCM: 2130, 4450

B4154 Enteral formula, nutritionally complete, for special metabolic needs, excludes inherited disease of metabolism, includes altered composition of proteins, fats, carbohydrates, vitamins and/or minerals, may include fiber, administered through an enteral feeding tube, 100 calories = 1 unit
CIM: 65-10 MCM: 2130, 4450

B4155 Enteral formula, nutritionally incomplete/modular nutrients, includes specific nutrients, carbohydrates (e.g. glucose polymers), proteins/amino acids (e.g. glutamine, arginine), fat (e.g. medium chain triglycerides) or combination, administered through an enteral feeding tube, 100 calories = 1 unit
CIM: 65-10 MCM: 2130, 4450

B4157 Enteral formula, nutritionally complete, for special metabolic needs for inherited disease of metabolism, includes proteins, fats, carbohydrates, vitamins and minerals, may include fiber, administered through an enteral feeding tube, 100 calories = 1 unit
CIM: 65-10

B4158 Enteral formula, for pediatrics, nutritionally complete with intact nutrients, includes proteins, fats, carbohydrates, vitamins and minerals, may include fiber and/or iron, administered through an enteral feeding tube, 100 calories = 1 unit
CIM: 65-10

B4159 Enteral formula, for pediatrics, nutritionally complete soy based with intact nutrients, includes proteins, fats, carbohydrates, vitamins and minerals, may include fiber and/or iron, administered through an enteral feeding tube, 100 calories = 1 unit
CIM: 65-10

B4160 Enteral formula, for pediatrics, nutritionally complete calorically dense (equal to or greater than 0.7 Kcal/ml) with intact nutrients, includes proteins, fats, carbohydrates, vitamins and minerals, may include fiber, administered through an enteral feeding tube, 100 calories = 1 unit
CIM: 65-10

B4161 Enteral formula, for pediatrics, hydrolyzed/amino acids and peptide chain proteins, includes fats, carbohydrates, vitamins and minerals, may include fiber, administered through an enteral feeding tube, 100 calories = 1 unit
CIM: 65-10

B4162 Enteral formula, for pediatrics, special metabolic needs for inherited disease of metabolism, includes proteins, fats, carbohydrates, vitamins and minerals, may include fiber, administered through an enteral feeding tube, 100 calories = 1 unit
CIM: 65-10

NOTE: For solution codes for other than parenteral nutrition therapy use, see J7060, J7070 and J7042.

PARENTERAL NUTRITION

B4164 Parenteral nutrition solution; carbohydrates (dextrose), 50% or less (500 ml = 1 unit)—homemix
CIM: 65-10 MCM: 2130, 4450

B4168 amino acid, 3.5% (500 ml = 1 unit)—homemix
CIM: 65-10 MCM: 2130, 4450

B4172 amino acid, 5.5% Thru 7%, (500 ml = 1 unit)—homemix
CIM: 65-10 MCM: 2130, 4450

B4176 amino acid, 7% thru 8.5% (500 ml = 1 unit)—homemix
CIM: 65-10 MCM: 2130, 4450

B4178 amino acid, greater than 8.5% (500 ml = 1 unit)—homemix
CIM: 65-10 MCM: 2130, 4450

B4180 carbohydrates (dextrose), greater than 50% (500 ml = 1 unit)—homemix
CIM: 65-10 MCM: 2130, 4450

B4185 Parenteral nutrition solution, per 10 grams lipids

B4189 compounded amino acids and carbohydrates with electrolytes, trace elements, and vitamins, including preparation, any strength, 10 to 51 grams of protein-premix
CIM: 65-10 MCM: 2130, 4450

B4193 compounded amino acid and carbohydrates with electrolytes, trace elements, and vitamins, including preparation, any strength, 52 to 73 grams of protein-premix
CIM: 65-10 MCM: 2130, 4450

B4197 compounded amino acid and carbohydrates with electrolytes, trace elements and vitamins, including preparation, any strength, 74 to 100 grams of protein - premix
CIM: 65-10 MCM: 2130, 4450

B4199 compounded amino acid and carbohydrates with electrolytes, trace elements and vitamins, including preparation, any strength, over 100 grams of protein - premix
CIM: 65-10 MCM: 2130, 4450

B4216 Parenteral nutrition; additives (vitamins, trace elements, heparin, electrolytes) homemix per day
CIM: 65-10 MCM: 2130, 4450

B4220 Parenteral nutrition supply kit; premix, per day
CIM: 65-10 MCM: 2130, 4450

B4222 home mix, per day
CIM: 65-10 MCM: 2130, 4450

B4224 Parenteral nutrition administration kit, per day
CIM: 65-10 MCM: 2130, 4450

B5000 Parenteral nutrition solution: compounded amino acid and carbohydrates with electrolytes, trace elements, and vitamins, including preparation, any strength; renal - amirosyn RF, nephramine, renamine - premix
CIM: 65-10 MCM: 2130, 4450

B5100 hepatic - freamine HBC, hepatamine - premix
CIM: 65-10 MCM: 2130, 4450

B5200 stress - branch chain amino acids - premix
CIM: 65-10 MCM: 2130, 4450

ENTERAL AND PARENTERAL PUMPS

B9000 Enteral nutrition infusion pump; without alarm
CIM: 65-10 MCM: 2130, 4450

B9002 with alarm
CIM: 65-10 MCM: 2130, 4450

B9004 Parenteral nutrition infusion pump; portable
CIM: 65-10 MCM: 2130, 4450

B9006 stationary
CIM: 65-10 MCM: 2130, 4450

B9998 NOC for enteral supplies
CIM: 65-10 MCM: 2130, 4450

B9999 NOC for parenteral supplies
CIM: 65-10 MCM: 2130, 4450

HOSPITAL OUTPATIENT PPS CODES

Guidelines

The "C" codes are unique temporary codes established by CMS for use under the Hospital Outpatient Prospective Payment System (OPPS). Non-OPPS use of these codes for Medicare is not valid.

The purpose of the "C" codes is to provide hospitals with a list of codes and long descriptors for drugs, biologicals and devices eligible for transitional pass-through payments, and for items classified in "new technology" ambulatory payment classifications (APCs) under the new Hospital Outpatient Prospective Payment System (OPPS).

The listing of HCPCS codes in this section does not assure coverage of the specific item or service in a given case. To be eligible for pass-through and new technology payments, the items reported with "C" codes must be considered reasonable and necessary.

All of the "C" codes are used exclusively for services paid under the Hospital Outpatient Prospective Payment System and may not be used to bill for services paid under other Medicare payment systems.

In addition to the information presented above, several other items unique to this section are defined here:

1. SPECIAL REPORT: A service, material or supply that is rarely provided, unusual, variable or new may require a special report in determining medical appropriateness for reimbursement purposes. Pertinent information should include an adequate definition or description of the nature, extent, and need for the service, material or supply.

2. MODIFIERS: Listed services may be modified under certain circumstances. When appropriate, the modifying circumstance is identified by adding a modifier to the basic procedure code. CPT and HCPCS National Level II modifiers may be used with CPT and HCPCS National Level II procedure codes.

Hospital Outpatient PPS Codes

(**C1204** Code deleted December 31, 2013. Use A9520.)

C1300 Hyperbaric oxygen under pressure, full body chamber, per 30 minute interval

C1713 Anchor/screw for opposing bone-to-bone or soft tissue-to-bone (implantable)

C1714 Catheter, transluminal atherectomy, directional

C1715 Brachytherapy needle

C1716 Brachytherapy source, non-stranded, gold-198, per source

C1717 Brachytherapy source, non-stranded, high dose rate iridium-192, per source

C1719 Brachytherapy source, non-stranded, non-high dose rate iridium-192, per source

C1721 Cardioverter-defibrillator, dual chamber (implantable)

C1722 Cardioverter-defibrillator, single chamber (implantable)

C1724 Catheter, transluminal atherectomy, rotational

C1725 Catheter, transluminal angioplasty, non-laser (may include guidance, infusion/perfusion capability)

C1726 Catheter, balloon dilatation, non-vascular

C1727 Catheter, balloon tissue dissector, non-vascular (insertable)

C1728 Catheter, brachytherapy seed administration

C1729 Catheter, drainage

C1730 Catheter, electrophysiology, diagnostic, other than 3d mapping (19 or fewer electrodes)

C1731 Catheter, electrophysiology, diagnostic, other than 3d mapping (20 or more electrodes)

C1732 Catheter, electrophysiology, diagnostic/ablation, 3d or vector mapping

C1733 Catheter, electrophysiology, diagnostic/ablation, other than 3d or vector mapping, other than cool-tip

C1749 Endoscope, retrograde imaging/illumination colonoscope device (implantable)

C1750 Catheter, hemodialysis/peritoneal, long-term

C1751 Catheter, infusion, inserted peripherally, centrally or midline (other than hemodialysis)

C1752 Catheter, hemodialysis/peritoneal, short-term

C1753 Catheter, intravascular ultrasound

C1754 Catheter, intradiscal

C1755 Catheter, intraspinal

C1756 Catheter, pacing, transesophageal

C1757 Catheter, thrombectomy/embolectomy

C1758 Catheter, ureteral

C1759 Catheter, intracardiac echocardiography

C1760 Closure device, vascular (implantable/insertable)

C1762 Connective tissue, human (includes fascia lata)

C1763 Connective tissue, non-human (includes synthetic)

C1764 Event recorder, cardiac (implantable)

C1765 Adhesion barrier

C1766 Introducer/sheath, guiding, intracardiac electrophysiological, steerable, other than peel-away

C1767 Generator, neurostimulator (implantable), non-rechargeable

C1768 Graft, vascular

C1769 Guide wire

C1770 Imaging coil, magnetic resonance (insertable)

C1771 Repair device, urinary, incontinence, with sling graft

C1772 Infusion pump, programmable (implantable)

C1773 Retrieval device, insertable (used to retrieve fractured medical devices)

C1776 Joint device (implantable)

C1777 Lead, cardioverter-defibrillator, endocardial single coil (implantable)

C1778 Lead, neurostimulator (implantable)

C1779 Lead, pacemaker, transvenous vdd single pass

C1780 Lens, intraocular (new technology)

C1781 Mesh (implantable)

C1782 Morcellator

C1783 Ocular implant, aqueous drainage assist device

C1784 Ocular device, intraoperative, detached retina

C1785 Pacemaker, dual chamber, rate-responsive (implantable)

C1786 Pacemaker, single chamber, rate-responsive (implantable)

C1787 Patient programmer, neurostimulator

C1788 Port, indwelling (implantable)

C1789 Prosthesis, breast (implantable)

C1813 Prosthesis, penile, inflatable

C1814 Retinal tamponade device, silicone oil

C1815 Prosthesis, urinary sphincter (implantable)

C1816 Receiver and/or transmitter, neurostimulator (implantable)

C1817 Septal defect implant system, intracardiac

C1818 Integrated keratoprosthesis

C1819 Surgical tissue localization and excision device (implantable)

C1820 Generator, neurostimulator (implantable), with rechargeable battery and charging system

C1821 Interspinous process distraction device (implantable)

C1830 Powered bone marrow biopsy needle

C1840 Lens, intraocular (telescopic)

● **C1841** Retinal prosthesis, includes all internal and external components

C1874 Stent, coated/covered, with delivery system

C1875 Stent, coated/covered, without delivery system

C1876 Stent, non-coated/non-covered, with delivery system

C1877 Stent, non-coated/non-covered, without delivery system

C1878 Material for vocal cord medialization, synthetic (implantable)

(C1879 Code deleted 6/30/2012. Use A4648)

C1880 Vena cava filter

C1881 Dialysis access system (implantable)

C1882 Cardioverter-defibrillator, other than single or dual chamber (implantable)

C1883 Adaptor/extension, pacing lead or neurostimulator lead (implantable)

C1884 Embolization protective system

C1885 Catheter, transluminal angioplasty, laser

C1886 Catheter, extravascular tissue ablation, any modality (insertable)

C1887 Catheter, guiding (may include infusion/perfusion capability)

C1888 Catheter, ablation, non-cardiac, endovascular (implantable)

C1891 Infusion pump, non-programmable, permanent (implantable)

C1892 Introducer/sheath, guiding, intracardiac electrophysiological, fixed-curve, peel-away

C1893 Introducer/sheath, guiding, intracardiac electrophysiological, fixed-curve, other than peel-away

C1894 Introducer/sheath, other than guiding, other than intracardiac electrophysiological, non-laser

C1895 Lead, cardioverter-defibrillator, endocardial dual coil (implantable)

C1896 Lead, cardioverter-defibrillator, other than endocardial single or dual coil (implantable)

C1897 Lead, neurostimulator test kit (implantable)

C1898 Lead, pacemaker, other than transvenous vdd single pass

C1899 Lead, pacemaker/cardioverter-defibrillator combination (implantable)

C1900 Lead, left ventricular coronary venous system

C2614 Probe, percutaneous lumbar discectomy

C2615 Sealant, pulmonary, liquid

C2616 Brachytherapy source, non-stranded, yttrium-90, per source

C2617 Stent, non-coronary, temporary, without delivery system

▲ **C2618** Probe/needle, cryoablation

C2619 Pacemaker, dual chamber, non rate-responsive (implantable)

C2620 Pacemaker, single chamber, non rate-responsive (implantable)

C2621 Pacemaker, other than single or dual chamber (implantable)

C2622 Prosthesis, penile, non-inflatable

C2625 Stent, non-coronary, temporary, with delivery system

C2626 Infusion pump, non-programmable, temporary (implantable)

C2627 Catheter, suprapubic/cystoscopic

C2628 Catheter, occlusion

C2629 Introducer/sheath, other than guiding, intracardiac electrophysiological, laser

C2630 Catheter, electrophysiology, diagnostic/ablation, other than 3d or vector mapping, cool-tip

C2631 Repair device, urinary, incontinence, without sling graft

C2634 Brachytherapy source, non-stranded, high activity, iodine-125, greater than 1.01 mci (nist), per source

C2635 Brachytherapy source, non-stranded, high activity, paladium-103, greater than 2.2 mci (nist), per source

C2636 Brachytherapy linear source, non-stranded, paladium-103, per 1mm

C2637 Brachytherapy source, non-stranded, ytterbium-169, per source

C2638 Brachytherapy source, stranded, iodine-125, per source

C2639 Brachytherapy source, non-stranded, iodine-125, per source

C2640 Brachytherapy source, stranded, palladium-103, per source

C2641 Brachytherapy source, non-stranded, palladium-103, per source

C2642 Brachytherapy source, stranded, cesium-131, per source

C2643 Brachytherapy source, non-stranded, cesium-131, per source

C2698 Brachytherapy source, stranded, not otherwise specified, per source

C2699 Brachytherapy source, non-stranded, not otherwise specified, per source

● **C5271** Application of low cost skin substitute graft to trunk, arms, legs, total wound surface area up to 100 sq cm; first 25 sq cm or less wound surface area

● **C5272** Application of low cost skin substitute graft to trunk, arms, legs, total wound surface area up to 100 sq cm; each additional 25 sq cm wound surface area, or part thereof (list separately in addition to code for primary procedure)

● **C5273** Application of low cost skin substitute graft to trunk, arms, legs, total wound surface area greater than or equal to 100 sq cm; first 100 sq cm wound surface area, or 1% of body area of infants and children

● **C5274** Application of low cost skin substitute graft to trunk, arms, legs, total wound surface area greater than or equal to 100 sq cm; each additional 100 sq cm wound surface area, or part thereof, or each additional 1% of body area of infants and children, or part thereof (list separately in addition to code for primary procedure)

● **C5275** Application of low cost skin substitute graft to face, scalp, eyelids, mouth, neck, ears, orbits, genitalia, hands, feet, and/or multiple digits, total wound surface area up to 100 sq cm; first 25 sq cm or less wound surface area

● **C5276** Application of low cost skin substitute graft to face, scalp, eyelids, mouth, neck, ears, orbits, genitalia, hands, feet, and/or multiple digits, total wound surface area up to 100 sq cm; each additional 25 sq cm wound surface area, or part thereof (list separately in addition to code for primary procedure)

● **C5277** Application of low cost skin substitute graft to face, scalp, eyelids, mouth, neck, ears, orbits, genitalia, hands, feet, and/or multiple digits, total wound surface area greater than or equal to 100 sq cm; first 100 sq cm wound surface area, or 1% of body area of infants and children

● **C5278** Application of low cost skin substitute graft to face, scalp, eyelids, mouth, neck, ears, orbits, genitalia, hands, feet, and/or multiple digits, total wound surface area greater than or equal to 100 sq cm; each additional 100 sq cm wound surface area, or part thereof, or each additional 1% of body area of infants and children, or part thereof (list separately in addition to code for primary procedure)

C8900 Magnetic resonance angiography with contrast, abdomen

C8901 Magnetic resonance angiography without contrast, abdomen

C8902 Magnetic resonance angiography without contrast followed by with contrast, abdomen

C8903 Magnetic resonance imaging with contrast, breast; unilateral

C8904 Magnetic resonance imaging without contrast, breast; unilateral

C8905 Magnetic resonance imaging without contrast followed by with contrast, breast; unilateral

C8906 Magnetic resonance imaging with contrast, breast; bilateral

C8907 Magnetic resonance imaging without contrast, breast; bilateral

C8908 Magnetic resonance imaging without contrast followed by with contrast, breast; bilateral

C8909 Magnetic resonance angiography with contrast, chest (excluding myocardium)

C8910 Magnetic resonance angiography without contrast, chest (excluding myocardium)

C8911 Magnetic resonance angiography without contrast followed by with contrast, chest (excluding myocardium)

C8912 Magnetic resonance angiography with contrast, lower extremity

C8913 Magnetic resonance angiography without contrast, lower extremity

C8914 Magnetic resonance angiography without contrast followed by with contrast, lower extremity

C8918 Magnetic resonance angiography with contrast, pelvis

C8919 Magentic resonance angiography without contrast, pelvis

C8920 Magnetic resonance angiography without contrast followed by with contrast, pelvis

C8921 Transthoracic echocardiography with contrast, or without contrast followed by with contrast, for congenital cardiac anomalies; complete

C8922 Transthoracic echocardiography with contrast, or without contrast followed by with contrast, for congenital cardiac anomalies; follow-up or limited study

C8923 Transthoracic echocardiography with contrast, or without contrast followed by with contrast, real-time with image documentation (2D) with or without m-mode recording; complete

C8924 Transthoracic echocardiography with contrast, or without contrast followed by with contrast, real-time with image documentation (2D) with or without m-mode recording; follow-up or limited study

C8925 Transesophageal echocardiography (TEE) with contrast, or without contrast followed by with contrast, real time with image documentation (2D) (with or without m-mode recording); including probe placement, image acquisition, interpretation and report

C8926 Transesophageal echocardiography (TEE) with contrast, or without contrast followed by with contrast, for congenital cardiac anomalies; including probe placement, image acquisition, interpretation and report

C8927 Transesophageal echocardiography (TEE) with contrast, or without contrast followed by with contrast, for monitoring purposes, including probe placement, real time 2-dimensional image acquisition and interpretation leading to ongoing (continuous) assessment of (dynamically changing) cardiac pumping function and to therapeutic measures on an immediate time basis

C8928 Transthoracic echocardiography with contrast, or without contrast followed by with contrast, real-time with image documentation (2D), with or without m-mode recording, during rest and cardiovascular stress test using treadmill, bicycle exercise and/or pharmacologically induced stress, with interpretation and report

C8929 Transthoracic echocardiography with contrast, or without contrast followed by with contrast, real-time with image documentation (2D), includes M-mode recording, when performed, complete, with spectral Doppler echocardiography, and with color flow Doppler echocardiography

C8930 Transthoracic echocardiography, with contrast, or without contrast followed by with contrast, real-time with image documentation (2D), includes m-mode recording, when performed, during rest and cardiovascular stress test using treadmill, bicycle exercise and/or pharmacologically induced stress, with interpretation and report; including performance of continuous electrocardiographic monitoring, with physician supervision

C8931 Magnetic resonance angiography without contrast followed by with contrast, spinal canal and contents

C8932 Magnetic resonance angiography without contrast, spinal canal and contents

C8933 Magnetic resonance angiography without contrast followed by with contrast, spinal canal and contents

C8934 Magnetic resonance angiography with contrast, upper extremity

C8935 Magnetic resonance angiography without contrast, upper extremity

C8936 Magnetic resonance angiography without contrast followed by with contrast, upper extremity

C8957 Intravenous infusion for therapy/diagnosis; initiation of prolonged infusion (more than 8 hours), requiring use of portable or implantable pump

C9113 Injection, pantoprazole sodium, per vial

C9121 Injection, argatroban, per 5 mg

(C9130 Code deleted December 31, 2013. Use J1556.)

(C9131 Code deleted December 31, 2013. Use J9354

● **C9132** Prothrombin complex concentrate (human), Kcentra, per IU of Factor IX activity

● **C9133** Factor IX (antihemophilic factor, recombinant), Rixibus, per IU

C9248 Injection, clevidipine butyrate, 1 mg

C9250 Human plasma fibrin sealant, vapor-heated, solvent-detergent (Artiss), 2 ml

C9254 Injection, lacosamide, 1 mg

C9257 Injection, bevacizumab, 0.25 mg

(C9270) Code deleted December 31, 2011. Use J1557

(C9272) Code deleted December 31, 2011. Use J0897

(C9273) Code deleted June 30, 2011. Use Q2043

(C9274) Code deleted December 31, 2011. Use J0840

C9275 Injection, hexaminolevulinate hydrochloride, 100 mg, per study dose

(C9276) Code deleted December 31, 2011. Use J9043

(C9277) Code deleted December 31, 2011. Use J0221

(C9278) Code deleted March 31, 2011. Use Q2040.

(C9279) Code deleted December 31, 2012. Use J1741

(C9280) Code deleted December 31, 2011. Use J9179

(C9281) Code deleted December 31, 2011. Use J2507

(C9282) Code deleted December 31, 2011. Use J0712

(C9283) Code deleted December 31, 2011. Use J0131

(C9284) Code deleted December 31, 2011. Use J9228

C9285 Lidocaine 70 mg / tetracaine 70 mg, per patch

(C9286) Code deleted December 31, 2012. Use J0485

(C9287) Code deleted December 31, 2012. Use J9042

(C9288) Code deleted December 31, 2012. Use J0716

(C9289) Code deleted December 31, 2012. Use J9019

C9290 Injection, bupivacaine liposome, 1 mg

(C9291) Code deleted June 30, 2012. Use J0178, Q2046.

(C9292 Code deleted December 31, 2013. Use J9306.)

C9293 Injection, glucarpidase, 10 units

(C9294 Code deleted December 31, 2013. Use J3060.)

(C9295 Code deleted December 31, 2013. Use J9047.)

(C9296 Code deleted December 31, 2013. Use J9400.)

(C9297 Code deleted December 31, 2013. Use J9262.)

(C9298 Code deleted December 31, 2013. Use J7316.)

C9352 Microporous collagen implantable tube (neuragen nerve guide), per centimeter length

C9353 Microporous collagen implantable slit tube (neurawrap nerve protector), per centimeter length

C9354 Acellular pericardial tissue matrix of non-human origin (veritas), per square centimeter

C9355 Collagen nerve cuff (neuromatrix), per 0.5 centimeter length

C9356 Tendon, porous matrix of cross-linked collagen and glycosaminoglycan matrix (tenoglide tendon protector sheet), per square centimeter

C9358 Dermal substitute, native, non-denatured collagen, fetal bovine origin, (Surgimend collagen matrix), per 0.5 square centimeters

C9359 Porous purified collagen matrix bone void filler (Integra Mozaik osteoconductive scaffold putty, Integra Os osteoconductive scaffold putty), per 0.5 cc

C9360 Dermal substitute, native, non-denatured collagen, neonatal bovine origin (Surgimend collagen matrix), per 0.5 square centimeters

C9361 Collagen matrix nerve wrap (Neuromend collagen nerve wrap), per 0.5 centimeter length

C9362 Porous purified collagen matrix bone void filler (Integra Mozaik osteoconductive scaffold strip), per 0.5 cc

C9363 Skin substitute, Integra meshed bilayer wound matrix, per square centimeter

C9364 Porcine implant, permacol, per square centimeter

(C9365) Code deleted December 31, 2011. Use Q4124

(C9366) Code deleted December 31, 2012. Use Q4131

C9367 Skin substitute, endoform dermal template, per square centimeter

(C9368) Code deleted December 31, 2012. Use Q4132

(C9369) Code deleted December 31, 2012. Use Q4133

C9399 Unclassified drugs or biologicals

(C9406) Code deleted December 31, 2011. Use A9584

● **C9441** Injection, ferric carboxymaltose, 1 mg

● **C9497** Loxapine, inhalation powder, 10 mg

C9600 Percutaneous transcatheter placement of drug eluting intracoronary stent(s), with coronary angioplasty when performed; single major coronary artery or branch

C9601 Percutaneous transcatheter placement of drug-eluting intracoronary stent(s), with coronary angioplasty when performed; each additional branch of a major coronary artery (list separately in addition to code for primary procedure)

C9602 Percutaneous transluminal coronary atherectomy, with drug eluting intracoronary stent, with coronary angioplasty when performed; single major coronary artery or branch

C9603 Percutaneous transluminal coronary atherectomy, with drug-eluting intracoronary stent, with coronary angioplasty when performed; each additional branch of a major coronary artery (list separately in addition to code for primary procedure

C9604 Percutaneous transluminal revascularization of or through coronary artery bypass graft (internal mammary, free arterial, venous), any combination of bypass graft (internal mammary, free arterial, venous), any combination of protection when performed; single vessel

C9605 Percutaneous transluminal revascularization of or through coronary artery bypass graft (internal mammary, free arterial, venous), any combination of drug-eluting intracoronary stent, atherectomy and angioplasty, including distal protection when performed; each additional branch subtended by the bypass graft (list separately in addition to code for primary procedure)

C9606 Percutaneous transluminal revascularization of acute total/subtotal occlusion during acute myocardial infarction, coronary artery or coronary artery bypass graft, any combination of drug-eluting intracoronary stent, atherectomy and angioplasty, including aspiration thrombectomy when performed, single vessel

C9607 Percutaneous transluminal revascularization of chronic total occlusion, coronary artery, coronary artery branch, or coronary artery bypass graft, any combination of drug-eluting intracoronary stent, atherectomy and angioplasty; single vessel

C9608 Percutaneous transluminal revascularization of chronic total occlusion, coronary artery, coronary artery branch, or coronary artery bypass graft, any combination of drug-eluting intracoronary stent, atherectomy and angioplasty; each additional coronary artery, coronary artery branch, or bypass graft (list separately in addition to code for primary procedure)

C9724 Endoscopic full-thickness plication in the gastric cardia using endoscopic plication system (eps); includes endoscopy

C9725 Placement of endorectal intracavitary applicator for high intensity brachytherapy

C9726 Placement and removal (if performed) of applicator into breast for radiation therapy

C9727 Insertion of implants into the soft palate; minimum of three implants

C9728 Placement of interstitial device(s) for radiation therapy/ surgery guidance (eg, fiducial markers, dosimeter), for other than the following sites (any approach): abdomen, pelvis, prostate, retroperitoneum, thorax, single or multiple

(C9729) Code deleted June 30, 2011. Use CPT 0275T.

(C9730) Code deleted December 31, 2011. Use CPT 0276T.

(C9731) Code deleted December 31, 2011. Use CPT 0277T

(C9732) Code deleted June 30, 2012. Use CPT 0308T

C9733 Non-ophthalmic fluorescent vascular angiography

● **C9734** Focused ultrasound ablation/therapeutic intervention, other than uterine leiomyomata, with magnetic resonance (MR) guidance

● **C9735** Anoscopy; with directed submucosal injection(s), any substance

(C9736 Code deleted December 31, 2013.

● **C9737** Laparoscopy, surgical, esophageal sphincter augmentation with device (eg, magnetic band)

C9800 Dermal injection procedure(s) for facial lipodystrophy syndrome (LDS) and provision of radiesse or sculptra dermal filler, including all items and supplies

C9898 Radiolabeled product provided during a hospital inpatient stay

C9899 Implanted prosthetic device, payable only for inpatients who do not have inpatient coverage

This page intentionally left blank.

DURABLE MEDICAL EQUIPMENT

Guidelines

In addition to the information presented in the INTRODUCTION, several other items unique to this section are defined or identified here:

1. DEFINITION OF DURABLE MEDICAL EQUIPMENT: Durable medical equipment (DME) can withstand repeated use and is used primarily to serve a medical purpose. It generally is not useful in the absence of an illness or injury, and is appropriate for use in the home. Expendable medical supplies, such as incontinent pads, lamb's wool pads, catheters, ace bandages, elastic stockings, surgical face masks, irrigating kits, sheets and bags, are not considered to be DME.

2. REASONABLE AND NECESSARY: DME may not be covered in every instance. The equipment must be reasonable and necessary for the illness or injury being treated or for improving the functioning of a malformed body part. A physician's prescription is normally sufficient to establish that the equipment is necessary. To determine reasonableness, the following conditions must be met: the expense must be proportionate to the therapeutic benefits of using the equipment; the cost must not substantially exceed a medically appropriate care plan; and, the item must not serve the same purpose as equipment already available to the patient. Claims for items that are not reasonable will be denied except when it is determined that no alternative plan of care is available for which payment could be made.

3. SUBSECTION INFORMATION: Some of the listed subheadings or subsections have special needs or instructions unique to that section. Where these are indicated, special "notes" will be presented preceding or following the listings. Those subsections within the DURABLE MEDICAL EQUIPMENT section that have "notes" are as follows:

Subsection	Code Numbers
Artificial kidney machines and accessories	E1510-E1699

4. UNLISTED SERVICE OR PROCEDURE: A service or procedure may be provided that is not listed in this edition of HCPCS. When reporting such a service, the appropriate "unlisted procedure" code may be used to indicate the service, identifying it by "special report"

as defined below. HCPCS terminology is inconsistent in defining unlisted procedures. The procedure definition may include the term(s) "unlisted", "not otherwise classified", "unspecified", "unclassified", "other" and "miscellaneous". Prior to using these codes, try to determine if a Local Level III code or CPT code is available. The "unlisted procedures" and accompanying codes for DURABLE MEDICAL EQUIPMENT are as follows:

E1399 Durable medical equipment, miscellaneous
E1699 Dialysis equipment, not otherwise specified

5. SPECIAL REPORT: A service, material or supply that is rarely provided, unusual, variable or new may require a special report in determining medical appropriateness for reimbursement purposes. Pertinent information should include an adequate definition or description of the nature, extent, and need for the service, material or supply.

6. MODIFIERS: Listed services may be modified under certain circumstances. When appropriate, the modifying circumstance is identified by adding a modifier to the basic procedure code. CPT and HCPCS National Level II modifiers may be used with CPT and HCPCS National Level II procedure codes. Modifiers commonly used with DURABLE MEDICAL EQUIPMENT are as follows:

-CC Procedure code change (use "CC" when the procedure code submitted was changed either for administrative reasons or because an incorrect code was filed)

-LL Lease/rental (used the "LL" modifier when DME rental is to be applied against the purchase price)

-LT Left side (used to identify procedures performed on the left sideof the body)

-MS Six-month maintenance and servicing fee for reasonable and necessary parts and labor which are not covered under any manufacturer or supplier warranty

-NR New when rented (use the "NR" modifier when DME which was new at the time of rental is subsequently purchased)

-NU New equipment

-QE Prescribed amount of oxygen is less than 1 liter per minute (LPM)

-QF Prescribed amount of oxygen exceeds 4 liters per minute (LPM) and portable oxygen is prescribed

-QG Prescribed amount of oxygen is greater than 4 liters per minute (LPM)

-QH Oxygen conserving device is being used with an oxygen delivery system

-QT Recording and storage on tape by an analog tape recorder

-RP Replacement and repair (may be used to indicate replacement of DME, orthotic and prosthetic devices which have been in use for some time. The claim shows the code for the part, followed by the "RP" modifier and the charge for the part.)

-RR Rental (used when DME is to be rented)

-RT Right side (used to identify procedures performed on the right side of the body)

-TC Technical component. Under certain circumstances, a charge may be made for the technical component alone. Under those circumstances, the technical component charge is identified by adding modifier -TC to the usual procedure code. Technical component charges are institutional charges and are not billed separately by physicians. However, portable x-ray suppliers bill only for technical component and should utilize modifier -TC. The charge data from portable x-ray suppliers will then be used to build customary and prevailing profiles.

-UE Used durable medical equipment

7. CPT CODE CROSS-REFERENCE: Unless otherwise specified, the equivalent CPT code for all listings in this section is 99070.

8. DURABLE MEDICAL EQUIPMENT REGIONAL CARRIERS (DMERCS): Effective October 1, 1993 claims for durable medical equipment (DME) must be billed to one of four regional carriers depending upon the residence of the beneficiary. The transition dates for DMERC claims is from November 1, 1993 to March 1, 1994 depending upon the state you practice in. See the Introduction for a complete discussion of DMERCs.

DURABLE MEDICAL EQUIPMENT

CANES

E0100 Cane, includes canes of all materials, adjustable or fixed, with tip
CIM: 60-3, 60-9 MCM: 2100.1

E0105 Cane, quad or three prong, includes canes of all materials, adjustable or fixed, with tips
CIM: 60-15, 60-9 MCM: 2100.1

CRUTCHES

E0110 Crutches, forearm, includes crutches of various materials, adjustable or fixed; pair, complete with tips and handgrip
CIM: 60-9 MCM: 2100.1

E0111 each, with tip and handgrip
CIM: 60-9 MCM: 2100.1

E0112 Crutches, underarm, wood, adjustable or fixed; pair, with pads, tips and handgrip
CIM: 60-9 MCM: 2100.1

E0113 each, with pad, tip and handgrip
CIM: 60-9 MCM: 2100.1

E0114 Crutches, underarm, other than wood, adjustable or fixed; pair, with pads, tips and handgrips
CIM: 60-9 MCM: 2100.1

E0116 Crutch, underarm, other than wood, adjustable or fixed, with pad, tip, handgrip, with or without shock absorber, each
CIM: 60-9 MCM: 2100.1

E0117 Crutch, underarm, articulating, spring assisted, each
MCM: 2100.1

E0118 Crutch substitute, lower leg platform, with or without wheels, each

WALKERS

E0130 Walker, rigid (pickup), adjustable or fixed height
CIM: 60-9 MCM: 2100.1

E0135 Walker, folding (pickup), adjustable or fixed height
CIM: 60-9 MCM: 2100.1

E0140 Walker, with trunk support, adjustable or fixed height, any type
CIM: 60-9 MCM: 2100.1

E0141 Walker, rigid, wheeled, adjustable or fixed height
CIM: 60-9 MCM: 2100.1

E0143 Walker, folding, wheeled, adjustable or fixed height
CIM: 60-9 MCM: 2100.1

E0144 Walker, enclosed, four-sided frame, rigid or folding, wheeled with posterior seat
CIM: 60-9 MCM: 2100.1

E0147 Walker, heavy duty, multiple braking system, variable wheel resistance
CIM: 60-15 MCM: 2100.1

E0148 Walker, heavy duty, without wheels, rigid or folding, any type, each

E0149 Walker, heavy duty, wheeled, rigid or folding, any type

ATTACHMENTS

E0153 Platform attachment; forearm crutch, each

E0154 walker, each

E0155 Wheel attachment, rigid pick-up walker, per pair

E0156 Seat attachment, walker

E0157 Crutch attachment, walker, each

E0158 Leg extensions for a walker, per set of four (4)

E0159 Brake attachment for wheeled walker, replacement, each

COMMODES

E0160 Sitz type bath or equipment, portable, used with or without commode;
CIM: 60-9

E0161 with faucet attachments
CIM: 60-9

E0162 Sitz bath chair
CIM: 60-9

E0163 Commode chair; mobile or stationary, with fixed arms
CIM: 60-9 MCM: 2100.1

E0165 Commode chair, mobile or stationary, with detachable arms
CIM: 60-9 MCM: 2100.1

E0167 Pail or pan for use with commode chair, replacement only
CIM: 60-9

E0168 Commode chair, extra wide and/or heavy duty, stationary or mobile, with or without arms, any type, each

E0170 Commode chair with integrated seat lift mechanism, electric, any type

E0171 Commode chair with integrated seat lift mechanism, non-electric, any type

E0172 Seat lift mechanism placed over or on top of toilet, any type

E0175 Foot rest, for use with commode chair, each

DECUBITUS CARE EQUIPMENT

E0181 Powered pressure reducing mattress overlay/pad, alternating, with pump, includes heavy duty
CIM: 60-9 MCM: 4107.6

E0182 Pump for alternating pressure pad, for replacement only
CIM: 60-9 MCM: 4107.6

E0184 Dry pressure mattress
CIM: 60-9 MCM: 4107.6

E0185 Gel or gel-like pressure pad for mattress, standard mattress length and width
CIM: 60-9 MCM: 4107.6

E0186 Air pressure mattress
CIM: 60-9

E0187 Water pressure mattress
CIM: 60-9

E0188 Synthetic sheepskin pad
CIM: 60-9 MCM: 4107.6

E0189 Lambswool sheepskin pad, any size
CIM: 60-9 MCM: 4107.6

E0190 Positioning cushion/pillow/wedge, any shape or size, includes all components
MCM: 2100.1

E0191 Heel or elbow protector, each

E0193 Powered air floatation bed (low air loss therapy)

E0194 Air fluidized bed
CIM: 60-19

E0196 Gel pressure mattress
CIM: 60-9

E0197 Air pressure pad for mattress, standard mattress length and width
CIM: 60-9

E0198 Water pressure pad for mattress, standard mattress length and width
CIM: 60-9

E0199 Dry pressure pad for mattress, standard mattress length and width
CIM: 60-9

HEAT/COLD APPLICATION

E0200 Heat lamp, without stand (table model), includes bulb, or infrared element
CIM: 60-9 MCM: 2100.1

E0202 Phototherapy (bilirubin) light with photometer

E0203 Therapeutic lightbox, minimum 10,000 lux, table top model
CIM: 60-9

E0205 Heat lamp, with stand, includes bulb, or infrared element
CIM: 60-9 MCM: 2100.1

E0210 Electric heat pad; standard
CIM: 60-9

E0215 moist
CIM: 60-9

E0217 Water circulating heat pad with pump
CIM: 60-9

E0218 Water circulating cold pad with pump
CIM: 60-9

E0221 Infrared heating pad system

E0225 Hydrocollator unit, includes pads
CIM: 60-9 MCM: 2210.3

E0231 Non-contact wound warming device (temperature control unit, AC adapter and power cord) for use with warming card and wound cover
MCM: 2303

E0232 Warming card for use with the non-contact wound warming device and non-contact wound warming wound cover
MCM: 2303

E0235 Paraffin bath unit, portable (see medical supply code A4265 for paraffin)
CIM: 60-9 MCM: 2210.3

E0236 Pump for water circulating pad
CIM: 60-9

E0239 Hydrocollator unit, portable
CIM: 60-9 MCM: 2210.3

BATH AND TOILET AIDS

E0240 Bath/shower chair, with or without wheels, any size
CIM: 60-9

E0241 Bath tub wall rail, each
CIM: 60-9 MCM: 2100.1

E0242 Bath tub rail, floor base
CIM: 60-9 MCM: 2100.1

E0243 Toilet rail, each
CIM: 60-9 MCM: 2100.1

E0244 Raised toilet seat
CIM: 60-9

E0245 Tub stool or bench
CIM: 60-9

E0246 Transfer tub rail attachment

E0247 Transfer bench for tub or toilet with or without commode opening
CIM: 60-9

E0248 Transfer bench, heavy duty, for tub or toilet with or without commode opening
CIM: 60-9

E0249 Pad for water circulating heat unit, for replacement only
CIM: 60-9

HOSPITAL BEDS AND ACCESSORIES

E0250 Hospital bed, fixed height, with any type side rails; with mattress
CIM: 60-18 MCM: 2100.1

E0251 without mattress
CIM: 60-18 MCM: 2100.1

E0255 Hospital bed, variable height, hi-lo, with any type side rails; with mattress
CIM: 60-18 MCM: 2100.1

E0256 without mattress
CIM: 60-18 MCM: 2100.1

E0260 Hospital bed, semi-electric (head and foot adjustment), with any type side rails; with mattress
CIM: 60-18 MCM: 2100.1

E0261 without mattress
CIM: 60-18 MCM: 2100.1

E0265 Hospital bed, total electric (head, foot and height adjustments), with any type side rails; with mattress
CIM: 60-18 MCM: 2100.1

E0266 without mattress
CIM: 60-18 MCM: 2100.1

E0270 Hospital bed, institutional type includes: oscillating, circulating and stryker frame, with mattress
CIM: 60-9

E0271 Mattress; innerspring
CIM: 60-18, 60-9

E0272 foam rubber
CIM: 60-18, 60-9

E0273 Bed board
CIM: 60-9

E0274 Over-bed table
CIM: 60-9

E0275 Bed pan; standard, metal or plastic
CIM: 60-9

E0276 fracture, metal or plastic
CIM: 60-9

E0277 Powered pressure-reducing air mattress
CIM: 60-9

E0280 Bed cradle, any type

E0290 Hospital bed; fixed-height, without side rails; with mattress
CIM: 60-18 MCM: 2100.1

E0291 without mattress
CIM: 60-18 MCM: 2100.1

E0292 Hospital variable height, hi-lo, without side rails; with mattress
CIM: 60-18 MCM: 2100.1

E0293 without mattress
CIM: 60-18 MCM: 2100.1

E0294 Hospital bed, semi-electric (head and foot adjustment), without side rails; with mattress
CIM: 60-18 MCM: 2100.1

E0295 without mattress
CIM: 60-18 MCM: 2100.1

E0296 Hospital bed, total electric (head, foot and height adjustments), without side rails; with mattress
CIM: 60-18 MCM: 2100.1

E0297 without mattress
CIM: 60-18 MCM: 2100.1

HOSPITAL BED ACCESSORIES

E0300 Pediatric crib, hospital grade, fully enclosed

E0301 Hospital bed, heavy duty, extra wide, with weight capacity greater than 350 pounds, but less than or equal to 600 pounds, with any type side rails, without mattress
CIM: 60-18

E0302 Hospital bed, extra heavy duty, extra wide, with weight capacity greater than 600 pounds, with any type side rails, without mattress
CIM: 60-18

E0303 Hospital bed, heavy duty, extra wide, with weight capacity greater than 350 pounds, but less than or equal to 600 pounds, with any type side rails, with mattress
CIM: 60-18

E0304 Hosptial bed, extra heavy duty, extra wide, with weight capacity greater than 600 pounds, with any type side rails, with mattress
CIM: 60-18

E0305 Bed side rails; half length
CIM: 60-18

E0310 full length
CIM: 60-18

E0315 Bed accessory: board, table, or support device, any type
CIM: 60-9

E0316 Safety enclosure frame/canopy for use with hospital bed, any type

E0325 Urinal; male, jug/type, any material
CIM: 60-9

E0326 female, jug/type, any material
CIM: 60-9

E0328 Hospital bed, pediatric, manual, 360 degree side enclosures, top of headboard, footboard and side rails up to 24 inches above the spring, includes mattress

E0329 Hospital bed, pediatric, electric or semi-electric, 360 degree side enclosures, top of headboard, footboard and side rails up to 24 inches above the spring, includes mattress

E0350 Control unit for electronic bowel irrigation/evacuation system

E0352 Disposable pack (water reservoir bag, speculum, valving mechanism and collection bag/box) for use with the electronic bowel irrigation/evacuation system

E0370 Air pressure elevator for heel

E0371 Nonpowered advanced pressure reducing overlay for mattress, standard mattress length and width

E0372 Powered air overlay for mattress, standard mattress length and width

E0373 Nonpowered advanced pressure reducing mattress

OXYGEN AND RELATED RESPIRATORY EQUIPMENT

E0424 Stationary compressed gaseous oxygen system, rental; includes container, contents, regulator, flowmeter, humidifier, nebulizer, cannula or mask, and tubing
CIM: 60-4 MCM: 4107.9

E0425 Stationary compressed gas system, purchase; includes regulator, flowmeter, humidifier, nebulizer, cannula or mask, and tubing
CIM: 60-4 MCM: 4107.9

E0430 Portable gaseous oxygen system, purchase; includes regulator flowmeter, humidifier, cannula or mask, and tubing
CIM: 60-4 MCM: 4107.9

E0431 Portable gaseous oxygen system, rental; includes portable container, regulator, flowmeter, humidifier, cannula or mask, and tubing
CIM: 60-4 MCM: 4107.9

E0433 Portable liquid oxygen system, rental; home liquefier used to fill portable liquid oxygen containers, includes portable containers, regulator, flowmeter, humidifier, cannula or mask and tubing, with or without supply reservoir and contents gauge

E0434 Portable liquid oxygen system, rental; includes portable container, supply reservoir, humidifier, flowmeter, refill adaptor, contents gauge, cannula or mask, and tubing
CIM: 60-4 MCM: 4107.9

E0435 Portable liquid oxygen system, purchase; includes portable container, supply reservoir, flowmeter, humidifier, contents gauge, cannula or masks, tubing and refill adaptor
CIM: 60-4 MCM: 4107.9

E0439 Stationary liquid oxygen system; rental, includes container, contents, regulator, flowmeter, humidifier, nebulizer, cannula or mask, and tubing
CIM: 60-4 MCM: 4107.9

E0440 purchase, includes use of reservoir, contents indicator, regulator, flowmeter, humidifier, nebulizer, cannula or mask, and tubing
CIM: 60-4 MCM: 4107.9

E0441 Stationary oxygen contents, gaseous, 1 month's supply = 1 unit
CIM: 60-4 MCM: 4107.9

E0442 Stationary oxygen contents, liquid, 1 month's supply = 1 unit
CIM: 60-4 MCM: 4107.9

E0443 Portable oxygen contents, gaseous, 1 month's supply = 1 unit
CIM: 60-4 MCM: 4107.9

E0444 Portable oxygen contents, liquid, 1 month's supply = 1 unit
CIM: 60-4 MCM: 4107.9

E0445 Oximeter device for measuring blood oxygen levels non-invasively

E0446 Topical oxygen delivery system, not otherwise specified, includes all supplies and accessories

E0450 Volume control ventilator, without pressure support mode, may include pressure control mode, used with invasive interface (e.g., tracheostomy tube)
CIM: 60-9

E0455 Oxygen tent, excluding croup or pediatric tents
CIM: 60-4 MCM: 4107.9

E0457 Chest shell (cuirass)

E0459 Chest wrap

E0460 Negative pressure ventilator, portable or stationary
CIM: 60-9

E0461 Volume control ventilator, without pressure support mode, may include pressure control mode, used with non-invasive interface (e.g. mask)
CIM: 60-9

E0462 Rocking bed with or without side rails

E0463 Pressure support ventilator with volume control mode, may include pressure control mode, used with invasive interface (e.g. tracheostomy tube)

E0464 Pressure support ventilator with volume control mode, may include pressure control mode, used with non-invasive interface (e.g. mask)

E0470 Respiratory assist device, bi-level pressure capability, without backup rate feature, used with noninvasive interface, eg., nasal or facial mask (intermittent assist device with continuous positive airway pressure device)
CIM: 60-9

E0471 Respiratory assist device, bi-level pressure capability, with backup rate feature, used with noninvasive interface, eg., nasal or facial mask (intermittent assist device with continuous positive airway pressure device)
CIM: 60-9

E0472 Respiratory assist device, bi-level pressure capability, with backup rate feature, used with invasive interface, eg., tracheostomy tube (intermittent assist device with continuous positive airway pressure device
CIM: 60-9

E0480 Percussor, electric or pneumatic, home model
CIM: 60-9

E0481 Intrapulmonary percussive ventilation system and related accessories
CIM: 60-21

E0482 Cough stimulating device, alternating positive and negative airway pressure

E0483 High frequency chest wall oscillation air-pulse generator system, (includes hoses and vest), each

E0484 Oscillatory positive expiratory pressure device, non-electric, any type, each

E0485 Oral device/appliance used to reduce upper airway collapsibility, adjustable or non-adjustable, prefabricated, includes fitting and adjustment

E0486 Oral device/appliance used to reduce upper airway collapsibility, adjustable or non-adjustable, custom fabricated, includes fitting and adjustment

E0487 Spirometer, electronic, includes all accessories

IPPB MACHINES

E0500 IPPB machine, all types, with built-in nebulization; manual or automatic valves; internal or external power source
CIM: 60-9

HUMIDIFIERS/NEBULIZERS FOR USE WITH OXYGEN IPPB EQUIPMENT

COMPRESSORS

E0550 Humidifier, durable for extensive supplemental humidification during IPPB treatments or oxygen delivery
CIM: 60-9

E0555 Humidifier, durable, glass or autoclavable plastic bottle type, for use with regulator or flowmeter
CIM: 60-9 MCM: 4107.9

E0560 Humidifier, durable for supplemental humidification during IPPB treatment or oxygen delivery
CIM: 60-9

E0561 Humidifier, non-heated, used with positive airway pressure device

E0562 Humidifier, heated, used with positive airway pressure device

E0565 Compressor, air power source for equipment which is not self-contained or cylinder driven

E0570 Nebulizer; with compressor
CIM: 60-9 MCM: 4107.9

(E0571) Code deleted December 31, 2011

E0572 Aerosol compressor, adjustable pressure, light duty for intermittent use

E0574 Ultrasonic/electronic aerosol generator with small volume nebulizer

E0575 Nebulizer, ultrasonic, large volume
CIM: 60-9

E0580 Nebulizer, with compressor, durable, glass or autoclavable plastic, bottle type, for use with regulator or flowmeter
CIM: 60-9 MCM: 4107.9

E0585 Nebulizer with compressor and heater
CIM: 60-9 MCM: 4107.9

SUCTION PUMP/ROOM VAPORIZERS

E0600 Respiratory suction pump, home model, portable or stationary, electric
CIM: 60-9

▲**E0601** Continuous positive airway pressure (CPAP) device
CIM: 60-17

E0602 Breast pump, manual, any type

E0603 Breast pump, electric (AC and/or DC), any type

E0604 Breast pump, hospital grade, electric (AC and/or DC), any type

E0605 Vaporizer, room type
CIM: 60-9

E0606 Postural drainage board
CIM: 60-9

MONITORING EQUIPMENT

E0607 Home blood glucose monitor
CIM: 60-11

PACEMAKER MONITOR

E0610 Pacemaker monitor, self-contained; (checks battery depletion, included audible and visible check systems)
CIM: 60-7, 50-1

E0615 (checks battery depletion and other pacemaker components, includes digital/visible check systems)
CIM: 60-7, 50-1

E0616 Implantable cardiac event recorder with memory, activator and programmer

E0617 External defibrillator with integrated electrocardiogram analysis

E0618 Apnea monitor, without recording feature

E0619 Apnea monitor, with recording feature

E0620 Skin piercing device for collection of capillary blood, laser, each

PATIENT LIFTS

E0621 Sling or seat, patient lift, canvas or nylon
CIM: 60-9

E0625 Patient lift, bathroom or toilet, not otherwise classified
CIM: 60-9

E0627 Seat lift mechanism incorporated into a combination lift-chair mechanism
CIM: 60-8 MCM: 4107.8

E0628 Separate seat life mechanism for use with patient owned furniture; electric
CIM: 60-8 MCM: 4107.8

E0629 non-electric
MCM: 4107.8

E0630 Patient lift; hydraulic or mechanical, includes any seat, sling, strap(s) or pad(s)
CIM: 60-9

E0635 electric, with seat or sling
CIM: 60-9

E0636 Multipositional patient support system, with integrated lift, patient accessible controls

E0637 Combination sit to stand frame/table system, any size including pediatric, with seat lift feature, with or without wheels
CIM: 60-9

E0638 Standing frame/table system, one position (e.g. upright, supine or prone stander), any size including pediatric, with or without wheels
CIM: 60-9

E0639 Patient lift, moveable from room to room with disassembly and reassembly, includes all components/accessories

E0640 Patient lift, fixed system, includes all components/accessories

E0641 Standing frame/table system, multi-position (e.g. Three-way stander), any size including pediatric, with or without wheels
CIM: 60-9

E0642 Standing frame/table system, mobile (dynamic stander), any size including pediatric
CIM: 60-9

PNEUMATIC COMPRESSOR AND APPLIANCES (LYMPHEDEMA PUMP)

E0650 Pneumatic compressor; non-segmental home model
CIM: 60-16

E0651 segmental home model without calibrated gradient pressure
CIM: 60-16

E0652 segmental home model with calibrated gradient pressure
CIM: 60-16

E0655 Non-segmental pneumatic appliance for use with pneumatic compressor; half arm
CIM: 60-16

E0656 Segmental pneumatic appliance for use with pneumatic compressor, trunk

E0657 Segmental pneumatic appliance for use with pneumatic compressor, chest

E0660 Non-segmental pneumatic appliance for use with pneumatic compressor; full leg
CIM: 60-16

E0665 full arm
CIM: 60-16

E0666 half leg
CIM: 60-16

E0667 Segmental pneumatic appliance for use with pneumatic compressor; full leg
CIM: 60-16

E0668 full arm
CIM: 60-16

E0669 half leg
CIM: 60-16

E0670 Segmental pneumatic appliance for use with pneumatic compressor, integrated, 2 full legs and trunk

E0671 Segmental gradient pressure pneumatic appliance, full leg
CIM: 60-16

E0672 full arm
CIM: 60-16

E0673 half leg
CIM: 60-16

E0675 Pneumatic compression device, high pressure, rapid inflation/deflation cycle, for arterial insufficiency (unilateral or bilateral system)

E0676 Intermittent limb compression device (includes all accessories), not otherwise specified

ULTRAVIOLET CABINET

E0691 Ultraviolet light therapy system, includes bulbs/lamps, timer and eye protection; treatment area 2 square feet or less

E0692 Ultraviolet light therapy system panel, includes bulbs/lamps, timer and eye protection, 4 foot panel

E0693 Ultraviolet light therapy system panel, includes bulbs/lamps, timer and eye protection, 6 foot panel

E0694 Ultraviolet multidirectional light therapy system in 6 foot cabinet, includes bulbs/lamps, timer and eye protection

SAFETY EQUIPMENT

E0700 Safety equipment, device or accessory, any type

RESTRAINTS

E0705 Transfer device, any type, each

E0710 Restraints, any type (body, chest, wrist or ankle)

TRANSCUTANEOUS AND/OR NEUROMUSCULAR ELECTRICAL NERVE STIMULATORS - TENS

E0720 TENS device; two lead, localized stimulation
CIM: 35-20, 35-46 MCM: 4107.6

E0730 four or more leads, for multiple nerve stimulation
CIM: 35-20, 35-46 MCM: 4107.6

E0731 Form fitting conductive garment for delivery of TENS or NMES (with conductive fibers separated from the patient's skin by layers of fabric)
CIM: 45-25

E0740 Incontinence treatment system, pelvic floor stimulator, monitor, sensor and/or trainer
CIM: 60.24

E0744 Neuromuscular stimulator for scoliosis

E0745 Neuromuscular stimulator, electronic shock unit
CIM: 35-77

E0746 Electromyography (EMG), biofeedback device
CIM: 35-27

E0747 Osteogenesis stimulator; electrical, non-invasive, other than spinal applications
CIM: 35-48

E0748 Osteogenesis stimulator; electrical, noninvasive, spinal applications
CIM: 35-48

E0749 Osteogenesis stimulator, electrical, surgically implanted
CIM: 35-48

E0755 Electronic salivary reflex stimulator (intra-oral/non-invasive)

E0760 Ostogenesis stimulator, low intensity ultrasound, non-invasive
MCM: 35-48

E0761 Non-thermal pulsed high frequency radiowaves, high peak power electromagnetic energy treatment device
CIM: 35-102

E0762 Transcutaneous electrical joint stimulation device system, includes all accessories

E0764 Functional neuromuscular stimulator, transcutaneous stimulation of muscles of ambulation with computer control, used for walking by spinal cord injured, entire system, after completion of training program
CIM: 35-77

E0765 FDA approved nerve stimulator with replaceable batteries for treatment of nausea and vomiting

● **E0766** Electrical stimulation device used for cancer treatment, includes all accessories, any type

E0769 Electrical stimulation or electromagnetic wound treatment device, not otherwise classified
CIM: 35-102

E0770 Functional electrical stimulator, transcutaneous stimulation of nerve and/or muscle groups, any type, complete system, not otherwise specified

E0776 IV pole

E0779 Ambulatory infusion pump, mechanical, reusable, for infusion 8 hours or greater

E0780 Ambulatory infusion pump, mechanical, reusable, for infusion less than 8 hours

E0781 Ambulatory infusion pump, single or multiple channels, electric or battery operated, with administrative equipment, worn by patient
CIM: 60-14

E0782 Infusion pump, implantable, non-programmable (includes all components, e.g., pump, catheter, connectors, etc.)
CIM: 60-14

E0783 Infusion pump system, implantable, programmable (includes all components, e.g., pump, catheter, connectors, etc.)
CIM: 60-14

E0784 External ambulatory infusion pump, insulin
CIM: 60-14

E0785 Implantable intraspinal (epidural/intrathecal) catheter used with implantable infusion pump, replacement
MCM: 60-14

E0786 Implantable programmable infusion pump, replacement (excludes implantable intraspinal catheter)
CIM: 60-14

E0791 Parenteral infusion pump, stationary, single or multi-channel
CIM: 65-10 MCM: 2130, 4450

TRACTION EQUIPMENT

TRACTION - CERVICAL

E0830 Ambulatory traction device, all types, each
CIM: 60-9

E0840 Traction frame, attached to headboard, cervical traction
CIM: 60-9

E0849 Traction equipment, cervical, free-standing stand/frame, pneumatic, applying traction force to other than mandible

E0850 Traction stand, free standing, cervical traction
CIM: 60-9

E0855 Cervical traction equipment not requiring additional stand or frame

E0856 Cervical traction device, cervical collar with inflatable air bladder

TRACTION - OVERDOOR

E0860 Traction equipment, overdoor, cervical
CIM: 60-9

TRACTION - EXTREMITY

E0870 Traction frame, attached to footboard, extremity traction, (e.g., Buck's)
CIM: 60-9

E0880 Traction stand, free standing, extremity traction, (e.g., Buck's)
CIM: 60-9

TRACTION - PELVIC

E0890 Traction frame, attached to footboard, pelvic traction
CIM: 60-9

E0900 Traction stand, free standing, pelvic traction (e.g., Buck's)
CIM: 60-9

TRAPEZE EQUIPMENT, FRACTURE FRAME, AND OTHER ORTHOPEDIC DEVICES

E0910 Trapeze bars, A/K/A patient helper, attached to bed, with grab bar
CIM: 60-9

E0911 Trapeze bar, heavy duty, for patient weight capacity greater than 250 pounds, attached to bed, with grab bar
CIM: 60-9

E0912 Trapeze bar, heavy duty, for patient weight capacity greater than 250 pounds, free standing, complete with grab bar
CIM: 60-9

E0920 Fracture frame; attached to bed, includes weights
CIM: 60-9

E0930 free standing, includes weights
CIM: 60-9

E0935 Continuous passive motion exercise device for use on knee only
CIM: 60-9

E0936 Continuous passive motion exercise device for use other than knee

E0940 Trapeze bar, free standing, complete with grab bar
CIM: 60-9

E0941 Gravity assisted traction device, any type
CIM: 60-9

E0942 Cervical head harness/halter

E0944 Pelvic belt/harness/boot

E0945 Extremity belt/harness

E0946 Fracture frame; dual with cross bars, attached to bed, (e.g., Balken, 4 poster)
CIM: 60-9

E0947 attachments for complex pelvic traction
CIM: 60-9

E0948 attachments for complex cervical traction
CIM: 60-9

WHEELCHAIRS AND WHEELCHAIR ACCESSORIES

E0950 Wheelchair accessory, tray, each
CIM: 60-9

E0951 Heel loop/holder, any type, with or without ankle strap, each

E0952 Toe loop/holder, any type, each
CIM: 60-9

E0955 Wheelchair accessory, headrest, cushioned, any type, including fixed mounting hardware, each

E0956 Wheelchair accessory, lateral trunk or hip support, any type, including fixed mounting hardware, each

E0957 Wheelchair accessory, medial thigh support, any type, including fixed mounting hardware, each

E0958 Manual wheelchair accessory, one-arm drive attachment, each
CIM: 60-9

E0959 Manual wheelchair accessory, adapter for amputee, each
CIM: 60-9

E0960 Wheelchair accessory, shoulder harness/straps or chest strap, including any type mounting hardware

E0961 Manual wheelchair accessory, wheel lock brake extension (handle), each
CIM: 60-9

E0966 Manual wheelchair accessory, headrest extension, each
CIM: 60-9

E0967 Manual wheelchair accessory, hand rim with projections, any type, each
CIM: 60-9

E0968 Commode seat, wheelchair
CIM: 60-9

E0969 Narrowing device, wheelchair
CIM: 60-9

E0970 No. 2 Footplates, except for elevating leg rest
CIM: 60-9

E0971 Manual wheelchair accessory, anti-tipping device, each
CIM: 60-9

E0973 Wheelchair accessory, adjustable height, detachable armrest, complete assembly, each
CIM: 60-9

E0974 Manual wheelchair accessory, anti-rollback device, each
CIM: 60-9

E0978 Wheelchair accessory, positioning belt/safety belt/pelvic strap, each

E0980 Safety vest, wheelchair

E0981 Wheelchair accessory, seat upholstery, replacement only, each

E0982 Wheelchair accessory, back upholstery, replacement only, each

E0983 Manual wheelchair accessory, power add-on to convert manual wheelchair to motorized wheelchair, joystick control

E0984 Manual wheelchair accessory, power add-on to convert manual wheelchair to motorized wheelchair, tiller control

E0985 Wheelchair accessory, seat lift mechanism

E0986 Manual wheelchair accessory, push activated power assist, each

E0988 Manual wheelchair accessory, lever-activated, wheel drive, pair

E0990 Wheelchair accessory, elevating leg rest, complete assembly, each
CIM: 60-9

E0992 Manual wheelchair accessory, solid seat insert

E0994 Arm rest, each
CIM: 60-9

E0995 Wheelchair accessory, calf rest/pad, each
CIM: 60-9

E1002 Wheelchair accessory, power seating system, tilt only

E1003 Wheelchair accessory, power seating system, recline only, without shear reduction

E1004 Wheelchair accessory, power seating system, recline only, with mechanical shear reduction

E1005 Wheelchair accessory, power seating system, recline only, with power shear reduction

E1006 Wheelchair accessory, power seating system, combination tilt and recline, without shear reduction

E1007 Wheelchair accessory, power seating system, combination tilt and recline, with mechanical shear reduction

E1008 Wheelchair accessory, power seating system, combination tilt and recline, with power shear reduction

E1009 Wheelchair accessory, addition to power seating system, mechanically linked leg elevation system, including pushrod and leg rest, each

E1010 Wheelchair accessory, addition to power seating system, power leg elevation system, including leg rest, pair

E1011 Modification to pediatric size wheelchair, width adjustment package (not to be dispensed with initial chair)
CIM: 60-9

E1014 Reclining back, addition to pediatric size wheelchair
CIM: 60-9

E1015 Shock absorber for manual wheelchair, each
MCM: 60.9

E1016 Shock absorber for power wheelchair, each
MCM: 60.9

E1017 Heavy duty shock absorber for heavy duty or extra heavy duty manual wheelchair, each
MCM: 60.9

E1018 Heavy duty shock absorber for heavy duty or extra heavy duty power wheelchair, each
MCM: 60.9

E1020 Residual limb support system for wheelchair
MCM: 60-6

E1028 Wheelchair accessory, manual swingaway, retractable or removable mounting hardware for joystick, other control interface or positioning accessory

E1029 Wheelchair accessory, ventilator tray, fixed

E1030 Wheelchair accessory, ventilator tray, gimbaled

ROLLABOUT CHAIR

E1031 Rollabout chair, any and all types with castors 5 inches or greater
CIM: 60-9

E1035 Multi-positional patient transfer system, with integrated seat, operated by care giver, patient weight capacity up to and including 300 lbs.
MCM: 2100

E1036 Multi-positional patient transfer system, extra-wide, with integrated seat, operated by care giver, patient weight capacity greater than 300 lbs.

E1037 Transport chair, pediatric size
CIM: 60-9

E1038 Transport chair, adult size, patient weight capacity up to and including 300 pounds
CIM: 60-9

E1039 Transport chair, adult size, heavy duty, patient weight capacity greater than 300 pounds

WHEELCHAIR - FULLY-RECLINING

E1050 Fully-reclining wheelchair; fixed full length arms, swing away detachable elevating leg rests
CIM: 60-9

E1060 Fully-reclining wheelchair; detachable arms, desk or full length, swing away detachable elevating leg rests
CIM: 60-9

E1070 Fully-reclining wheelchair, detachable arms (desk or full length) swing away detachable footrest
CIM: 60-9

E1083 Hemi-wheelchair; fixed full length arms, swing away detachable elevating leg rest
CIM: 60-9

E1084 detachable arms desk or full length arms, swing away detachable elevating leg rests
CIM: 60-9

E1085 fixed full length arms, swing away detachable footrests
CIM: 60-9

E1086 detachable arms desk or full length, swing away detachable footrests
CIM: 60-9

E1087 High strength lightweight wheelchair; fixed full length arms, swing away detachable elevating leg rests
CIM: 60-9

E1088 detachable arms desk or full length, swing away detachable elevating leg rests
CIM: 60-9

E1089 fixed length arms, swing away detachable footrest
CIM: 60-9

E1090 detachable arms desk or full length, swing away detachable footrests
CIM: 60-9

E1092 Wide heavy duty wheelchair, detachable arms (desk or full length); swing away detachable elevating leg rests
CIM: 60-9

E1093 swing away detachable footrests
CIM: 60-9

WHEELCHAIR - SEMI-RECLINING

E1100 Semi-reclining wheelchair; fixed full length arms, swing away detachable elevating leg rests
CIM: 60-9

E1110 detachable arms (desk or full length), elevating leg rest
CIM: 60-9

WHEELCHAIR - STANDARD

E1130 Standard wheelchair, fixed full length arms, fixed or swing away detachable footrests
CIM: 60-9

E1140 Wheelchair, detachable arms, desk or full length; swing away detachable footrests
CIM: 60-9

E1150 swing away detachable elevating leg rests
CIM: 60-9

E1160 Wheelchair, fixed full length arms, swing away detachable elevating leg rests
CIM: 60-9

E1161 Manual adult size wheelchair, includes tilt in space

WHEELCHAIR - AMPUTEE

E1170 Amputee wheelchair; fixed full length arms, swing away detachable elevating leg rests
CIM: 60-9

E1171 fixed full length arms, without foot rests or leg rest
CIM: 60-9

E1172 detachable arms (desk or full length), without foot rests or leg rest
CIM: 60-9

E1180 detachable arms (desk or full length), swing away detachable foot rests
CIM: 60-9

E1190 detachable arms (desk or full length), swing away detachable elevating leg rests
CIM: 60-9

E1195 Heavy duty wheelchair, fixed full length arms, swing away detachable elevating leg rests
CIM: 60-9

E1200 Amputee wheelchair, fixed full length arms, swing away detachable foot rest
CIM: 60-9

WHEELCHAIR - SPECIAL SIZE

E1220 Wheelchair specially sized or constructed (indicate brand name, model number, if any, and justification)
CIM: 60-6

E1221 Wheelchair with fixed arm; footrests
CIM: 60-6

E1222 elevating leg rests
CIM: 60-6

E1223 Wheelchair with detachable arms; foot rests
CIM: 60-6

E1224 elevating leg rests
CIM: 60-6

E1225 Wheelchair accessory, manual semi-reclining back, (recline greater than 15 degrees, but less than 80 degrees), each
CIM: 60-6

E1226 Wheelchair accessory, manual fully reclining back, (recline greater than 80 degrees), each
CIM: 60-9

E1227 Special height arms for wheelchair
CIM: 60-6

E1228 Special back height for wheelchair
CIM: 60-6

E1229 Wheelchair, pediatric size, not otherwise specified

POWER OPERATED VEHICLE

E1230 Power operated vehicle (3 or 4 wheel non-highway) specify brand name and model number
CIM: 60-5 MCM: 4107.6

E1231 Wheelchair, pediatric size, tilt-in-space, rigid, adjustable, with seating system
CIM: 60-9

E1232 Wheelchair, pediatric size, tilt-in-space, folding, adjustable, with seating system
CIM: 60-9

E1233 Wheelchair, pediatric size, tilt-in-space, rigid, adjustable, without seating system
CIM: 60-9

E1234 Wheelchair, pediatric size, tilt-in-space, folding, adjustable, without seating system
CIM: 60-9

E1235 Wheelchair, pediatric size, rigid, adjustable, with seating system
CIM: 60-9

E1236 Wheelchair, pediatric size, folding, adjustable, with seating system
CIM: 60-9

E1237 Wheelchair, pediatric size, rigid, adjustable, without seating system
CIM: 60-9

E1238 Wheelchair, pediatric size, folding, adjustable, without seating system
CIM: 60-9

E1239 Power wheelchair, pediatric size, not otherwise specified

WHEELCHAIR - LIGHTWEIGHT

E1240 Lightweight wheelchair; detachable arms, (desk or full length) swing away detachable, elevating leg rest
CIM: 60-9

E1250 fixed full length arms, swing away detachable footrest
CIM: 60-9

E1260 detachable arms (desk or full length) swing away detachable footrest
CIM: 60-9

E1270 fixed full length arms, swing away detachable elevating leg rests
CIM: 60-9

WHEELCHAIR - HEAVY DUTY

E1280 Heavy duty wheelchair; detachable arms (desk or full length) elevating leg rests
CIM: 60-9

E1285 fixed full length arms, swing away detachable foot rest
CIM: 60-9

E1290 detachable arms (desk or full length) swing away detachable foot rest
CIM: 60-9

E1295 fixed full length arms, elevating leg rest
CIM: 60-9

E1296 Special wheelchair; seat height from floor
CIM: 60-6

E1297 seat depth, by upholstery
CIM: 60-6

E1298 seat depth and/or width, by construction
CIM: 60-6

WHIRLPOOL EQUIPMENT

E1300 Whirlpool; portable (overtub type)
CIM: 60-9

E1310 non-portable (built-in type)
CIM: 60-9

ADDITIONAL OXYGEN RELATED SUPPLIES AND EQUIPMENT

● **E1352** Oxygen accessory, flow regulator capable of positive inspiratory pressure

E1353 Regulator
CIM: 60-4 MCM: 4107.9

E1354 Oxygen accessory, wheeled cart for portable cylinder or portable concentrator, any type, replacement only, each

E1355 Stand/Rack
CIM: 60-4

E1356 Oxygen accessory, battery pack/cartridge for portable concentrator, any type, replacement only, each

E1357 Oxygen accessory, battery charger for portable concentrator, any type, replacement only, each

E1358 Oxygen accessory, dc power adapter for portable concentrator, any type, replacement only, each

E1372 Immersion external heater for nebulizer
CIM: 60-4

E1390 Oxygen concentrator, single delivery port, capable of delivering 85 percent or greater oxygen concentration at the prescribed flow rate
CIM: 60-4

E1391 Oxygen concentrator, dual delivery port, capable of delivering 85 percent or greater oxygen concentration at the prescribed flow rate
CIM: 60-4

E1392 Portable oxygen concentrator, rental
CIM: 60-4

E1399 Durable medical equipment, miscellaneous

E1405 Oxygen and water vapor enriching system; with heated delivery
CIM: 60-4 MCM: 4107

E1406 without heated delivery
CIM: 60-4 MCM: 4107

ARTIFICIAL KIDNEY MACHINES AND ACCESSORIES

NOTE: For supplies for ESRD, see codes A4650-A4999.

E1500 Centrifuge, for dialysis

E1510 Kidney dialysate delivery system; kidney machine, pump recirculating, air removal system, flowrate meter, power off, heater and temp control with alarm, I.V. poles, pressure gauge, concentrate container

E1520 Heparin infusion pump for hemodialysis

E1530 Air bubble detector for hemodialysis, each, replacement

E1540 Pressure alarm for hemodialysis, each, replacement

E1550 Bath conductivity meter for hemodialysis, each

E1560 Blood leak detector for hemodialysis, each, replacement

E1570 Adjustable chair, for ESRD patients

E1575 Transducer protectors/fluid barriers, for hemodialysis, any size, per 10

E1580 Unipuncture control system for hemodialysis

E1590 Hemodialysis machine

E1592 Automatic intermittent peritoneal dialysis system

E1594 Cycler dialysis machine for peritoneal dialysis

E1600 Delivery and/or installation charges for hemodialysis equipment

E1610 Reverse osmosis water purification system, for hemodialysis
CIM: 55-1A

E1615 Deionizer water purification system, for hemodialysis
CIM: 55-1A

E1620 Blood pump for hemodialysis, replacement

E1625 Water softening system, for hemodialysis
CIM: 55-1B

E1630 Reciprocating peritoneal dialysis system

E1632 Wearable artificial kidney, each

E1634 Peritoneal dialysis clamps, each
MCM: 4270

E1635 Compact (portable) travel hemodialyzer system

E1636 Sorbent cartridges, for hemodialysis, per 10

E1637 Hemostats, each

E1639 Scale, each

E1699 Dialysis equipment, not otherwise specified

E1700 Jaw motion rehabilitation system

E1701 Replacement cushions for jaw motion rehabilitation system, pkg. of 6

E1702 Replacement measuring scales for jaw motion rehabilitation system, pkg. of 200

E1800 Dynamic adjustable elbow extension/flexion device, includes soft interface material

E1801 Static progressive stretch elbow device, extension and/or flexion, with or without range of motion adjustment, includes all components and accessories

E1802 Dynamic adjustable forearm pronation/supination device, includes soft interface material

E1805 Dynamic adjustable wrist extension/flexion device, includes soft interface material

E1806 Static progressive stretch wrist device, flexion and/or extension, with or without range of motion adjustment, includes all components and accessories

E1810 Dynamic adjustable knee extension/flexion device, includes soft interface material

E1811 Static progressive stretch knee device, extension and/or flexion, with or without range of motion adjustment, includes all components and accessories

E1812 Dynamic knee, extension/flexion device with active resistance control

E1815 Dynamic adjustable ankle extension/flexion device, includes soft interface material

E1816 Static progressive stretch ankle device, flexion and/or extension, with or without range of motion adjustment, includes all components and accessories

E1818 Static progressive stretch forearm pronation / supination device, with or without range of motion adjustment, includes all components and accessories

E1820 Replacement soft interface material, dynamic adjustable extension/flexion device

E1821 Replacement soft interface material/cuffs for bi-directional static progressive stretch device

E1825 Dynamic adjustable finger extension/flexion device, includes soft interface material

E1830 Dynamic adjustable toe extension/flexion device, includes soft interface material

E1831 Static progressive stretch toe device, extension and/or flexion, with or without range of motion adjustment, includes all components and accessories

E1840 Dynamic adjustable shoulder flexion/abduction/rotation device, includes soft interface material

E1841 Static progressive stretch shoulder device, with or without range of motion adjustment, includes all components and accessories

E1902 Communication board, non-electronic augmentative or alternative communication device

E2000 Gastric suction pump, home model, portable or stationary, electric

E2100 Blood glucose monitor with integrated voice synthesizer
CIM: 60-11

E2101 Blood glucose monitor with integrated lancing/blood sample
CIM: 60-11

E2120 Pulse generator system for tympanic treatment of inner ear endolymphatic fluid

WHEELCHAIR ACCESSORIES

E2201 Manual wheelchair accessory, nonstandard seat frame, width greater than or equal to 20 inches and less than 24 inches

E2202 Manual wheelchair accessory, nonstandard seat frame width, 24-27 inches

E2203 Manual wheelchair accessory, nonstandard seat frame depth, 20 to less than 22 inches

E2204 Manual wheelchair accessory, nonstandard seat frame depth, 22 to 25 inches

E2205 Manual wheelchair accessory, handrim without projections (includes ergonomic or contoured), any type, replacement only, each

E2206 Manual wheelchair accessory, wheel lock assembly, complete, each

E2207 Wheelchair accessory, crutch and cane holder, each

E2208 Wheelchair accessory, cylinder tank carrier, each

E2209 Arm trough, with or without hand support, each

E2210 Wheelchair accessory, bearings, any type, replacement only, each

E2211 Manual wheelchair accessory, pneumatic propulsion tire, any size, each

E2212 Manual wheelchair accessory, tube for pneumatic propulsion tire, any size, each

E2213 Manual wheelchair accessory, insert for pneumatic propulsion tire (removable), any type, any size, each

E2214 Manual wheelchair accessory, pneumatic caster tire, any size, each

E2215 Manual wheelchair accessory, tube for pneumatic caster tire, any size, each

E2216 Manual wheelchair accessory, foam filled propulsion tire, any size, each

E2217 Manual wheelchair accessory, foam filled caster tire, any size, each

E2218 Manual wheelchair accessory, foam propulsion tire, any size, each

E2219 Manual wheelchair accessory, foam caster tire, any size, each

E2220 Manual wheelchair accessory, solid (rubber/plastic) propulsion tire, any size, each

E2221 Manual wheelchair accessory, solid (rubber/plastic) caster tire (removable), any size, each

E2222 Manual wheelchair accessory, solid (rubber/plastic) caster tire with integrated wheel, any size, each

E2224 Manual wheelchair accessory, propulsion wheel excludes tire, any size, each

E2225 Manual wheelchair accessory, caster wheel excludes tire, any size, replacement only, each

E2226 Manual wheelchair accessory, caster fork, any size, replacement only, each

E2227 Manual wheelchair accessory, gear reduction drive wheel, each

E2228 Manual wheelchair accessory, wheel braking system and lock, complete, each

E2230 Manual wheelchair accessory, manual standing system

E2231 Manual wheelchair accessory, solid seat support base (replaces sling seat), includes any type mounting hardware

E2291 Back, planar, for pediatric size wheelchair including fixed attaching hardware

E2292 Seat, planar, for pediatric size wheelchair including fixed attaching hardware

E2293 Back, contoured, for pediatric size wheelchair including fixed attaching hardware

E2294 Seat, contoured, for pediatric size wheelchair including fixed attaching hardware

E2295 Manual wheelchair accessory, for pediatric size wheelchair, dynamic seating frame, allows coordinated movement of multiple positioning features

▲**E2300** Wheelchair accessory, power seat elevation system, any type

▲**E2301** Wheelchair accessory, power standing system, any type

E2310 Power wheelchair accessory, electronic connection between wheelchair controller and one power seating system motor, including all related electronics, indicator feature, mechanical function selection switch, and fixed mounting hardware

E2311 Power wheelchair accessory, electronic connection between wheelchair controller and two or more power seating system motors, including all related electronics, indicator feature, mechanical function selection switch, and fixed mounting hardware

E2312 Power wheelchair accessory, hand or chin control interface, mini-proportional remote joystick, proportional, including fixed mounting hardware

E2313 Power wheelchair accessory, harness for upgrade to expandable controller, including all fasteners, connectors and mounting hardware, each

E2321 Power wheelchair accessory, hand control interface, remote joystick, nonproportional, including all related electronics, mechanical stop switch, and fixed mounting hardware

E2322 Power wheelchair accessory, hand control interface, multiple mechanical switches, nonproportional, including all related electronics, mechanical stop switch, and fixed mounting hardware

E2323 Power wheelchair accessory, specialty joystick handle for hand control interface, prefabricated

E2324 Power wheelchair accessory, chin cup for chin control interface

E2325 Power wheelchair accessory, sip and puff interface, nonproportional, including all related electronics, mechanical stop switch, and manual swingaway mounting hardware

E2326 Power wheelchair accessory, breath tube kit for sip and puff interface

E2327 Power wheelchair accessory, head control interface, mechanical, proportional, including all related electronics, mechanical direction change switch, and fixed mounting hardware

E2328 Power wheelchair accessory, head control or extremity control interface, electronic, proportional, including all related electronics and fixed mounting hardware

E2329 Power wheelchair accessory, head control interface, contact switch mechanism, nonproportional, including all related electronics, mechanical stop switch, mechanical direction change switch, head array, and fixed mounting hardware

E2330 Power wheelchair accessory, head control interface, proximity switch mechanism, nonproportional, including all related electronics, mechanical stop switch, mehcanical direction change switch, head array, and fixed mounting hardware

E2331 Power wheelchair accessory, attendant control, proportional, including all related electronics and fixed mounting hardware

E2340 Power wheelchair accessory, nonstandard seat frame width, 20-23 inches

E2341 Power wheelchair accessory, nonstandard seat frame width, 24-27 inches

E2342 Power wheelchair accessory, nonstandard seat frame depth, 20 or 21 inches

E2343 Power wheelchair accessory, nonstandard seat frame depth, 22-25 inches

E2351 Power wheelchair accessory, electronic interface to operate speech generating device using power wheelchair control interface

E2358 Power wheelchair accessory, group 34 non-sealed lead acid battery, each

E2359 Power wheelchair accessory, group 34 sealed lead acid battery, each (e.g. gel cell, absorbed glass mat)

E2360 Power wheelchair accessory, 22 NF non-sealed lead acid battery, each

E2361 Power wheelchair accessory, 22 NF sealed lead acid battery, each (eg., gel cell, absorbed glassmat)

E2362 Power wheelchair accessory, group 24 non-sealed lead acid battery, each

E2363 Power wheelchair accessory, group 24 sealed lead acid battery, each (eg., gel cell, absorbed glassmat)

E2364 Power wheelchair accessory, U-1 non-sealed lead acid battery, each

E2365 Power wheelchair accessory, U-1 sealed lead acid battery, each (eg., gel cell, absorbed glassmat)

E2366 Power wheelchair accessory, battery charger, single mode, for use with only one battery type, sealed or non-sealed, each

E2367 Power wheelchair accessory, battery charger, dual mode, for use with either battery type, sealed or non-sealed, each

E2368 Power wheelchair component, motor, replacement only

E2369 Power wheelchair component, gear box, replacement only

E2370 Power wheelchair component, motor and gear box combination, replacement only

E2371 Power wheelchair accessory, group 27 sealed lead acid battery, (e.g. Gel cell, absorbed glassmat), each

E2372 Power wheelchair accessory, group 27 non-sealed lead acid battery, each

E2373 Power wheelchair accessory, hand or chin control interface, compact remote joystick, proportional, including fixed mounting hardware

E2374 Power wheelchair accessory, hand or chin control interface, standard remote joystick (not including controller), proportional, including all related electronics and fixed mounting hardware, replacement only

E2375 Power wheelchair accessory, non-expandable controller, including all related electronics and mounting hardware, replacement only

E2376 Power wheelchair accessory, expandable controller, including all related electronics and mounting hardware, replacement only

E2377 Power wheelchair accessory, expandable controller, including all related electronics and mounting hardware, upgrade provided at initial issue

E2378 Power wheelchair component, actuator, replacement only

E2381 Power wheelchair accessory, pneumatic drive wheel tire, any size, replacement only, each

E2382 Power wheelchair accessory, tube for pneumatic drive wheel tire, any size, replacement only, each

E2383 Power wheelchair accessory, insert for pneumatic drive wheel tire (removable), any type, any size, replacement only, each

E2384 Power wheelchair accessory, pneumatic caster tire, any size, replacement only, each

E2385 Power wheelchair accessory, tube for pneumatic caster tire, any size, replacement only, each

E2386 Power wheelchair accessory, foam filled drive wheel tire, any size, replacement only, each

E2387 Power wheelchair accessory, foam filled caster tire, any size, replacement only, each

E2388 Power wheelchair accessory, foam drive wheel tire, any size, replacement only, each

E2389 Power wheelchair accessory, foam caster tire, any size, replacement only, each

E2390 Power wheelchair accessory, solid (rubber/plastic) drive wheel tire, any size, replacement only, each

E2391 Power wheelchair accessory, solid (rubber/plastic) caster tire (removable), any size, replacement only, each

E2392 Power wheelchair accessory, solid (rubber/plastic) caster tire with integrated wheel, any size, replacement only, each

E2394 Power wheelchair accessory, drive wheel excludes tire, any size, replacement only, each

E2395 Power wheelchair accessory, caster wheel excludes tire, any size, replacement only, each

E2396 Power wheelchair accessory, caster fork, any size, replacement only, each

E2397 Power wheelchair accessory, lithium-based battery, each

E2402 Negative pressure wound therapy electrical pump, stationary or portable

E2500 Speech generating device, digitized speech, using pre-recorded messages, less than or equal to 8 minutes recording time
CIM: 60-23

E2502 Speech generating device, digitized speech, using pre-recorded messages, greater than 8 minutes but less than or equal to 20 minutes recording time
CIM: 60-23

E2504 Speech generating device, digitized speech, using pre-recorded messages, greater than 20 minutes but less than or equal to 40 minutes recording time
CIM: 60-23

E2506 Speech generating device, digitized speech, using pre-recorded messages, greater than 40 minutes recording time
CIM: 60-23

E2508 Speech generating device, synthesized speech, requiring message formulation by spelling and access by physical contact with the device
CIM: 60-23

E2510 Speech generating device, synthesized speech, permitting multiple methods of message formulation and multiple methods of device access
CIM: 60-23

E2511 Speech generating software program, for personal computer or personal digital assistant
CIM: 60-23

E2512 Accessory for speech generating device, mounting system
CIM: 60-23

E2599 Accessory for speech generating device, not otherwise classified
CIM: 60-23

E2601 General use wheelchair seat cushion, width less than 22 inches, any depth

E2602 General use wheelchair seat cushion, width 22 inches or greater, any depth

E2603 Skin protection wheelchair seat cushion, width less than 22 inches, any depth

E2604 Skin protection wheelchair seat cushion, width 22 inches or greater, any depth

E2605 Positioning wheelchair seat cushion, width less than 22 inches, any depth

E2606 Positioning wheelchair seat cushion, width 22 inches or greater, any depth

E2607 Skin protection and positioning wheelchair seat cushion, width less than 22 inches, any depth

E2608 Skin protection and positioning wheelchair seat cushion, width 22 inches or greater, any depth

E2609 Custom fabricated wheelchair seat cushion, any size

E2610 Wheelchair seat cushion, powered

E2611 General use wheelchair back cushion, width less than 22 inches, any height, including any type mounting hardware

E2612 General use wheelchair back cushion, width 22 inches or greater, any height, including any type mounting hardware

E2613 Positioning wheelchair back cushion, posterior, width less than 22 inches, any height, including any type mounting hardware

E2614 Positioning wheelchair back cushion, posterior, width 22 inches or greater, any height, including any type mounting hardware

E2615 Positioning wheelchair back cushion, posterior-lateral, width less than 22 inches, any height, including any type mounting hardware

E2616 Positioning wheelchair back cushion, posterior-lateral, width 22 inches or greater, any height, including any type mounting hardware

E2617 Custom fabricated wheelchair back cushion, any size, including any type mounting hardware

E2619 Replacement cover for wheelchair seat cushion or back cushion, each

E2620 Positioning wheelchair back cushion, planar back with lateral supports, width less than 22 inches, any height, including any type mounting hardware

E2621 Positioning wheelchair back cushion, planar back with lateral supports, width 22 inches or greater, any height, including any type mounting hardware

E2622 Skin protection wheelchair seat cushion, adjustable, width less than 22 inches, any depth

E2623 Skin protection wheelchair seat cushion, adjustable, width 22 inches or greater, any depth

E2624 Skin protection and positioning wheelchair seat cushion, adjustable, width less than 22 inches, any depth

E2625 Skin protection and positioning wheelchair seat cushion, adjustable, width 22 inches or greater, any depth

E2626 Wheelchair accessory, shoulder elbow, mobile arm support attached to wheelchair, balanced, adjustable

E2627 Wheelchair accessory, shoulder elbow, mobile arm support attached to wheelchair, balanced, adjustable rancho type

E2628 Wheelchair accessory, shoulder elbow, mobile arm support attached to wheelchair, balanced, reclining

E2629 Wheelchair accessory, shoulder elbow, mobile arm support attached to wheelchair, balanced, friction arm support (friction dampening to proximal and distal joints)

E2630 Wheelchair accessory, shoulder elbow, mobile arm support, monosuspension arm and hand support, overhead elbow forearm hand sling support, yoke type suspension support

E2631 Wheelchair accessory, addition to mobile arm support, elevating proximal arm

E2632 Wheelchair accessory, addition to mobile arm support, offset or lateral rocker arm with elastic balance control

E2633 Wheelchair accessory, addition to mobile arm support, supinator

GAIT TRAINER

E8000 Gait trainer, pediatric size, posterior support, includes all accessories and components

E8001 Gait trainer, pediatric size, upright support, includes all accessories and components

E8002 Gait trainer, pediatric size, anterior support, includes all accessories and components

PROCEDURES AND PROFESSIONAL SERVICES

Guidelines

In addition to the information presented in the INTRODUCTION, several other items unique to this section are defined or identified here:

1. TEMPORARY CODES: The codes listed in this section are assigned by CMS on a temporary basis to identify procedures/services.

PROCEDURES/PROFESSIONAL SERVICES

G0008 Administration of influenza virus vaccine

G0009 Administration of pneumococcal vaccine

G0010 Administration of hepatitis B vaccine

G0027 Semen analysis; presence and/or motility of sperm excluding huhner

G0101 Cervical or vaginal cancer screening; pelvic and clinical breast examination

G0102 Prostate cancer screening; digital rectal examination
CIM: 50-55 MCM: 4182

G0103 Prostate cancer screening; prostate specific antigen test (PSA)
CIM: 50-55 MCM: 4182

G0104 Colorectal cancer screening; flexible sigmoidoscopy

G0105 colonoscopy on individual at high risk

G0106 alternative to G0104, screening sigmoidoscopy, barium enema

G0108 Diabetes outpatient self-management training services, individual, per 30 minutes

G0109 Diabetes outpatient self-management training services, group session (2 or more), per 30 minutes

G0117 Glaucoma screening for high risk patients furnished by an optometrist or ophthalmologist

G0118 Glaucoma screening for high risk patient furnished under the direct supervision of an optometrist or ophthalmologist

G0120 Colorectal cancer screening; alternative to G0105, screening colonoscopy, barium enema

G0121 colonoscopy on individual not meeting criteria for high risk

G0122 barium enema

G0123 Screening cytopathology, cervical or vaginal (any reporting system), collected in preservative fluid, automated thin layer preparation; screening by cytotechnologist under physician supervision
CIM: 50-20

G0124 requiring interpretation by physician
CIM: 50-20

G0127 Trimming of dystrophic nails, any number
MCM: 2323, 4120

G0128 Direct (fact-to-face with patient) skilled nursing services of a registered nurse provided in a comprehensive outpatient rehabilitation facility, each 10 minutes beyond the first 5 minutes

G0129 Occupational therapy services requiring the skills of a qualified occupational therapist, furnished as a component of a partial hospitalization treatment program, per session (45 minutes or more)

G0130 Single energy X-ray absorptiometry (sexa) bone density study, one or more sites; appendicular skeleton (peripheral) (e.g., radius, wrist, heel)
CIM: 50-44

G0141 Screening cytopathology smears, cervical or vaginal, performed by automated system, with manual rescreening, requiring interpretation by physician

G0143 Screening cytopathology, cervical or vaginal (any reporting system), collected in preservative fluid, automated thin layer preparation; with manual screening and rescreening by cytotechnologist under physician supervision

G0144 with screening by automated system, under physician supervision

G0145 with screening by automated system and manual rescreening under physician supervision

G0147 Screening cytopathology smears, cervical or vaginal; performed by automated system under physician supervision

G0148 performed by automated system with manual rescreening

G0151 Services performed by a qualified physical therapist in the home health or hospice setting, each 15 minutes

G0152 Services performed by a qualified occupational therapist in the home health or hospice setting, each 15 minutes

G0153 Services performed by a qualified speech-language pathologist in the home health or hospice setting, each 15 minutes

G0154 Direct skilled nursing services of a licensed nurse (LPN or RN) in the home health or hospice setting, each 15 minutes

G0155 Services of clinical social worker in home health or hospice setting, each 15 minutes

G0156 Services of home health/hospice aide in home health or hospice setting, each 15 minutes

G0157 Services performed by a qualified physical therapist assistant in the home health or hospice setting, each 15 minutes

G0158 Services performed by a qualified occupational therapist assistant in the home health or hospice setting, each 15 minutes

G0159 Services performed by a qualified physical therapist, in the home health setting, in the establishment or delivery of a safe and effective therapy maintenance program, each 15 minutes

G0160 Services performed by a qualified occupational therapist, in the home health setting, in the establishment or delivery of a safe and effective therapy maintenance program, each 15 minutes

G0161 Services performed by a qualified speech-language pathologist, in the home health setting, in the establishment or delivery of a safe and effective therapy maintenance program, each 15 minutes

G0162 Skilled services by a registered nurse (RN) in the delivery of management & evaluation of the plan of care; each 15 minutes (the patient's underlying condition or complication requires an RN to ensure that essential non-skilled care achieve its purpose in the home health or hospice setting)

G0163 Skilled services of a licensed nurse (lpn or rn) in the delivery of observation & assessment of the patient's condition, each 15 minutes (when the likelihood of change in the patient's condition requires skilled nursing personnel to identify and evaluate the patient's need for possible modification of treatment in the home health or hospice setting)

G0164 Skilled services of a licensed nurse, in the training and/or education of a patient or family member, in the home health or hospice setting, each 15 minutes

G0166 External counterpulsation, per treatment session
CIM: 35-74

G0168 Wound closure utilizing tissue adhesive(s) only

G0173 Linear accelerator based stereotactic radiosurgery, complete course of therapy in one session

G0175 Scheduled interdisciplinary team conference (minimum of three exclusive of patient care nursing staff) with patient present

G0176 Activity therapy, such as music, dance, art or play therapies not for recreation, related to the care and treatment of patient's disabling mental health problems, per session (45 minutes or more)

G0177 Training and education services related to the care and treatment of patient's disabling mental health problems per session (45 minutes or more)

G0179 Physician recertification services for Medicare-covered services provided by a participating home health agency (patient not present) including review of subsequent reports of patient status, review of patient's responses to the Oasis assessment instrument, contact with the home health agency to ascertain the follow-up implementation plan of care, and documentation in the patient's office record, per certification period

G0180 Physician certification services for Medicare-covered services provided by a participating home health agency (patient not present), including review of initial or subsequent reports of patient status, review of patient's responses to the oasis assessment instrument, contact with the home health agency to ascertain the initial implementation plan of care, and documentation in the patient's office record, per certification period

G0181 Physician supervision of a patient receiving Medicare-covered services provided by a participating home health agency (patient not present), requiring complex and multidisciplinary care modalities involving regular physician development and/or revision of care plans, review of subsequent reports of patient status, review of laboratory and other studies, communication (including telephone calls) with other health care professionals involved in the patient's care, integration of new information into the medical treatment plan and/or adjustment of medical therapy, within a calendar month, 30 minutes or more

G0182 Physician supervision of a patient under a Medicare-approved hospice (patient not present) requiring complex and multidisciplinary care modalities involving regular physician development and/or revision of care plans, review of subsequent reports of patient status, review of laboratory and other studies, communication (including telephone calls) with other health care professionals involved in the patient's care, integration of new information into the medical treatment plan and/or adjustment of medical therapy, within a calendar month, 30 minutes or more

G0186 Destruction of localized lesion of choroid (for example, choroidal neovascularization); photocoagulation, feeder vessel technique (one or more sessions)

G0202 Screening mammography, producing direct digital image, bilateral, all views

G0204 Diagnostic mammography, producing direct digital image, bilateral, all views

G0206 Diagnostic mammography, producing direct digital image, unilateral, all views

G0219 PET imaging whole body; full and partial ring PET scanners only, for non-covered indications
CIM: 50-36 MCM: 4173

G0235 Pet imaging, any site, not otherwise specified
CIM: 50-36

G0237 Therapeutic procedures to increase strength or endurance of respiratory muscles, face to face, one on one, each 15 minutes (includes monitoring)

G0238 Therapeutic procedures to improve respiratory function, other than described by G0237, one on one, face to face, per 15 minutes (includes monitoring)

G0239 Therapeutic procedures to improve respiratory function or increase strength or endurance of respiratory muscles, two or more individuals (includes monitoring)

G0245 Initial physician evaluation of a diabetic patient with diabetic sensory neuropathy resulting in a loss of protective sensation (LOPS) which must include the diagnosis of LOPS; a patient history; a physical examination that consists of at least the following elements: (a) visual inspection of the forefoot, hindfoot and toe web spaces, (b) evaluation of a protective sensation, (c) evaluation of foot structure and biomechanics, (d) evaluation of vascular status and skin integrity, (e) evaluation and recommendation of footwear, (f) patient education
CIM: 50.81

G0246 Follow up evaluation of a diabetic patient with diabetic sensory neuropathy resulting in a loss of protective sensation (LOPS) to include at least the following, a patient history and physical examination that includes: (a) visual inspection of the forefoot, hindfoot and toe web spaces, (b) evaluation of protective sensation, (c) evaluation of foot structure and biomechanics, (d) evaluation of vascular status and skin integrity, (e) evaluation and recommendation of footwear, (f) patient education
CIM: 50.81

G0247 Routine foot care by a physician of a diabetic patient with diabetic sensory neuropathy resulting in a loss of protective sensation (LOPS) to include, the local care of superficial wounds (i.e., superficial to muscle and fascia) and at least the following if present: (1) local care of superficial wounds, (2) debridement of corns and callouses, and (3) trimming and debridement of nails
CIM: 50.81

G0248 Demonstration, prior to initial use, of home INR (international normalized ratio) monitoring for patient with either mechanical heart valve(s), chronic atrial fibrillation, or venous thromboembolism who meets Medicare coverage criteria, under the direction of a physician; includes: face-to-face demonstration of use and care of the INR monitor, obtaining at least one blood sample, provision of instructions for reporting home INR test results, and documentation of patient ability to perform testing prior to its use.
CIM: 50.55

G0249 Provision of test materials and equipment for home INR monitoring to patient with either mechanical heart valve(s), chronic atrial fibrillation or venous thromboembolism who meets Medicare coverage criteria. Includes provision of materials for use in the home and reporting of test results to physician; not occurring more frequently than once a week
CIM: 50.55

G0250 Physician review, interpretation and patient management of home INR testing for a patient with either mechanical heart valve(s), chronic atrial fibrillation, or venous thromboembolism who meets other coverage criteria; includes face-to-face verification by the physician at least once a year (e.g. during an evaluation and management service) that the patient uses the device in the context of

the management of the anticoagulation therapy following initiation of the home inr monitoring; not occurring more frequently than once a week
CIM: 50.55

G0251 Linear accelerator based stereotactic radiosurgery, delivery including collimator changes and custom plugging, fractionated treatment, all lesions, per session, maximum five sessions per course of treatment

G0252 PET imaging, full and partial-ring PET scanners only, for initial diagnosis of breast cancer and/or surgical planning for beast cancer (e.g., initial staging of axillary lymph nodes)
CIM: 50-36

G0255 Current perception threshold/sensory nerve conduction test, (SNCT) per limb, any nerve
CIM: 50-57

G0257 Unscheduled or emergency dialysis treatment for an ESRD patient in a hospital outpatient department that is not certified as an ESRD facility

G0259 Injection procedure for sacroiliac joint; arthrography

G0260 Injection procedure for sacroiliac joint; provision of anesthetic, steroid and/or other therapeutic agent, with or without arthrography

G0268 Removal of impacted cerumen (one or both ears) by physician on same date of service as audiologic function testing

G0269 Placement of occlusive device into either a venous or arterial access site, post surgical or interventional procedure (e.g. angioseal plug, vascular plug)

Ⓟ **G0270** Medical nutrition therapy; reassessment and subsequent intervention(s) following second referral in same year for change in diagnosis, medical condition or treatment regimen (including additional hours needed for renal disease), individual, face to face with the patient, each 15 minutes

Ⓟ **G0271** Medical nutrition therapy, reassessment and subsequent intervention(s) following second referral in same year for change in diagnosis, medical condition, or treatment regimen (including additional hours needed for renal disease), group (2 or more individuals), each 30 minutes

(G0275) Code deleted December 31, 2013.

G0278 Iliac artery angiography performed at the same time of cardiac catheterization, includes catheter placement, injection of dye, radiologic supervision and interpretation, and production of images (list separately in addition to primary procedure)

G0281 Electrical stimulation, (unattended), to one or more areas, for chronic stage iii and stage iv pressure ulcers, arterial ulcers, diabetic ulcers, and venous stasis ulcers not demonstrating measurable signs of healing after 30 days of conventional care, as part of a therapy plan of care

G0282 Electrical stimulation, (unattended), to one or more areas, for wound care other than described in G0281
MCM: 35-98

G0283 Electrical stimulation (unattended), to one or more areas for indication(s) other than wound care, as part of a therapy plan of care

G0288 Reconstruction, computed tomographic angiography of aorta for surgical planning for vascular surgery

G0289 Arthroscopy, knee, surgical, for removal of loose body, foreign body, debridement/shaving of articular cartilage (chondroplasty) at the time of other surgical knee arthroscopy in a different compartment of the same knee

(G0290) Code deleted December 31, 2012. Use C9600-C9604

(G0291) Code deleted December 31, 2012. Use C9605-9608

G0293 Noncovered surgical procedure(s) using conscious sedation, regional, general or spinal anesthesia in a Medicare qualifying clinical trial, per day

G0294 Noncovered procedure(s) using either no anesthesia or local anesthesia only, in a Medicare qualifying clinical trial, per day

G0295 Electromagnetic therapy, to one or more areas, for wound care other than described in G0329 or for other uses
CIM: 35-98

G0302 Pre-operative pulmonary surgery services for preparation for LVRS, complete course of services, to include a minimum of 16 days of services

G0303 Pre-operative pulmonary surgery services for preparation for LVRS, 10 to 15 days of services

G0304 Pre-operative pulmonary surgery services for preparation for LVRS, 1 to 9 days of services

G0305 Post-discharge pulmonary surgery services after LVRS, minimum of 6 days of services

G0306 Complete CBC, automated (HGB, HCT, RBC, WBC, without platelet count) and automated WBC differential count

G0307 Complete (CBC), automated (HGB, HCT, RBC, WBC, without platelet count)

G0328 Colorectal cancer screening; fecal occult blood test, immunoassay, 1-3 simultaneous

G0329 Electromagnetic therapy, to one or more areas for chronic stage III and stage IV pressure ulcers, arterial ulcers, diabetic ulcers and venous stasis ulcers not demonstrating measurable signs of healing after 30 days of conventional care as part of a therapy plan of care

G0333 Pharmacy dispensing fee for inhalation drug(s); initial 30-day supply as a beneficiary

G0337 Hospice evaluation and counseling services, pre-election

G0339 Image-guided robotic linear accelerator-based stereotactic radiosurgery, complete course of therapy in one session or first session of fractionated treatment

G0340 Image-guided robotic linear accelerator-based sterotactic radiosurgery, delivery including collimator changes and custom plugging, fractionated treatment, all lesions, per session, second through fifth sessions, maximum five sessions per course of treatment

G0341 Percutaneous islet cell transplant, includes portal vein catheterization and infusion
CIM: 260.3, 35-82

G0342 Laparoscopy for islet cell transplant, includes portal vein catheterization and infusion
CIM: 35-82

G0343 Laparotomy for islet cell transplant, includes portal vein catheterization and infusion
CIM: 35-82

G0364 Bone marrow aspiration performed with bone marrow biopsy through the same incision on the same date of service

G0365 Vessel mapping of vessels for hemodialysis access (services for preoperative vessel mapping prior to creation of hemodialysis access using an autogenous hemodialysis conduit, including arterial inflow and venous outflow)

G0372 Physician service required to establish and document the need for a power mobility device

G0378 Hospital observation service, per hour

G0379 Direct admission of patient for hospital observation care

G0380 Level 1 hospital emegency department visit provided in a type B emergency department; (the ED must meet at least one of the following requirements: (1) it is licensed by the state in which it is located under applicable state law as an emergency room or emergency department; (2) it is held out to the public (by name, posted signs, advertising, or other means) as a place that provides care for emergency medical conditions on an urgent basis without requiring a previously scheduled appointment; or (3) during the calendar year immediately preceding the calendar year in which a determination under 42 cfr ¤489.24 is being made, based on a representative sample of patient visits that occurred during that calendar year, it provides at least one-third of all of its outpatient visits for the treatment of emergency medical conditions on an urgent basis without requiring a previously scheduled appointment)

G0381 Level 2 hospital emergency department visit provided in a type B emergency department; (the ED must meet at least one of the following requirements: (1) it is licensed by the state in which it is located under applicable state law as an emergency room or emergency department; (2) it is held out to the public (by name, posted signs, advertising, or other means) as a place that provides care for emergency medical conditions on an urgent basis without requiring a previously scheduled appointment; or (3) during the calendar year immediately preceding the calendar year in which a determination under 42 cfr ¤489.24 is being made, based on a representative sample of patient visits that occurred during that calendar year, it provides at least one-third of all of its outpatient visits for the treatment of emergency medical conditions on an urgent basis without requiring a previously scheduled appointment)

G0382 Level 3 hospital emergency department visit provided in a type B emergency department; (the ED must meet at least one of the following requirements: (1) it is licensed by the state in which it is located under applicable state law as an emergency room or emergency department; (2) it is held out to the public (by name, posted signs, advertising, or other means) as a place that provides care for emergency medical conditions on an urgent basis without requiring a previously scheduled appointment; or (3) during the calendar year immediately preceding the calendar year in which a determination under 42 cfr ¤489.24 is being made, based on a representative sample of patient visits that occurred during that calendar year, it provides at least one-third of all of its outpatient visits for the treatment of emergency medical conditions on an urgent basis without requiring a previously scheduled appointment)

G0383 Level 4 hospital emergency department visit provided in a type B emergency department; (the ED must meet at least one of the following requirements: (1) it is licensed by the state in which it is located under applicable state law as an emergency room or emergency department; (2) it is held out to the public (by name, posted signs, advertising, or other means) as a place that provides care for emergency medical conditions on an urgent basis without requiring a previously scheduled appointment; or (3) during the calendar year immediately preceding the calendar year in which a determination under 42 cfr ¤489.24 is being made, based on a representative sample of patient visits that occurred during that calendar year, it provides at least one-third of all of its outpatient visits for the treatment of emergency medical conditions on an urgent basis without requiring a previously scheduled appointment)

G0384 Level 5 hospital emergency department visit provided in a type B emergency department; (the ED must meet at least one of the following requirements: (1) it is licensed by the state in which it is located under applicable state law as an emergency room or emergency department; (2) it is held out to the public (by name, posted signs, advertising, or other means) as a place that provides care for emergency medical conditions on an urgent basis without requiring a previously scheduled appointment; or (3) during the calendar year immediately preceding the calendar year in which a determination under 42 cfr §489.24 is being made, based on a representative sample of patient visits that occurred during that calendar year, it provides at least one-third of all of its outpatient visits for the treatment of emergency medical conditions on an urgent basis without requiring a previously scheduled appointment)

G0389 Ultrasound B-scan and/or real time with image documentation; for abdominal aortic aneurysm (AAA) screening

G0390 Trauma response team associated with hospital critical care service

G0396 Alcohol and/or substance (other than tobacco) abuse structured assessment (e.g., audit, dast), and brief intervention 15 to 30 minutes

G0397 Alcohol and/or substance (other than tobacco) abuse structured assessment (e.g., audit, dast), and intervention, greater than 30 minutes

G0398 Home sleep study test (HST) with type II portable monitor, unattended; minimum of 7 channels: EEG, EOG, EMG, ECG/heart rate, airflow, respiratory effort and oxygen saturation

G0399 Home sleep test (HST) with type III portable monitor, unattended; minimum of 4 channels: 2 respiratory movement/airflow, 1 ECG/heart rate and 1 oxygen saturation

G0400 Home sleep test (HST) with typeIVv portable monitor, unattended; minimum of 3 channels

Ⓟ **G0402** Initial preventive physical examination; face-to-face visit, services limited to new beneficiary during the first 12 months of Medicare enrollment

G0403 Electrocardiogram, routine ECG with 12 leads; performed as a screening for the initial preventive physical examination with interpretation and report

G0404 Electrocardiogram, routineECGg with 12 leads; tracing only, without interpretation and report, performed as a screening for the initial preventive physical examination

G0405 Electrocardiogram, routine ECG with 12 leads; interpretation and report only, performed as a screening for the initial preventive physical examination

G0406 Follow-up inpatient consultation, limited, physicians typically spend 15 minutes communicating with the patient via telehealth

G0407 Follow-up inpatient consultation, intermediate, physicians typically spend 25 minutes communicating with the patient via telehealth

G0408 Follow-up inpatient consultation, complex, physicians typically spend 35 minutes communicating with the patient via telehealth

G0409 Social work and psychological services, directly relating to and/or furthering the patient's rehabilitation goals, each 15 minutes, face-to-face; individual (Services provided by a CORF-qualified social worker or psychologist in a CORF)

G0410 Group psychotherapy other than of a multiple-family group, in a partial hospitalization setting, approximately 45 to 50 minutes

G0411 Interactive group psychotherapy, in a partial hospitalization setting, approximately 45 to 50 minutes

G0412 Open treatment of iliac spine(s), tuberosity avulsion, or iliac wing fracture(s), unilateral or bilateral for pelvic bone fracture patterns which do not disrupt the pelvic ring includes internal fixation, when performed

G0413 Percutaneous skeletal fixation of posterior pelvic bone fracture and/or dislocation, for fracture patterns which disrupt the pelvic ring, unilateral or bilateral, (includes ilium, sacroiliac joint and/or sacrum)

G0414 Open treatment of anterior pelvic bone fracture and/or dislocation for fracture patterns which disrupt the pelvic ring, unilateral or bilateral, includes internal fixation when performed (includes pubic symphysis and/or superior/inferior rami)

G0415 Open treatment of posterior pelvic bone fracture and/or dislocation, for fracture patterns which disrupt the pelvic ring, unilateral or bilateral, includes internal fixation, when performed (includes ilium, sacroiliac joint and/or sacrum)

▲**G0416** Surgical pathology, gross and microscopic examinations, for prostate needle biopsy, any method, 10-20 specimens

▲**G0417** Surgical pathology, gross and microscopic examination, for prostate needle biopsy, any method, 21-40 specimens

▲**G0418** Surgical pathology, gross and microscopic examination, for prostate needle biopsy, any method, 41-60 specimens

▲**G0419** Surgical pathology, gross and microscopic examination, for prostate needle biopsy, any method, >60 specimens

G0420 Face-to-face educational services related to the care of chronic kidney disease; individual, per session, per 1 hour

G0421 Face-to-face educational services related to the care of chronic kidney disease; group, per session, per 1 hour

G0422 Intensive cardiac rehabilitation; with or without continuous ECG monitoring; with exercise, per session

G0423 without exercise, per session

G0424 Pulmonary rehabilitation, including exercise (includes monitoring), one hour, per session, up to 2 sessions per day

G0425 Telehealth consultation, emergency department or initial inpatient, typically 30 minutes communicating with the patient via telehealth

Not valid for Medicare | Non-covered by Medicare | Special coverage instructions | Carrier discretion

G0426 Telehealth consultation, emergency department or initial inpatient, typically 50 minutes communicating with the patient via telehealth

G0427 Telehealth consultation, emergency department or initial inpatient, typically 70 minutes or more communicating with the patient via telehealth

G0428 Collagen meniscus implant procedure for filling meniscal defects (e.g., CMI, collagen scaffold, menaflex)

G0429 Dermal filler injection(s) for the treatment of facial lipodystrophy syndrome (LDS) (e.g., as a result of highly active antiretroviral therapy)

G0431 Drug screen, qualitative; multiple drug classes by high complexity test method (e.g., immunoassay, enzyme assay), per patient encounter

G0432 Infectious agent antibody detection by enzyme immunoassay (EIA) technique, HIV-1 and/or HIV-2, screening

G0433 Infectious agent antibody detection by enzyme-linked immunosorbent assay (ELISA) technique, HIV-1 and/or HIV-2, screening

G0434 Drug screen, other than chromatographic; any number of drug classes, by CLIA-waived test or moderate complexity test, per patient encounter

G0435 Infectious agent antibody detection by rapid antibody test, HIV-1 and/or HIV-2, screening

G0436 Smoking and tobacco cessation counseling visit for the asymptomatic patient; intermediate, greater than 3 minutes, up to 10 minutes

G0437 intermediate, greater than 10 minutes

G0438 Annual wellness visit; includes a personalized prevention plan of service (PPS); initial visit

G0439 subsequent visit

(G0440) Code deleted December 31, 2011

(G0441) Code deleted December 31, 2011

G0442 Annual alcohol misuse screening, 15 minutes

G0443 Brief face-to-face behavioral counseling for alcohol misuse, 15 minutes

G0444 Annual depression screening, 15 minutes

G0445 High intensity behavioral counseling to prevent sexually transmitted infection; face-to-face, individual, includes: education, skills training and guidance on how to change sexual behavior; performed semi-annually, 30 minutes

G0446 Intensive behavioral therapy to reduce cardiovascular disease risk, individual, face-to-face, bi-annual, 15 minutes

G0447 Face-to-face behavioral counseling for obesity, 15 minutes

G0448 Insertion or replacement of a permanent pacing cardioverter-defibrillator system with transvenous lead(s), single or dual chamber with insertion of pacing electrode, cardiac venous system, for left ventricular pacing

G0449 Annual face-to-face obesity screening, 15 minutes

G0450 Screening for sexually transmitted infections, includes laboratory tests for chlamydia, gonorrhea, syphilis and hepatitis B

G0451 Development testing, with interpretation and report, per standardized instrument form

G0452 Molecular pathology procedure; physician interpretation and report

G0453 Continuous intraoperative neurophysiology monitoring, from outside the operating room (remote or nearby), per patient, (attention directed exclusively to one patient) each 15 minutes (list in addition to primary procedure)

G0454 Physician documentation of face-to-face visit for durable medical equipment determination performed by nurse practitioner, physician assistant or clinical nurse specialist

G0455 Preparation with instillation of fecal microbiota by any method, including assessment of donor specimen

G0456 Negative pressure wound therapy, (e. G. Vacuum assisted drainage collection) using a mechanically-powered device, not durable medical equipment, including provision of cartridge and dressing(s), topical application(s), wound assessment, and instructions for ongoing care, per session; total wounds(s) surface area less than or equal to 50 square centimeters

G0457 Negative pressure wound therapy, (e. G. Vacuum assisted drainage collection) using a mechanically-powered device, not durable medical equipment, including provision of cartridge and dressing(s), topical application(s), wound assessment, and instructions for ongoing care, per session; total wounds(s) surface area greater than 50 square centimeters

G0458 Low dose rate (ldr) prostate brachytherapy services, composite rate

● **G0461** Immunohistochemistry or immunocytochemistry, per specimen; first single or multiplex antibody stain

● **G0462** Immunohistochemistry or immunocytochemistry, per specimen; each additional single or multiplex antibody stain (list separately in addition to code for primary procedure)

● **G0463** Hospital outpatient clinic visit for assessment and management of a patient

Ⓟ **G0908** Most recent hemoglobin (hgb) level > 12.0 g/dl

Ⓟ **G0909** Hemoglobin level measurement not documented, reason not otherwise specified

Ⓟ **G0910** Most recent hemoglobin level <= 12.0 g/dl

(G0911) Code deleted December 31, 2012.

(G0912) Code deleted December 31, 2012.

Ⓟ **G0913** Improvement in visual function achieved within 90 days following cataract surgery

Ⓟ **G0914** Patient care survey was not completed by patient

Ⓟ **G0915** Improvement in visual function not achieved within 90 days following cataract surgery

Ⓟ **G0916** Satisfaction with care achieved within 90 days following cataract surgery

Ⓟ **G0917** Patient satisfaction survey was not completed by patient

Ⓟ **G0918** Satisfaction with care not achieved within 90 days following cataract surgery

Ⓟ **G0919** Influenza immunization ordered or recommended (to be given at alternate location or alternate provider); vaccine not available at time of visit

Ⓟ **G0920** Type, anatomic location, and activity all documented

Ⓟ **G0921** Documentation of patient reason(s) for not being able to assess

Ⓟ **G0922** No documentation of disease type, anatomic location, and activity, reason not otherwise specified

G3001 Administration and supply of Tositumomab, 450 mg

PHYSICIAN'S VOLUNTARY REPORTING PROGRAM CODES

These HCPCS codes are to be used for the physician's voluntary reporting program in which CMS seeks to analyze the quality of care provided to Medicare beneficiaries. Reporting of these codes is voluntary. Physicians should not charge for these codes. Unless otherwise indicated, report these codes in addition to office visit, home visit, nursing facility and domiciliary evaluation and management codes. For additional information, please visit the following website: http://www.cms.hhs.gov/ providers/p4p/.

▲**G8126** Patient with a diagnosis of major depression documented as being treated with antidepressant medication during the entire 84 day (12 week) acute treatment phase

▲**G8127** Patient with a diagnosis of major depression not documented as being treated with antidepressant medication during the entire 84 day (12 week) acute treatment phase

G8128 Clinician documented that patient was not an eligible candidate for antidepressant medication during the entire 12 week acute treatment phase measure

G8395 Left ventricular ejection fraction (LVEF) >= 40% or documentation as normal or mildly depressed left ventricular systolic function

Ⓟ **G8396** Left ventricular ejection fraction (LVEF) not performed or documented

G8397 Dilated macular or fundus exam performed, including documentation of the presence or absence of macular edema and level of severity of retinopathy

G8398 Dilated macular or fundus exam not performed

Ⓟ **G8399** Patient with central dual-energy x-ray absorptiometry (dxa) results documented or ordered or pharmacologic therapy (other than minerals/vitamins) for osteoporosis prescribed)

Ⓟ **G8400** Patient with central dual-energy x-ray absorptiometry (dxa) results not documented or not ordered or pharmacologic therapy (other than minerals/vitamins) for osteoporosis not prescribed

Ⓟ **G8401** Clinician documented that patient was not an eligible candidate for screening or therapy for osteoporosis for women measure

G8404 Lower extremity neurological exam performed and documented

G8405 Lower extremity neurological exam not performed

G8406 Clinician documented that patient was not an eligible candidate for lower extremity neurological exam measure

G8410 Footwear evaluation performed and documented

G8415 Footwear evaluation was not performed

G8416 Clinician documented that patient was not an eligible candidate for footwear evaluation measure

Ⓟ ▲ **G8417** BME is documented above normal parameters and a follow-up plan is documented

Ⓟ ▲ **G8418** BME is documented below normal parameters and a follow-up plan is documented

Ⓟ ▲ **G8419** BME documented outside normal parameters, no follow-up plan documented, no reason given

Ⓟ ▲ **G8420** BME is documented within normal parameters and no follow-up plan is required

Ⓟ ▲ **G8421** BME not documented and no reason is given

Ⓟ ▲ **G8422** BME not documented, documentation the patient is not eligible for BEI calculation

Ⓟ ▲ **G8427** Eligible professional attests to documenting in the medical record they obtained, updated, or reviewed the patient's current medications

Ⓟ ▲ **G8428** Current list of medications not documented as obtained, updated, or reviewed by the eligible professional, reason not given

Ⓟ ▲ **G8430** Eligible professional attests to documenting in the medical record the patient is not eligible for a current list of medications being obtained, updated, or reviewed by the eligible professional

▲ **G8431** Screening for clinical depression is documented as being positive and a follow-up plan is documented

G8432 No documentation of clinical depression screening using an age-appropriate standardized tool

▲ **G8433** Screening for clinical depression not documented, documentation stating the patient is not eligible

(G8440) Code deleted December 31, 2011

(G8441) Code deleted December 31, 2011

▲ **G8442** Pain assessment not documented as being performed, documentation the patient is not eligible for a pain assessment using a standardized tool

Not valid for Medicare | Non-covered by Medicare | Special coverage instructions | Carrier discretion

(G8447) Code deleted December 31, 2012.

(G8448) Code deleted December 31, 2012.

Ⓟ **G8450** Beta-blocker therapy prescribed for patients with left ventricular ejection fraction (LVEF) <40% or documentation as moderately or severely depressed left ventricular systolic function

▲ **G8451** Beta-blocker therapy for LVEF < 40% not prescribed for reasons documented by the clinician (e.g., low blood pressure, fluid overload, asthma, patients recently treated with an intravenous positive inotropic agent, allergy, intolerance, other medical reasons, patient declined, other patient reasons, or other reasons attributable to the healthcare system)

Ⓟ **G8452** Beta-blocker therapy not prescribed for patients with left ventricular ejection fraction (LVEF) <40% or documentation as moderately or severely depressed left ventricular systolic function

Ⓟ **G8458** Clinician documented that patient is not an eligible candidate for genotype testing; patient not receiving antiviral treatment for hepatitis C

(G8459) Code deleted December 31, 2013.

Ⓟ **G8460** Clinician documented that patient is not an eligible candidate for quantitative RNA testing at week 12; patient not receiving antiviral treatment for hepatitis C

Ⓟ **G8461** Patient receiving antiviral treatment for hepatitis C

(G8462) Code deleted December 31, 2013.

(G8463) Code deleted December 31, 2013.

G8464 Clinician documented that prostate cancer patient is not an eligible candidate for adjuvant hormonal therapy; low or intermediate risk of recurrence or risk of recurrence not determined

G8465 High risk of recurrence of prostate cancer

(G8468) Code deleted December 31, 2012.

(G8469) Code deleted December 31, 2012.

(G8470) Code deleted December 31, 2012.

(G8471) Code deleted December 31, 2012.

(G8472) Code deleted December 31, 2012.

G8473 Angiotensin converting enzyme (ACE) inhibitor or angiotensin receptor blocker (ARB) therapy prescribed

G8474 Angiotensin converting enzyme (ACE) inhibitor or angiotensin receptor blocker (ARB) therapy not prescribed for reasons documented by the clinician

G8475 Angiotensin converting enzyme (ACE) inhibitor or angiotensin receptor blocker (ARB) therapy not prescribed, reason not specified

Ⓟ **G8476** Most recent blood pressure has a systolic measurement of <130 mm/hg and a diastolic measurement of <80 mm/hg

Ⓟ **G8477** Most recent blood pressure has a systolic measurement of >=130 mm/hg and/or a diastolic measurement of >=80 mm/hg

Ⓟ **G8478** Blood pressure measurement not performed or documented, reason not specified

Ⓟ **G8482** Influenza immunization administered or previously received

Ⓟ **G8483** Influenza immunization was not ordered or administered for reasons documented by clinician

Ⓟ **G8484** Influenza immunization was not ordered or administered, reason not specified

Ⓟ **G8485** I intend to report the diabetes mellitus measures group

Ⓟ **G8486** I intend to report the preventive care measures group

Ⓟ **G8487** I intend to report the chronic kidney disease (CKD) measures group

Ⓟ **G8489** I intend to report the coronary artery disease (CAD) measures group

Ⓟ **G8490** I intend to report the rheumatoid arthritis measures group

Ⓟ **G8491** I intend to report the HIV/AIDS measures group

Ⓟ **G8492** I intend to report the perioperative care measures group

Ⓟ **G8493** I intend to report the back pain measures group

Ⓟ **G8494** All quality actions for the applicable measures in the diabetes mellitus measures group have been performed for this patient

Ⓟ **G8495** All quality actions for the applicable measures in the CKD measures group have been performed for this patient

Ⓟ **G8496** All quality actions for the applicable measures in the preventive care measures group have been performed for this patient

Ⓟ **G8497** All quality actions for the applicable measures in the coronary artery bypass graft (CABG) measures group have been performed for this patient

Ⓟ **G8498** All quality actions for the applicable measures in the coronary artery disease (CAD) measures group have been performed for this patient

Ⓟ **G8499** All quality actions for the applicable measures in the rheumatoid arthritis measures group have been performed for this patient

G8500 All quality actions for the applicable measures in the HIV/AIDS measures group have been performed for this patient

Ⓟ **G8501** All quality actions for the applicable measures in the perioperative care measures group have been performed for this patient

Ⓟ **G8502** All quality actions for the applicable measures in the back pain measures group have been performed for this patient

Ⓟ **G8506** Patient receiving angiotensin converting enzyme (ACE) inhibitor or angiotensin receptor blocker (ARB) therapy

(G8508) Code deleted December 31, 2011

▲**G8509** Pain assessment documented as positive using a standardized tool, follow-up plan not documented, reason not given

▲**G8510** Screening for clinical depression is documented as negative, a follow-up plan is not required

▲**G8511** Screening for clinical depression documented as positive, follow up plan not documented, reason not given

(G8524) Code deleted December 31, 2012.

(G8525) Code deleted December 31, 2012.

(G8526) Code deleted December 31, 2012.

G8530 Autogenous AV fistula received

G8531 Clinician documented that patient was not an eligible candidate for autogenous AV fistula

G8532 Clinician documented that patient received vascular access other than autogenous AV fistula, reason not specified

(G8534) Code deleted December 31, 2011

▲**G8535** Elder maltreatment screen not documented; documentation that patient not eligible for the elder maltreatment screen

G8536 No documentation of an elder maltreatment screen, reason not specified

(G8537) Code deleted December 31, 2011

(G8538) Code deleted December 31, 2011

▲**G8539** Functional outcome assessment documented as positive using a standardized tool and a care plan based on identified deficiencies on the date of functional outcome assessment, is documented

▲**G8540** Functional outcome assessment not documented as being performed, documentation the patient is not eligible for a functional outcome assessment using a standardized tool

G8541 No documentation of a current functional outcome assessment using a standardized tool, reason not specified

▲**G8542** Functional outcome assessment using a standardized tool is documented; no functional deficiencies identified, care plan not required

▲**G8543** Documentation of a positive functional outcome assessment using a standardized tool; care plan not documented, reason not given

Ⓟ **G8544** I intend to report the coronary artery bypass graft (CABG) measures group

Ⓟ **G8545** I intend to report the hepatitis C measures group

(G8546) Code deleted December 31, 2012.

Ⓟ **G8547** I intend to report the ischemic vascular disease (IVD) measures group

Ⓟ **G8548** I intend to report the heart failure (HF) measures group

Ⓟ **G8549** All quality actions for the applicable measures in the hepatitis C measures group have been performed for this patient

(G8550) Code deleted December 31, 2012.

G8551 All quality actions for the applicable measures in the heart failure (HF) measures group have been perfomed for this patient

Ⓟ **G8552** All quality actions for the applicable measures in the ischemic vascular disease (IVD) measures group have been performed for this patient

(G8553) Code deleted December 31, 2013.

(G8556) Code deleted December 31, 2013.

(G8557) Code deleted December 31, 2013.

(G8558) Code deleted December 31, 2013.

G8559 Patient referred to a physician (preferably a physician with training in disorders of the ear) for an otologic evaluation

G8560 Patient has a history of active drainage from the ear within the previous 90 days

G8561 Patient is not eligible for the referral for otologic evaluation for patients with a history of active drainage measure

G8562 Patient does not have a history of active drainage from the ear within the previous 90 days

G8563 Patient not referred to a physician (preferably a physician with training in disorders of the ear) for an otologic evaluation, reason not specified

G8564 Patient was referred to a physician (preferably a physician with training in disorders of the ear) for an otologic evaluation, reason not specified

G8565 Verification and documentation of sudden or rapidly progressive hearing loss

G8566 Patient is not eligible for the "referral for otologic evaluation for sudden or rapidly progressive hearing loss" measure

G8567 Patient does not have verification and documentation of sudden or rapidly progressive hearing loss

G8568 Patient was not referred to a physician (preferably a physician with training in disorders of the ear) for an otologic evaluation, reason not specified

▲**G8569** Prolonged postoperative intubation (> 24 hrs) required

▲**G8570** Prolonged postoperative intubation (> 24 hrs) not required

Ⓟ **G8571** Development of deep sternal wound infection within 30 days postoperatively

Ⓟ **G8572** No deep sternal wound infection

Ⓟ **G8573** Stroke following isolated CABG surgery

Ⓟ **G8574** No stroke following isolated CABG surgery

Ⓟ **G8575** Developed postoperative renal failure or required dialysis

Ⓟ **G8576** No postoperative renal failure/dialysis not required

Ⓟ **G8577** Reexploration required due to mediastinal bleeding with or without tamponade, graft occlusion, valve dysfunction or other cardiac reason

Ⓟ **G8578** Reexploration not required due to mediastinal bleeding with or without tamponade, graft occlusion, valve dysfunction or other cardiac reason

Ⓟ **G8579** Antiplatelet medication at discharge

Ⓟ **G8580** Antiplatelet medication contraindicated

Ⓟ **G8581** No antiplatelet medication at discharge

Ⓟ **G8582** Beta-blocker at discharge

Ⓟ **G8583** Beta-blocker contraindicated

Ⓟ **G8584** No beta-blocker at discharge

Ⓟ **G8585** Anti-lipid treatment at discharge

Ⓟ **G8586** Anti-lipid treatment contraindicated

Ⓟ **G8587** No anti-lipid treatment at discharge

(G8588) Code deleted December 31, 2013.

(G8589) Code deleted December 31, 2013.

(G8590) Code deleted December 31, 2013.

(G8591) Code deleted December 31, 2013.

(G8592) Code deleted December 31, 2013.

Ⓟ **G8593** Lipid profile results documented and reviewed (must include total cholesterol, HDL-C, triglycerides, and calculated LDL-C)

Ⓟ **G8594** Lipid profile not performed, reason not otherwise specified

Ⓟ **G8595** Most recent LDL-C < 100 mg/dl

(G8596) Code deleted December 31, 2013.

Ⓟ **G8597** Most recent LDL-C ≥ 100 mg/dl

Ⓟ **G8598** Aspirin or another antithrombotic therapy used

Ⓟ **G8599** Aspirin or another antithrombotic therapy not used, reason not otherwise specified

G8600 IV T-PA initiated within three hours (≤ 180 minutes) of time last known well

G8601 IV T-PA not initiated within three hours (≤ 180 minutes) of time last known well for reasons documented by clinician

G8602 I T-PA not initiated within three hours (≤ 180 minutes) of time last known well, reason not specified

(G8603) Code deleted December 31, 2013.

(G8604) Code deleted December 31, 2013.

(G8605) Code deleted December 31, 2013.

(G8606) Code deleted December 31, 2013.

(G8607) Code deleted December 31, 2013.

(G8608) Code deleted December 31, 2013.

(G8609) Code deleted December 31, 2013.

(G8610) Code deleted December 31, 2013.

(G8611) Code deleted December 31, 2013.

(G8612) Code deleted December 31, 2013.

(G8613) Code deleted December 31, 2013.

(G8614) Code deleted December 31, 2013.

(G8615) Code deleted December 31, 2013.

(G8616) Code deleted December 31, 2013.

(G8617) Code deleted December 31, 2013.

(G8618) Code deleted December 31, 2013.

(G8619) Code deleted December 31, 2013.

(G8620) Code deleted December 31, 2013.

(G8621) Code deleted December 31, 2013.

(G8622) Code deleted December 31, 2013.

(G8623) Code deleted December 31, 2013.

(G8624) Code deleted December 31, 2013.

(G8625) Code deleted December 31, 2013.

(G8626) Code deleted December 31, 2013.

G8627 Surgical procedure performed within 30 days following cataract surgery for major complications (e.g., retained nuclear fragments, endophthalmitis, dislocated or wrong power IOL, retinal detachment, or wound dehiscence)

G8628 Surgical procedure not performed within 30 days following cataract surgery for major complications (e.g., retained nuclear fragments, endophthalmitis, dislocated or wrong power IOL, retinal detachment, or wound dehiscence)

G8629 Documentation of order for prophylactic parenteral antibiotic to be given within one hour (if fluoroquinolone or vancomycin, two hours) prior to surgical incision (or start of procedure when no incision is required)

G8630 Documentation that administration of prophylactic parenteral antibiotics was initiated within one hour (if fluoroquinolone or vancomycin, two hours) prior to surgical incision (or start of procedure when no incision is required), as ordered

Ⓟ **G8631** Clinician documented that patient was not an eligible candidate for ordering prophylactic parenteral antibiotics to be given within one hour (if fluoroquinolone or vancomycin, two hours) prior to surgical incision (or start of procedure when no incision is required)

Ⓟ **G8632** Prophylactic parenteral antibiotics were not ordered to be given or given within one hour (if fluoroquinolone or vancomycin, two hours) prior to the surgical incision (or start of procedure when no incision is required), reason not otherwise specified)

G8633 Pharmacologic therapy (other than minierals/vitamins) for osteoporosis prescribed

G8634 Clinician documented patient not an eligible candidate to receive pharmacologic therapy for osteoporosis

G8635 Pharmacologic therapy for osteoporosis was not prescribed, reason not otherwise specified

(G8636) Code deleted December 31, 2011

(G8637) Code deleted December 31, 2011

(G8638) Code deleted December 31, 2011

(G8639) Code deleted December 31, 2011

(G8640) Code deleted December 31, 2011

(G8641) Code deleted December 31, 2011

(G8642) Code deleted December 31, 2013.

(G8643) Code deleted December 31, 2013.

(G8644) Code deleted December 31, 2013.

Ⓟ **G8645** I intend to report the asthma measures group

Ⓟ **G8646** All quality actions for the applicable measures in the asthma measures group have been performed for this patient

G8647 Risk-adjusted functional status change residual score for the knee successfully calculated and the score was equal to zero (0) or greater than zero (>0)

G8648 Risk-adjusted functional status change residual score for the knee successfully calculated and the score was less than zero (<0)

G8649 Risk-adjusted functional status change residual scores for the knee not measured because the patient did not complete foto's functional intake on admission and/or follow up status survey near discharge, patient not eligible/not appropriate

G8650 Risk-adjusted functional status change residual scores for the knee not measured because the patient did not complete foto's functional intake on admission and/or follow up status survey near discharge, reason not specified

G8651 Risk-adjusted functional status change residual score for the hip successfully calculated and the score was equal to zero (0) or greater than zero (>0)

G8652 Risk-adjusted functional status change residual score for the hip successfully calculated and the score was less than zero (<0)

G8653 Risk-adjusted functional status change residual scores for the hip not measured because the patient did not complete foto's functional intake on admission and/or follow up status survey near discharge, patient not eligible/not appropriate

G8654 Risk-adjusted functional status change residual scores for the hip not measured because the patient did not complete foto's functional intake on admission and/or follow up status survey near discharge, reason not specified

G8655 Risk-adjusted functional status change residual score for the lower leg, foot or ankle successfully calculated and the score was equal to zero (0) or greater than zero(>0)

G8656 Risk-adjusted functional status change residual score for the lower leg, foot or ankle successfully calculated and the score was less than zero (<0)

G8657 Risk-adjusted functional status change residual scores for the lower leg, foot or ankle not measured because the patient did not complete foto's functional intake on admission and/or follow up status survey near discharge, patient not eligible/not appropriate

G8658 Risk-adjusted functional status change residual scores for the lower leg, foot or ankle not measured because the patient did not complete foto's functional intake on admission and/or follow up status survey near discharge, reason not specified

G8659 Risk-adjusted functional status change residual score for the lumbar spine successfully calculated and the score was equal to zero (0) or greater than zero (>0)

G8660 Risk-adjusted functional status change residual score for the lumbar spine successfully calculated and the score was less than zero (<0)

G8661 Risk-adjusted functional status change residual scores for the lumbar spine not measured because the patient did not complete foto's functional intake on admission and/or follow up status survey near discharge, patient not eligible/not appropriate

G8662 Risk-adjusted functional status change residual scores for the lumbar spine not measured because the patient did not complete foto's functional intake on admission and/or follow up status survey near discharge, reason not specified

G8663 Risk-adjusted functional status change residual score for the shoulder successfully calculated and the score was equal to zero (0) or greater than zero (>0)

G8664 Risk-adjusted functional status change residual score for the shoulder successfully calculated and the score was less than zero (<0)

G8665 Risk-adjusted functional status change residual scores for the shoulder not measured because the patient did not complete foto's functional intake on admission and/or follow up status survey near discharge, patient not eligible/not appropriate

G8666 Risk-adjusted functional status change residual scores for the shoulder not measured because the patient did not complete foto's functional intake on admission and/or follow up status survey near discharge, reason not specified

G8667 Risk-adjusted functional status change residual score for the elbow, wrist or hand successfully calculated and the score was equal to zero (0) or greater than zero (>0)

G8668 Risk-adjusted functional status change residual score for the elbow, wrist or hand successfully calculated and the score was less than zero (<0)

G8669 Risk-adjusted functional status change residual scores for the elbow, wrist or hand not measured because the patient did not complete foto's functional intake on admission and/or follow up status survey near discharge, patient not eligible/not appropriate

G8670 Risk-adjusted functional status change residual scores for the elbow, wrist or hand not measured because the patient did not complete foto's functional intake on admission and/or follow up status survey near discharge, reason not specified

G8671 Risk-adjusted functional status change residual score for the neck, cranium, mandible, thoracic spine, ribs, or other general orthopedic impairment successfully calculated and the score was equal to zero (0) or greater than zero (>0)

G8672 Risk-adjusted functional status change residual score for the neck, cranium, mandible, thoracic spine, ribs, or other general orthopedic impairment successfully calculated and the score was less than zero (<0)

G8673 Risk-adjusted functional status change residual scores for the neck, cranium, mandible, thoracic spine, ribs, or other general orthopedic impairment not measured because the patient did not complete foto's functional intake on admission and/or follow up status survey near discharge, patient not eligible/not appropriate

G8674 Risk-adjusted functional status change residual scores for the neck, cranium, mandible, thoracic spine, ribs, or other general orthopedic impairment not measured because the patient did not complete foto's functional intake on admission and/or follow up status survey near discharge, reason not specified

(G8675) Code deleted December 31, 2012

(G8676) Code deleted December 31, 2012

(G8677) Code deleted December 31, 2012

(G8678) Code deleted December 31, 2012

(G8679) Code deleted December 31, 2012

(G8680) Code deleted December 31, 2012

(G8681) Code deleted December 31, 2011

▲**G8682** LVF testing documented as being performed prior to discharge or in the previous 12 months

▲**G8683** LVF testing not performed prior to discharge or in the previous 12 months for a medical or patient documented reason

(G8684) Code deleted December 31, 2011

▲**G8685** LVF testing not documented as being performed prior to discharge or in the previous 12 months, reason not given

(G8686) Code deleted December 31, 2011

(G8687) Code deleted December 31, 2011

(G8688) Code deleted December 31, 2011

(G8689) Code deleted December 31, 2011

(G8690) Code deleted December 31, 2011

(G8691) Code deleted December 31, 2011

(G8692) Code deleted December 31, 2011

(G8693) Code deleted December 31, 2011

G8694 Left ventricular ejection fraction (LVEF) < 40%

(G8695) Code deleted December 31, 2012.

G8696 Antithrombotic therapy prescribed at discharge

G8697 Antithrombotic therapy not prescribed for documented reasons

G8698 Antithrombotic therapy was not prescribed at discharge, reason not otherwise specified

G8699 Rehabilitation services (occupational, physical or speech) ordered at or prior to discharge

G8700 Rehabilitation services (occupational, physical or speech) not indicated at or prior to discharge

G8701 Rehabilitation services were not ordered, reason not otherwise specified

G8702 Documentation that prophylactic antibiotics were given within 4 hours prior to surgical incision or intraoperatively

G8703 Documentation that prophylactic antibiotics were neither given within 4 hours prior to surgical incision nor intraoperatively

G8704 12-lead electrocardiogram (ECG) performed

G8705 Documentation of medical reason(s) for not performing a 12-lead electrocardiogram (ECG)

G8706 Documentation of patient reason(s) for not performing a 12-lead electrocardiogram (ECG)

G8707 12-lead electrocardiogram (ECG) not performed, reason not otherwise specified

G8708 Patient not prescribed or dispensed antibiotic

▲G8709 Patient prescribed or dispensed antibiotic for documented medical reason(s) (e.g. intestinal infection, pertussis, bacterial infection, lyme disease, otitis media, acute sinusitis, acute pharyngitis, acute tonsillitis, chronic sinusitis, infection of the pharynx/larynx/tonsils/adenoids, prostatitis, cellulitis, mastoiditis, or bone infections, acute lymphadenitis, impetigo, skin staph infections, pneumonia/gonococcal infections, venereal disease (syphilis, chlamydia, inflammatory diseases (female reproductive organs)), infections of the kidney, cystitis or UTI, and acne)

G8710 Patient prescribed or dispensed antibiotic

G8711 Prescribed or dispensed antibiotic

G8712 Antibiotic not prescribed or dispensed

G8713 Spkt/v greater than or equal to 1.2 (single?pool clearance of urea [kt] / volume [v])

G8714 Hemodialysis treatment performed exactly three times per week

(G8715) Code deleted December 31, 2012.

(G8716) Code deleted December 31, 2012.

G8717 Spkt/v less than 1.2 (single-pool clearance of urea [kt] / volume [v]), reason not specified

G8718 Total kt/v greater than or equal to 1.7 per week (total clearance of urea [kt] / volume [v])

G8720 Total kt/v less than 1.7 per week (total clearance of urea [kt] / volume [v]), reason not specified

G8721 PT category (primary tumor), PN category (regional lymph nodes), and histologic grade were documented in pathology report

▲**G8722** Documentation of medical reason(s) for not including the pt category, the PN category or the histologic grade in the pathology report (e.g., re-excision without residual tumor; non-carcinomas anal canal)

G8723 Specimen site is other than anatomic location of primary tumor

G8724 PT category, PN category and histologic grade were not documented in the pathology report, reason not otherwise specified

Ⓟ **G8725** Fasting lipid profile performed (triglycerides, LDL?c, HDL?c and total cholesterol)

Ⓟ **G8726** Clinician has documented reason for not performing fasting lipid profile

(G8727) Code deleted December 31, 2012.

Ⓟ **G8728** Fasting lipid profile not performed, reason not otherwise specified

▲**G8730** Pain assessment documented as positive using a standardized tool and a follow-up plan is documented

▲**G8731** Pain assessment using a standardized tool is documented as negative, no follow-up plan required

G8732 No documentation of pain assessment

▲**G8733** Elder maltreatment screen documented as positive and a follow-up plan is documented

G8734 Elder maltreatment screen documented as negative, no follow-up required

G8735 Elder maltreatment screen documented as positive, follow-up plan not documented, reason not specified

Ⓟ **G8736** Most current LDL <100mg/dl

Ⓟ **G8737** Most current LDL?c >=100mg/dl

Ⓟ **G8738** Left ventricular ejection fraction (LVEF) < 40% or documentation of severely or moderately depressed left ventricular systolic function

Ⓟ **G8739** Left ventricular ejection fraction (LVEF) >= 40% or documentation as normal or mildly depressed left ventricular systolic function

Ⓟ **G8740** Left ventricular ejection fraction (LVEF) not performed or assessed, reason not specified

(G8741) Code deleted December 31, 2013

(G8742) Code deleted December 31, 2013

(G8743) Code deleted December 31, 2013

(G8744) Code deleted December 31, 2013

(G8745) Code deleted December 31, 2013

(G8746) Code deleted December 31, 2013

(G8747) Code deleted December 31, 2013

(G8748) Code deleted December 31, 2013

G8749 Absence of signs of melanoma (cough, dyspnea, tenderness, localized neurologic signs such as weakness, jaundice or any other sign suggesting systemic spread) or absence of symptoms of melanoma (pain, paresthesia, or any other symptom suggesting the possibility of systemic spread of melanoma)

(G8750) Code deleted December 31, 2012.

Ⓟ **G8751** Smoking status and exposure to secondhand smoke in the home not assessed, reason not specified

Ⓟ **G8752** Most recent systolic blood pressure < 140mmHg

Ⓟ **G8753** Most recent systolic blood pressure >= 140mmHg

Ⓟ **G8754** Most recent diastolic blood pressure < 90mmHg

Ⓟ **G8755** Most recent diastolic blood pressure >= 90mmHg

Ⓟ **G8756** No documentation of blood pressure measurement, reason not otherwise specified

Ⓟ **G8757** All quality actions for the applicable measures in the chronic obstructive pulmonary disease measures group have been performed for this patient

Ⓟ **G8758** All quality actions for the applicable measures in the inflammatory bowel disease measures group have been performed for this patient

Ⓟ **G8759** All quality actions for the applicable measures in the obstructive sleep apnea measures group have been performed for this patient

(G8760) Code deleted December 31, 2012.

Ⓟ **G8761** All quality actions for the applicable measures in the dementia measures group have been performed for this patient

Ⓟ **G8762** All quality actions for the applicable measures in the Parkinson's disease measures group have been performed for this patient

Ⓟ **G8763** All quality actions for the applicable measures in the hypertension measures group have been performed for this patient

Ⓟ **G8764** All quality actions for the applicable measures in the cardiovascular prevention measures group have bee performed for this patient

Ⓟ **G8765** All quality actions for the applicable measures in the cataract measures group have been performed for this patient

Ⓟ **G8767** Lipid panel results documented and reviewed (must include total cholesterol, HDL, triglycerides and calculated LDL)

Ⓟ ▲ **G8768** Documentation of medical reason(s) for not performing lipid profile (e.g., patients with palliative goals or for whom treatment of hypertension with standard treatment goals is not clinically appropriate)

Ⓟ **G8769** Lipid profile not performed, reason not otherwise specified

Ⓟ **G8770** Urine protein test result documented and reviewed

Ⓟ **G8771** Documentation of diagnosis of chronic kidney disease

Ⓟ ▲ **G8772** Documentation of medical reason(s) for not performing urine protein test (e.g., patients with palliative goals or for whom treatment of hypertension with standard treatment goals is not clinically appropriate)

Ⓟ **G8773** Urine protein test was not performed, reason not otherwise specified

Ⓟ **G8774** Serum creatinine test result documented and reviewed

Ⓟ ▲ **G8775** Documentation of medical reason(s) for not performing serum creatinine test (e.g., patients with palliative goals or for whom treatment of hypertension with standard treatment goals is not clinically appropriate)

Ⓟ **G8776** Serum creatinine test not performed, reason not otherwise specified

Ⓟ **G8777** Diabetes screening test performed

Ⓟ ▲ **G8778** Documentation of medical reason(s) for not performing diabetes screening test (e.g., patients with a diagnosis of diabetes, or with palliative goals or for whom treatment of hypertension with standard treatment goals is not clinically appropriate)

Ⓟ **G8779** Diabetes screening test not performed, reason not otherwise specified

Ⓟ **G8780** Counseling for diet and physical activity performed

Ⓟ ▲ **G8781** Documentation of medical reason(s) for patient not receiving counseling for diet and physical activity (e.g., patients with palliative goals or for whom treatment of hypertension with standard treatment goals is not clinically appropriate)

Ⓟ **G8782** Counseling for diet and physical activity not performed, reason not otherwise specified

Ⓟ **G8783** Blood pressure screening performed as recommended by the defined screening interval

Ⓟ ▲ **G8784** Blood pressure reading not documented, documentation the patient is not eligible

Ⓟ **G8785** Blood pressure screening not performed as recommended by screening interval, reason not otherwise specified

(G8786) Code deleted December 31, 2012.

(G8787) Code deleted December 31, 2012.

(G8788) Code deleted December 31, 2012.

(G8789) Code deleted December 31, 2012.

(G8790) Code deleted December 31, 2013

(G8791) Code deleted December 31, 2013

(G8792) Code deleted December 31, 2013

(G8793) Code deleted December 31, 2013

(G8794) Code deleted December 31, 2013

(G8795) Code deleted December 31, 2013

(G8796) Code deleted December 31, 2013

G8797 Specimen site other than anatomic location of esophagus

G8798 Specimen site other than anatomic location of prostate

(G8799) Code deleted December 31, 2013

(G8800) Code deleted December 31, 2013

(G8801) Code deleted December 31, 2013

(G8802) Code deleted December 31, 2012.

(G8803) Code deleted December 31, 2012.

(G8805) Code deleted December 31, 2012.

G8806 Performance of transabdominal or transvaginal ultrasound

G8807 Transabdominal or transvaginal ultrasound not performed for reasons documented by clinician

▲**G8808** Performance of trans-abdominal or trans-vaginal ultrasound not ordered, reason not given (e.g., patient has visited the ed multiple times with no documentation of a trans-abdominal or trans-vaginal ultrasound within ed or from referring eligible professional)

G8809 Rh immunoglobulin (RhoGAM) ordered

▲**G8810** Rh-immunoglobulin (RhoGAM) not ordered for reasons documented by clinician (e.g., patient had prior documented receipt of RhoGAM within 12 weeks, patient refusal)

G8811 Documentation Rh immunoglobulin (RhoGAM) was not ordered, reason not specified

(G8812) Code deleted December 31, 2013

(G8813) Code deleted December 31, 2013

(G8814) Code deleted December 31, 2013

G8815 Statin therapy not prescribed for documented reasons

G8816 Statin medication prescribed at discharge

G8817 Statin therapy not prescribed at discharge, reason not specified

G8818 Patient discharge to home no later than post-operative day #7

(G8819) Code deleted December 31, 2012.

(G8820) Code deleted December 31, 2012.

(G8821) Code deleted December 31, 2012.

(G8822) Code deleted December 31, 2012.

(G8823) Code deleted December 31, 2012.

(G8824) Code deleted December 31, 2012.

G8825 Patient not discharged to home by post-operative day #7

G8826 Patient discharge to home no later than post-operative day #2 following EVAR

(G8827) Code deleted December 31, 2013

(G8828) Code deleted December 31, 2012.

(G8829) Code deleted December 31, 2012.

(G8830) Code deleted December 31, 2012.

(G8831) Code deleted December 31, 2012.

(G8832) Code deleted December 31, 2012.

G8833 Patient not discharge to home by post-operative day #2 following EVAR

G8834 Patient discharged to home no later than post-operative day #2 following CEA

(G8835) Code deleted December 31, 2013

(G8836) Code deleted December 31, 2012.

(G8837) Code deleted December 31, 2012.

G8838 Patient not discharged to home by post-operative day #2

Ⓟ **G8839** Sleep apnea symptoms assessed, including presence or absence of snoring and daytime sleepiness

Ⓟ **G8840** Documentation of reason(s) for not performing an assessment of sleep symptoms (e.g., patient didn't have initial daytime sleepiness, patient visits between initial testing and initiation of therapy)

Ⓟ **G8841** Sleep apnea symptoms not assessed, reason not otherwise specified

Ⓟ **G8842** Apnea hypopnea index (AHI) or respiratory disturbance index (RDI) measured at the time of initial diagnosis

Ⓟ **G8843** Documentation of reason(s) for not measuring an apnea hypopnea index (AHI) or a respiratory disturbance index (RDI) at the time of initial diagnosis

Ⓟ **G8844** Apnea hypopnea index (AHI) or respiratory disturbance index (RDI) not measured at the time of initial diagnosis, reason not specified

Ⓟ **G8845** Positive airway pressure therapy prescribed

Ⓟ **G8846** Moderate or severe obstructive sleep apnea (apnea hypopnea index (AHI) or respiratory disturbance index (RDI) of 15 or greater)

(G8847) Code deleted December 31, 2012.

Ⓟ **G8848** Mild obstructive sleep apnea (apnea hypopnea index (AHI) or respiratory disturbance index (RDI) of less than 15)

Ⓟ **G8849** Documentation of reason(s) for not prescribing positive airway pressure therapy

Ⓟ **G8850** Positive airway pressure therapy not prescribed, reason not otherwise specified

Ⓟ **G8851** Objective measurement of adherence to positive airway pressure therapy, documented

Ⓟ **G8852** Positive airway pressure therapy prescribed

Ⓟ **G8853** Positive airway pressure therapy not prescribed

Ⓟ **G8854** Documentation of reason(s) for not objectively measuring adherence to positive airway pressure therapy

Ⓟ **G8855** Objective measurement of adherence to positive airway pressure therapy not performed, reason not otherwise specified

G8856 Referral to a physician for an otologic evaluation performed

G8857 Patient is not eligible for the referral for otologic evaluation measure (e.g., patients who are already under the care of a physician for acute or chronic dizziness)

G8858 Referral to a physician for an otologic evaluation not performed, reason not specified

Ⓟ **G8859** Patient receiving corticosteroids greater than or equal to 10mg/day for 60 or greater consecutive days

Ⓟ **G8860** Patients who have received dose of corticosteroids greater than or equal to 10mg/day for 60 or greater consecutive days

Ⓟ **G8861** Central dual-energy x-ray absorptiometry (DXA) ordered or documented, review of systems and medication history or pharmacologic therapy (other than minerals/vitamins) for osteoporosis prescribed

Ⓟ **G8862** Patients not receiving corticosteroids greater than or equal to 10mg/day for 60 or greater consecutive days

Ⓟ **G8863** Patients not assessed for risk of bone loss, reason not otherwise specified

Ⓟ **G8864** Pneumococcal vaccine administered or previously received

Ⓟ **G8865** Documentation of medical reason(s) for not administering or previously receiving pneumococcal vaccine (e.g., patient allergic reaction, potential adverse drug reaction)

Ⓟ **G8866** Documentation of patient reason(s) for not administering or previously receiving pneumococcal vaccine (e.g., patient refusal)

Ⓟ **G8867** Pneumococcal vaccine not administered or previously received, reason not otherwise specified

Ⓟ **G8868** Patients receiving a first course of anti-TNF therapy

Ⓟ **G8869** Patient has documented immunity to hepatitis B and is receiving a first course of anti-TNF therapy

Ⓟ **G8870** Hepatitis B vaccine injection administered or previously received and is receiving a first course of anti-TNF therapy

G8871 Patient not receiving a first course of anti-TNF therapy

G8872 Excised tissue evaluated by imaging intraoperatively to confirm successful inclusion of targeted lesion

G8873 Patients with needle localization specimens which are not amenable to intraoperative imaging such as MRI needle wire localization, or targets which are tentatively identified on mammogram or ultrasound which do not contain a biopsy marker but which can be verified on intraoperative inspection or pathology

G8874 Excised tissue not evaluated by imaging intraoperatively to confirm successful inclusion of targeted lesion

G8875 Clinician diagnosed breast cancer preoperatively by a minimally invasive biopsy method

G8876 Documentation of reason(s) for not performing minimally invasive biopsy to diagnose breast cancer preoperatively

G8877 Clinician did not attempt to achieve the diagnosis of breast cancer preoperatively by a minimally invasive biopsy method, reason not otherwise specified

G8878 Sentinel lymph node biopsy procedure performed

G8879 Clinically node negative (t1n0m0) or t2n0m0) invasive breast cancer

▲ **G8880** Documentation of reason(s) sentinel lymph node biopsy not performed (e.g., reasons could include but not limited to; non-invasive cancer, incidental discovery of breast cancer on prophylactic mastectomy, incidental discovery of breast cancer on reduction mammoplasty, pre-operative biopsy proven lymph node (ln) metastases, inflammatory carcinoma, stage 3 locally advanced cancer, recurrent invasive breast cancer, patient refusal after informed consent)

G8881 Stage of breast cancer is greater than t1n0m0 or t2n0m0

▲ **G8882** Sentinel lymph node biopsy procedure not performed, reason not given

G8883 Biopsy results reviewed, communicated, tracked and documented

G8884 Clinician documented reason that patient's biopsy results were not reviewed

G8885 Biopsy results not reviewed, communicated, tracked or documented

Ⓟ **G8886** Most recent blood pressure under control

Ⓟ ▲ **G8887** Documentation of medical reason(s) for most recent blood pressure not being under control (e.g., patients with palliative goals or for whom treatment of hypertension with standard treatment goals is not clinically appropriate)

Ⓟ **G8888** Most recent blood pressure not under control, results documented and reviewed

Ⓟ **G8889** No documentation of blood pressure measurement, reason not otherwise specified

Ⓟ **G8890** Most recent LDL under control, results documented and reviewed

Ⓟ ▲ **G8891** Documentation of medical reason(s) for most recent LDL-c not under control (e.g., patients with palliative goals for whom treatment of hypertension with standard treatment goals is not clinically appropriate)

Ⓟ ▲ **G8892** Documentation of medical reason(s) for not performing LDL-c test (e.g. patients with palliative goals or for whom treatment of hypertension with standard treatment goals is not clinically appropriate)

Ⓟ **G8893** Most recent LDL?c not under control, results documented and reviewed

Ⓟ **G8894** LDL-c not performed, reason not specified

Ⓟ **G8895** Oral aspirin or other anticoagulant/antiplatelet therapy prescribed

Ⓟ **G8896** Documentation of medical reason(s) for not prescribing oral aspirin or other anticoagulant/antiplatelet therapy (e.g. under age 30, patient documented to be low risk, patient with terminal illness or treatment of hypertension with standard treatment goals is not clinically appropriate)

Ⓟ **G8897** Oral aspirin or other anticoagulant/antiplatelet therapy was not prescribed, reason not otherwise specified

Ⓟ **G8898** I intend to report the chronic obstructive pulmonary disease measures group

Ⓟ **G8899** I intend to report the inflammatory bowel disease measures group

Ⓟ **G8900** I intend to report the obstructive sleep apnea measures group

(G8901) Code deleted December 31, 2012.

Ⓟ **G8902** I intend to report the dementia measures group

Ⓟ **G8903** I intend to report the Parkinson's disease measures group

Ⓟ **G8904** I intend to report the hypertension measures group

Ⓟ **G8905** I intend to report the cardiovascular prevention measures group

Ⓟ **G8906** I intend to report the cataract measures group

G8907 Patient documented not to have experienced any of the following events: a burn prior to discharge; a fall within the facility; wrong site/side/patient/procedure/implant event; or a hospital transfer or hospital admission upon discharge from the facility

G8908 Patient documented to have received a burn prior to discharge

G8909 Patient documented not to have received a burn prior to discharge

G8910 Patient documented to have experienced a fall within ambulatory surgical center (ASC)

G8911 Patient documented not to have experienced a fall within ambulatory surgical center (ASC)

G8912 Patient documented to have experienced a wrong site, wrong side, wrong patient, wrong procedure or wrong implant event

G8913 Patient documented not to have experienced a wrong site, wrong side, wrong patient, wrong procedure or wrong implant event

G8914 Patient documented to have experienced a hospital transfer or hospital admission upon discharge from ASC

G8915 Patient documented not to have experienced a hospital transfer or hospital admission upon discharge from ASC

G8916 Patient with preoperative order for IV antibiotic surgical site infection (SSI) prophylaxis, antibiotic initiated on time

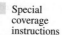

G8917 Patient with preoperative order for IV antibiotic surgical site infection (SSI) prophylaxis, antibiotic not initiated on time

G8918 Patient without preoperative order for IV antibiotic surgical site infection (SSI) prophylaxis

(G8919) Code deleted December 31, 2013

(G8920) Code deleted December 31, 2013

(G8921) Code deleted December 31, 2013

(G8922) Code deleted December 31, 2013

Ⓟ **G8923** Left ventricular ejection fraction (lvef) < 40% or documentation of moderately or severely depressed left ventricular systolic function

Ⓟ **G8924** Spirometry test results demonstrate fev1/fvc <60% with COPD symptoms (e. G. ,dyspnea, cough/sputum, wheezing)

Ⓟ **G8925** Spirometry test results demonstrate fev1/fvc >=60% or patient does not have COPD symptoms

Ⓟ **G8926** Spirometry test not performed or documented, reason not given

Ⓟ **G8927** Adjuvant chemotherapy referred, prescribed or previously received for AJCC stage III, colon cancer

Ⓟ ▲ **G8928** Adjuvant chemotherapy not prescribed or previously received for documented reasons (e.g., medical co-morbidities, diagnosis date more than 5 years prior to the current visit date, patient's cancer has metastasized, medical contraindication/allergy, poor performance status, other medical reasons, patient refusal, other patient reasons, patient is currently enrolled in a clinical trial that precludes prescription of chemotherapy, other system reasons)

Ⓟ ▲ **G8929** Adjuvant chemotherapy not prescribed or previously received, reason not specified

G8930 Assessment of depression severity not documented, reason not given

G8931 Assessment of depression severity not documented, reason not given

G8932 Suicide risk assessed at the initial evaluation

G8933 Suicide risk not assessed at the initial evaluation, reason not given

G8934 Left ventricular ejection fraction (lvef) <40% or documentation of moderately or severely depressed left ventricular systolic function

G8935 Clinician prescribed angiotensin converting enzyme (ACE) inhibitor or angiotensin receptor blocker (ARB) therapy

G8936 Clinician documented that patient was not an eligible candidate for angiotensin converting enzyme (ACE) inhibitor or angiotensin receptor blocker (ARB) therapy

G8937 Clinician did not prescribe angiotensin converting enzyme (ACE) inhibitor or angiotensin receptor blocker (ARB) therapy, reason not given

Ⓟ ▲ **G8938** BME is documented as being outside of normal limits, follow-up plan is not documented, documentation the patient is not eligible

▲ **G8939** Pain assessment documented as positive, follow-up plan not documented, documentation the patient is not eligible

▲ **G8940** Screening for clinical depression documented as positive, a follow-up plan not documented, documentation stating the patient is not eligible

▲ **G8941** Elder maltreatment screen documented as positive, follow-up plan not documented, documentation the patient is not eligible

▲ **G8942** Functional outcomes assessment using a standardized tool is documented within the previous 30 days and care plan, based on identified deficiencies on the date of the functional outcome assessment, is documented

Ⓟ **G8943** LDL-C result not present or not within 12 months prior

G8944 AJCC melanoma cancer stage 0 through IIc melanoma

(G8945) Code deleted December 31, 2013

▲**G8946** Minimally invasive biopsy method attempted but not diagnostic of breast cancer (e.g., high risk lesion of breast such as atypical ductal hyperplasia, lobular neoplasia, atypical lobular hyperplasia, lobular carcinoma in situ, atypical columnar hyperplastica, flat epithelial atypia, radial scar, complex sclerosing lesion, papillary lesion, or any lesion with spindle cells)

Ⓟ **G8947** One or more neuropsychiatric symptoms

Ⓟ **G8948** No neuropsychiatric symptoms

Ⓟ **G8949** Documentation of patient reason(s) for patient not receiving counseling for diet and physical activity (e. G. , patient is not willing to discuss diet or exercise interventions to help control blood pressure, or the patient said he/she refused to make these changes)

Ⓟ ▲ **G8950** Pre-hypertensive or hypertensive blood pressure reading documented, and the indicated follow-up is documented

Ⓟ ▲ **G8951** Pre-hypertensive or hypertensive blood pressure reading documented, indicated follow-up not documented, documentation the patient is not eligible

Ⓟ **G8952** Pre-hypertensive or hypertensive blood pressure reading documented, indicated follow-up not documented, reason not given

Ⓟ **G8953** All quality actions for the applicable measures in the oncology measures group have been performed for this patient

(G8954) Code deleted December 31, 2013

G8955 Most recent assessment of adequacy of volume management

G8956 Patient receiving maintenance hemodialysis in an outpatient dialysis facility

G8957 Patient not receiving maintenance hemodialysis in an outpatient dialysis facility

G8958 Assessment of adequacy of volume management not documented, reason not given

G8959 Clinician treating major depressive disorder communicates to clinician treating comorbid condition

G8960 Clinician treating major depressive disorder did not communicate to clinician treating comorbid condition, reason not given

G8961 Cardiac stress imaging test primarily performed on low-risk surgery patient for preoperative evaluation within 30 days preceding this surgery

G8962 Cardiac stress imaging test performed on patient for any reason including those who did not have low risk surgery or test that was performed more than 30 days preceding low risk surgery

G8963 Cardiac stress imaging performed primarily for monitoring of asymptomatic patient who had PCI within 2 years

G8964 Cardiac stress imaging test performed primarily for any other reason than monitoring of asymptomatic patient who had PCI wthin 2 years (e. G. ,symptomatic patient, patient greater than 2 years since PCI, initial evaluation, etc)

G8965 Cardiac stress imaging test primarily performed on low CHD risk patient for initial detection and risk assessment

G8966 Cardiac stress imaging test performed on symptomatic or higher than low CHD risk patient or for any reason other than initial detection and risk assessment

G8967 Warfarin or another oral anticoagulant that is FDA approved prescribed

▲**G8968** Documentation of medical reason(s) for not prescribing warfarin or another oral anticoagulant that is fad approved for the prevention of thromboembolism (e.g. patients with mitral stenosis or prosthetic heart valves, patients with transient or reversible causes of af (e.g., pneumonia or hyperthyroidism), postoperative patients, patients who are pregnant, allergy, risk of bleeding, other medical reasons)

▲**G8969** Documentation of patient reason(s) for not prescribing warfarin or another oral anticoagulant that is fad approved (e.g., economic, social, and/or religious impediments, noncompliance patient refusal, other patient reasons)

G8970 No risk factors or one moderate risk factor for thromboembolism

G8971 Warfarin or another oral anticoagulant that is FDA approved not prescribed, reason not given

G8972 One or more high risk factors for thromboembolism or more than one moderate risk factor for thromboembolism

G8973 Most recent hemoglobin (hgb) level < 10 g/dl

G8974 Hemoglobin level measurement not documented, reason not given

G8975 Documentation of medical reason(s) for patient having a hemoglobin level < 10 g/dl (e. G. , patients who have non-renal etiologies of anemia [e. G. , sickle cell anemia or other hemoglobinopathies, hypersplenism, primary bone marrow disease, anemia related to chemotherapy for diagnosis of malignancy, postoperative bleeding, active bloodstream or peritoneal infection], other medical reasons)

G8976 Most recent hemoglobin (hgb) level >= 10 g/dl

Ⓟ **G8977** I intend to report the oncology measures group

G8978 Mobility: walking & moving around functional limitation, current status, at therapy episode outset and at reporting intervals

G8979 Mobility: walking & moving around functional limitation, projected goal status, at therapy episode outset, at reporting intervals, and at discharge or to end reporting

G8980 Mobility: walking & moving around functional limitation, discharge status, at discharge from therapy or to end reporting

G8981 Changing & maintaining body position functional limitation, current status, at therapy episode outset and at reporting intervals

G8982 Changing & maintaining body position functional limitation, projected goal status, at therapy episode outset, at reporting intervals, and at discharge or to end reporting

G8983 Changing & maintaining body position functional limitation, discharge status, at discharge from therapy or to end reporting

G8984 Carrying, moving & handling objects functional limitation, current status, at therapy episode outset and at reporting intervals

▲ **G8985** Carrying, moving and handling objects, projected goal status, at therapy episode outset, at reporting intervals, and at discharge or to end reporting

G8986 Carrying, moving & handling objects functional limitation, discharge status, at discharge from therapy or to end reporting

G8987 Self care functional limitation, current status, at therapy episode outset and at reporting intervals

G8988 Self care functional limitation, projected goal status, at therapy episode outset, at reporting intervals, and at discharge or to end reporting

G8989 Self care functional limitation, discharge status, at discharge from therapy or to end reporting

▲ **G8990** Other physical or occupational therapy primary functional limitation, current status, at therapy episode outset and at reporting intervals

▲ **G8991** Other physical or occupational therapy primary functional limitation, projected goal status, at therapy episode outset, at reporting intervals, and at discharge or to end reporting

▲ **G8992** Other physical or occupational therapy primary functional limitation, discharge status, at discharge from therapy or to end reporting

▲ **G8993** Other physical or occupational therapy subsequent functional limitation, current status, at therapy episode outset and at reporting intervals

▲ **G8994** Other physical or occupational therapy subsequent functional limitation, projected goal status, at therapy episode outset, at reporting intervals, and at discharge or to end reporting

▲**G8995** Other physical or occupational therapy subsequent functional limitation, discharge status, at discharge from therapy or to end reporting

▲**G8996** Swallowing functional limitation, current status at therapy episode outset and at reporting intervals

▲**G8997** Swallowing functional limitation, projected goal status, at therapy episode outset, at reporting intervals, and at discharge or to end reporting

▲**G8998** Swallowing functional limitation, discharge status, at discharge from therapy or to end reporting

▲**G8999** Motor speech functional limitation, current status at therapy episode outset and at reporting intervals

G9001 Coordinated care fee; initial rate

G9002 maintenance rate

G9003 risk adjusted high, initial

G9004 risk adjusted low, initial

G9005 risk adjusted maintenance

G9006 home monitoring

G9007 scheduled team conference

G9008 physician coordinated care oversight services

G9009 risk adjusted maintenance, level 3

G9010 risk adjusted maintenance, level 4

G9011 risk adjusted maintenance, level 5

G9012 Other specified case management service not elsewhere classified

G9013 ESRD demo basic bundle level I

G9014 ESRD demo expanded bundle including venous access and related services

G9016 Smoking cessation counseling, individual, in the absence of or in addition to any other evaluation and management service, per session (6-10 minutes) [DEMO PROJECT CODE ONLY]

G9017 Amantadine hydrochloride, oral, per 100 mg (for use as a Medicare approved demonstration project)

G9018 Zanamivir, inhalation powder administered through inhaler, per 10 mg (for use as a Medicare approved demonstration project)

G9019 Oseltamivir phosphate, oral, per 75 mg (for use as a Medicare approved demonstration project)

G9020 Rimantadine hydrochloride, oral, per 100 mg (for use as a Medicare approved demonstration project)

G9033 Amantadine hydrochloride, oral brand, per 100 mg (for use in a Medicare-approved demonstration project)

G9034 Zanamivir, inhalation powder, administered through inhaler, brand, per 10 mg (for use in a Medicare-approved demonstration project)

G9035 Oseltamivir phosphate, oral, brand, per 75 mg (for use in a Medicare-approved demonstration project)

G9036 Rimantadine HCl, oral, brand, per 100 mg (for use in a Medicare-approved demonstration project)

(G9041) Code deleted December 31, 2011

(G9042) Code deleted December 31, 2011

(G9043) Code deleted December 31, 2011

(G9044) Code deleted December 31, 2011

ONCOLOGY

G9050 Oncology; primary focus of visit; work-up, evaluation, or staging at the time of cancer diagnosis or recurrence (for use in a Medicare-approved demonstration project)

G9051 Oncology; primary focus of visit; treatment decision-making after disease is staged or restaged, discussion of treatment options, supervising/coordinating active cancer directed therapy or managing consequences of cancer directed therapy (for use in a Medicare-approved demonstration project)

G9052 Oncology; primary focus of visit; surveillance for disease recurrence for patient who has completed definitive cancer-directed therapy and currently lacks evidence of recurrent disease; cancer directed therapy might be considered in the future (for use in a Medicare-approved demonstration project)

G9053 Oncology; primary focus of visit; expectant management of patient with evidence of cancer for whom no cancer directed therapy is being administered or arranged at present; cancer directed therapy might be considered in the future (for use in a Medicare-approved demonstration project)

G9054 Oncology; primary focus of visit; supervising, coordinating or managing care of patient with terminal cancer or for whom other medical illness prevents further cancer treatment; includes symptom management, end-of-life care planning, management of palliative therapies (for use in a Medicare-approved demonstration project)

G9055 Oncology; primary focus of visit; other, unspecified service not otherwise listed (for use in a Medicare-approved demonstration project)

G9056 Oncology; practice guidelines; management adheres to guidelines (for use in a Medicare-approved demonstration project)

G9057 Oncology; practice guidelines; management differs from guidelines as a result of patient enrollment in an institutional review board approved clinical trial (for use in a Medicare-approved demonstration project)

G9058 Oncology; practice guidelines; management differs from guidelines because the treating physician disagrees with guideline recommendations (for use in a Medicare-approved demonstration project)

G9059 Oncology; practice guidelines; management differs from guidelines because the patient, after being offered treatment consistent with guidelines, has opted for alternative treatment or management, including no treatment (for use in a Medicare-approved demonstration project)

G9060 Oncology; practice guidelines; management differs from guidelines for reason(s) associated with patient comorbid illness or performance status not factored into guidelines (for use in a Medicare-approved demonstration project)

G9061 Oncology; practice guidelines; patient's condition not addressed by available guidelines (for use in a Medicare-approved demonstration project)

G9062 Oncology; practice guidelines; management differs from guidelines for other reason(s) not listed (for use in a Medicare-approved demonstration project)

G9063 Oncology; disease status; limited to non-small cell lung cancer; extent of disease initially established as stage I (prior to neo-adjuvant therapy, if any) with no evidence of disease progression, recurrence, or metastases (for use in a Medicare-approved demonstration project)

G9064 Oncology; disease status; limited to non-small cell lung cancer; extent of disease initially established as stage II (prior to neo-adjuvant therapy, if any) with no evidence of disease progression, recurrence, or metastases (for use in a Medicare-approved demonstration project)

G9065 Oncology; disease status; limited to non-small cell lung cancer; extent of disease initially established as stage III A (prior to neo-adjuvant therapy, if any) with no evidence of disease progression, recurrence, or metastases (for use in a Medicare-approved demonstration project)

G9066 Oncology; disease status; limited to non-small cell lung cancer; stage III B- IV at diagnosis, metastatic, locally recurrent, or progressive (for use in a Medicare-approved demonstration project)

G9067 Oncology; disease status; limited to non-small cell lung cancer; extent of disease unknown, under evaluation, not yet determined, or not listed (for use in a Medicare-approved demonstration project)

G9068 Oncology; disease status; limited to small cell and combined small cell/non-small cell; extent of disease initially established as limited with no evidence of disease progression, recurrence, or metastases (for use in a Medicare-approved demonstration project)

G9069 Oncology; disease status; small cell lung cancer, limited to small cell and combined small cell/non-small cell; extensive stage at diagnosis, metastatic, locally recurrent, or progressive (for use in a Medicare-approved demonstration project)

G9070 Oncology; disease status; small cell lung cancer, limited to small cell and combined small cell/non-small; extent of disease unknown, under evaluation, pre-surgical, or not listed (for use in a Medicare-approved demonstration project)

G9071 Oncology; disease status; invasive female breast cancer (does not include ductal carcinoma in situ); adenocarcinoma as predominant cell type; stage I or stage IIA-IIB; or T3, N1, M0; and ER and/or PR positive; with no evidence of disease progression, recurrence, or metastases (for use in a Medicare-approved demonstration project)

G9072 Oncology; disease status; invasive female breast cancer (does not include ductal carcinoma in situ); adenocarcinoma as predominant cell type; stage I, or stage IIA-IIB; or T3, N1, M0; and ER and PR negative; with no evidence of disease progression, recurrence, or metastases (for use in a Medicare-approved demonstration project)

G9073 Oncology; disease status; invasive female breast cancer (does not include ductal carcinoma in situ); adenocarcinoma as predominant cell type; stage IIIA-IIIB; and not T3, N1, M0; and ER and/or PR positive; with no evidence of disease progression, recurrence, or metastases (for use in a Medicare-approved demonstration project)

G9074 Oncology; disease status; invasive female breast cancer (does not include ductal carcinoma in situ); adenocarcinoma as predominant cell type; stage IIIA-IIIB; and not T3, N1, M0; and ER and PR negative; with no evidence of disease progression, recurrence, or metastases (for use in a Medicare-approved demonstration project)

G9075 Oncology; disease status; invasive female breast cancer (does not include ductal carcinoma in situ); adenocarcinoma as predominant cell type; M1 at diagnosis, metastatic, locally recurrent, or progressive (for use in a Medicare-approved demonstration project)

G9077 Oncology; disease status; prostate cancer, limited to adenocarcinoma as predominant cell type; T1-T2C and Gleason 2-7 and PSA < or equal to 20 at diagnosis with no evidence of disease progression, recurrence, or metastases (for use in a Medicare-approved demonstration project)

G9078 Oncology; disease status; prostate cancer, limited to adenocarcinoma as predominant cell type; T2 or Gleason 8-10 or PSA > 20 at diagnosis with no evidence of disease progression, recurrence, or metastases (for use in a Medicare-approved demonstration project)

G9079 Oncology; disease status; prostate cancer, limited to adenocarcinoma as predominant cell type; T3B-T4, any N; any T, N1 at diagnosis with no evidence of disease progression, recurrence, or metastases (for use in a Medicare-approved demonstration project)

G9080 Oncology; disease status; prostate cancer, limited to adenocarcinoma; after initial treatment with rising PSA or failure of PSA decline (for use in a Medicare-approved demonstration project)

G9083 Oncology; disease status; prostate cancer, limited to adenocarcinoma; extent of disease unknown, under evaluation or not listed (for use in a Medicare-approved demonstration project)

G9084 Oncology; disease status; colon cancer, limited to invasive cancer, adenocarcinoma as predominant cell type; extent of disease initially established as T1-3, N0, M0 with no evidence of disease progression, recurrence, or metastases (for use in a Medicare-approved demonstration project)

G9085 Oncology; disease status; colon cancer, limited to invasive cancer, adenocarcinoma as predominant cell type; extent of disease initially established as T4, N0, M0 with no evidence of disease progression, recurrence, or metastases (for use in a Medicare-approved demonstration project)

G9086 Oncology; disease status; colon cancer, limited to invasive cancer, adenocarcinoma as predominant cell type; extent of disease initially established as T1-4, N1-2, M0 with no evidence of disease progression, recurrence, or metastases (for use in a Medicare-approved demonstration project)

G9087 Oncology; disease status; colon cancer, limited to invasive cancer, adenocarcinoma as predominant cell type; M1 at diagnosis, metastatic, locally recurrent, or progressive with current clinical, radiologic, or biochemical evidence of disease (for use in a Medicare-approved demonstration project)

G9088 Oncology; disease status; colon cancer, limited to invasive cancer, adenocarcinoma as predominant cell type; M1 at diagnosis, metastatic, locally recurrent, or progressive without current clinical, radiologic, or biochemical evidence of disease (for use in a Medicare-approved demonstration project)

G9089 Oncology; disease status; colon cancer, limited to invasive cancer, adenocarcinoma as predominant cell type; extent of disease unknown, not yet determined, under evaluation, pre-surgical, or not listed (for use in a Medicare-approved demonstration project)

G9090 Oncology; disease status; rectal cancer, limited to invasive cancer, adenocarcinoma as predominant cell type; extent of disease initially established as T1-2, N0, M0 (prior to neo-adjuvant therapy, if any) with no evidence of disease progression, recurrence, or metastases (for use in a Medicare-approved demonstration project)

G9091 Oncology; disease status; rectal cancer, limited to invasive cancer, adenocarcinoma as predominant cell type; extent of disease initially established as T3, N0, M0 (prior to neo-adjuvant therapy, if any) with no evidence of disease progression, recurrence, or metastases (for use in a Medicare-approved demonstration project)

G9092 Oncology; disease status; rectal cancer, limited to invasive cancer, adenocarcinoma as predominant cell type; extent of disease initially established as T1-3, N1-2, M0 (prior to neo-adjuvant therapy, if any) with no evidence of disease progression, recurrence or metastases (for use in a Medicare-approved demonstration project)

G9093 Oncology; disease status; rectal cancer, limited to invasive cancer, adenocarcinoma as predominant cell type; extent of disease initially established as T4, any N, M0 (prior to neo-adjuvant therapy, if any) with no evidence of disease progression, recurrence, or metastases (for use in a Medicare-approved demonstration project)

G9094 Oncology; disease status; rectal cancer, limited to invasive cancer, adenocarcinoma as predominant cell type; M1 at diagnosis, metastatic, locally recurrent, or progressive (for use in a Medicare-approved demonstration project)

G9095 Oncology; disease status; rectal cancer, limited to invasive cancer, adenocarcinoma as predominant cell type; extent of disease unknown, not yet determined, under evaluation, pre-surgical, or not listed (for use in a Medicare-approved demonstration project)

G9096 Oncology; disease status; esophageal cancer, limited to adenocarcinoma or squamous cell carcinoma as predominant cell type; extent of disease initially established as T1-T3, N0-N1 or NX (prior to neo-adjuvant therapy, if any) with no evidence of disease progression, recurrence, or metastases (for use in a Medicare-approved demonstration project)

G9097 Oncology; disease status; esophageal cancer, limited to adenocarcinoma or squamous cell carcinoma as predominant cell type; extent of disease initially established as T4, any N, M0 (prior to neo-adjuvant therapy, if any) with no evidence of disease progression, recurrence, or metastases (for use in a Medicare-approved demonstration project)

G9098 Oncology; disease status; esophageal cancer, limited to adenocarcinoma or squamous cell carcinoma as predominant cell type; M1 at diagnosis, metastatic, locally recurrent, or progressive (for use in a Medicare-approved demonstration project)

G9099 Oncology; disease status; esophageal cancer, limited to adenocarcinoma or squamous cell carcinoma as predominant cell type; extent of disease unknown, not yet determined, under evaluation, pre-surgical, or not listed (for use in a Medicare-approved demonstration project)

G9100 Oncology; disease status; gastric cancer, limited to adenocarcinoma as predominant cell type; post R0 resection (with or without neoadjuvant therapy) with no evidence of disease recurrence, progression, or metastases (for use in a Medicare-approved demonstration project)

G9101 Oncology; disease status; gastric cancer, limited to adenocarcinoma as predominant cell type; post R1 or R2 resection (with or without neoadjuvant therapy) with no evidence of disease progression, or metastases (for use in a Medicare-approved demonstration project)

G9102 Oncology; disease status; gastric cancer, limited to adenocarcinoma as predominant cell type; clinical or pathologic M0, unresectable with no evidence of disease progression, or metastases (for use in a Medicare-approved demonstration project)

G9103 Oncology; disease status; gastric cancer, limited to adenocarcinoma as predominant cell type; clinical or pathologic M1 at diagnosis, metastatic, locally recurrent, or progressive (for use in a Medicare-approved demonstration project)

G9104 Oncology; disease status; gastric cancer, limited to adenocarcinoma as predominant cell type; extent of disease unknown, under evaluation, not yet determined, pre-surgical, or not listed (for use in a Medicare-approved demonstration project)

G9105 Oncology; disease status; pancreatic cancer, limited to adenocarcinoma as predominant cell type; post R0 resection without evidence of disease progression, recurrence, or metastases (for use in a Medicare-approved demonstration project)

G9106 Oncology; disease status; pancreatic cancer, limited to adenocarcinoma; post R1 or R2 resection with no evidence of disease progression, or metastases (for use in a Medicare-approved demonstration project)

G9107 Oncology; disease status; pancreatic cancer, limited to adenocarcinoma; unresectable at diagnosis, M1 at diagnosis, metastatic, locally recurrent, or progressive (for use in a Medicare-approved demonstration project)

G9108 Oncology; disease status; pancreatic cancer, limited to adenocarcinoma; extent of disease unknown, under evaluation, not yet determined, pre-surgical, or not listed (for use in a Medicare-approved demonstration project)

G9109 Oncology; disease status; head and neck cancer, limited to cancers of oral cavity, pharynx and larynx with squamous cell as predominant cell type; extent of disease initially established as T1-T2 and N0, M0 (prior to neo-adjuvant therapy, if any) with no evidence of disease progression, recurrence, or metastases (for use in a Medicare-approved demonstration project)

G9110 Oncology; disease status; head and neck cancer, limited to cancers of oral cavity, pharynx and larynx with squamous cell as predominant cell type; extent of disease initially established as T3-4 and/or N1-3, M0 (prior to neo-adjuvant therapy, if any) with no evidence of disease progression, recurrence, or metastases (for use in a Medicare-approved demonstration project)

G9111 Oncology; disease status; head and neck cancer, limited to cancers of oral cavity, pharynx and larynx with squamous cell as predominant cell type; M1 at diagnosis, metastatic, locally recurrent, or progressive (for use in a Medicare-approved demonstration project)

G9112 Oncology; disease status; head and neck cancer, limited to cancers of oral cavity, pharynx and larynx with squamous cell as predominant cell type; extent of disease unknown, not yet determined, pre-surgical, or not listed (for use in a Medicare-approved demonstration project)

G9113 Oncology; disease status; ovarian cancer, limited to epithelial cancer; pathologic stage IA-B (grade 1) without evidence of disease progression, recurrence, or metastases (for use in a Medicare-approved demonstration project)

G9114 Oncology; disease status; ovarian cancer, limited to epithelial cancer; pathologic stage IA-B (grade 2-3); or stage IC (all grades); or stage II; without evidence of disease progression, recurrence, or metastases (for use in a Medicare-approved demonstration project)

G9115 Oncology; disease status; ovarian cancer, limited to epithelial cancer; pathologic stage III-IV; without evidence of progression, recurrence, or metastases (for use in a Medicare-approved demonstration project)

G9116 Oncology; disease status; ovarian cancer, limited to epithelial cancer; evidence of disease progression, or recurrence, and/or platinum resistance (for use in a Medicare-approved demonstration project)

G9117 Oncology; disease status; ovarian cancer, limited to epithelial cancer; extent of disease unknown, under evaluation, incomplete surgical staging, pre-surgical staging, or not listed (for use in a Medicare-approved demonstration project)

G9123 Oncology; disease status; non-Hodgkin's lymphoma, limited to follicular lymphoma, mantle cell lymphoma, diffuse large B-cell lymphoma, or histologically transformed from follicular lymphoma to diffuse large B-cell lymphoma; relapsed or refractory (for use in a Medicare-approved demonstration project)

G9124 Oncology; disease status; non-Hodgkin's lymphoma, limited to follicular lymphoma, mantle cell lymphoma, diffuse large B-cell lymphoma, peripheral T cell lymphoma or small lympocytic lymphoma; relapsed and refractory (for use in a Medicare-approved demonstration project)

G9125 Oncology; disease status; non-Hodgkin's lymphoma, limited to follicular lymphoma, mantle cell lymphoma, diffuse large B-cell lymphoma, peripheral T cell lymphoma or small lymphocytic lymphoma; diagnostic evaluation, stage not determined, evaluation of possible relapse or non-response to therapy, or not listed (for use in a Medicare-approved demonstration project)

G9126 Oncology; disease status; ovarian cancer, limited to pathologically stage patients with epithelial cancer; stage IA/IB (for use in a Medicare-approved demonstration project)

G9128 Oncology; disease status; limited to multiple myeloma, systemic disease; stage II or higher (for use in a Medicare-approved demonstration project)

G9129 Oncology; disease status; chronic myelogenous leukemia, limited to Philadelphia chromosome positive and/or BCR-ABL positive; extent of disease unknown, under evaluation, not listed, or treatment options being considered (for use in a Medicare-approved demonstration project)

G9130 Oncology; disease status; limited to multiple myeloma, systemic disease; extent of disease unknown, under evaluation, or not listed (for use in a Medicare-approved demonstration project)

G9131 Oncology; disease status; invasive female breast cancer (does not include ductal carcinoma in situ); adenocarcinoma as predominant cell type; extent of disease unknown, staging in progress, or not listed (for use in a Medicare-approved demonstration project)

G9132 Oncology; disease status; prostate cancer, limited to adenocarcinoma hormone-refractory/androgen-independent (e.g., rising PSA on anti-androgen therapy or post-orchiectomy); clinical metastases (for use in a Medicare-approved demonstration project)

G9133 Ooncology; disease status; prostate cancer, limited to adenocarcinoma; hormone-responsive; clinical metastases or M1 at diagnosis (for use in a Medicare-approved demonstration project)

G9134 Oncology; disease status; non-Hodgkin's lymphoma, any cellular classification; stage I, II at diagnosis, not relapsed, not refractory (for use in a Medicare-approved demonstration project)

G9135 Oncology; disease status; non-Hodgkin's lymphoma, any cellular classification; stage III, IV, not relapsed, not refractory (for use in a Medicare-approved demonstration project)

G9136 Oncology; disease status; non-Hodgkin's lymphoma, transformed from original cellular diagnosis to a second cellular classification (for use in a Medicare-approved demonstration project)

G9137 Oncology; disease status; non-Hodgkin's lymphoma, any cellular classification; relapsed/refractory (for use in a Medicare-approved demonstration project)

G9138 Oncology; disease status; non-Hodgkin's lymphoma, any cellular classification; diagnostic evaluation, stage not determined, evaluation of possible relapse or non-response to therapy, or not listed (for use in a Medicare-approved demonstration project)

G9139 Oncology; disease status; chronic myelogenous leukemia, limited to Philadelphia chromosome positive and/or BCr-abl positive; extent of disease unknown, staging in progress, not listed (for use in a Medicare-approved demonstration project)

G9140 Frontier extended stay clinic demonstration; for a patient stay in a clinic approved for the cms demonstration project; the following measures should be present: the stay must be equal to or greater than 4 hours; weather or other conditions must prevent transfer or the case falls into a category of monitoring and observation cases that are permitted by the rules of the demonstration; there is a maximum frontier extended stay clinic (FESC) visit of 48 hours, except in the case when weather or other conditions prevent transfer; payment is made on each period up to 4 hours, after the first 4 hours

(G9141) Code deleted December 31, 2012

(G9142) Code deleted December 31, 2012

G9143 Warfarin responsiveness testing by genetic technique using any method, any number of specimen(s)

G9147 Outpatient intravenous insulin treatment (Oivit) either pulsatile or continuous, by any means, guided by the results of measurements for: respiratory quotient; and/or, urine urea nitrogen (uun); and/or, arterial, venous or capillary glucose; and/or potassium concentration

G9148 National committee for quality assurance - level I medical home

G9149 National committee for quality assurance - level 2 medical home

G9150 National committee for quality assurance - level 3 medical home

G9151 Mapcp demonstration - state provided services

G9152 Mapcp demonstration - community health teams

G9153 Mapcp demonstration - physician incentive pool

G9156 Evaluation for wheelchair requiring face to face visit with physician

G9157 Transesophageal doppler use for cardiac monitoring

▲**G9158** Motor speech functional limitation, discharge status, at discharge from therapy or to end reporting

▲**G9159** Spoken language comprehension functional limitation, current status at therapy episode outset and at reporting intervals

▲**G9160** Spoken language comprehension functional limitation, projected goal status at therapy episode outset, at reporting intervals, and at discharge from or to end reporting

▲**G9161** Spoken language comprehension functional limitation, discharge status, at discharge from therapy or to end reporting

▲**G9162** Spoken language expression functional limitation, current status at therapy episode outset and at reporting intervals

▲**G9163** Spoken language expression functional limitation, projected goal status at therapy episode outset, at reporting intervals, and at discharge from or to end reporting

▲**G9164** Spoken language expression functional limitation, discharge status at discharge from therapy or to end reporting

▲**G9165** Attention functional limitation, current status at therapy episode outset and at reporting intervals

▲**G9166** Attention functional limitation, projected goal status at therapy episode outset, at reporting intervals, and at discharge from or to end reporting

▲**G9167** Attention functional limitation, discharge status at discharge from therapy or to end reporting

▲**G9168** Memory functional limitation, current status at therapy episode outset and at reporting intervals

▲**G9169** Memory functional limitation, projected goal status at therapy episode outset, at reporting intervals, and at discharge from or to end reporting

▲**G9170** Memory functional limitation, discharge status at discharge from therapy or to end reporting

▲**G9171** Voice functional limitation, current status at therapy episode outset and at reporting intervals

▲**G9172** Voice functional limitation, projected goal status at therapy episode outset, at reporting intervals, and at discharge from or to end reporting

▲**G9173** Voice functional limitation, discharge status at discharge from therapy or to end reporting

▲**G9174** Other speech language pathology functional limitation, current status at therapy episode outset and at reporting intervals

▲**G9175** Other speech language pathology functional limitation, projected goal status at therapy episode outset, at reporting intervals, and at discharge from or to end reporting

▲**G9176** Other speech language pathology functional limitation, discharge status at discharge from therapy or to end reporting

▲**G9186** Motor speech functional limitation, projected goal status at therapy episode outset, at reporting intervals, and at discharge from or to end reporting

●**G9187** Bundled payments for care improvement initiative home visit for patient assessment performed by a qualified health care professional for individuals not considered homebound including, but not limited to, assessment of safety, falls, clinical status, fluid status, medication reconciliation/management, patient compliance with orders/plan of care, performance of activities of daily living, appropriateness of care setting; (for use only in the Medicare-approved bundled payments for care improvement initiative); may not be billed for a 30-day period covered by a transitional care management code

●**G9188** Beta-blocker therapy not prescribed, reason not given

●**G9189** Beta-blocker therapy prescribed or currently being taken

● **G9190** Documentation of medical reason(s) for not prescribing beta-blocker therapy (eg, allergy, intolerance, other medical reasons)

● **G9191** Documentation of patient reason(s) for not prescribing beta-blocker therapy (eg, patient declined, other patient reasons)

● **G9192** Documentation of system reason(s) for not prescribing beta-blocker therapy (eg, other reasons attributable to the health care system)

● **G9193** Clinician documented that patient with a diagnosis of major depression was not an eligible candidate for antidepressant medication treatment or patient did not have a diagnosis of major depression

● **G9194** Patient with a diagnosis of major depression documented as being treated with antidepressant medication during the entire 180 day (6 month) continuation treatment phase

● **G9195** Patient with a diagnosis of major depression not documented as being treated with antidepressant medication during the entire 180 day (6 months) continuation treatment phase

● **G9196** Documentation of medical reason(s) for not ordering first or second generation cephalosporin for antimicrobial prophylaxis

● **G9197** Documentation of order for first or second generation cephalosporin for antimicrobial prophylaxis

● **G9198** Order for first or second generation cephalosporin for antimicrobial prophylaxis was not documented, reason not given

● **G9199** Venous thromboembolism (vote) prophylaxis not administered the day of or the day after hospital admission for documented reasons (eg, patient is ambulatory, patient expired during inpatient stay, patient already on warfarin or another anticoagulant, other medical reason(s) or eg, patient left against medical advice, other patient reason(s))

● **G9200** Venous thromboembolism (vote) prophylaxis was not administered the day of or the day after hospital admission, reason not given

● **G9201** Venous thromboembolism (vote) prophylaxis administered the day of or the day after hospital admission

● **G9202** Patients with a positive hepatitis C antibody test

● **G9203** RNA testing for hepatitis C documented as performed within 12 months prior to initiation of antiviral treatment for hepatitis C

● **G9204** RNA testing for hepatitis C was not documented as performed within 12 months prior to initiation of antiviral treatment for hepatitis C, reason not given

● **G9205** Patient starting antiviral treatment for hepatitis C during the measurement period

● **G9206** Patient starting antiviral treatment for hepatitis C during the measurement period

● **G9207** Hepatitis C genotype testing documented as performed within 12 months prior to initiation of antiviral treatment for hepatitis C

● **G9208** Hepatitis C genotype testing was not documented as performed within 12 months prior to initiation of antiviral treatment for hepatitis C, reason not given

● **G9209** Hepatitis C quantitative RNA testing documented as performed between 4-12 weeks after the initiation of antiviral treatment

● **G9210** Hepatitis C quantitative RNA testing not performed between 4-12 weeks after the initiation of antiviral treatment for reasons documented by clinician (eg, patients whose treatment was discontinued during the testing period prior to testing, other medical reasons, patient declined, other patient reasons)

● **G9211** Hepatitis C quantitative rna testing was not documented as performed between 4-12 weeks after the initiation of antiviral treatment, reason not given

● **G9212** DSM-IV criteria for major depressive disorder documented at the initial evaluation

● **G9213** DSMT-IV-TR criteria for major depressive disorder not documented at the initial evaluation, reason not otherwise specified

● **G9214** CD4+ cell count or CD4+ cell percentage results documented

● **G9215** CD4+ cell count or percentage not documented as performed, reason not given

● **G9216** (No Suggestions) prophylaxis was not prescribed at time of diagnosis of HIV, reason not given

● **G9217** (No Suggestions) prophylaxis was not prescribed within 3 months of low CD4+ cell count below 200 cells/mm^3, reason not given

● **G9218** (No Suggestions) prophylaxis was not prescribed within 3 months of low CD4+ cell count below 500 cells/mm^3 or a CD4 percentage below 15%, reason not given

● **G9219** Pneumocystis jiroveci pneumonia prophylaxis not prescribed within 3 months of low CD4+ cell count below 200 cells/mm^3 for medical reason (i.e., patient's CD4+ cell count above threshold within 3 months after CD4+ cell count below threshold, indicating that the patient's CD4+ levels are within an acceptable range and the patient does not require pcx prophylaxis)

● **G9220** Pneumocystis jiroveci pneumonia prophylaxis not prescribed within 3 months of low CD4+ cell count below 500 cells/mm^3 or a CD4 percentage below 15% for medical reason (i.e., patient's CD4+ cell count above threshold within 3 months after CD4+ cell count below threshold, indicating that the patient's CD4+ levels are within an acceptable range and the patient does not require pcx prophylaxis)

● **G9221** Pneumocystis jiroveci pneumonia prophylaxis prescribed

● **G9222** Pneumocystis jiroveci pneumonia prophylaxis prescribed within 3 months of low CD4+ cell count below 200 cells/mm^3

● **G9223** Pneumocystis jiroveci pneumonia prophylaxis prescribed within 3 months of low CD4+ cell count below 500 cells/mm^3 or a CD4 percentage below 15%

● **G9224** Documentation of medical reason for not performing foot exam (e.g., patient with bilateral foot/leg amputation)

● **G9225** Foot exam was not performed, reason not given

● **G9226** Foot examination performed (includes examination through visual inspection, sensory exam with monofilament, and pulse exam - report when all of the 3 components are completed)

● **G9227** Functional outcome assessment documented, care plan not documented, documentation the patient is not eligible for a care plan

● **G9228** Chlamydia, gonorrhea and syphilis screening results documented (report when results are present for all of the 3 screenings)

● **G9229** Chlamydia, gonorrhea, and syphilis not screened, due to documented reason (patient refusal is the only allowed exclusion)

● **G9230** Chlamydia, gonorrhea, and syphilis not screened, reason not given

● **G9231** Documentation of end stage renal disease (esrd), dialysis, renal transplant or pregnancy

● **G9232** Clinician treating major depressive disorder did not communicate to clinician treating comorbid condition for specified patient reason

● **G9233** All quality actions for the applicable measures in the total knee replacement measures group have been performed for this patient

● **G9234** I intend to report the total knee replacement measures group

● **G9235** All quality actions for the applicable measures in the general surgery measures group have been performed for this patient

● **G9236** All quality actions for the applicable measures in the optimizing patient exposure to ionizing radiation measures group have been perform

● **G9237** I intend to report the general surgery measures group

● **G9238** I intend to report the optimizing patient exposure to ionizing radiation measures group

● **G9239** Documentation of reasons for patient initiating maintenance hemodialysis with a catheter as the mode of vascular access (eg, patient has a maturing aVF/avg, time-limited trial of hemodialysis, patients undergoing palliative dialysis, other medical reasons, patient declined aVF/avg, other patient reasons, patient followed by reporting nephrologist for fewer than 90 days, other system reasons)

● **G9240** Patient whose mode of vascular access is a catheter at the time maintenance hemodialysis is initiated

● **G9241** Patient whose mode of vascular access is not a catheter at the time maintenance hemodialysis is initiated

● **G9242** Documentation of viral load equal to or greater than 200 copies/ml

● **G9243** Documentation of viral load less than 200 copies/ml

● **G9244** Antiretroviral therapy not prescribed

● **G9245** Antiretroviral therapy prescribed

● **G9246** Patient did not have at least one medical visit in each 6 month period of the 24 month measurement period, with a minimum of 60 days between medical visits

● **G9247** Patient had at least one medical visit in each 6 month period of the 24 month measurement period, with a minimum of 60 days between medical visits

● **G9248** Patient did not have a medical visit in the last 6 months

● **G9249** Patient had a medical visit in the last 6 months

● **G9250** Documentation of patient pain brought to a comfortable level within 48 hours from initial assessment

● **G9251** Documentation of patient with pain not brought to a comfortable level within 48 hours from initial assessment

● **G9252** Adenoma(s) or other neoplasm detected during screening colonoscopy

● **G9253** Adenoma(s) or other neoplasm not detected during screening colonoscopy

● **G9254** Documentation of patient discharged to home later than post-operative day 2 following CAS

● **G9255** Documentation of patient discharged to home no later than post operative day 2 following CAS

● **G9256** Documentation of patient death following CAS

● **G9257** Documentation of patient stroke following CAS

● **G9258** Documentation of patient stroke following CEA

● **G9259** Documentation of patient survival and absence of stroke following CAS

● **G9260** Documentation of patient death following CEA

● **G9261** Documentation of patient survival and absence of stroke following CEA

● **G9262** Documentation of patient death in the hospital following endovascular AAA repair

● **G9263** Documentation of patient survival in the hospital following endovascular AAA repair

● **G9264** Documentation of patient receiving maintenance hemodialysis for greater than or equal to 90 days with a catheter for documented reasons (eg, patient is undergoing palliative dialysis with a catheter, patient approved by a qualified transplant program and scheduled to receive a living donor kidney transplant, other medical reasons, patient declined aVF/avg, other patient reasons)

● **G9265** Patient receiving maintenance hemodialysis for greater than or equal to 90 days with a catheter as the mode of vascular access

● **G9266** Patient receiving maintenance hemodialysis for greater than or equal to 90 days without a catheter as the mode of vascular access

● **G9267** Documentation of patient with one or more complications or mortality within 30 days

● **G9268** Documentation of patient with one or more complications within 90 days

● **G9269** Documentation of patient without one or more complications and without mortality within 30 days

● **G9270** Documentation of patient without one or more complications within 90 days

● **G9271** LDL value < 100

● **G9272** LDL value >= 100

● **G9273** Blood pressure has a systolic value of < 140 and a diastolic value of < 90

● **G9274** Blood pressure has a systolic value of =140 and a diastolic value of = 90 or systolic value < 140 and diastolic value = 90 or systolic value = 140 and diastolic value < 90

● **G9275** Documentation that patient is a current non-tobacco user

● **G9276** Documentation that patient is a current tobacco user

● **G9277** Documentation that the patient is on daily aspirin or has documentation of a valid contraindication to aspirin automatic contraindications include anti-coagulant use, allergy, and history of gastrointestinal bleed; additionally, any reason documented by the physician as a reason for not taking daily aspirin is acceptable (examples include non-steroidal anti-inflammatory agents, risk for drug interaction, or uncontrolled hypertension defined as > 180 systolic or > 110 diastolic)

● **G9278** Documentation that the patient is not on daily aspirin regimen

● **G9279** Pneumococcal screening performed and documentation of vaccination received prior to discharge

● **G9280** Pneumococcal vaccination not administered prior to discharge, reason not specified

● **G9281** Screening performed and documentation that vaccination not indicated/patient refusal

● **G9282** Documentation of medical reason(s) for not reporting the histological type or NSCLC-nos classification with an explanation (e.g., biopsy taken for other purposes in a patient with a history of non-small cell lung cancer or other documented medical reasons)

● **G9283** Non small cell lung cancer biopsy and cytology specimen report documents classification into specific histologic type or classified as NSCLC-nos with an explanation

● **G9284** Non small cell lung cancer biopsy and cytology specimen report does not document classification into specific histologic type or classified as NSCLC-nos with an explanation

● **G9285** Specimen site other than anatomic location of lung or is not classified as non small cell lung cancer

● **G9286** Documentation of antibiotic regimen prescribed within 7 days of diagnosis or within 10 days after onset of symptoms

● **G9287** No antibiotic regimen prescribed within 7 days of diagnosis or within 10 days after onset of symptoms

● **G9288** Documentation of medical reason(s) for not reporting the histological type or NSCLC-nos classification with an explanation (e.g., a solitary fibrous tumor in a person with a history of non-small cell carcinoma or other documented medical reasons)

● **G9289** Non small cell lung cancer biopsy and cytology specimen report documents classification into specific histologic type or classified as NSCLC-nos with an explanation

● **G9290** Non small cell lung cancer biopsy and cytology specimen report does not document classification into specific histologic type or classified as NSCLC-nos with an explanation

● **G9291** Specimen site other than anatomic location of lung, is not classified as non small cell lung cancer or classified as NSCLC-nos

● **G9292** Documentation of medical reason(s) for not reporting pt category and a statement on thickness and ulceration and for pt1, mitotic rate (e.g., negative skin biopsies in a patient with a history of melanoma or other documented medical reasons)

● **G9293** Pathology report does not include the pt category and a statement on thickness and ulceration and for pt1, mitotic rate

● **G9294** Pathology report includes the pt category and a statement on thickness and ulceration and for pt1, mitotic rate

● **G9295** Specimen site other than anatomic cutaneous location

● **G9296** Patients with documented shared decision-making including discussion of conservative (non-surgical) therapy prior to the procedure

● **G9297** Shared decision-making including discussion of conservative (non-surgical) therapy prior to the procedure not documented, reason not given

● **G9298** Patients who are evaluated for venous thromboembolic and cardiovascular risk factors within 30 days prior to the procedure including history of DVT, pe, mi, arrhythmia and stroke

● **G9299** Patients who are not evaluated for venous thromboembolic and cardiovascular risk factors within 30 days prior to the procedure including history of DVT, pe, mi, arrhythmia and stroke, reason not given

● **G9300** Documentation of medical reason(s) for not completely infusing the prophylactic antibiotic prior to the inflation of the proximal tourniquet (e.g., a tourniquet was not used)

● **G9301** Patients who had the prophylactic antibiotic completely infused prior to the inflation of the proximal tourniquet

● **G9302** Prophylactic antibiotic not completely infused prior to the inflation of the proximal tourniquet, reason not given

● **G9303** Operative report does not identify the prosthetic implant specifications including the prosthetic implant manufacturer, the brand name of the prosthetic implant and the size of the prosthetic implant, reason not given

● **G9304** Operative report identifies the prosthetic implant specifications including the prosthetic implant manufacturer, the brand name of the prosthetic implant and the size of the prosthetic implant

● **G9305** Intervention for presence of leak of endoluminal contents through an anastomosis not required

● **G9306** Intervention for presence of leak of endoluminal contents through an anastomosis required

● **G9307** No return to the operating room for a surgical procedure, for any reason, within 30 days of the principal operative procedure

● **G9308** Unplanned return to the operating room for a surgical procedure, for any reason, within 30 days of the principal operative procedure

● **G9309** No unplanned hospital readmission within 30 days of principal procedure

● **G9310** Unplanned hospital readmission within 30 days of principal procedure

● **G9311** No surgical site infection

● **G9312** Surgical site infection

● **G9313** Amoxicillin, with or without clavulanate, not prescribed as first line antibiotic at the time of diagnosis for documented reason (eg, cystic fibrosis, immotile cilia disorders, ciliary dyskinesia, immune deficiency, prior history of sinus surgery within the past 12 months, and anatomic abnormalities, such as deviated nasal septum, resistant organisms, allergy to medication, recurrent sinusitis, chronic sinusitis, or other reasons)

● **G9314** Amoxicillin, with or without clavulanate, not prescribed as first line antibiotic at the time of diagnosis, reason not given

● **G9315** Documentation amoxicillin, with or without clavulanate, prescribed as a first line antibiotic at the time of diagnosis

● **G9316** Documentation of patient-specific risk assessment with a risk calculator based on multi-institutional clinical data, the specific risk calculator used, and communication of risk assessment from risk calculator with the patient or family

● **G9317** Documentation of patient-specific risk assessment with a risk calculator based on multi-institutional clinical data, the specific risk calculator used, and communication of risk assessment from risk calculator with the patient or family not completed

● **G9318** Imaging study named according to standardized nomenclature

● **G9319** Imaging study not named according to standardized nomenclature, reason not given

● **G9320** Documentation of medical reason(s) for not naming CT studies according to a standardized nomenclature provided (eg, ct studies performed for radiation treatment planning or image-guided radiation treatment delivery)

● **G9321** Count of previous CT (any type of CT) and cardiac nuclear medicine (myocardial perfusion) studies documented in the 12-month period prior to the current study

● **G9322** Count of previous CT and cardiac nuclear medicine (myocardial perfusion) studies not documented in the 12-month period prior to the current study, reason not given

● **G9323** Documentation of medical reason(s) for not counting previous CT and cardiac nuclear medicine (myocardial perfusion) studies (eg, CT studies performed for radiation treatment planning or image-guided radiation treatment delivery)

● **G9324** All necessary data elements not included, reason not given

● **G9325** CT studies not reported to a radiation dose index registry due to medical reasons (eg, CT studies performed for radiation treatment planning or image-guided radiation treatment delivery)

● **G9326** CT studies performed not reported to a radiation dose index registry, reason not given

● **G9327** CT studies performed reported to a radiation dose index registry with all necessary data elements

● **G9328** DICOM format image data availability not documented in final report due to medical reasons (eg, CT studies performed for radiation treatment planning or image-guided radiation treatment delivery)

● **G9329** DICOM format image data available to non-affiliated external entities on a secure, media free, reciprocally searchable basis with patient authorization for at least a 12-month period after the study not documented in final report, reason not given

● **G9340** Final report documented that DICOM format image data available to non-affiliated external entities on a secure, media free, reciprocally searchable basis with patient authorization for at least a 12-month period after the study

● **G9341** Search conducted for prior patient CT imaging studies completed at non-affiliated external entities within the past 12-months and are available through a secure, authorized, media-free, shared archive prior to an imaging study being performed

● **G9342** Search conducted for prior patient imaging studies completed at non-affiliated external entities within the past 12-months and are available through a secure, authorized, media-free, shared archive prior to an imaging study being performed not completed, reason not given

● **G9343** Search for prior patient completed DICOM format images not completed due to medical reasons (eg, CT studies performed for radiation treatment planning or image-guided radiation treatment delivery)

● **G9344** Search for prior patient completed DICOM format images not completed due to system reasons (ie, facility does not have archival abilities through a shared archival system)

● **G9345** Follow-up recommendations according to recommended guidelines for incidentally detected pulmonary nodules (eg, follow-up CT imaging studies needed or that no follow-up is needed) based at a minimum on nodule size and patient risk factors documented

● **G9346** Follow-up recommendations according to recommended guidelines for incidentally detected pulmonary nodules not documented due to medical reasons (eg, patients with known malignant disease, patients with unexplained fever, CT studied performed for radiation treatment planning or image-guided radiation treatment delivery)

● **G9347** Follow-up recommendations according to recommended guidelines for incidentally detected pulmonary nodules not documented, reason not given

● **G9348** CT scan of the paranasal sinuses ordered at the time of diagnosis for documented reasons (eg, persons with sinusitis symptoms lasting at least 7 to 10 days, antibiotic resistance, immunocompromised, recurrent sinusitis, acute frontal sinusitis, acute sphenoid sinusitis, periorbital cellulitis, or other medical)

● **G9349** Documentation of a CT scan of the paranasal sinuses ordered at the time of diagnosis or received within 28 days after date of diagnosis

● **G9350** CT scan of the paranasal sinuses not ordered at the time of diagnosis or received within 28 days after date of diagnosis

● **G9351** More than one CT scan of the paranasal sinuses ordered or received within 90 days after diagnosis

● **G9352** More than one CT scan of the paranasal sinuses ordered or received within 90 days after the date of diagnosis, reason not given

● **G9353** More than one CT scan of the paranasal sinuses ordered or received within 90 days after the date of diagnosis for documented reasons (eg, patients with complications, second CT obtained prior to surgery, other medical reasons)

● **G9354** More than one CT scan of the paranasal sinuses not ordered within 90 days after the date of diagnosis

● **G9355** Elective delivery or early induction not performed

● **G9356** Elective delivery or early induction performed

● **G9357** Post-partum screenings, evaluations and education performed

● **G9358** Post-partum screenings, evaluations and education not performed

● **G9359** Documentation of negative or managed positive t.b. screen with further evidence that t.b. is not active

● **G9360** No documentation of negative or managed positive t.b. screen

REHABILITATIVE SERVICES

Rehabilitative Services

H0001 Alcohol and/or drug assessment

H0002 Behavioral health screening to determine eligibility for admission to treatment program

H0003 Alcohol and/or drug screening; laboratory analysis of specimens for presence of alcohol and/or drugs

H0004 Behavioral health counseling and therapy, per 15 minutes

H0005 Alcohol and/or drug services; group counseling by a clinician

H0006 Alcohol and/or drug services; case management

H0007 Alcohol and/or drug services; crisis intervention (outpatient)

H0008 Alcohol and/or drug services; sub-acute detoxification (hospital inpatient)

H0009 Alcohol and/or drug services; acute detoxification (hospital inpatient)

H0010 Alcohol and/or drug services; sub-acute detoxification (residential addiction program inpatient)

H0011 Alcohol and/or drug services; acute detoxification (residential addiction program inpatient)

H0012 Alcohol and/or drug services; sub-acute detoxification (residential addiction program outpatient)

H0013 Alcohol and/or drug services; acute detoxification (residential addiction program outpatient)

H0014 Alcohol and/or drug services; ambulatory detoxification

H0015 Alcohol and/or drug services; intensive outpatient (treatment program that operates at least 3 hours/day and at least 3 days/week and is based on an individualized treatment plan), including assessment, counseling, crisis intervention, and activity therapies or education

H0016 Alcohol and/or drug services; medical/somatic (medical intervention in ambulatory setting)

H0017 Behavioral health; residential (hospital residential treatment program), without room and board, per diem

H0018 Behavioral health; short-term residential (non-hospital residential treatment program), without room and board, per diem

H0019 Behavioral health; long-term residential (non-medical, non-acute care in residential treatment program where stay is typically longer than 30 days), without room and board, per diem

H0020 Alcohol and/or drug services; methadone administration and/or service (provision of the drug by a licensed program)

H0021 Alcohol and/or drug training service (for staff and personnel not employed by providers)

H0022 Alcohol and/or drug intervention service (planned facilitation)

H0023 Behavioral health outreach service (planned approach to reach a targeted population)

H0024 Behavioral health prevention information dissemination service (one-way direct or non-direct contact with service audiences to affect knowledge and attitude)

H0025 Behavioral health prevention education service (delivery of services with target population to affect knowledge, attitude and/or behavior)

H0026 Alcohol and/or drug prevention process services, community-based (delivery of services to develop skills of impactors)

H0027 Alcohol and/or drug prevention environmental services (broad range of external activities geared toward modifying systems in order to mainstream prevention through policy and law)

H0028 Alcohol and/or drug prevention problem identification and referral service (e.g., student assistance and employee assistance programs), does not include assessment

H0029 Alcohol and/or drug prevention alternatives service (services for populations that exclude alcohol and other drug use, e.g. alcohol-free social events)

H0030 Behavioral health hotline service

H0031 Mental health assessment, by non-physician

H0032 Mental health service plan development by non-physician

H0033 Oral medication administration, direct observation

H0034 Medication training and support, per 15 minutes

H0035 Mental health partial hospitalization, treatment, less than 24 hours

H0036 Community psychiatric supportive treatment, face-to-face, per 15 minutes

H0037 Community psychiatric supportive treatment program, per diem

H0038 Self-help/peer services, per 15 minutes

H0039 Assertive community treatment, face-to-face, per 15 minutes

H0040 Assertive community treatment program, per diem

H0041 Foster care, child, non-therapeutic, per diem

H0042 Foster care, child, non-therapeutic, per month

H0043 Supported housing, per diem

H0044 Supported housing, per month

H0045 Respite care services, not in the home, per diem

H0046 Mental health services, not otherwise specified

H0047 Alcohol and/or other drug abuse services, not otherwise specified

H0048 Alcohol and/or other drug testing: collection and handling only, specimens other than blood

H0049 Alcohol and/or drug screening

H0050 Alcohol and/or drug service, brief intervention, per 15 minutes

H1000 Prenatal care, at-risk assessment

H1001 Prenatal care, at-risk enhanced service; antepartum management

H1002 Prenatal care, at-risk enhanced service; care coordination

H1003 Prenatal care, at-risk enhanced service; education

H1004 Prenatal care, at-risk enhanced service; follow-up home visit

H1005 Prenatal care, at-risk enhanced service package (includes H1001-H1004)

H1010 Non-medical family planning education, per session

H1011 Family assessment by licensed behavioral health professional for state defined purposes

H2000 Comprehensive multidisciplinary evaluation

H2001 Rehabilitation program, per 1/2 day

H2010 Comprehensive medication services, per 15 minutes

H2011 Crisis intervention service, per 15 minutes

H2012 Behavioral health day treatment, per hour

H2013 Psychiatric health facility service, per diem

H2014 Skills training and development, per 15 minutes

H2015 Comprehensive community support services, per 15 minutes

H2016 Comprehensive community support services, per diem

H2017 Psychosocial rehabilitation services, per 15 mintues

H2018 Psychosocial rehabilitation services, per diem

H2019 Therapeutic behavioral services, per 15 minutes

H2020 Therapeutic behavioral services, per diem

H2021 Community-based wrap-around services, per 15 minutes

H2022 Community-based wrap-around services, per diem

H2023 Supported employment, per 15 minutes

H2024 Supported employment, per diem

H2025 Ongoing support to maintain employment, per 15 minutes

H2026 Ongoing support to maintain employment, per diem

H2027 Psychoeducational service, per 15 minutes

H2028 Sexual offender treatment service, per 15 minutes

H2029 Sexual offender treatment service, per diem

H2030 Mental health clubhouse services, per 15 minutes

H2031 Mental health clubhouse services, per diem

H2032 Activity therapy, per 15 minutes

H2033 Multisystemic therapy for juveniles, per 15 minutes

H2034 Alcohol and/or drug abuse halfway house services, per diem

H2035 Alcohol and/or other drug treatment program, per hour

H2036 Alcohol and/or other drug treatment program, per diem

H2037 Developmental delay prevention activities, dependent child of client, per 15 minutes

DRUGS ADMINISTERED OTHER THAN ORAL METHOD

(EXCEPTION: ORAL IMMUNOSUPPRESSIVE DRUGS)

Guidelines

In addition to the information presented in the INTRODUCTION, several other items unique to this section are defined or identified here:

1. EXCEPTION: Oral immunosuppressive drugs are not included in this section.

2. ROUTE OF ADMINISTRATION: Unless otherwise specified, the drugs listed in this section may be injected either subcutaneously, intramuscularly or intravenously.

3. SUBSECTION INFORMATION: Some of the listed subheadings or subsections have special needs or instructions unique to that section. Where these are indicated, special "notes" will be presented preceding or following the listings. Those subsections within the DRUGS ADMINISTERED OTHER THAN ORAL METHOD section that have "notes" are as follows:

Subsection	Code Numbers
Drugs administered other than oral method	J0000-J8999
Immunosuppressive drugs	J7500-J7506
Chemotherapy drugs	J9000-J9999

4. UNLISTED SERVICE OR PROCEDURE: A service or procedure may be provided that is not listed in this edition of HCPCS. When reporting such a service, the appropriate "unlisted procedure" code may be used to indicate the service, identifying it by "special report" as defined below. HCPCS terminology is inconsistent in defining unlisted procedures. The procedure definition may include the term(s) "unlisted", "not otherwise classified", "unspecified", "unclassified", "other" and "miscellaneous". Prior to using these codes, try to determine if a Local Level III code or CPT code is available. The "unlisted procedures" and accompanying codes for DRUGS ADMINISTERED OTHER THAN ORAL METHOD are as follows:

J CODES

J3490	Unclassified drugs
J9999	Not otherwise classified, antineoplastic drugs

5. SPECIAL REPORT: A service, material or supply that is rarely provided, unusual, variable or new may require a special report in determining medical appropriateness for reimbursement purposes. Pertinent information should include an adequate definition or description of the nature, extent, and need for the service, material or supply.

6. MODIFIERS: Listed services may be modified under certain circumstances. When appropriate, the modifying circumstance is identified by adding a modifier to the basic procedure code. CPT and HCPCS National Level II modifiers may be used with CPT and HCPCS National Level II procedure codes. Modifiers commonly used with DRUGS ADMINISTERED OTHER THAN ORAL METHOD are as follows:

   -AA Anesthesia services performed personally by anesthesiologist

   -AD Medical supervision by a physician: more than four concurrent anesthesia procedures.

   -CC Procedure code change (use "CC" when the procedure code submitted was changed either for administrative reasons or because an incorrect code was filed)

   -G8 Monitored anesthesia care (MAC) for deep complex, complicated, or markedly invasive surgical procedure

   -G9 Monitored anesthesia care (MAC) for patient who has history of severe cardio-pulmonary condition

   -TC Technical component. Under certain circumstances, a charge may be made for the technical component alone. Under those circumstances, the technical component charge is identified by adding modifier -TC to the usual procedure code. Technical component charges are institutional charges and are not billed separately by physicians. However, portable x-ray suppliers bill only for the technical component and should use modifier -TC. The charge data from portable x-ray suppliers will then be used to build customary and prevailing profiles.

7. CPT CODE CROSS-REFERENCE: Unless otherwise specified, the equivalent CPT codes for all listings in this section fall within the range 90701-90799.

Drugs Administered Other Than Oral Method

The following list of drugs can be injected either subcutaneous, intramuscular, or intravenous. The brand name(s) of the drugs has been included as bold-type in brackets [ ] in some cases.

NOTE: Third party payers may wish to determine a threshold and pay up to a certain dollar limit before developing for the drug. Use procedure code J0110 for processing these cases.

J0120 Injection, tetracycline, up to 250 mg
MCM: 2049

Ⓟ **J0129** Injection, abatacept, 10 mg (code may be used for Medicare when drug administered under the direct supervision of a physician, not for use when drug is self administered)

J0130 Injection abciximab, 10 mg
MCM: 2049

J0131 Injection, acetaminophen, 10 mg

J0132 Injection, acetylcysteine, 100 mg

J0133 Injection, acyclovir, 5 mg

Ⓟ **J0135** Injection, adalimumab, 20 mg

J0150 Injection, adenosine for therapeutic use, 6 mg (not to be used to report any adenosine phosphate compounds, instead use A9270)
MCM: 2049

● **J0151** Injection, adenosine for diagnostic use, 1 mg (not to be used to report any adenosine phosphate compounds, instead use A9270)

(J0152) Code deleted December 31, 2013

J0171 Injection, adrenalin, epinephrine, 0.1 mg
MCM: 2049

J0178 Injection, aflibercept, 1 mg

J0180 Injection, agalsidase beta, 1 mg

J0190 Injection, biperiden lactate, per 5 mg
MCM: 2049

J0200 Injection, alatrofloxacin mesylate, 100 mg
MCM: 2049.5

J0205 Injection, alglucerase, per 10 units
MCM: 2049

J0207 Injection, amifostine, 500 mg
MCM: 2049

J0210 Injection, methyldopate HCl, [Aldomet], up to 250 mg
MCM: 2049

J0215 Injection, alefacept, 0.5 mg

J0220 Injection, alglucosidase alfa, 10 mg, not otherwise specified

J0221 Injection, alglucosidase alfa, (lumizyme), 10 mg

J0256 Injection, alpha 1 proteinase inhibitor (human), not otherwise specified, 10 mg
MCM: 2049

J0257 Injection, alpha 1 proteinase inhibitor (human), (glassia), 10 mg
MCM: 2049

J0270 Injection, alprostadil, 1.25 mcg (code may be used for Medicare when drug administered under the direct supervision of a physician, not for use when drug is self administered)
MCM: 2049

J0275 Alprostadil urethral suppository (code may be used for Medicare when drug administered under the direct supervision of a physician, not for use when drug is self administered)
MCM: 2049

J0278 Injection, amikacin sulfate, 100 mg

J0280 Injection, aminophylline, up to 250 mg
MCM: 2049

J0282 Injection, amiodarone hydrochloride, 30 mg
MCM: 2049

J0285 Injection, amphotericin B, 50 mg
MCM: 2049

J0287 Injection, amphotericin b lipid complex, 10 mg
MCM: 2049

J0288 Injection, amphotericin b cholesteryl sulfate complex, 10 mg
MCM: 2049

J0289 Injection, amphotericin b liposome, 10 mg
MCM: 2049

J0290 Injection, ampicillin sodium, 500 mg
MCM: 2049

J0295 Injection, ampicillin sodium/sulbactam sodium, per 1.5 gram
MCM: 2049

J0300 Injection, amobarbital, up to 125 mg
MCM: 2049

J0330 Injection, succinylcholine chloride, [Anectine], up to 20 mg
MCM: 2049

J0348 Injection, anidulafungin, 1 mg

J0350 Injection, anistreplase, per 30 units
MCM: 2049

J0360 Injection, hydralazine HCl, [Apresoline], up to 20 mg
MCM: 2049

J0364 Injection, apomorphine hydrochloride, 1 mg

J0365 Injection, aprotonin, 10,000 kiu
MCM: 2049

J0380 Injection, metaraminol bitartrate, per 10 mg
MCM: 2049

J0390 Injection, chloroquine HCl, [Aralen HCl], up to 250 mg
MCM: 2049

J0395 Injection, arbutamine HCl, 1 mg
MCM: 2049

J0400 Injection, aripiprazole, intramuscular, 0.25 mg

● **J0401** Injection, aripiprazole, extended release, 1 mg

J0456 Injection, azithromycin, 500 mg
MCM: 2049.5

J0461 Injection, atropine sulfate, 0.01 mg
MCM: 2049

J0470 Injection, dimercaprol, per 100 mg
MCM: 2049

J0475 Injection, baclofen, 10 mg
MCM: 2049

J0476 Injection, baclofen, 50 mcg for intrathecal trial
MCM: 2049

J0480 Injection, basiliximab, 20 mg
MCM: 2049

J0485 Injection, belatacept, 1 mg

J0490 Injection, belimumab, 10 mg

J0500 Injection, dicyclomine HCl, [Bentyl, Spasmoject], up to 20 mg
MCM: 2049

J0515 Injection, benztropine mesylate, [Cogentin], per 1 mg
MCM: 2049

J0520 Injection, bethanechol chloride, myotonachol or urecholine, up to 5 mg
MCM: 2049

J0558 Injection, penicillin G benzathine and penicillin G procaine, 100,000 units

J0561 Injection, penicillin G benzathine, 100,000 units
MCM: 2049

J0583 Injection, bivalirudin, 1 mg

J0585 Injection, onabotulinumtoxinA, 1 unit
MCM: 2049

J0586 Injection, abobotulinumtoxinA, 5 units

J0587 Injection, rimabotulinumtoxinB, 100 units
MCM: 2049

J0588 Injection, incobotulinumtoxinA, 1 unit

J0592 Injection, buprenorphine hydrochloride, 0.1 mg
MCM: 2049

J0594 Injection, busulfan, 1 mg

J0595 Injection, butorphanol tartrate, 1 mg

J0597 Injection, C-1 esterase inhibitor (human), Berinert, 10 units

J0598 Injection, C-1 esterase inhibitor (human), Cinryze, 10 units

J0600 Injection, edetate calcium disodium, [calcium disodium versenate], up to 1,000 mg
MCM: 2049

J0610 Injection, calcium gluconate, per 10 ml
MCM: 2049

J0620 Injection, calcium glycerophosphate and calcium lactate, per 10 ml
MCM: 2049

J0630 Injection, calcitonin salmon, up to 400 units
MCM: 2049

J0636 Injection, calcitriol, 0.1 mcg
MCM: 2049

J0637 Injection, caspofungin acetate, 5 mg

J0638 Injection, canakinumab, 1 mg

J0640 Injection, leucovorin calcium, per 50 mg
MCM: 2049

J0641 Injection, levoleucovorin calcium, 0.5 mg

J0670 Injection, mepivacaine HCl, [Carbocaine], per 10 ml
MCM: 2049

J0690 Injection, cefazolin sodium, 500 mg
MCM: 2049

J0692 Injection, cefepime hydrochloride, 500 mg

J0694 Injection, cefoxitin sodium, [Mefoxin], 1 gram
MCM: 2049

J0696 Injection, ceftriaxone sodium, [Rocephin], per 250 mg
MCM: 2049

J0697 Injection sterile cefuroxime sodium, [Ceftin, Kefurox, Zihacef injection], per 750 mg
MCM: 2049

J0698 Injection, cefotaxime sodium, [Claforan], per gram
MCM: 2049

J0702 Injection, betamethasone acetate 3mg and betamethasone sodium phosphate 3mg
MCM: 2049

J0706 Injection, caffeine citrate, 5 mg

J0710 Injection, cephapirin sodium, [Cefadyl], up to 1 gram
MCM: 2049

J0712 Injection, ceftaroline fosamil, 10 mg

J0713 Injection, ceftazidime, per 500 mg
MCM: 2049

J0715 Injection, ceftizoxime sodium, per 500 mg
MCM: 2049

J0716 Injection, centruroides immune f(ab)2, up to 120 milligrams

● **J0717** Injection, Certolizumab pegol, 1 mg (code may be used for medicare when drug administered under the direct supervision of a physician, not for use when drug is self administered)

(J0718) Code deleted December 31, 2013

J0720 Injection, chloramphenicol sodium succinate, [Chloromycetin Sodium Succinate], up to 1 gram
MCM: 2049

J0725 Injection, chorionic gonadotropin, per 1,000 USP units
MCM: 2049

J0735 Injection, clonidine hydrochloride, 1 mg
MCM: 2049

J0740 Injection, cidofovir, 375 mg
MCM: 2049

J0743 Injection, cilastatin sodium/imipenem, [Primaxin], per 250 mg
MCM: 2049

J0744 Injection, ciprofloxacin for intravenous infusion, 200 mg

J0745 Injection, codeine phosphate, per 30 mg
MCM: 2049

J0760 Injection, colchicine, per 1 mg
MCM: 2049

J0770 Injection, colistimethate sodium, [Coly-Mycin M], up to 150 mg
MCM: 2049

J0775 Injection, collagenase, clostridium histolyticum, 0.01 mg

J0780 Injection, prochlorperazine, [Compazine], up to 10 mg
MCM: 2049

J0795 Injection, corticorelin ovine triflutate, 1 microgram
MCM: 2049

J0800 Injection, corticotropin, up to 40 units
MCM: 2049

J0833 Injection, cosyntropin, not otherwise specified, 0.25 mg

J0834 Injection, cosyntropin (Cortrosyn), 0.25 mg

J0840 Injection, crotalidae polyvalent immune fab (ovine), up to 1 gram

J0850 Injection, cytomegalovirus immune globulin intravenous (human), per vial
MCM: 2049

J0878 Injection, daptomycin, 1 mg

J0881 Injection, darbepoetin alfa, 1 microgram (non-ESRD use)

J0882 Injection, darbepoetin alfa, 1 microgram (for ESRD on dialysis)
MCM: 4273.1

J0885 Injection, epoetin alfa, (for non-ESRD use), 1000 units

MCM: 2049

J0886 Injection, epoetin alfa, 1000 units (for ESRD on dialysis)
MCM: 4273.1

J0890 Injection, peginesatide, 0. 1 mg (for esrd on dialysis)

J0894 Injection, decitabine, 1 mg

J0895 Injection, deferoxamine mesylate, [Desferal] 500 mg
MCM: 2049

J0897 Injection, denosumab, 1 mg

J0900 Injection, testosterone enanthate and estradiol valerate, up to 1 cc
MCM: 2049

J0945 Injection, brompheniramine maleate, per 10 mg
MCM: 2049

J1000 Injection, depo-estradiol cypionate, up to 5 mg
MCM: 2049

J1020 Injection, methylprednisolone acetate; 20 mg
MCM: 2049

J1030 40 mg
MCM: 2049

J1040 80 mg
MCM: 2049

J1050 Injection, medroxyprogesterone acetate, 1 mg

(J1051) Code deleted December 31, 2012

(J1055) Code deleted December 31, 2012

(J1056) Code deleted December 31, 2012

J1060 Injection, testosterone cypionate and estradiol cypionate, up to 1 ml
MCM: 2049

J1070 Injection, testosterone cypionate, up to 100 mg
MCM: 2049

J1080 Injection, testosterone cypionate, 1 cc, 200 mg
MCM: 2049

J1094 Injection, dexamethasone acetate, 1 mg
MCM: 2049

J1100 Injection, dexamethasone sodium phosphate, 1mg
MCM: 2049

J1110 Injection, dihydroergotamine mesylate, per 1 mg
MCM: 2049

J1120 Injection, acetazolamide sodium, [Diamox Sodium], up to 500 mg
MCM: 2049

J1160 Injection, digoxin, up to 0.5 mg
MCM: 2049

J1162 Injection, digoxin immune fab (ovine), per vial
MCM: 2049

J1165 Injection, phenytoin sodium, [Dilantin], per 50 mg
MCM: 2049

J1170 Injection, hydromorphone, up to 4 mg
MCM: 2049

J1180 Injection, dyphylline, [Dilor, Lufyllin], up to 500 mg
MCM: 2049

J1190 Injection, dexrazoxane hydrochloride, per 250 mg
MCM: 2049

J1200 Injection, diphenhydramine HCl, [Benadryl], up to 50 mg
MCM: 2049

J1205 Injection, chlorothiazide sodium [Diuril], per 500 mg
MCM: 2049

J1212 Injection, DMSO, dimethyl sulfoxide, 50%, 50 ml
CIM: 45-23 MCM: 2049

J1230 Injection, methadone HCl, [Dolophine HCl], up to 10 mg
MCM: 2049

J1240 Injection, dimenhydrinate, [Dramamine], up to 50 mg
MCM: 2049

J1245 Injection, dipyridamole, per 10 mg
MCM: 15030, 2049

J1250 Injection, dobutamine hydrochloride, per 250 mg
MCM: 2049

J1260 Injection, dolasetron mesylate, 10 mg
MCM: 2049

J1265 Injection, dopamine hcl, 40 mg

J1267 Injection, doripenem, 10 mg

J1270 Injection, doxercalciferol, 1 mcg

J1290 Injection, ecallantide, 1 mg

J1300 Injection, eculizumab, 10 mg

J1320 Injection, amitriptyline HCl, [Elavil HCl], up to 20 mg
MCM: 2049

J1324 Injection, enfuvirtide, 1 mg

J1325 Injection, epoprostenol, 0.5 mg
MCM: 2049

J1327 Injection, eptifibatide, 5 mg
MCM: 2049

J1330 Injection, ergonovine maleate, up to 0.2 mg
MCM: 2049

J1335 Injection, ertapenem sodium, 500 mg

J1364 Injection, erythromycin lactobionate, per 500 mg
MCM: 2049

J1380 Injection, estradiol valerate, up to 10 mg
MCM: 2049

(J1390) Code deleted December 31, 2010

J1410 Injection, estrogen conjugated, per 25 mg
MCM: 2049

J1430 Injection, ethanolamine oleate, 100 mg
MCM: 2049

J1435 Injection, estrone, per 1 mg
MCM: 2049

J1436 Injection, etidronate disodium per 300 mg
MCM: 2049

Ⓟ **J1438** Injection, etanercept, 25 mg (code may be used for Medicare when drug administered under the direct supervision of a physician, not for use when drug is self administered)
MCM: 2049

(J1440) Code deleted December 31, 2013

(J1441) Code deleted December 31, 2013

● **J1442** Injection, filgrastim (G-CSF), 1 microgram

● **J1446** Injection, to-filgrastim, 5 micrograms

J1450 Injection, fluconazole, 200 mg
MCM: 2049.5

J1451 Injection, fomepizole, 15 mg
MCM: 2049

J1452 Injection, fomivirsen sodium, intraocular, 1.65 mg
MCM: 2049.3

J1453 Injection, fosaprepitant, 1 mg

J1455 Injection, foscarnet sodium, [Foscavir], per 1000 mg
MCM: 2049

J1457 Injection, gallium nitrate, 1 mg

J1458 Injection, galsulfase, 1 mg

J1459 Injection, immune globulin (privigen), intravenous, non-lyophilized (eg., liquid), 500 mg

J1460 Injection, gamma globulin; intramuscular 1 cc
MCM: 2049

● **J1556** Injection, immune globulin(bivigam), 500 mg

J1557 Injection, immune globulin, (gammaplex), intravenous, non-lyophilized (e.g. liquid), 500 mg

J1559 Injection, immune globulin (Hizentra), 100 mg

J1560 Injection, gamma globulin; intramuscular over 10 cc
MCM: 2049

J1561 Injection, immune globulin, (Gamunex/Gamunex-c/gammaked), non-lyophilized (e.g. liquid), 500 mg
MCM: 2049

J1562 Injection, immune globulin (Vivaglobin), 100 mg

J1566 Injection, immune globulin, intravenous, lyophilized (e.g. powder), not otherwise specified, 500 mg
MCM: 2049

J1568 Injection, immune globulin, (octagam), intravenous, non-lyophilized (e.g. liquid), 500 mg

J1569 Injection, immune globulin, (gammagard liquid), intravenous, non-lyophilized, (e.g. liquid), 500 mg
MCM: 2049

J1570 Injection, ganciclovir sodium, [Cytovene], 500 mg
MCM: 2049

J1571 Injection, hepatitis B immune globulin (hepagam b), intramuscular, 0.5 ml
MCM: 2049

J1572 Injection, immune globulin, (flebogamma/flebogamma dif), intravenous, non-lyophilized (e.g. liquid), 500 mg
MCM: 2049

J1573 Injection, hepatitis b immune globulin (hepagam b), intravenous, 0.5 ml

J1580 Injection, garamycin, gentamicin, up to 80 mg
MCM: 2049

J1590 Injection, gatifloxacin, 10 mg

J1595 Injection, glatiramer acetate, 20 mg
MCM: 2049

J1599 Injection, immune globulin, intravenous, non-lyophilized (e.g. liquid), not otherwise specified, 500 mg

Ⓟ **J1600** Injection, gold sodium thiomalate, up to 50 mg
MCM: 2049

● **J1602** Injection, golimumab, 1 mg, for intravenous use

J1610 Injection, glucagon hydrochloride, per 1 mg
MCM: 2049

J1620 Injection, gonadorelin hydrochloride, per 100 mcg
MCM: 2049

J1626 Injection, granisetron hydrochloride, 100 mcg
MCM: 2049

J1630 Injection, haloperidol, up to 5 mg
MCM: 2049

J1631 Injection, haloperidol decanoate, per 50 mg
MCM: 2049

J1640 Injection, hemin, 1 mg
MCM: 2049

J1642 Injection, heparin sodium, (heparin lock flush), per 10 units
MCM: 2049

J1644 Injection, heparin sodium, per 1,000 units
MCM: 2049

J1645 Injection, dalteparin sodium, per 2500 IU
MCM: 2049

J1650 Injection, enoxaparin sodium, 10 mg

J1652 Injection, fondaparinux sodium, 0.5 mg
MCM: 2049

J1655 Injection, tinzaparin sodium, 1000 IU

J1670 Injection, tetanus immune globulin, human, up to 250 units
MCM: 2049

J1675 Injection, histrelin acetate, 10 micrograms
MCM: 2049

(J1680) Code deleted December 31, 2012

J1700 Injection, hydrocortisone acetate, [Analpram HC, Hydrocortone Acetate], up to 25 mg
MCM: 2049

J1710 Injection, hydrocortisone sodium phosphate, [Hydrocortone Phosphate], up to 50 mg
MCM: 2049

J1720 Injection, hydrocortisone sodium succinate, [Solu-Cortef], up to 100 mg
MCM: 2049

J1725 Injection, hydroxyprogesterone caproate, 1 mg

J1730 Injection, diazoxide, [Hyperstat], up to 300 mg
MCM: 2049

J1740 Injection, ibandronate sodium, 1 mg

J1741 Injection, ibuprofen, 100 mg

J1742 Injection, ibutilide fumarate, 1 mg
MCM: 2049

J1743 Injection, idursulfase, 1 mg

J1744 Injection, icatibant, 1 mg

Ⓟ **J1745** Injection, infliximab, 10 mg
MCM: 2049

J1750 Injection, iron dextran, 50 mg
MCM: 2049.5

J1756 Injection, iron sucrose, 1 mg

J1786 Injection, imiglucerase, 10 units
MCM: 2049

J1790 Injection, droperidol, [Inapsine], up to 5 mg
MCM: 2049

J1800 Injection, propranolol HCl, [Inderal], up to 1 mg
MCM: 2049

J1810 Injection, droperidol and fentanyl citrate, [Innovar], up to 2 ml ampule
MCM: 2049

J1815 Injection, insulin, per 5 units
CIM: 60-14 MCM: 2049

J1817 Insulin for administration through DME (i.e., Insulin pump) per 50 units

J1826 Injection, interferon beta-1a, 30 mcg

J1830 Injection, interferon beta-1b, 0.25 mg (code may be used for Medicare when drug administered under the direct supervision of a physician, not for use when drug is self administered)
MCM: 2049

J1835 Injection, itraconazole, 50 mg

J1840 Injection, kanamycin sulfate, [Kantrex], up to 500 mg
MCM: 2049

J1850 Injection, kanamycin sulfate, [Kantrex Pediatric], up to 75 mg
MCM: 2049

J1885 Injection, ketorolac tromethamine, [Toradol IM], per 15 mg
MCM: 2049

J1890 Injection, cephalothin sodium, [Keflin], up to 1 gram
MCM: 2049

J1930 Injection, lanreotide, 1 mg

J1931 Injection, laronidase, 0.1 Mg

J1940 Injection, furosemide, [Lasix], up to 20 mg
MCM: 2049

J1945 Injection, lepirudin, 50 mg
MCM: 2049

J1950 Injection, leuprolide acetate (for depot suspension), per 3.75 mg
MCM: 2049

J1953 Injection, levetiracetam, 10 mg

J1955 Injection, levocarnitine, per 1 gram
MCM: 2049

J1956 Injection, levofloxacin, 250 mg
MCM: 2049

J1960 Injection, levorphanal tartrate, up to 2 mg
MCM: 2049

J1980 Injection, hyoscyamine sulfate, [Levsin], up to 0.25 mg
MCM: 2049

J1990 Injection, chlordiazepoxide HCl, [Librium], up to 100 mg

MCM: 2049

J2001 Injection, lidocaine HCl for intravenous infusion, 10 mg
MCM: 2049

J2010 Injection, lincomycin HCl, up to 300 mg
MCM: 2049

J2020 Injection, linezolid, 200 mg

J2060 Injection, lorazepam, [Ativan], 2 mg
MCM: 2049

J2150 Injection, mannitol, 25% in 50 ml
MCM: 2049

J2170 Injection, mecasermin, 1 mg

J2175 Injection, meperidine HCl, per 100 mg
MCM: 2049

J2180 Injection, meperidine and promethazine HCl, [Mepergan], up to 50 mg
MCM: 2049

J2185 Injection, meropenem, 100 mg

J2210 Injection, methylergonovine maleate, [Methergine Maleate], up to 0.2 mg
MCM: 2049

J2212 Injection, methylnaltrexone, 0.1 mg

J2248 Injection, micafungin sodium, 1 mg

J2250 Injection, midazolam hydrochloride, per 1 mg
MCM: 2049

J2260 Injection, milrinone lactate, 5 mg
MCM: 2049

J2265 Injection, minocycline hydrochloride, 1 mg

J2270 Injection, morphine sulfate, up to 10 mg
MCM: 2049

J2271 Injection, morphine sulfate, 100 mg
CIM: 60-14A MCM: 2049

J2275 Injection, morphine sulfate (preservative-free sterile solution), per 10 mg
CIM: 60-14B MCM: 2049

J2278 Injection, ziconotide, 1 microgram

J2280 Injection, moxifloxacin, 100 mg

J2300 Injection, nalbuphine HCl, per 10 mg
MCM: 2049

J2310 Injection, naloxone hydrochloride, per 1 mg
MCM: 2049

J2315 Injection, naltrexone, depot form, 1 mg

J2320 Injection, nandrolone deconoate; up to 50 mg
MCM: 2049

J2323 Injection, natalizumab, 1 mg

J2325 Injection, nesiritide, 0.1 mg
MCM: 2049

J2353 Injection, octreotide, depot form for intramuscular injection, 1 mg

J2354 Injection, octreotide, non-depot form for subcutaneous or intravenous injection, 25 mcg

J2355 Injection, oprelvekin, 5 mg
MCM: 2049

J2357 Injection, omalizumab, 5 mg

J2358 Injection, olanzapine, long-acting, 1 mg

J2360 Injection, orphenadrine citrate, [Norflex, Norgesic], up to 60 mg
MCM: 2049

J2370 Injection, phenylephrine HCl, [Neo-Synephrine], up to 1 ml
MCM: 2049

J2400 Injection, chloroprocaine HCl [Nesacaine and Nesacaine-MPF], per 30 ml
MCM: 2049

J2405 Injection, ondansetron hydrochloride, per 1 mg
MCM: 2049

J2410 Injection, oxymorphone HCl [Numorphan], up to 1 mg
MCM: 2049

J2425 Injection, palifermin, 50 micrograms

J2426 Injection, paliperidone palmitate extended release, 1 mg

J2430 Injection, pamidronate disodium, per 30 mg
MCM: 2049

J2440 Injection, papaverine HCl, up to 60 mg
MCM: 2049

J2460 Injection, oxytetracycline HCl, up to 50 mg
MCM: 2049

J2469 Injection, palonosetron hcl, 25 mcg

J2501 Injection, paricalcitol, 1 mcg
MCM: 2049

J2503 Injection, pegaptanib sodium, 0.3 mg

J2504 Injection, pegademase bovine, 25 iu
MCM: 2049

J2505 Injection, pegfilgrastim, 6 mg

J2507 Injection, pegloticase, 1 mg

J2510 Injection, penicillin G procaine, aqueous, up to 600,000 units
MCM: 2049

J2513 Injection, pentastarch, 10% solution, 100 ml
MCM: 2049

J2515 Injection, pentobarbital sodium, per 50 mg
MCM: 2049

J2540 Injection, penicillin G potassium, [Pfizerpen], up to 600,000 units
MCM: 2049

J2543 Injection, piperacillin sodium/tazobactam sodium, 1 gram/0.125 grams (1.125 grams)
MCM: 2049

J2545 Pentamidine isethionate, inhalation solution, FDA-approved final product, non-compounded, administered through DME, unit dose form, per 300 mg

J2550 Injection, promethazine HCl, [Phenergan], up to 50 mg
MCM: 2049

J2560 Injection, phenobarbital sodium, [Phenobarbital], up to 120 mg
MCM: 2049

J2562 Injection, plerixafor, 1 mg

J2590 Injection, oxytocin, [Pitocin], up to 10 units
MCM: 2049

J2597 Injection, desmopressin acetate, per 1 mcg
MCM: 2049

J2650 Injection, prednisolone acetate, up to 1 ml
MCM: 2049

J2670 Injection, tolazoline HCl, [Priscoline HCl], up to 25 mg
MCM: 2049

J2675 Injection, progesterone, per 50 mg
MCM: 2049

J2680 Injection, fluphenazine deconoate, [Prolixin Deconoate], up to 25 mg
MCM: 2049

J2690 Injection, procainamide HCl, [Proenstyl], up to 1 gram
MCM: 2049

J2700 Injection, oxacillin sodium, [Prostaphlin], up to 250 mg
MCM: 2049

J2710 Injection, neostigmine methylsulfate, [Prostigmin Methylsulfate], up to 0.5 mg
MCM: 2049

J2720 Injection, protamine sulfate, per 10 mg
MCM: 2049

J2724 Injection, protein C concentrate, intravenous, human, 10 IU

J2725 Injection, protirelin, per 250 mcg
MCM: 2049

J2730 Injection, pralidoxime chloride, [Protopam Chloride], up to 1 gram
MCM: 2049

J2760 Injection, phentolamine mesylate, [Regitine], up to 5 mg
MCM: 2049

J2765 Injection, metoclopramide HCl [Reglan], up to 10 mg
MCM: 2049

J2770 Injection, quinupristin/dalfopristin, 500 mg (150/350)
MCM: 2049

J2778 Injection, ranibizumab, 0.1 mg

J2780 Injection, ranitidine hydrochloride, 25 mg
MCM: 2049

J2783 Injection, rasburicase, 0.5 mg

J2785 Injection, regadenoson, 0.1 mg

J2788 Injection, RHo(D) immune globulin, human, minidose, 50 mcg (250 IU)
MCM: 2049

J2790 Injection, RHo(D) immune globulin, human, full dose, 300 mcg (1500 IU)
MCM: 2049

J2791 Injection, RHo(D) immune globulin (human), (rhophylac), intramuscular or intravenous, 100 IU
MCM: 2049

J2792 Injection, RHo(D) immune globulin, intravenous, human, solvent detergent, 100 IU
MCM: 2049

J2793 Injection, rilonacept, 1 mg
MCM: 2049

J2794 Injection, risperidone, long acting, 0.5 Mg

J2795 Injection, ropivacaine hydrochloride, 1 mg

J2796 Injection, romiplostim, 10 micrograms

J2800 Injection, methocarbamol, [Robaxin], up to 10 ml
MCM: 2049

J2805 Injection, sincalide, 5 micrograms

J2810 Injection, theophylline, per 40 mg
MCM: 2049

J2820 Injection, sargramostim (GM-CSF), 50 mcg
MCM: 2049

J2850 Injection, secretin, synthetic, human, 1 microgram
MCM: 2049

J2910 Injection, aurothioglucose, [Solganal], up to 50 mg
MCM: 2049

J2916 Injection, sodium ferric gluconate complex in sucrose injection, 12.5 mg
MCM: 2049.2, 2049.4

J2920 Injection, methylprednisolone sodium succinate, [Solu-Medrol], up to 40 mg
MCM: 2049

J2930 Injection, methylprednisolone sodium succinate, [Solu-Medrol], up to 125 mg
MCM: 2049

J2940 Injection, somatrem, 1 mg
MCM: 2049

J2941 Injection, somatropin, 1 mg
MCM: 2049

J2950 Injection, promazine HCl, [Prozine, Sparine], up to 25 mg
MCM: 2049

J2993 Injection, reteplase, 18.1 mg
MCM: 2049

J2995 Injection, streptokinase, per 250,000 IU
MCM: 2049

J2997 Injection, alteplase recombinant, 1 mg
MCM: 2049

J3000 Injection, streptomycin, up to 1 gram
MCM: 2049

J3010 Injection, fentanyl citrate, 0.1 mg
MCM: 2049

J3030 Injection, sumatriptan succinate, 6 mg (code may be used for Medicare when drug administered under the direct supervision of a physician, not for use when drug is self administered)
MCM: 2049

● **J3060** Injection, taliglucerase alfa, 10 units

J3070 Injection, pentazocine, 30 mg
MCM: 2049

J3095 Injection, televancin, 10 mg

J3101 Injection, tenecteplase, 1 mg

J3105 Injection, terbutaline sulfate, up to 1 mg
MCM: 2049

J3110 Injection, teriparatide, 10 mcg

J3120 Injection, testosterone enanthate; up to 100 mg
MCM: 2049

J3130 up to 200 mg
MCM: 2049

J3140 Injection, testosterone suspension, up to 50 mg
MCM: 2049

J3150 Injection, testosterone propionate, up to 100 mg
MCM: 2049

J3230 Injection, chlorpromazine HCl, [Thorazine], up to 50 mg
MCM: 2049

J3240 Injection, thyrotropin alpha, 0.9 mg, provided in 1.1 mg vial
MCM: 2049

J3243 Injection, tigecycline, 1 mg

J3246 Injection, tirofiban HCl, 0.25 Mg

J3250 Injection, trimethobenzamide HCl, up to 200 mg
MCM: 2049

J3260 Injection, tobramycin sulfate, [Nebcin], up to 80 mg
MCM: 2049

Ⓟ **J3262** Injection, tocilizumab, 1 mg

J3265 Injection, torsemide, 10 mg/ml
MCM: 2049

J3280 Injection, thiethylperazine maleate, up to 10 mg
MCM: 2049

J3285 Injection, treprostinil, 1 mg

J3300 Injection, triamcinolone acetonide, preservative free, 1 mg

J3301 Injection, triamcinolone acetonide, not otherwise specified, 10 mg
MCM: 2049

J3302 Injection, triamcinolone diacetate, [Aristocort], per 5 mg
MCM: 2049

J3303 Injection, triamcinolone hexacetonide, [Aristospan], per 5 mg
MCM: 2049

J3305 Injection, trimetrexate glucoronate, per 25 mg
MCM: 2049

J3310 Injection, perphenazine, [Trilafon], up to 5 mg
MCM: 2049

J3315 Injection, triptorelin pamoate, 3.75 mg
MCM: 2049

J3320 Injection, spectinomycin hydrochloride, [Trobicin], up to 2 gram
MCM: 2049

J3350 Injection, urea, [Ureaphil], up to 40 grams
MCM: 2049

J3355 Injection, urofollitropin, 75 iu
MCM: 2049

J3357 Injection, ustekinumab, 1 mg

J3360 Injection, diazepam, [Valium], up to 5 mg
MCM: 2049

J3364 Injection, urokinase, 5000 IU vial
MCM: 2049

J3365 Injection, IV, urokinase, 250,000 IU vial
MCM: 2049

J3370 Injection, vancomycin HCl, 500 mg
CIM: 60-14 MCM: 2049

J3385 Injection, velaglucerase alfa, 100 units

J3396 Injection, verteporfin, 0.1 Mg
MCM: 35-100, 45-30

J3400 Injection, triflupromazine HCl, [Vesprin], up to 20 mg
MCM: 2049

J3410 Injection, hydroxyzine HCl, [Vistaril], up to 25 mg
MCM: 2049

J3411 Injection, thiamine HCl, 100 mg

J3415 Injection, pyridoxine HCl, 100 mg

J3420 Injection, vitamin B-12 cyanocobalamin, up to 1000 mcg
CIM: 45-4 MCM: 2049

J3430 Injection, phytonadione (vitamin K), per 1 mg
MCM: 2049

J3465 Injection, voriconazole, 10 mg
MCM: 2049

J3470 Injection, hyaluronidase, [Wydase], up to 150 units
MCM: 2049

J3471 Injection, hyaluronidase, ovine, preservative free, per 1 usp unit (up to 999 USP units)

J3472 Injection, hyaluronidase, ovine, preservative free, per 1000 usp units

J3473 Injection, hyaluronidase, recombinant, 1 USP unit
MCM: 2049

J3475 Injection, magnesium sulfate, per 500 mg
MCM: 2049

J3480 Injection, potassium chloride, per 2 mEq
MCM: 2049

J3485 Injection, zidovudine, 10 mg
MCM: 2049

J3486 Injection, ziprasidone mesylate, 10 mg

(J3487) Code deleted December 31, 2013

(J3488) Code deleted December 31, 2013

● **J3489** Injection, zoledronic acid, 1 mg

J3490 Unclassified drugs
MCM: 2049

J3520 Edetate disodium, per 150 mg
CIM: 35-64, 45-20

J3530 Nasal vaccine inhalation
MCM: 2049

J3535 Drug administered through a metered dose inhaler
MCM: 2050.5

J3570 Laetrile, amygdalin, vitamin B17
CIM: 45-10

J3590 Unclassified biologics

MISCELLANEOUS DRUGS AND SOLUTIONS

J7030 Infusion, normal saline solution, 1000 cc
MCM: 2049

J7040 Infusion, normal saline solution, sterile (500 ml = 1 unit)
MCM: 2049

J7042 5% dextrose/normal saline solution (500 ml = 1 unit)
MCM: 2049

J7050 Infusion, normal saline solution, 250 cc
MCM: 2049

J7060 5% dextrose/water (500 ml = 1 unit)
MCM: 2049

J7070 Infusion, D5W, 1000 cc
MCM: 2049

J7100 Infusion, dextran 40, 500 ml
MCM: 2049

J7110 Infusion, dextran 75, 500 ml
MCM: 2049

J7120 Ringers lactate infusion, up to 1000 cc

MCM: 2049

(J7130) Code deleted December 31, 2011. See J7131

J7131 Hypertonic saline solution, 1 ml
MCM: 2049

J7178 Injection, human fibrinogen concentrate, 1 mg

J7180 Injection, factor XIII (antihemophilic factor, human), 1 IU

J7183 Injection, von Willebrand factor complex (human), wilate, 1 IU vwf:rco
MCM: 2049

(J7184) Code deleted December 31, 2011

J7185 Injection, Factor VIII (antihemophilic factor, recombinant) (Xyntha), per IU

J7186 Injection, antihemophilic factor VIII/von Willebrand factor complex (human), per factor VIII IU
MCM: 2049

J7187 Injection, von willebrand factor complex (Humate-p), per IU VWF:RCO
MCM: 2049

J7189 Factor VIIA (antihemophilic factor, recombinant), per 1 microgram
MCM: 2049

J7190 Factor VIII (antihemophilic factor, human), per IU
MCM: 2049

J7191 Factor VIII (antihemophilic factor (porcine)), per IU
MCM: 2049

J7192 Factor VIII (antihemophilic factor, recombinant), per IU, not otherwise specified
MCM: 2049

J7193 Factor IX (antihemophilic factor, purified, non-recombinant) per IU
MCM: 2049

J7194 Factor IX, complex, per IU
MCM: 2049

J7195 Factor IX (antihemophilic factor, recombinant) per IU

MCM: 2049

J7196 Injection, antithrombin recombinant, 50 IU

J7197 Antithrombin III (human), per IU
MCM: 2049

J7198 Anti-inhibitor, per IU
CIM: 45-24 MCM: 2049

J7199 Hemophilia clotting factor, not otherwise classified
CIM: 45-24 MCM: 2049

J7300 Intrauterine copper contraceptive

● **J7301** Levonorgestrel-releasing intrauterine contraceptive system (Skylark), 13.5 mg

J7302 Levonorgestrel-releasing intrauterine contraceptive system, 52 mg

J7303 Contraceptive supply, hormone containing vaginal ring, each

J7304 Contraceptive supply, hormone containing patch, each

J7306 Levonorgestrel (contraceptive) implant system, including implants and supplies

J7307 Etonogestrel (contraceptive) implant system, including implant and supplies

J7308 Aminolevulinic acid HCL for topical administration, 20%, single unit dosage form (354 mg)

J7309 Methyl aminolevulinate (mal) for topical administration, 16.8%, 1 gram

J7310 Ganciclovir, 4.5 mg, long-acting implant
MCM: 2049

J7311 Fluocinolone acetonide, intravitreal implant

J7312 Injection, dexamethasone, intravitreal implant, 0.1 mg

J7315 Mitomycin, opthalmic, 0.2 mg

● **J7316** Injection, Ocriplasmin, 0.125 mg

Not valid for Medicare | Non-covered by Medicare | Special coverage instructions | Carrier discretion

J7321 Hyaluronan or derivative, Hyalgan or Supartz, for intra-articular injection, per dose

J7323 Hyaluronan or derivative, Euflexxa, for intra-articular injection, per dose

J7324 Hyaluronan or derivative, Orthovisc, for intra-articular injection, per dose

J7325 Hyaluronan or derivative, Synvisc or Synvisc-One, for intra-articular injection, 1 mg

J7326 Hyaluronan or derivative, gel-one, for intra-articular injection, per dose

J7330 Autologous cultured chondrocytes, implant

J7335 Capsaicin 8% patch, per 10 square centimeters

IMMUNOSUPPRESSIVE DRUGS (INCLUDES NON-INJECTIBLES)

J7500 Azathioprine, oral, 50 mg
MCM: 2049.5

J7501 Azathioprine, parenteral, 100 mg
MCM: 2049

Ⓟ **J7502** Cyclosporine, oral, 100 mg
MCM: 2049.5

J7504 Lymphocyte immune globulin, antithymocyte globulin, equine, parenteral, 250 mg
CIM: 45-22 MCM: 2049

J7505 muromonab-CD3, parenteral, 5 mg
MCM: 2049

J7506 Prednisone, oral, per 5 mg
MCM: 2049.5

▲ **J7507** Tacrolimus, immediate release, oral; 1 mg
MCM: 2049.5

● **J7508** Tacrolimus, extended release, oral, 0.1 mg
MCM:: 2049.5

J7509 Methylprednisolone, oral, per 4 mg
MCM: 2049.5

J7510 Prednisolone, oral, per 5 mg
MCM: 2049.5

J7511 Lymphocyte immune globulin, antithymocyte globulin, rabbit, parenteral, 25 mg

J7513 Daclizumab, parenteral, 25 mg
MCM: 2049.5

Ⓟ **J7515** Cyclosporine, oral, 25 mg

Ⓟ **J7516** Cyclosporine, parenteral, 250 mg

Ⓟ **J7517** Mycophenolate mofetil, oral, 250 mg

Ⓟ **J7518** Mycophenolic acid, oral, 180 mg
MCM: 2050.5, 4471, 5249

J7520 Sirolimus, oral, 1 mg
MCM: 2049.5

J7525 Tacrolimus, parenteral, 5 mg
MCM: 2049.5

J7527 Everolimus, oral, 0. 25 mg

J7599 Immunosuppressive drug, not otherwise classified
MCM: 2049.5

J7604 Acetylcysteine, inhalation solution, compounded product, administered through DME, unit dose form, per gram

J7605 Arformoterol, inhalation solution, FDA approved final product, non-compounded, administered through DME, unit dose form, 15 micrograms

J7606 Formoterol fumarate, inhalation solution, FDA approved final product, non-compounded, administered through DME, unit dose form, 20 micrograms

J7607 Levalbuterol, inhalation solution, compounded product, administered through DME, concentrated form 0.5 mg

J7608 Acetylcysteine, inhalation solution, FDA-approved final product, non-compounded, administered through DME, unit dose form, per gram

J7609 Albuterol, inhalation solution, compounded product, administered through DME, unit dose, 1 mg

J7610 Albuterol, inhalation solution, compounded product, administered through DME, concentrated form, 1 mg

J7611 Albuterol, inhalation solution, FDA-approved final product, non-compounded, administered through DME, concentrated form, 1 mg
MCM: 2100.5

J7612 Levalbuterol, inhalation solution, FDA-approved final product, non-compounded, administered through DME, concentrated form, 0.5 mg
MCM: 2100.5

J7613 Albuterol, inhalation solution, FDA-approved final product, non-compounded, administered through DME, unit dose, 1 mg
MCM: 2100.5

J7614 Levalbuterol, inhalation solution, FDA-approved final product, non-compounded, administered through DME, unit dose, 0.5 mg
MCM: 2100.5

J7615 Levalbuterol, inhalation solution, compounded product, administered through DME, unit dose, 0.5 Mg

J7620 Albuterol, up to 2.5 mg and ipratropium bromide, up to 0.5 mg, FDA-approved final product, non-compounded administered through DME
MCM: 2100.5

J7622 Beclomethasone, inhalation solution, compounded product, administered through DME, unit dose form, per milligram

J7624 Betamethasone, inhalation solution, compounded product, administered through DME, unit dose form, per milligram

J7626 Budesonide inhalation solution, FDA-approved final product, non-compounded, administered through DME, unit dose form, up to 0.5 mg

J7627 Budesonide, inhalation solution, compounded product, administered through DME, unit dose form, up to 0.5 mg

J7628 Bitolterol mesylate, inhalation solution, compounded product, administered through DME, concentrated form, per mg

J7629 Bitolterol mesylate, inhalation solution, compounded product, administered through DME, unit dose form, per mg

J7631 Cromolyn sodium, inhalation solution, FDA-approved final product, non-compounded, administered through DME, unit dose form, per 10 milligrams
MCM: 2100.5

J7632 Cromolyn sodium, inhalation solution, compounded product, administered through DME, unit dose form, per 10 milligrams

J7633 Budesonide, inhalation solution, FDA-approved final product, non-compounded, administered through DME, concentrated form, per 0.25 mg

J7634 Budesonide, inhalation solution, compounded product, administered through DME, concentrated form, per 0.25 mg

J7635 Atropine, inhalation solution, compounded product, administered through DME, concentrated form, per mg

J7636 Atropine, inhalation solution, compounded product, administered through DME, unit dose form, per mg

J7637 Dexamethasone, inhalation solution, compounded product, administered through DME, concentrated form, per mg

J7638 Dexamethasone, inhalation solution, compounded product, administered through DME, unit dose form, per mg

J7639 Dornase alfa, inhalation solution, FDA-approved final product, non-compounded, administered through DME, unit dose form, per milligram

J7640 Formoterol, inhalation solution, compounded product, administered through DME, unit dose form, 12 micrograms

J7641 Flunisolide, inhalation solution, compounded product, administered through DME, unit dose, per milligram

J7642 Glycopyrrolate, inhalation solution, compounded product, administered through DME, concentrated form, per mg

J7643 Glycopyrrolate, inhalation solution, compounded product, administered through DME, unit dose form, per mg

J7644 Ipratropium bromide, inhalation solution, FDA-approved final product, non-compounded, administered through DME, unit dose form, per mg

J7645 Ipratropium bromide, inhalation solution, compounded product, administered through DME, unit dose form, per mg

J7647 Isoetharine HCl, inhalation solution, compounded product, administered through DME, concentrated form, per mg

J7648 Isoetharine HCl, inhalation solution, FDA-approved final product, non-compounded, administered through DME, concentrated form, per mg

J7649 Isoetharine HCl, inhalation solution, FDA-approved final product, non-compounded, administered through DME, unit dose form, per mg

J7650 Isoetharine HCl, inhalation solution, compounded product, administered through DME, unit dose form, per mg

J7657 Isoproterenol HCl, inhalation solution, compounded product, administered through DME, concentrated form, per mg

J7658 Isoproterenol HCl, inhalation solution, FDA-approved final product, non-compounded, administered through DME, concentrated form, per mg

J7659 Isoproterenol HCl, inhalation solution, FDA-approved final product, non-compounded, administered through DME, unit dose form, per mg

J7660 Isoproterenol HCl, inhalation solution, compounded product, administered through DME, unit dose form, per mg

J7665 Mannitol, administered through an inhaler, 5 mg

J7667 Metaproterenol sulfate, inhalation solution, compounded product, concentrated form, per 10 mg

J7668 Metaproterenol sulfate, inhalation solution, FDA-approved final product, non-compounded, administered through DME, concentrated form, per 10 mg

J7669 Metaproterenol sulfate, inhalation solution, compounded product, administered through DME, unit dose form, per 10 mg

J7670 Metaproterenol sulfate, inhalation solution, FDA-approved final product, non-compounded, administered through DME, unit dose form, per 10 mg

J7674 Methacholine chloride administered as inhalation solution through a nebulizer, per 1 mg

J7676 Pentamidine isethionate, inhalation solution, compounded product, administered through DME, unit dose form, per 300 mg

J7680 Terbutaline sulfate, inhalation solution, compounded product, administered through DME, concentrated form, per mg

J7681 Terbutaline sulfate, inhalation solution, compounded product, administered through DME, unit dose form, per mg

J7682 Tobramycin, inhalation solution, FDA-approved final product, non-compounded, unit dose form, administered through DME, per 300 mg

J7683 Triamcinolone, inhalation solution, compounded product, administered through DME, concentrated form, per mg

J7684 Triamcinolone, inhalation solution, compounded product, administered through DME, unit dose form, per mg

J7685 Tobramycin, inhalation solution, compounded product, administered through DME, unit dose form, per 300 mg

J7686 Treprostinil, inhalation solution, FDA-approved final product, non-compounded, administered through DME, unit dose form, 1.74 mg

J7699 NOC drugs, inhalation solution administered through DME

J7799 NOC drugs, other than inhalation drugs, administered through DME
MCM: 2100.5

J8498 Antiemetic drug, rectal/suppository, not otherwise specified

J8499 Prescription drug, oral, non-chemotherapeutic, NOS
MCM: 2049

J8501 Aprepitant, oral, 5 mg

J8510 Busulfan, oral, 2 mg
MCM: 2049.5

J8515 Cabergoline, oral, 0.25 mg
MCM: 2049.5

J8520 Capecitabine, oral, 150 mg
MCM: 2049.5

J8521 Capecitabine, oral, 500 mg
MCM: 2049.5

J8530 Cyclophosphamide, oral, 25 mg
MCM: 2049.5

J8540 Dexamethasone, oral, 0.25 mg

J8560 Etoposide, oral, 50 mg
MCM: 2049.5

(J8561) Code deleted December 31, 2012

J8562 Fludarabine phosphate, oral, 10 mg

J8565 Gefitinib, oral, 250 mg

J8597 Antiemetic drug, oral, not otherwise specified

J8600 Melphalan, oral, 2 mg
MCM: 2049.5

J8610 Methotrexate, oral, 2.5 mg
MCM: 2049.5

J8650 Nabilone, oral, 1 mg

J8700 Temozolmide, oral, 5 mg
MCM: 2049.5C

J8705 Topotecan, oral, 0.25 mg

J8999 Prescription drug, oral, chemotherapeutic, NOS
MCM: 2049.5

This page intentionally left blank

CHEMOTHERAPY DRUGS

Guidelines

In addition to the information presented in the INTRODUCTION, several other items unique to this section are defined or identified here:

1. EXCEPTION: Oral immunosuppressive drugs are not included in this section.

2. ROUTE OF ADMINISTRATION: Unless otherwise specified, the drugs listed in this section may be injected either subcutaneously, intramuscularly or intravenously.

3. DRUG COST ONLY: The codes listed in this section include the cost of the chemotherapy drug only and do not include the administration of the drug.

4. SUBSECTION INFORMATION: Some of the listed subheadings or subsections have special needs or instructions unique to that section. Where these are indicated, special "notes" will be presented preceding or following the listings. Those subsections within the CHEMOTHERAPY DRUGS section that have "notes" are as follows:

Subsection	Code Numbers
Chemotherapy drugs	J9000-J9999

5. UNLISTED SERVICE OR PROCEDURE: A service or procedure may be provided that is not listed in this edition of HCPCS. When reporting such a service, the appropriate "unlisted procedure" code may be used to indicate the service, identifying it by "special report" as defined below. HCPCS terminology is inconsistent in defining unlisted procedures. The procedure definition may include the term(s) "unlisted", "not otherwise classified", "unspecified", "unclassified", "other" and "miscellaneous". Prior to using these codes, try to determine if a Local Level III code or CPT code is available. The "unlisted procedures" and accompanying codes for CHEMOTHERAPY DRUGS are as follows:

J9999	Not otherwise classified, antineoplastic drugs

6. SPECIAL REPORT: A service, material or supply that is rarely provided, unusual, variable or new may require a special report in determining medical appropriateness for reimbursement purposes. Pertinent information should include an adequate definition or description of the nature, extent, and need for the service, material or supply.

7. MODIFIERS: Listed services may be modified under certain circumstances. When appropriate, the modifying circumstance is identified by adding a modifier to the basic procedure code. CPT and HCPCS National Level II modifiers may be used with CPT and HCPCS National Level II procedure codes. Modifiers commonly used with CHEMOTHERAPY DRUGS are as follows:

   -CC Procedure code change (used when the procedure code submitted was changed either for administrative reasons or because an incorrect code was filed)

   -TC Technical component. Under certain circumstances, a charge may be made for the technical component alone. Under these circumstances, the technical component charge is identified by adding the modifier -TC to the usual procedure code. Technical component charges are institutional charges and are not billed separately by physicians. Portable x-ray suppliers bill only for the technical component however, and should use modifier -TC.

8. CPT CODE CROSS-REFERENCE: Unless otherwise specified, the equivalent CPT code for all listings in this section is 96545.

Chemotherapy Drugs

J9000 Injection, doxorubicin hydrochloride, 10 mg
MCM: 2049

(J9001) Code deleted December 31, 2012

(J9002) Code deleted December 31, 2013

J9010 Injection, alemtuzumab, 10 mg

J9015 Injection, aldesleukin, per single use vial
MCM: 2049

J9017 Injection, arsenic trioxide, 1 mg

J9019 Injection, asparaginase (erwinaze), 1,000 IU
MCM: 2049

J9020 Injection, asparaginase, 10,000 units
MCM: 2049

J9025 Injection, azacitidine, 1 mg

J9027 Injection, clofarabine, 1 mg

J9031 BCG (intravesical), per installation
MCM: 2049

J9033 Injection, bendamustine HCl, 1 mg

J9035 Injection, bevacizumab, 10 mg

J9040 Injection, bleomycin sulfate, 15 units
MCM: 2049

J9041 Injection, bortezomib, 0.1 Mg

J9042 Injection, brentuximab vedotin, 1 mg

J9043 Injection, cabazitaxel, 1 mg

J9045 Injection, carboplatin, 50 mg
MCM: 2049

● **J9047** Injection, carfilzomib, 1 mg

J9050 Injection, carmustine, 100 mg
MCM: 2049

J9055 Injection, cetuximab, 10 mg

J9060 Injection, cisplatin, powder or solution, 10 mg
MCM: 2049

J9065 Injection, cladribine, per 1 mg
MCM: 2049

J9070 Cyclophosphamide, 100 mg
MCM: 2049

J9098 Injection, cytarabine liposome, 10 mg

J9100 Injection, cytarabine, 100 mg
MCM: 2049

J9120 Injection, dactinomycin, 0.5 mg
MCM: 2049

J9130 Dacarbazine, 100 mg
MCM: 2049

J9150 Injection, daunorubicin, 10 mg
MCM: 2049

J9151 Injection, daunorubicin citrate, liposomal formulation, 10 mg
MCM: 2049

J9155 Injection, degarelix, 1 mg

J9160 Injection, denileukin diftitox, 300 mcg

J9165 Injection, diethylstilbestrol diphosphate, 250 mg
MCM: 2049

J9171 Injection, docetaxel, 1 mg
MCM: 2049

J9175 Injection, Elliott's' b solution, 1 ml
MCM: 2049

J9178 Injection, epirubicin HCl, 2 mg

J9179 Injection, eribulin mesylate, 0.1 mg

J9181 Injection, etoposide, 10 mg
MCM: 2049

J9185 Injection, fludarabine phosphate, 50 mg
MCM: 2049

J9190 Injection, fluorouracil, 500 mg
MCM: 2049

J9200 Injection, floxuridine, 500 mg
MCM: 2049

J9201 Injection, gemcitabine HCl, 200 mg
MCM: 2049

J9202 Goserelin acetate implant, per 3.6 mg
MCM: 2049

J9206 Injection, irinotecan, 20 mg
MCM: 2049

J9207 Injection, ixabepilone, 1 mg

J9208 Injection, ifosfomide, 1 gram

MCM: 2049

J9209 Injection, mesna, 200 mg
MCM: 2049

J9211 Injection, idarubicin hydrochloride, 5 mg
MCM: 2049

J9212 Injection, interferon alfacon-1, recombinant, 1 mcg
MCM: 2049

J9213 Injection, interferon, alfa-2A, recombinant, 3 million units
MCM: 2049

J9214 Injection, interferon, alfa-2B, recombinant, 1 million units
MCM: 2049

J9215 Injection, interferon, alfa-N3, (human leukocyte derived), 250,000 IU
MCM: 2049

J9216 Injection, interferon, gamma 1-B, 3 million units
MCM: 2049

J9217 Leuprolide acetate, [Lupron Depot], (for depot suspension), 7.5 mg
MCM: 2049

J9218 Leuprolide acetate, [Lupron], per 1 mg
MCM: 2049

J9219 Leuprolide acetate implant, 65 mg
MCM: 2049

J9225 Histrelin implant (Vantas), 50 mg
MCM: 2049

J9226 Histrelin implant (Supprelin lA), 50 mg
MCM: 2049

J9228 Injection, ipilimumab, 1 mg

J9230 Injection, mechlorethamine HCl, (nitrogen mustard), 10 mg
MCM: 2049

J9245 Injection, melphalan HCl, 50 mg
MCM: 2049

Ⓟ **J9250** Methotrexate sodium; 5 mg
MCM: 2049

Ⓟ **J9260** 50 mg
MCM: 2049

J9261 Injection, nelarabine, 50 mg

● **J9262** Injection, omacetaxine mepesuccinate, 0.01 mg

J9263 Injection, oxaliplatin, 0.5 mg

J9264 Injection, paclitaxel protein-bound particles, 1 mg

J9265 Injection, paclitaxel, 30 mg
MCM: 2049

J9266 Injection, pegaspargase, per single dose vial
MCM: 2049

J9268 Injection, pentostatin, 10 mg
MCM: 2049

J9270 Injection, plicamycin, 2.5 mg
MCM: 2049

J9280 Mitomycin; 5 mg
MCM: 2049

J9293 Injection, mitoxantrone HCl, per 5 mg
MCM: 2049

J9300 Injection, gemtuzumab ozogamicin, 5 mg

J9302 Injection, ofatumumab, 10 mg

J9303 Injection, panitumumab, 10 mg

J9305 Injection, pemetrexed, 10 mg

● **J9306** Injection, pertuzumab, 1 mg

J9307 Injection, pralatrexate, 1 mg

Ⓟ **J9310** Injection, rituximab, 100 mg
MCM: 2049

J9315 Injection, romidepsin, 1 mg

J9320 Injection, streptozocin, 1 gram
MCM: 2049

J9328 Injection, temozolomide, 1 mg

J9330 Injection, temsirolimus, 1 mg

J9340 Injection, thiotepa, 15 mg
MCM: 2049

J9351 Injection, topotecan, 0.1 mg

● **J9354** Injection, ado-trastuzumab emtansine, 1 mg

J9355 Injection, trastuzumab, 10 mg

J9357 Injection, valrubicin, intravesical, 200 mg
MCM: 2049

J9360 Injection, vinblastine sulfate, 1 mg
MCM: 2049

J9370 Vincristine sulfate; 1 mg
MCM: 2049

● **J9371** Injection, vincristine sulfate liposome, 1 mg

J9390 Injection, vinorelbine tartrate, 10 mg
MCM: 2049

J9395 Injection, fulvestrant, 25 mg

● **J9400** Injection, Ziv-aflibercept, 1 mg

J9600 Injection, porfimer sodium, 75 mg
MCM: 2049

J9999 Not otherwise classified, antineoplastic drugs
CIM: 45-16 MCM: 2049

This page intentionally left blank

K CODES: FOR DME-MACs USE ONLY

Guidelines

In addition to the information presented in the INTRODUCTION, several other items unique to this section are defined or identified here:

1. EXCLUSIVE USE BY DME-MACs: The codes listed in this section are assigned by CMS on a temporary basis and are for the exclusive use of the Durable Medical Equipment Medicare Administrative Contractors (DME-MACs). These codes are not to be used by providers for reporting purposes unless specifically instructed to do so by the local carrier.

2. UNLISTED SERVICE OR PROCEDURE: A service or procedure may be provided that is not listed in this edition of HCPCS. When reporting such a service, the appropriate "unlisted procedure" code may be used to indicate the service, identifying it by "special report" as defined below. HCPCS terminology is inconsistent in defining unlisted procedures. The procedure definition may include the term(s) "unlisted", "not otherwise classified", "unspecified", "unclassified", "other" and "miscellaneous". Prior to using these codes, try to determine if a Local Level III code or CPT code is available.

3. SPECIAL REPORT: A service, material or supply that is rarely provided, unusual, variable or new may require a special report in determining medical appropriateness for reimbursement purposes. Pertinent information should include an adequate definition or description of the nature, extent, and need for the service, material or supply.

4. CPT CODE CROSS-REFERENCE: Unless otherwise specified, the equivalent CPT code for all listings in this section is 99070.

Temporary Codes for DMERCS

WHEELCHAIRS

K0001 Standard wheelchair

K0002 Standard hemi (low seat) wheelchair

K0003 Lightweight wheelchair

K0004 High strength, lightweight wheelchair

K0005 Ultralightweight wheelchair

K0006 Heavy duty wheelchair

K0007 Extra heavy duty wheelchair

● **K0008** Custom manual wheelchair/base

K0009 Other manual wheelchair/base

K0010 Standard - weight frame motorized/power wheelchair

K0011 Standard - weight frame motorized/power wheelchair with programmable control parameters for speed adjustment, tremor dampening, acceleration control and braking

K0012 Lightweight portable motorized/power wheelchair

● **K0013** Custom motorized/power wheelchair/base

K0014 Other motorized/power wheelchair base

K0015 Detachable, non-adjustable height armrest, each

K0017 Detachable, adjustable height armrest; base, each

K0018 upper portion each

K0019 Arm pad, each

K0020 Fixed, adjustable height armrest, pair

K0037 High mount flip-up foot rest, each

K0038 Leg strap, each

K0039 Leg strap, H style, each

K0040 Adjustable angle footplate, each

K0041 Large size footplate, each

K0042 Standard size footplate, each

K0043 Foot rest, lower extension tube, each

K0044 Foot rest, upper hanger bracket, each

K0045 Foot rest, complete assembly

K0046 Elevating leg rest; lower extension tube, each

K0047 upper hanger bracket, each

K0050 Ratchet assembly

K0051 Cam release assembly, foot rest or leg rest, each

K0052 Swingaway, detachable foot rests, each

K0053 Elevating foot rests, articulating (telescoping), each

K0056 Seat height less than 17" or equal to or greater than 21" for a high strength, lightweight, or ultralightweight wheelchair

K0065 Spoke protectors, each

K0069 Rear wheel assembly, complete; with solid tire, spokes or molded, each

K0070 with pneumatic tire, spokes or molded, each

K0071 Front caster assembly, complete; with pneumatic tire, each

K0072 with semi-pneumatic tire, each

K0073 Caster pin lock, each

K0077 Front caster assembly, complete, with solid tire, each

K0098 Drive belt for power wheelchair

K0105 IV hanger, each

K0108 Wheelchair component or accessory, not otherwise specified

TRACHEOSTOMY CARE SUPPLIES

K0195 Elevating leg rests, pair (for use with capped rental wheelchair base)
CIM: 60-9

K0455 Infusion pump used for uninterrupted parenteral administration of medication, (eg., epoprostenol or treprostinol)
CIM: 60-14

K0462 Temporary replacement for patient owned equipment being repaired, any type
MCM: 5102.3

K0552 Supplies for external drug infusion pump, syringe type cartridge, sterile, each
CIM: 60-14

K0601 Replacement battery for external infusion pump owned by patient, silver oxide, 1.5 volt, each

K0602 Replacement battery for external infusion pump owned by patient, silver oxide, 3 volt, each

K0603 Replacement battery for external infusion pump owned by patient, alkaline, 1.5 volt, each

K0604 Replacement battery for external infusion pump owned by patient, lithium, 3.6 volt, each

K0605 Replacement battery for external infusion pump owned by patient, lithium, 4.5 volt, each

K0606 Automatic external defibrillator, with integrated electrocardiogram analysis, garment type

K0607 Replacement battery for automated external defibrillator, garment type only, each

K0608 Replacement garment for use with automated external defibrillator, each

K0609 Replacement electrodes for use with automated external defibrillator, garment type only, each

K0669 Wheelchair accessory, wheelchair seat or back cushion, does not meet specific code criteria or no written coding verification from DME PDAC

K0672 Addition to lower extremity orthosis, removable soft interface, all components, replacement only, each

K0730 Controlled dose inhalation drug delivery system

K0733 Power wheelchair accessory, 12 to 24 amp hour sealed lead acid battery, each (e.g., gel cell, absorbed glassmat)

K0738 Portable gaseous oxygen system, rental; home compressor used to fill portable oxygen cylinders, includes portable oxygen containers, regulator, flowmeter, humidifier, cannula or mask, and tubing

K0739 Repair or nonroutine service for durable medical equipment other than oxygen equipment requiring the skill of a technician, labor component, per 15 minutes

K0740 Repair or nonroutine service for oxygen equipment requiring the skill of a technician, labor component, per 15 minutes

(K0741) Code deleted December 31, 2012

(K0742) Code deleted December 31, 2012

K0743 Suction pump, home model, portable, for use on wounds

K0744 Absorptive wound dressing for use with suction pump, home model, portable, pad size 16 square inches or less

K0745 Absorptive wound dressing for use with suction pump, home model, portable, pad size more than 16 square inches but less than or equal to 48 square inches

K0746 Absorptive wound dressing for use with suction pump, home model, portable, pad size greater than 48 square inches.

K0800 Power operated vehicle, group 1 standard, patient weight capacity up to and including 300 pounds

K0801 Power operated vehicle, group 1 heavy duty, patient weight capacity 301 to 450 pounds

K0802 Power operated vehicle, group 1 very heavy duty, patient weight capacity 451 to 600 pounds

K0806 Power operated vehicle, group 2 standard, patient weight capacity up to and including 300 pounds

K0807 Power operated vehicle, group 2 heavy duty, patient weight capacity 301 to 450 pounds

K0808 Power operated vehicle, group 2 very heavy duty, patient weight capacity 451 to 600 pounds

K0812 Power operated vehicle, not otherwise classified

K0813 Power wheelchair, group 1 standard, portable, sling/solid seat and back, patient weight capacity up to and including 300 pounds

K0814 Power wheelchair, group 1 standard, portable, captains chair, patient weight capacity up to and including 300 lbs.

K0815 Power wheelchair, group 1 standard, sling/solid seat and back, patient weight capacity up to and including 300 lbs.

K0816 Power wheelchair, group 1 standard, captains chair, patient weight capacity up to and including 300 lbs.

K0820 Power wheelchair, group 2 standard, portable, sling/solid seat/back, patient weight capacity up to and including 300 pounds

K0821 Power wheelchair, group 2 standard, portable, captains chair, patient weight capacity up to and including 300 pounds

K0822 Power wheelchair, group 2 standard, sling/solid seat/back, patient weight capacity up to and including 300 lbs.

K0823 Power wheelchair, group 2 standard, captains chair, patient weight capacity up to and inlcuding 300 pounds

K0824 Power wheelchair, group 2 heavy duty, sling/solid seat/back, patient weight capacity 301 to 450 pounds

K0825 Power wheelchair, group 2 heavy duty, captains chair, patient weight capacity 301 to 450 pounds

K0826 Power wheelchair, group 2 very heavy duty, sling/solid seat/back, patient weight capacity 451 to 600 pounds

K0827 Power wheelchair, group 2 very heavy duty, captains chair, patient weight capacity 451 to 600 pounds

K0828 Power wheelchair, group 2 extra heavy duty, sling/solid seat/back, patient weight capacity 601 pounds or more

K0829 Power wheelchair, group 2 extra heavy duty, captains chair, patient weight capacity 601 pounds or more

K0830 Power wheelchair, group 2 standard, seat elevator, sling/solid seat/back, patient weight capacity up to and including 300 lbs.

K0831 Power wheelchair, group 2 standard, seat elevator, captains chair, patient weight capacity up to and including 300 pounds

K0835 Power wheelchair, group 2 standard, single power option, sling/solid seat/back, patient weight capacity up to and including 300 pounds

K0836 Power wheelchair, group 2 standard, single power option, captains chair, patient weight capacity up to and including 300 pounds

K0837 Power wheelchair, group 2 heavy duty, single power option, sling/solid seat/back, patient weight capacity 301 to 450 pounds

K0838 Power wheelchair, group 2 heavy duty, single power option, captains chair, patient weight capacity 301 to 450 pounds

K0839 Power wheelchair, grou 2 very heavy duty, single power option, sling/solid seat/back, patient weight capacity 451 to 600 pounds

K0840 Power wheelchair, group 2 extra heavy duty, single power option, sling/solid seat/back, patient weight capacity 601 pounds or more

K0841 Power wheelchair, group 2 standard, multiple power option, sling/solid seat/back, patient weight capacity up to and including 300 pounds

K0842 Power wheelchair, group 2 standard, multiple power option, captains chair, patient weight capacity up to and including 300 pounds

K0843 Power wheelchair, group 2 heavy duty, multiple power option, sling/solid seat/back, patient weight capacity 301 to 450 pounds

K0848 Power wheelchair, group 3 standard, sling/solid seat/back, patient weight capacity up to and inlcuding 300 pounds

K0849 Power wheelchair, group 3 standard, captains chair, patient weight capacity up to and including 300 pounds

K0850 Power wheelchair, group 3 heavy duty, sling/solid seat/back, patient weight capacity 301 to 450 pounds

K0851 Power wheelchair, group 3 heavy duty, captains chair, patient weight capacity 301 to 450 pounds

K0852 Power wheelchair, group 3 very heavy duty, sling/solid seat/back, patient weight capacity 451 to 600 pounds

K0853 Power wheelchair, group 3 very heavy duty, captains chair, patient weight capacity 451 to 600 pounds

K0854 Power wheelchair, group 3 extra heavy duty, sling/solid seat/back, patient weight capacity 601 pounds or more

K0855 Power wheelchair, group 3 extra heavy duty, captains chair, patient weight capacity 601 pounds or more

K0856 Power wheelchair, group 3 standard, single power option, sling/solid seat/back, patient weight capacity up to and including 300 pounds

K0857 Power wheelchair, group 3 standard, single power option, captains chair, patient weight capacity up to and inlcuding 300 pounds

K0858 Power wheelchair, group 3 heavy duty, single power option, sling/solid seat/back, patient weight capacity 301 to 450 pounds

K0859 Powe wheelchair, group 3 heavy duty, single power option, captains chair, patient weight capacity 301 to 450 pounds

K0860 Power wheelchair, group 3 very heavy duty, single power option, sling/solid seat/back, patient weight capacity 451 to 600 pounds

K0861 Power wheelchair, group 3 standard, multiple power option, sling/solid seat/back, patient weight capacity up to and including 300 pounds

K0862 Power wheelchair, group 3 heavy duty, multiple power option, sling/solid seat/back, patient weight capacity 301 to 450 pounds

K0863 Power wheelchair, group 3 very heavy duty, multiple power option, sling/solid seat/back, patient weight capacity 451 to 600 pounds

K0864 Power wheelchair, group 3 extra heavy duty, multiple power option, sling/solid seat/back, patient weight capacity 601 pounds or more

K0868 Power wheelchair, group 4 standard, sling/solid seat/back, patient weight capacity up to and including 300 pounds

K0869 Power wheelchair, group 4 standard, captains chair, patient weight capacity up to and including 300 pounds

K0870 Power wheelchair, group 4 heavy duty, sling/solid seat/back, patient weight capacity 301 to 450 pounds

K0871 Power wheelchair, group 4 very heavy duty, sling/solid seat/back, patient weight capacity 451 to 600 pounds

K0877 Power wheelchair, group 4 standard, single power option, sling/solid seat/back, patient weight capacity up to and including 300 pounds

K0878 Power wheelchair, group 4 standard, single power option, captains chair, patient weight capacity up to and including 300 pounds

K0879 Power wheelchair, group 4 heavy duty, single power option, sling/solid seat/back, patient weight capacity 301 to 450 pounds

K0880 Power wheelchair, group 4 very heavy duty, single power option, sling/solid seat/back, patient weight 451 to 600 pounds

K0884 Power wheelchair, group 4 standard, multiple power option, sling/solid seat/back, patient weight capacity up to and including 300 pounds

K0885 Power wheelchair, group 4 standard, multiple power option, captains chair, patient weight capacity up to and including 300 pounds

K0886 Power wheelchair, group 4 heavy duty, multiple power option, sling/solid seat/back, patient weight capacity 301 to 450 pounds

K0890 Power wheelchair, group 5 pediatric, single power option, sling/solid seat/back, patient weight capacity up to and including 125 pounds

K0891 Power wheelchair. group 5 pediatric, multiple power option, sling/solid seat/back, patient weight capacity up to and including 125 pounds

K0898 Power wheelchair, not otherwise classified

K0899 Power mobility device, not coded by DME PDAC or does not meet criteria

● **K0900** Customized durable medical equipment, other than wheelchair

ORTHOTIC PROCEDURES

L

Guidelines

In addition to the information presented in the INTRODUCTION, several other items unique to this section are defined or identified here:

1. SUBSECTION INFORMATION: Some of the listed subheadings or subsections have special needs or instructions unique to that section. Where these are indicated, special "notes" will be presented preceding or following the listings. Those subsections within the ORTHOTIC PROCEDURES section that have "notes" are as follows:

Subsection	Code Numbers
Scoliosis procedures	L1000-L1499
Orthotic devices-lower limb	L1600-L2999
Lower limb-hip-knee-angle-foot (or any combination)	L2000-L2199
Orthotic devices-upper limb	L3650-L3999

2. UNLISTED SERVICE OR PROCEDURE: A service or procedure may be provided that is not listed in this edition of HCPCS. When reporting such a service, the appropriate "unlisted procedure" code may be used to indicate the service, identifying it by "special report" as defined below. HCPCS terminology is inconsistent in defining unlisted procedures. The procedure definition may include the term(s) "unlisted", "not otherwise classified", "unspecified", "unclassified", "other" and "miscellaneous". Prior to using these codes, try to determine if a Local Level III code or CPT code is available. The "unlisted procedures" and accompanying codes for ORTHOTIC PROCEDURES are as follows:

L0999	Addition to spinal orthosis, not otherwise specified
L1499	Spinal orthosis, not otherwise specified
L2999	Lower extremity orthosis, not otherwise specified
L3649	Orthopedic shoe, modification, addition or transfer, not otherwise specified
L3999	Upper limb orthosis, not otherwise specified

3. SPECIAL REPORT: A service, material or supply that is rarely provided, unusual, variable or new may require a special report in determining medical appropriateness for reimbursement purposes.

Pertinent information should include an adequate definition or description of the nature, extent, and need for the service, material or supply.

4. MODIFIERS: Listed services may be modified under certain circumstances. When appropriate, the modifying circumstance is identified by adding a modifier to the basic procedure code. CPT and HCPCS National Level II modifiers may be used with CPT and HCPCS National Level II procedure codes. Modifiers commonly used with ORTHOTIC PROCEDURES are as follows:

   -CC Procedure code change (use "CC" when the procedure code submitted was changed either for administrative reasons or because an incorrect code was filed)

   -LT Left side (used to identify procedures performed on the left side of the body)

   -RT Right side (used to identify procedures performed on the right side of the body)

   -TC Technical component. Under certain circumstances, a charge may be made for the technical component alone. Under those circumstances, the technical component charge is identified by adding modifier -TC to the usual procedure number. Technical component charges are institutional charges and are not billed separately by physicians. However, portable x-ray suppliers bill only for the technical component and should use modifier -TC. The change data from portable x-ray suppliers will then be used to build customary and prevailing profiles.

5. CPT CODE CROSS-REFERENCE: Unless otherwise specified, the equivalent CPT code for all listings in this section is 99070.

6. DURABLE MEDICAL EQUIPMENT REGIONAL CARRIERS (DMERCS): Effective October 1, 1993, claims orthotics must be billed to one of four regional carriers depending upon the residence of the beneficiary. The transition dates for DMERC claims is from November 1, 1993 to March 1, 1994, depending upon the state you practice in. See the Introduction for a complete discussion of DMERCs.

ORTHOTIC DEVICES

SPINAL - CERVICAL

L0112 Cranial cervical orthosis, congenital torticollis type, with or without soft interface material, adjustable range of motion joint, custom fabricated

L0113 Cranial cervical orthosis, torticollis type, with or without joint, with or without soft interface material, prefabricated, includes fitting and adjustment

▲**L0120** Cervical, flexible; non-adjustable, prefabricated, off-the-shelf (foam collar)

L0130 thermoplastic collar, molded to patient

L0140 Cervical, semi-rigid; adjustable (plastic collar)

L0150 adjustable molded chin cup (plastic collar with mandibular/occipital piece)

▲**L0160** wire frame occipital/mandibular support, prefabricated, off-the-shelf

L0170 Cervical collar; molded to patient model

▲**L0172** semi-rigid thermoplastic foam, two-piece, prefabricated, off-the-shelf

▲**L0174** semi-rigid, thermoplastic foam, two piece with thoracic extension, prefabricated, off-the-shelf

L0180 Cervical, multiple post collar, occipital/mandibular supports; adjustable

L0190 adjustable cervical bars (somi, guilford, taylor types)

L0200 adjustable cervical bars, and thoracic extension

SPINAL - THORACIC

L0220 Thoracic, rib belt, custom fabricated

SPINAL - THORACIC-LUMBAR-SACRAL

(L0430) Code deleted December 31, 2013.

▲**L0450** TLSO, flexible, provides trunk support, upper thoracic region, produces intracavitary pressure to reduce load on the intervertebral disks with rigid stays or panel(s), includes shoulder straps and closures, prefabricated, off-the-shelf

L0452 TLSO, flexible, provides trunk support, upper thoracic region, produces intracavitary pressure to reduce load on the intervertebral disks with rigid stays or panel(s), includes shoulder straps and closures, custom fabricated

▲**L0454** TLSO flexible, provides trunk support, extends from sacrococcygeal junction to above t-9 vertebra, restricts gross trunk motion in the sagittal plane, produces intracavitary pressure to reduce load on the intervertebral disks with rigid stays or panel(s), includes shoulder straps and closures, prefabricated item that has been trimmed, bent, molded, assembled, or otherwise customized to fit a specific patient by an individual with expertise

●**L0455** TLSO, flexible, provides trunk support, extends from sacrococcygeal junction to above T-9 vertebra, restricts gross trunk motion in the sagittal plane, produces intracavitary pressure to reduce load on the intervertebral disks with rigid stays or panel(s), includes shoulder straps and closures, prefabricated, off-the-shelf

▲**L0456** TLSO, flexible, provides trunk support, thoracic region, rigid posterior panel and soft anterior apron, extends from the sacrococcygeal junction and terminates just inferior to the scapular spine, restricts gross trunk motion in the sagittal plane, produces intracavitary pressure to reduce load on the intervertebral disks, includes straps and closures, prefabricated item that has been trimmed, bent, molded, assembled, or otherwise customized to fit a specific patient by an individual with expertise

●**L0457** TLSO, flexible, provides trunk support, thoracic region, rigid posterior panel and soft anterior apron, extends from the sacrococcygeal junction and terminates just inferior to the scapular spine, restricts gross trunk motion in the sagittal plane, produces intracavitary pressure to reduce load on the intervertebral disks, includes straps and closures, prefabricated, off-the-shelf

L0458 TLSO, triplanar control, modular segmented spinal system, two rigid plastic shells, posterior extends from the sacrococcygeal junction and terminates just inferior to the scapular spine, anterior extends from the symphysis pubis to the xiphoid, soft liner, restricts gross trunk motion in the sagittal, coronal, and transverse planes, lateral strength is provided by overlapping plastic and stabilizing closures, includes straps and closures, prefabricated, includes fitting and adjustment

▲**L0460** TLSO, triplanar control, modular segmented spinal system, two rigid plastic shells, posterior extends from the sacrococcygeal junction and terminates just inferior to the scapular spine, anterior extends from the symphysis pubis to the sternal notch, soft liner, restricts gross trunk motion in the sagittal, coronal, and transverse planes, lateral strength is provided by overlapping plastic and stabilizing closures, includes straps and closures, prefabricated item that has been trimmed, bent, molded, assembled, or otherwise customized to fit a specific patient by an individual with expertise

L0462 TLSO, triplanar control, modular segmented spinal system, three rigid plastic shells, posterior extends from the sacrococcygeal junction and terminates just inferior to the scapular spine, anterior extends from the symphysis pubis to the sternal notch, soft liner, restricts gross trunk motion in the sagittal, coronal, and transverse planes, lateral strength is provided by overlapping plastic and stabilizing closures, includes straps and closures, prefabricated, includes fitting and adjustment

L0464 TLSO, triplanar control, modular segmented spinal system, four rigid plastic shells, posterior extends from sacrococcygeal junction and terminates just inferior to scapular spine, anterior extends from symphysis pubis to the sternal notch, soft liner, restricts gross trunk motion in sagittal, coronal, and transverse planes, lateral strength is provided by overlapping plastic and stabilizing closures, includes straps and closures, prefabricated, includes fitting and adjustment

▲**L0466** TLSO, sagittal control, rigid posterior frame and flexible soft anterior apron with straps, closures and padding, restricts gross trunk motion in sagittal plane, produces intracavitary pressure to reduce load on intervertebral disks, prefabricated item that has been trimmed, bent, molded, assembled, or otherwise customized to fit a specific patient by an individual with expertise

● **L0467** TLSO, sagittal control, rigid posterior frame and flexible soft anterior apron with straps, closures and padding, restricts gross trunk motion in sagittal plane, produces intracavitary pressure to reduce load on intervertebral disks, prefabricated, off-the-shelf

▲**L0468** TLSO, sagittal-coronal control, rigid posterior frame and flexible soft anterior apron with straps, closures and padding, extends from sacrococcygeal junction over scapulae, lateral strength provided by pelvic, thoracic, and lateral frame pieces, restricts gross trunk motion in sagittal, and coronal planes, produces intracavitary pressure to reduce load on intervertebral disks, prefabricated item that has been trimmed, bent, molded, assembled, or otherwise customized to fit a specific patient by an individual with expertise

● **L0469** TLSO, sagittal-coronal control, rigid posterior frame and flexible soft anterior apron with straps, closures and padding, extends from sacrococcygeal junction over scapulae, lateral strength provided by pelvic, thoracic, and lateral frame pieces, restricts gross trunk motion in sagittal and coronal planes, produces intracavitary pressure to reduce load on intervertebral disks, prefabricated, off-the-shelf

L0470 TLSO, triplanar control, rigid posterior frame and flexible soft anterior apron with straps, closures and padding, extends from sacrococcygeal junction to scapula, lateral strength provided by pelvic, thoracic, and lateral frame pieces, rotational strength provided by subclavicular extensions, restricts gross trunk motion in sagittal, coronal, and transverse planes, produces intracavitary pressure to reduce load on the intervertebral disks, includes fitting and shaping the frame, prefabricated, includes fitting and adjustment

L0472 TLSO, triplanar control, hyperextension, rigid anterior and lateral frame extends from symphysis pubis to sternal notch with two anterior components (one pubic and one sternal), posterior and lateral pads with straps and closures, limits spinal flexion, restricts gross trunk motion in sagittal, coronal, and transverse planes, includes fitting and shaping the frame, prefabricated, includes fitting and adjustment

L0480 TLSO, triplanar control, one piece rigid plastic shell without interface liner, with multiple straps and closures, posterior extends from sacrococcygeal junction and terminates just inferior to scapular spine, anterior extends from symphysis pubis to sternal notch, anterior or posterior opening, restricts gross trunk motion in sagittal, coronal, and transverse planes, includes a carved plaster or cad-cam model, custom fabricated

L0482 TLSO, triplanar control, one piece rigid plastic shell with interface liner, multiple straps and closures, posterior extends from sacrococcygeal junction and terminates just inferior to scapular spine, anterior extends from symphysis pubis to sternal notch, anterior or posterior opening, restricts gross trunk motion in sagittal, coronal, and transverse planes, includes a carved plaster or cad-cam model, custom fabricated

L0484 TLSO, triplanar control, two piece rigid plastic shell without interface liner, with multiple straps and closures, posterior extends from sacrococcygeal junction and terminates just inferior to scapular spine, anterior extends from symphysis pubis to sternal notch, lateral strength is enhanced by overlapping plastic, restricts gross trunk motion in the sagittal, coronal, and transverse planes, includes a carved plaster or cad-cam model, custom fabricated

L0486 TLSO, triplanar control, two piece rigid plastic shell with interface liner, multiple straps and closures, posterior extends from sacrococcygeal junction and terminates just inferior to scapular spine, anterior extends from symphysis pubis to sternal notch, lateral strength is enhanced by overlapping plastic, restricts gross trunk motion in the sagittal, coronal, and transverse planes, includes a carved plaster or cad-cam model, custom fabricated

L0488 TLSO, triplanar control, one piece rigid plastic shell with interface liner, multiple straps and closures, posterior extends from sacrococcygeal junction and terminates just inferior to scapular spine, anterior extends from symphysis pubis to sternal notch, anterior or posterior opening, restricts gross trunk motion in sagittal, coronal, and transverse planes, prefabricated, includes fitting and adjustment

L0490 TLSO, sagittal-coronal control, one piece rigid plastic shell, with overlapping reinforced anterior, with multiple straps and closures, posterior extends from sacrococcygeal junction and terminates at or before the t-9 vertebra, anterior extends from symphysis pubis to xiphoid, anterior opening, restricts gross trunk motion in sagittal and coronal planes, prefabricated, includes fitting and adjustment

L0491 TLSO, sagittal-coronal control, modular segmented spinal system, two rigid plastic shells, posterior extends from the sacrococcygeal junction and terminates just inferior to the scapular spine, anterior extends from the symphysis pubis to the xiphoid, soft liner, restricts gross trunk motion in the sagittal and coronal planes, lateral strength is provided by overlapping plastic and stabilizing closures, includes straps and closures, prefabricated, includes fitting and adjustment

L0492 TLSO, sagittal-coronal control, modular segmented spinal system, three rigid plastic shells, posterior extends from the sacrococcygeal junction and terminates just inferior to the scapular spine, anterior extends from the symphysis pubis to the xiphoid, soft liner, restricts gross trunk motion in the sagittal and coronal planes, lateral strength is provided by overlapping plastic and stabilizing closures, includes straps and closures, prefabricated, includes fitting and adjustment

SPINAL - SACROILIAC

SEMI-RIGID

▲**L0621** Sacroiliac orthosis, flexible, provides pelvic-sacral support, reduces motion about the sacroiliac joint, includes straps, closures, may include pendulous abdomen design, prefabricated, off-the-shelf

L0622 Sacroiliac orthosis, flexible, provides pelvic-sacral support, reduces motion about the sacroiliac joint, includes straps, closures, may include pendulous abdomen design, custom fabricated

▲**L0623** Sacroiliac orthosis, provides pelvic-sacral support, with rigid or semi-rigid panels over the sacrum and abdomen, reduces motion about the sacroiliac joint, includes straps, closures, may include pendulous abdomen design, prefabricated, off-the-shelf

L0624 Sacroiliac orthosis, provides pelvic-sacral support, with rigid or semi-rigid panels placed over the sacrum and abdomen, reduces motion about the sacroiliac joint, includes straps, closures, may include pendulous abdomen design, custom fabricated

▲**L0625** Lumbar orthosis, flexible, provides lumbar support, posterior extends from l-1 to below l-5 vertebra, produces intracavitary pressure to reduce load on the intervertebral discs, includes straps, closures, may include pendulous abdomen design, shoulder straps, stays, prefabricated, off-the-shelf

▲**L0626** Lumbar orthosis, sagittal control, with rigid posterior panel(s), posterior extends from l-1 to below l-5 vertebra, produces intracavitary pressure to reduce load on the intervertebral discs, includes straps, closures, may include padding, stays, shoulder straps, pendulous abdomen design, prefabricated item that has been trimmed, bent, molded, assembled, or otherwise customized to fit a specific patient by an individual with expertise

▲**L0627** Lumbar orthosis, sagittal control, with rigid anterior and posterior panels, posterior extends from l-1 to below l-5 vertebra, produces intracavitary pressure to reduce load on the intervertebral discs, includes straps, closures, may include padding, shoulder straps, pendulous abdomen design, prefabricated item that has been trimmed, bent, molded, assembled, or otherwise customized to fit a specific patient by an individual with expertise

▲**L0628** Lumbar-sacral orthosis, flexible, provides lumbo-sacral support, posterior extends from sacrococcygeal junction to t-9 vertebra, produces intracavitary pressure to reduce load on the intervertebral discs, includes straps, closures, may include stays, shoulder straps, pendulous abdomen design, prefabricated, off-the-shelf

L0629 Lumbar-sacral orthosis, flexible, provides lumbo-sacral support, posterior extends from sacrococcygeal junction to T-9 vertebra, produces intracavitary pressure to reduce load on the intervertebral discs, includes straps, closures, may include stays, shoulder straps, pendulous abdomen design, custom fabricated

▲**L0630** Lumbar-sacral orthosis, sagittal control, with rigid posterior panel(s), posterior extends from sacrococcygeal junction to t-9 vertebra, produces intracavitary pressure to reduce load on the intervertebral discs, includes straps, closures, may include padding, stays, shoulder straps, pendulous abdomen design, prefabricated item that has been trimmed, bent, molded, assembled, or otherwise customized to fit a specific patient by an individual with expertise

▲**L0631** Lumbar-sacral orthosis, sagittal control, with rigid anterior and posterior panels, posterior extends from sacrococcygeal junction to t-9 vertebra, produces intracavitary pressure to reduce load on the intervertebral discs, includes straps, closures, may include padding, shoulder straps, pendulous abdomen design, prefabricated item that has been trimmed, bent, molded, assembled, or otherwise customized to fit a specific patient by an individual with expertise

L0632 Lumbar-sacral orthosis, sagittal control, with rigid anterior and posterior panels, posterior extends from sacrococcygeal junction to T-9 vertebra, produces intracavitary pressure to reduce load on the intervertebral discs, includes straps, closures, may include padding, shoulder straps, pendulous abdomen design, custom fabricated

▲**L0633** Lumbar-sacral orthosis, sagittal-coronal control, with rigid posterior frame/panel(s), posterior extends from sacrococcygeal junction to t-9 vertebra, lateral strength provided by rigid lateral frame/panels, produces intracavitary pressure to reduce load on intervertebral discs, includes straps, closures, may include padding, stays, shoulder straps, pendulous abdomen design, prefabricated item that has been trimmed, bent, molded, assembled, or otherwise customized to fit a specific patient by an individual with expertise

L0634 Lumbar-sacral orthosis, sagittal-coronal control, with rigid posterior frame/panel(s), posterior extends from sacrococcygeal junction to T-9 vertebra, lateral strength provided by rigid lateral frame/panel(s), produces intracavitary pressure to reduce load on intervertebral discs, includes straps, closures, may include padding, stays, shoulder straps, pendulous abdomen design, custom fabricated

L0635 Lumbar-sacral orthosis, sagittal-coronal control, lumbar flexion, rigid posterior frame/panel(s), lateral articulating design to flex the lumbar spine, posterior extends from sacrococcygeal junction to T-9 vertebra, lateral strength provided by rigid lateral frame/panel(s), produces intracavitary pressure to reduce load on intervertebral discs, includes straps, closures, may include padding, anterior panel, pendulous abdomen design, prefabricated, includes fitting and adjustment

L0636 Lumbar sacral orthosis, sagittal-coronal control, lumbar flexion, rigid posterior frame/panels, lateral articulating design to flex the lumbar spine, posterior extends from sacrococcygeal junction to T-9 vertebra, lateral strength provided by rigid lateral frame/panels, produces intracavitary pressure to reduce load on intervertebral discs, includes straps, closures, may include padding, anterior panel, pendulous abdomen design, custom fabricated

▲**L0637** Lumbar-sacral orthosis, sagittal-coronal control, with rigid anterior and posterior frame/panels, posterior extends from sacrococcygeal junction to t-9 vertebra, lateral strength provided by rigid lateral frame/panels, produces intracavitary pressure to reduce load on intervertebral discs, includes straps, closures, may include padding, shoulder straps, pendulous abdomen design, prefabricated item that has been trimmed, bent, molded, assembled, or otherwise customized to fit a specific patient by an individual with expertise

L0638 Lumbar-sacral orthosis, sagittal-coronal control, with rigid anterior and posterior frame/panels, posterior extends from sacrococcygeal junction to T-9 vertebra, lateral strength provided by rigid lateral frame/panels, produces intracavitary pressure to reduce load on intervertebral discs, includes straps, closures, may include padding, shoulder straps, pendulous abdomen design, custom fabricated

▲**L0639** Lumbar-sacral orthosis, sagittal-coronal control, rigid shell(s)/panel(s), posterior extends from sacrococcygeal junction to t-9 vertebra, anterior extends from symphysis pubis to xyphoid, produces intracavitary pressure to reduce load on the intervertebral discs, overall strength is provided by overlapping rigid material and stabilizing closures, includes straps, closures, may include soft interface, pendulous abdomen design, prefabricated item that has been trimmed, bent, molded, assembled, or otherwise customized to fit a specific patient by an individual with expertise

L0640 Lumbar-sacral orthosis, sagittal-coronal control, rigid shell(s)/panel(s), posterior extends from sacrococcygeal junction to T-9 vertebra, anterior extends from symphysis pubis to xyphoid, produces intracavitary pressure to reduce load on the intervertebral discs, overall strength is provided by overlapping rigid material and stabilizing closures, includes straps, closures, may include soft interface, pendulous abdomen design, custom fabricated

● **L0641** Lumbar orthosis, sagittal control, with rigid posterior panel(s), posterior extends from l-1 to below l-5 vertebra, produces intracavitary pressure to reduce load on the intervertebral discs, includes straps, closures, may include padding, stays, shoulder straps, pendulous abdomen design, prefabricated, off-the-shelf

● **L0642** Lumbar orthosis, sagittal control, with rigid anterior and posterior panels, posterior extends from l-1 to below l-5 vertebra, produces intracavitary pressure to reduce load on the intervertebral discs, includes straps, closures, may include padding, shoulder straps, pendulous abdomen design, prefabricated, off-the-shelf

● **L0643** Lumbar-sacral orthosis, sagittal control, with rigid posterior panel(s), posterior extends from sacrococcygeal junction to t-9 vertebra, produces intracavitary pressure to reduce load on the intervertebral discs, includes straps, closures, may include padding, stays, shoulder straps, pendulous abdomen design, prefabricated, off-the-shelf

● **L0648** Lumbar-sacral orthosis, sagittal control, with rigid anterior and posterior panels, posterior extends from sacrococcygeal junction to t-9 vertebra, produces intracavitary pressure to reduce load on the intervertebral discs, includes straps, closures, may include padding, shoulder straps, pendulous abdomen design, prefabricated, off-the-shelf

● **L0649** Lumbar-sacral orthosis, sagittal-coronal control, with rigid posterior frame/panel(s), posterior extends from sacrococcygeal junction to t-9 vertebra, lateral strength provided by rigid lateral frame/panels, produces intracavitary pressure to reduce load on intervertebral discs, includes straps, closures, may include padding, stays, shoulder straps, pendulous abdomen design, prefabricated, off-the-shelf

● **L0650** Lumbar-sacral orthosis, sagittal-coronal control, with rigid anterior and posterior frame/panel(s), posterior extends from sacrococcygeal junction to t-9 vertebra, lateral strength provided by rigid lateral frame/panel(s), produces intracavitary pressure to reduce load on intervertebral discs, includes straps, closures, may include padding, shoulder straps, pendulous abdomen design, prefabricated, off-the-shelf

● **L0651** Lumbar-sacral orthosis, sagittal-coronal control, rigid shell(s)/panel(s), posterior extends from sacrococcygeal junction to t-9 vertebra, anterior extends from symphysis pubis to xyphoid, produces intracavitary pressure to reduce load on the intervertebral discs, overall strength is provided by overlapping rigid material and stabilizing closures, includes straps, closures, may include soft interface, pendulous abdomen design, prefabricated, off-the-shelf

SPINAL - CERVICAL-THORACIC-LUMBAR-SACRAL-HALO PROCEDURE

ANTERIOR-POSTERIOR-LATERAL CONTROL

L0700 Cervical-thoracic-lumber-sacral-orthoses (CTLSO), anterior-posterior-lateral control, molded to patient model; (Minerva type)

L0710 with interface material, (Minerva type)

HALO PROCEDURE

L0810 Halo procedure; cervical halo incorporated into jacket vest

L0820 cervical halo incorporated into plaster body jacket

L0830 cervical halo incorporated into Milwaukee type orthosis

L0859 Addition to halo procedure, magnetic resonance image compatible systems, rings and pins, any material

SPINAL - TORSO SUPPORTS

PTOSIS SUPPORTS

L0861 Addition to halo procedure, replacement liner/interface material

ADDITIONS TO SPINAL ORTHOSES

L0970 TLSO, corset front

L0972 LSO, corset front

L0974 TLSO, full corset

L0976 LSO, full corset

L0978 Axillary crutch extension

▲**L0980** Peroneal straps, prefabricated, off-the-shelf, pair

▲**L0982** Stocking supporter grips, prefabricated, off-the-shelf, set of four (4)

▲**L0984** Protective body sock, prefabricated, off-the-shelf, each

L0999 Addition to spinal orthosis, not otherwise specified

ORTHOTIC DEVICES - SCOLIOSIS PROCEDURES

NOTE: The orthotic care of scoliosis differs from other orthotic care in that the treatment is more dynamic in nature and utilizes ongoing, continual modification of the orthosis to the patient's changing condition. This coding structure uses the proper names or eponyms of the procedures because they have historic and universal acceptance in the profession. It should be recognized that variations to the basic procedures described by the founders/developers are accepted in various medical and orthotic practices throughout the country. All procedures include model of patient when indicated.

SCOLIOSIS - CERVICAL-THORACIC-LUMBAR-SACRAL (MILWAUKEE)

L1000 Cervical-thoracic-lumbar-sacral orthosis (CTLSO) (Milwaukee), inclusive of furnishing initial orthosis, including model

L1001 Cervical-thoracic-lumbar-sacral orthosis, immobilizer, infant size, prefabricated, includes fitting and adjustment

L1005 Tension based scoliosis orthosis and accessory pads, includes fitting and adjustment

CORRECTION PADS

L1010 Additions to cervical-thoracic-lumber-sacral orthosis (CTLSO) or scoliosis orthosis; axilla sling

L1020 kyphosis pad

L1025 kyphosis pad, floating

L1030 lumbar bolster pad

L1040 lumbar or lumbar rib pad

L1050 sternal pad

L1060 thoracic pad

L1070 trapezius sling

L1080 outrigger

L1085 outrigger, bilateral with vertical extensions

L1090 lumbar sling

L1100 ring flange, plastic or leather

L1110 ring flange, plastic or leather, molded to patient model

L1120 covers for upright, each

SCOLIOSIS - THORACIC-LUMBAR-SACRAL (LOW PROFILE)

L1200 Thoracic-lumbar-sacral-orthosis (TLSO), inclusive of furnishing initial orthosis only

L1210 Addition to TLSO, (low profile); lateral thoracic extension

L1220 anterior thoracic extension

L1230 Milwaukee type superstructure

L1240 lumbar derotation pad

L1250 anterior asis pad

L1260 anterior thoracic derotation pad

L1270 abdominal pad

L1280 rib gusset (elastic), each

L1290 lateral trochanteric pad

OTHER SCOLIOSIS PROCEDURES

L1300 Other scoliosis procedure; body jacket molded to patient model

L1310 post-operative body jacket

L1499 Spinal orthosis, not otherwise specified

THORACIC-HIP-KNEE-ANKLE

(L1500) Code deleted December 31, 2011

(L1510) Code deleted December 31, 2011

(L1520) Code deleted December 31, 2011

ORTHOTIC DEVICES - LOWER LIMB

NOTE: The procedures L1600-L2999 are considered as "base" or the "basic procedures" and may be modified by listing other procedures from the "additions" (L2200-L2999) section and adding them to the base procedure.

LOWER LIMB-HIP

FLEXIBLE

▲**L1600** Hip orthosis, abduction control of hip joints, flexible, Frejka type with cover, prefabricated item that has been trimmed, bent, molded, assembled, or otherwise customized to fit a specific patient by an individual with expertise

▲**L1610** Hip orthosis, abduction control of hip joints, flexible, (Frejka cover only), prefabricated item that has been trimmed, bent, molded, assembled, or otherwise customized to fit a specific patient by an individual with expertise

▲**L1620** Hip orthosis, abduction control of hip joints, flexible, (Pavlik harness), prefabricated item that has been trimmed, bent, molded, assembled, or otherwise customized to fit a specific patient by an individual with expertise

L1630 HO, abduction control of hip joints; semi-flexible (Von Rosen type), custom fabricated

L1640 HO, abduction control of hip joints; static, pelvic band or spreader bar, thigh cuffs, custom fabricated

L1650 HO, abduction control of hip joints; static, adjustable, (Ilfled type), prefabricated, includes fitting and adjustment

L1652 Hip orthosis, bilateral thigh cuffs with adjustable abductor spreader bar, adult size, prefabricated, includes fitting and adjustment, any type

L1660 HO, abduction control of hip joints; static, plastic, prefabricated, includes fitting and adjustment

L1680 HO, abduction control of hip joints; dynamic, pelvic control, adjustable hip motion control, thigh cuffs (Rancho hip action type), custom fabricated

L1685 HO, abduction control of hip joints; postoperative hip abduction type, custom fabricated

L1686 HO, abduction control of hip joints; postoperative hip abduction type, prefabricated, includes fitting and adjustment

L1690 Combination, bilateral, lumbo-sacral, hip, femur orthosis providing adduction and internal rotation control, prefabricated, includes fitting and adjustment

LOWER LIMB-LEGG PERTHES

L1700 Legg Perthes orthosis; (Toronto type), custom fabricated

L1710 (Newington type), custom fabricated

L1720 trilateral, (Tachidijan type), custom fabricated

L1730 (Scottish Rite type), custom fabricated

L1755 (Patten Bottom type), custom fabricated

LOWER LIMB-KNEE

▲**L1810** Knee orthosis, elastic with joints, prefabricated item that has been trimmed, bent, molded, assembled, or otherwise customized to fit a specific patient by an individual with expertise

●**L1812** elastic with joints, prefabricated, off-the-shelf

L1820 elastic with condylar pads and joints, with or without patellar control, prefabricated, includes fitting and adjustment

▲**L1830** Knee orthosis, immobilizer, canvas longitudinal, prefabricated, off-the-shelf

L1831 Knee orthosis (KO); locking knee joint(s), positional orthosis, prefabricated, includes fitting and adjustment

▲**L1832** Knee orthosis; adjustable knee joints (unicentric or polycentric), positional orthosis, rigid support, prefabricated item that has been trimmed, bent, molded, assembled, or otherwise customized to fit a specific patient by an individual with expertise

●**L1833** adjustable knee joints (unicentric or polycentric), positional orthosis, rigid support, prefabricated, off-the shelf

L1834 without knee joint, rigid, custom fabricated

▲**L1836** Knee orthosis, rigid, without joint(s), includes soft interface material, prefabricated, off-the-shelf

L1840 Knee orthosis, derotation, medial-lateral, anterior cruciate ligament, custom fabricated

▲**L1843** Knee orthosis, single upright, thigh and calf, with adjustable flexion and extension joint (unicentric or polycentric), medial-lateral and rotation control, with or without varus/valgus adjustment, prefabricated item that has been trimmed, bent, molded, assembled, or otherwise customized to fit a specific patient by an individual with expertise

L1844 Knee orthosis, single upright, thigh and calf, with adjustable flexion and extension joint (unicentric or polycentric), medial-lateral and rotation control, with or without varus/valgus adjustment, custom fabricated

▲**L1845** Knee orthosis, double upright, thigh and calf, with adjustable flexion and extension joint (unicentric or polycentric), medial-lateral and rotation control, with or without varus/valgus adjustment, prefabricated item that has been trimmed, bent, molded, assembled, or otherwise customized to fit a specific patient by an individual with expertise

L1846 Knee orthosis, double upright, thigh and calf, with adjustable flexion and extension joint (unicentric or polycentric), medial-lateral and rotation control, with or without varus/valgus adjustment, custom fabricated

▲**L1847** Knee orthosis, double upright with adjustable joint, with inflatable air support chamber(s), prefabricated item that has been trimmed, bent, molded, assembled, or otherwise customized to fit a specific patient by an individual with expertise

●**L1848** Knee orthosis, double upright with adjustable joint, with inflatable air support chamber(s), prefabricated, off-the-shelf

▲**L1850** Knee orthosis, Swedish type, prefabricated, off-the-shelf

L1860 modification of supracondylar prosthetic socket, custom fabricated (SK)

LOWER LIMB-ANKLE-FOOT

L1900 Ankle-foot orthosis (AFO); spring wire, dorsiflexion assist calf band, custom fabricated

▲**L1902** AFO; ankle gauntlet, prefabricated, off-the-shelf

▲**L1904** Ankle orthosis, ankle gauntlet, custom-fabricated

▲**L1906** Ankle foot orthosis, multiligamentous ankle support, prefabricated, off-the-shelf

▲**L1907** Ankle orthosis, supramalleolar with straps, with or without interface/pads, custom fabricated

L1910 posterior, single bar, clasp attachment to shoe counter, prefabricated, includes fitting and adjustment

L1920 single upright with static or adjustable stop (Phelps or Perlstein type), custom fabricated

L1930 Ankle foot orthosis; plastic or other material, prefabricated, includes fitting and adjustment

L1932 AFO, rigid anterior tibial section, total carbon fiber or equal material, prefabricated, includes fitting and adjustment

L1940 Ankle foot orthosis; plastic or other material, custom-fabricated

L1945 plastic, rigid anterior tibial section (floor reaction), custom fabricated

L1950 spiral, (Institute of Rehabilitative Medicine type), plastic, custom-fabricated

L1951 spiral, (Institute of Rehabilitative Medicine type), plastic or other material, prefabricated, includes fitting and adjustment

L1960 posterior solid ankle, plastic, custom fabricated

L1970 plastic with ankle joint, custom fabricated

L1971 plastic or other material with ankle joint, prefabricated, includes fitting and adjustment

L1980 single upright free plantar dorsiflexion, solid stirrup, calf band/cuff (single bar "BK" orthosis), custom fabricated

L1990 double upright free plantar dorsiflexion, solid stirrup, calf band/cuff (double bar "BK" orthosis), custom fabricated

LOWER LIMB-HIP-KNEE-ANKLE-FOOT (OR ANY COMBINATION)

NOTE: L2000, L2020, and L2036 are base procedures to be used with any knee joint. L2010 and L2030 are to used only with no knee joint.

L2000 Knee-ankle-foot-orthosis (KAFO); single upright, free knee, free ankle, solid stirrup, thigh and calf bands/cuffs (single bar "AK" orthosis), custom fabricated

L2005 Knee ankle foot orthosis; any material, single or double upright, stance control, automatic lock and swing phase release, any type activation, includes ankle joint, any type, custom fabricated

L2010 single upright, free ankle, solid stirrup, thigh and calf bands/cuffs (single bar "AK" orthosis), without knee joint, custom fabricated

L2020 double upright, free ankle, solid stirrup, thigh and calf bands/cuffs (double bar "AK" orthosis), custom fabricated

L2030 double upright, free ankle, solid stirrup, thigh and calf bands/cuffs, (double bar "AK" orthosis), without knee joint, custom fabricated

L2034 full plastic, single upright, with or without free motion knee, medial lateral rotation control, with or without free motion ankle, custom fabricated

L2035 full plastic, static (pediatric size), without free motion ankle, prefabricated, includes fitting and adjustment

L2036 full plastic, double upright, with or without free motion knee, with or without free motion ankle, custom fabricated

L2037 full plastic, single upright, with or without free motion knee, with or without free motion ankle, custom fabricated

L2038 full plastic, with or without free motion knee, multiaxis ankle, custom fabricated

TORSION CONTROL

L2040 Hip-knee-ankle-foot orthosis (HKAFO); torsion control, bilateral rotation straps, pelvic band/belt, custom fabricated

L2050 torsion control, bilateral torsion cables, hip joint, pelvic band/belt, custom fabricated

L2060 torsion control, bilateral torsion cables, ball bearing hip joint, pelvic band/belt, custom fabricated

L2070 torsion control, unilateral rotation straps, pelvic band/belt, custom fabricated

L2080 torsion control, unilateral torsion cable, hip joint, pelvic band/belt, custom fabricated

L2090 torsion control, unilateral torsion cable, ball bearing hip joint, pelvic band/belt, custom fabricated

FRACTURE ORTHOSES

L2106 Ankle-foot-orthosis (AFO), fracture orthosis, tibial fracture cast orthosis; thermoplastic type casting material, custom fabricated

L2108 custom fabricated

L2112 soft, pre-fabricated, includes fitting and adjustment

L2114 semi-rigid, pre-fabricated, includes fitting and adjustment

L2116 rigid, pre-fabricated, includes fitting and adjustment

L2126 Knee-ankle-foot-orthosis (KAFO), fracture orthosis, femoral fracture cast orthosis; thermoplastic type casting material, custom fabricated

L2128 custom fabricated

L2132 soft, prefabricated, includes fitting and adjustment

L2134 semi-rigid, prefabricated, includes fitting and adjustment

L2136 rigid, prefabricated, includes fitting and adjustment

ADDITIONS TO FRACTURE ORTHOSIS

L2180 Addition to lower extremity fracture orthosis; plastic shoe insert with ankle joints

L2182 drop lock knee joint

L2184 limited motion knee joint

L2186 adjustable motion knee joint, Lerman type

L2188 quadrilateral brim

L2190 waist belt

L2192 hip joint, pelvic band, thigh flange, and pelvic belt

ADDITIONS TO LOWER EXTREMITY ORTHOSIS

ADDITIONS - SHOE-ANKLE-SHIN-KNEE

L2200 Addition to lower extremity; limited ankle motion, each joint

L2210 dorsiflexion assist (plantar flexion resist), each joint

L2220 dorsiflexion and plantar flexion assist/resist, each joint

L2230 split flat caliper stirrups and plate attachment

L2232 Addition to lower extremity orthosis, rocker bottom for total contact ankle foot orthosis, for custom fabricated orthosis only

L2240 round caliper and plate attachment

L2250 foot plate, molded to patient model, stirrup attachment

L2260 reinforced solid stirrup (Scott-Craig type)

L2265 long tongue stirrup

L2270 varus/valgus correction ("T") strap, padded/lined or malleolus pad

L2275 varus/valgus correction, plastic modification, padded/lined

L2280 molded inner boot

L2300 abduction bar (bilateral hip involvement), jointed, adjustable

L2310 abduction bar-straight

L2320 non-molded lacer, for custom fabricated orthosis only

L2330 lacer molded to patient model, for custom fabricated orthosis only

L2335 anterior swing band

L2340 pre-tibial shell, molded to patient model

L2350 prosthetic type, (BK) socket, molded to patient model, (used for "PTB" "AFO" orthoses)

L2360 extended steel shank

L2370 patten bottom

L2375 torsion control, ankle joint and half solid stirrup

L2380 torsion control, straight knee joint, each joint

L2385 straight knee joint, heavy duty, each joint

L2387 Addition to lower extremity, polycentric knee joint, for custom fabricated knee ankle foot orthosis, each joint

L2390 offset knee joint, each joint

L2395 offset knee joint, heavy duty, each joint

L2397 Addition to lower extremity orthosis, suspension sleeve

ADDITIONS TO STRAIGHT OR OFFSET KNEE JOINTS

L2405 Addition to knee joint, drop lock, each

L2415 Addition to knee lock with integrated release mechanism (bail, cable, or equal), any material, each joint

L2425 Addition to knee joint; disc or dial lock for adjustable knee flexion, each joint

L2430 ratchet lock for active and progressive knee extension, each joint

L2492 lift loop for drop lock ring

ADDITIONS - THIGH/WEIGHT BEARING

GLUTEAL/ISCHIAL WEIGHT

L2500 Addition to lower extremity, thigh/weight bearing; gluteal/ischial weight bearing, ring

L2510 quadrilateral brim, molded to patient model

L2520 quadrilateral brim, custom fitting

L2525 ischial containment/narrow M-L brim molded to patient model

L2526 ischial containment/narrow M-L brim, custom fitted

L2530 lacer, non-molded

L2540 lacer, molded to patient model

L2550 high roll cuff

ADDITIONS - PELVIC AND THORACIC CONTROL

L2570 Addition to lower extremity, pelvic control; hip joint, Clevis type two position joint; each

L2580 pelvic sling

L2600 hip joint, Clevis type, or thrust bearing, free, each

L2610 hip joint, Clevis or thrust bearing, lock, each

L2620 Addition to lower extremity, pelvic control, hip joint; heavy duty, each

L2622 adjustable flexion, each

L2624 adjustable flexion, extension, abduction control, each

L2627 Addition to lower extremity, pelvic control; plastic, molded to patient model, reciprocating hip joint and cables

L2628 metal frame, reciprocating hip joint and cables

L2630 band and belt, unilateral

L2640 band and belt, bilateral

L2650 Addition to lower extremity, pelvic and thoracic control, gluteal pad, each

L2660 Addition to lower extremity, thoracic control; thoracic band

L2670 paraspinal uprights

L2680 lateral support uprights

ADDITIONS - GENERAL

L2750 Addition to lower extremity orthosis; plating chrome or nickel, per bar

L2755 high strength, lightweight material, all hybrid lamination/prepreg composite, per segment, for custom fabricated orthosis only

L2760 extension, per extension, per bar (for lineal adjustment for growth)

L2768 orthotic side bar disconnect device, per bar

L2780 non-corrosive finish, per bar

L2785 drop lock retainer, each

L2795 knee control, full kneecap

L2800 knee control, knee cap, medial or lateral pull, for use with custom fabricated orthosis only

L2810 knee control, condylar pad

L2820 soft interface for molded plastic, below knee section

L2830 soft interface for molded plastic, above knee section

L2840 tibial length sock, fracture or equal, each

L2850 femoral length sock, fracture or equal, each

L2861 Addition to lower extremity joint, knee or ankle, concentric adjustable torsion style mechanism for custom fabricated orthotics only, each

L2999 Lower extremity orthosis, not otherwise specified

FOOT ORTHOPEDIC SHOES, SHOE MODIFICATIONS, TRANSFERS

FOOT, INSERT, REMOVABLE, MOLDED TO PATIENT MODEL

L3000 Foot, insert, removable, molded to patient model; "UCB" type, Berkeley Shell, each
MCM: 2323

L3001 Spenco, each
MCM: 2323

L3002 plastazote or equal, each
MCM: 2323

L3003 silicone gel, each
MCM: 2323

L3010 longitudinal arch support, each
MCM: 2323

L3020 longitudinal/metatarsal support, each
MCM: 2323

L3030 Foot, insert, removable, formed to patient foot, each
MCM: 2323

L3031 Foot, insert/plate, removable, addition to lower extremity orthosis, high strength, lightweight material, all hybrid lamination/prepreg composite, each

FOOT, ARCH SUPPORT, REMOVABLE, PREMOLDED

L3040 Foot, arch support, removable, premolded; longitudinal, each
MCM: 2323

L3050 metatarsal, each
MCM: 2323

L3060 longitudinal/metatarsal, each
MCM: 2323

FOOT, ARCH SUPPORT, NONREMOVABLE, ATTACHED TO SHOE

L3070 Foot, arch support, non-removable attached to shoe; longitudinal, each
MCM: 2323

L3080 metatarsal, each
MCM: 2323

L3090 longitudinal/metatarsal, each
MCM: 2323

▲**L3100** Hallus-valgus night dynamic splint, prefabricated, off-the-shelf
MCM: 2323

ABDUCTION AND ROTATION BARS

L3140 Foot, abduction rotation bar, including shoes
MCM: 2323

L3150 Foot, abduction rotation bars, without shoes
MCM: 2323

L3160 Foot, adjustable shoe-styled positioning device

▲**L3170** Foot, plastic, silicone or equal, heel stabilizer, prefabricated, off-the-shelf, each
MCM: 2323

ORTHOPEDIC FOOTWEAR

L3201 Orthopedic shoe, oxford with supinator or pronator; infant
MCM: 2323

L3202 child
MCM: 2323

L3203 junior
MCM: 2323

L3204 Orthopedic shoe, hightop with supinator or pronator; infant
MCM: 2323

L3206 child
MCM: 2323

L3207 junior

MCM: 2323

L3208 Surgical boot, each; infant
MCM: 2079

L3209 child
MCM: 2079

L3211 junior
MCM: 2079

L3212 Benesch boot, pair; infant
MCM: 2079

L3213 child
MCM: 2079

L3214 junior
MCM: 2079

L3215 Orthopedic footwear, ladies shoe, oxford, each

L3216 depth inlay, each

L3217 hightop, depth inlay, each

L3219 Orthopedic footwear, mens shoe, oxford, each

L3221 depth inlay, each

L3222 hightop, depth inlay, each

L3224 Orthopedic footwear, woman's shoe, oxford, used as an integral part of a brace (orthosis)
MCM: 2323D

L3225 Orthopedic footwear, man's shoe, oxford, used as an integral part of a brace (orthosis)
MCM: 2323D

L3230 Orthopedic footwear, custom shoe, depth inlay, each
MCM: 2323

L3250 Orthopedic footwear, custom molded shoe, removable inner mold, prosthetic shoe, each
MCM: 2323

L3251 Foot, shoe molded to patient model; silicone shoe, each
MCM: 2323

L3252 plastazote (or similar), custom fabricated, each
MCM: 2323

L3253 Foot, molded shoe plastazote (or similar) custom fitted, each
MCM: 2323

L3254 Non-standard size or width
MCM: 2323

L3255 Non-standard size or length
MCM: 2323

L3257 Orthopedic footwear, additional charge for split size
MCM: 2323

L3260 Surgical boot/shoe, each
MCM: 2079

L3265 Plastazote sandal, each

SHOE MODIFICATION

LIFTS

L3300 Lift, elevation; heel, tapered to metatarsal, per inch
MCM: 2323

L3310 heel and sole, neoprene, per inch
MCM: 2323

L3320 heel and sole, cork, per inch
MCM: 2323

L3330 metal extension (skate)
MCM: 2323

L3332 inside shoe, tapered, up to one-half inch
MCM: 2323

L3334 heel, per inch
MCM: 2323

WEDGES

L3340 Heel wedge, SACH
MCM: 2323

L3350 Heel wedge
MCM: 2323

L3360 Sole wedge; outside sole
MCM: 2323

L3370 between sole
MCM: 2323

L3380 Clubfoot wedge
MCM: 2323

L3390 Outflare wedge
MCM: 2323

L3400 Metatarsal bar wedge; rocker
MCM: 2323

L3410 between sole
MCM: 2323

L3420 Full sole and heel wedge, between sole
MCM: 2323

HEELS

L3430 Heel; counter, plastic reinforced
MCM: 2323

L3440 counter, leather reinforced
MCM: 2323

L3450 SACH cushion type
MCM: 2323

L3455 new leather, standard
MCM: 2323

L3460 new rubber, standard
MCM: 2323

L3465 Thomas with wedge
MCM: 2323

L3470 Thomas extended to ball
MCM: 2323

L3480 pad and depression for spur
MCM: 2323

L3485 pad, removable for spur
MCM: 2323

ORTHOPEDIC SHOE ADDITIONS

L3500 Orthopedic shoe addition; insole, leather
MCM: 2323

L3510 insole, rubber
MCM: 2323

L3520 insole, felt covered with leather
MCM: 2323

L3530 sole, half
MCM: 2323

L3540 sole, full
MCM: 2323

L3550 toe tap, standard
MCM: 2323

L3560 toe tap, horseshoe
MCM: 2323

L3570 special extension to instep (leather with eyelets)
MCM: 2323

L3580 convert instep to velcro closure
MCM: 2323

L3590 convert firm shoe counter to soft counter
MCM: 2323

L3595 march bar
MCM: 2323

TRANSFER OR REPLACEMENT

L3600 Transfer of an orthosis from one shoe to another; caliper plate, existing
MCM: 2323

L3610 caliper plate, new
MCM: 2323

L3620 solid stirrup, existing
MCM: 2323

L3630 solid stirrup, new
MCM: 2323

L3640 Dennis Browne splint (Riveton), both shoes

MCM: 2323

L3649 Orthopedic shoe, modification, addition or transfer, not otherwise specified
MCM: 2323

ORTHOTIC DEVICES - UPPER LIMB

NOTE: The procedures in this section are considered as "base" or "basic" procedures and may be modified by listing other procedures from the "additions" section, and adding them to the base procedure.

UPPER LIMB-SHOULDER

▲**L3650** Shoulder orthosis, (SO); figure of eight design abduction restrainer, prefabricated, off-the-shelf

▲**L3660** Shoulder orthosis, figure of eight design abduction restrainer, canvas and webbing, prefabricated, off-the-shelf

▲**L3670** Shoulder orthosis, acromio/clavicular (canvas and webbing type), prefabricated, off-the-shelf

L3671 Shoulder orthosis, shoulder joint design, without joints, may include soft interface, straps, custom fabricated, includes fitting and adjustment

L3674 Shoulder orthosis, abduction positioning (airplane design), thoracic component and support bar, with or without nontorsion joint/turnbuckle, may include soft interface, straps, custom fabricated, includes fitting and adjustment

▲**L3675** Shoulder orthosis, vest type abduction restrainer, canvas webbing type or equal, prefabricated, off-the-shelf

▲**L3677** Shoulder orthosis, shoulder joint design, without joints, may include soft interface, straps, prefabricated item that has been trimmed, bent, molded, assembled, or otherwise customized to fit a specific patient by an individual with expertise
MCM: 2130

●**L3678** Shoulder orthosis, shoulder joint design, without joints, may include soft interface, straps, prefabricated, off-the-shelf

UPPER LIMB-ELBOW

L3702 Elbow orthosis (EO); without joints, may include soft interface, straps, custom fabricated, includes fitting and adjustment

▲**L3710** elastic with metal joints, prefabricated, off-the-shelf

L3720 double upright with forearm/arm cuffs, free motion, custom fabricated

L3730 double upright with forearm/arm cuffs, extension/flexion assist, custom fabricated

L3740 double upright with forearm/arm cuffs, adjustable position lock with active control, custom fabricated

L3760 with adjustable position locking joint(s), prefabricated, includes fitting and adjustment

▲**L3762** Elbow orthosis, rigid, without joints, includes soft interface material, prefabricated, off-the-shelf

L3763 Elbow wrist hand orthosis; rigid, without joints, may include soft interface, straps, custom fabricated, includes fitting and adjustment

L3764 includes one or more nontorsion joints, elastic bands, turnbuckles, may include soft interface, straps, custom fabricated, includes fitting and adjustment

L3765 Elbow wrist hand finger orthosis, rigid, without joints, may include soft interface, straps, custom fabricated, includes fitting and adjustment

L3766 Elbow wrist hand finger orthosis, includes one or more nontorsion joints, elastic bands, turnbuckles, may include soft interface, straps, custom fabricated, includes fitting and adjustment

UPPER LIMB - WRIST-HAND-FINGER

L3806 Wrist-hand-finger-orthosis (WHFO); includes one or more nontorsion joint(s), turnbuckles, elastic bands/springs, may include soft interface material, straps, custom fabricated, includes fitting and adjustment

▲**L3807** without joint(s), prefabricated item that has been trimmed, bent, molded, assembled, or otherwise customized to fit a specific patient by an individual with expertise

L3808 rigid without joints, may include soft interface material; straps, custom fabricated, includes fitting and adjustment

●**L3809** without joint(s), prefabricated, off-the-shelf, any type

ADDITIONS

L3891 Addition to upper extremity joint, wrist or elbow, concentric adjustable torsion style mechanism for custom fabricated orthotics only, each

DYNAMIC FLEXOR HINGE, RECIPROCAL WRIST EXTENSION/FLEXION, FINGER FLEXION/EXTENSION

L3900 Wrist-hand-finger-orthosis, dynamic flexor hinge, reciprocal wrist extension/flexion, finger flexion/extension; wrist or finger driven, custom fabricated

L3901 cable driven, custom fabricated

EXTERNAL POWER

L3904 Wrist-hand-finger-orthosis, external powered; electric, custom fabricated

OTHER WRIST-HAND-FINGER ORTHOSES - CUSTOM FITTED

L3905 Wrist hand orthosis, includes one or more nontorsion joints, elastic bands, turnbuckles, may include soft interface, straps, custom fabricated, includes fitting and adjustment

L3906 Wrist hand orthosis, without joints, may include soft interface, straps, custom fabricated, includes fitting and adjustment

▲**L3908** Wrist hand orthosis, wrist extension control cock-up, non molded, prefabricated, off-the-shelf

▲**L3912** Hand finger orthosis (hof), flexion glove with elastic finger control, prefabricated, off-the-shelf

L3913 Hand finger orthosis, without joints, may include soft interface, straps, custom fabricated, includes fitting and adjustment

▲**L3915** Wrist hand orthosis, includes one or more non torsion joint(s), elastic bands, turnbuckles, may include soft interface, straps, prefabricated item that has been trimmed, bent, molded, assembled, or otherwise customized to fit a specific patient by an individual with expertise

●**L3916** Wrist hand orthosis, includes one or more non torsion joint(s), elastic bands, turnbuckles, may include soft interface, straps, prefabricated, off-the-shelf

▲**L3917** Hand orthosis, metacarpal fracture orthosis, prefabricated item that has been trimmed, bent, molded, assembled, or otherwise customized to fit a specific patient by an individual with expertise

●**L3918** Hand orthosis, metacarpal fracture orthosis, prefabricated, off-the-shelf

L3919 Hand orthosis, without joints, may include soft interface, straps, custom fabricated, includes fitting and adjustment

L3921 Hand finger orthosis, includes one or more nontorsion joints, elastic bands, turnbuckles, may include soft interface, straps, custom fabricated, includes fitting and adjustment

▲**L3923** Hand finger orthosis, without joints, may include soft interface, straps, prefabricated item that has been trimmed, bent, molded, assembled, or otherwise customized to fit a specific patient by an individual with expertise

●**L3924** Hand finger orthosis, without joints, may include soft interface, straps, prefabricated, off-the-shelf

▲**L3925** Finger orthosis, proximal interphalangeal (PIP)/distal interphalangeal (DIP), non torsion joint/spring, extension/flexion, may include soft interface material, prefabricated, off-the-shelf

▲**L3927** Finger orthosis, proximal interphalangeal (PIP)/distal interphalangeal (DIP), without joint/spring, extension/flexion (e.g. static or ring type), may include soft interface material, prefabricated, off-the-shelf

▲**L3929** Hand finger orthosis, includes one or more non torsion joint(s), turnbuckles, elastic bands/springs, may include soft interface material, straps, prefabricated item that has been trimmed, bent, molded, assembled, or otherwise customized to fit a specific patient by an individual with expertise

●**L3930** Hand finger orthosis, includes one or more non torsion joint(s), turnbuckles, elastic bands/springs, may include soft interface material, straps, prefabricated, off-the-shelf

L3931 Wrist hand finger orthosis, includes one or more nontorsion joint(s), turnbuckles, elastic bands/springs, may include soft interface material, straps, prefabricated, includes fitting and adjustment

L3933 Finger orthosis; without joints, may include soft interface, custom fabricated, includes fitting and adjustment

L3935 nontorsion joint, may include soft interface, custom fabricated, includes fitting and adjustment

L3956 Addition of joint to upper extremity orthosis, any material; per joint

UPPER LIMB - SHOULDER-ELBOW-WRIST-HAND

ABDUCTION POSITIONING - CUSTOM FITTED

L3960 Shoulder-elbow-wrist-hand orthoses, (SEWHO); abduction positioning, airplane design, prefabricated, includes fitting and adjustment

L3961 shoulder cap design, without joints, may include soft interface, straps, custom fabricated, includes fitting and adjustment

L3962 abduction positioning, Erbs palsey design, prefabricated, includes fitting and adjustment

(L3964) Code deleted December 31, 2011; see E2626

(L3965) Code deleted December 31, 2011; see E2627

(L3966) Code deleted December 31, 2011; see E2628

L3967 Shoulder elbow wrist hand orthosis, abduction positioning (airplane design), thoracic component and support bar, without joints, may include soft interface, straps, custom fabricated, includes fitting and adjustment

(L3968) Code deleted December 31, 2011; see E2629

(L3969) Code deleted December 31, 2011; see E2630

ADDITIONS TO MOBILE ARM SUPPORTS

(L3970) Code deleted December 31, 2011; see E2631

L3971 Shoulder elbow wrist hand orthosis, shoulder cap design, includes one or more nontorsion joints, elastic bands, turnbuckles, may include soft interface, straps, custom fabricated, includes fitting and adjustment

(L3972) Code deleted December 31, 2011; see E2632

L3973 abduction positioning (airplane design), thoracic component and support bar, includes one or more nontorsion joints, elastic bands, turnbuckles, may include soft interface, straps, custom fabricated, includes fitting and adjustment

(L3974) Code deleted December 31, 2011; see E2633

L3975 without joints, may include soft interface, straps, custom fabricated, includes fitting and adjustment

L3976 abduction positioning (airplane design), thoracic component and support bar, without joints, may include soft interface, straps, custom fabricated, includes fitting and adjustment

L3977 shoulder cap design, includes one or more nontorsion joints, elastic bands, turnbuckles, may include soft interface, straps, custom fabricated, includes fitting and adjustment

L3978 abduction positioning (airplane design), thoracic component and support bar, includes one or more nontorsion joints, elastic bands, turnbuckles, may include soft interface, straps, custom fabricated, includes fitting and adjustment

UPPER LIMB - FRACTURE ORTHOSES

L3980 Upper extremity fracture orthosis; humeral, prefabricated, includes fitting and adjustment

L3982 radius/ulnar, prefabricated, includes fitting and adjustment

L3984 wrist, prefabricated, includes fitting and adjustment

L3995 Addition to upper extremity orthosis, sock, fracture or equal, each

L3999 Upper limb orthosis, not otherwise specified

SPECIFIC REPAIR

L4000 Replace girdle for spinal orthosis (CTLSO or SO)

L4002 Replacement strap, any orthosis, includes all components, any length, any type

L4010 Replace trilateral socket brim

L4020 Replace quadrilateral socket brim; molded to patient model

L4030 custom fitted

L4040 Replace molded thigh lacer, for custom fabricated orthosis only

L4045 Replace non-molded thigh lacer, for custom fabricated orthosis only

L4050 Replace molded calf lacer, for custom fabricated orthosis only

L4055 Replace non-molded calf lacer, for custom fabricated orthosis only

L4060 Replace high roll cuff

L4070 Replace proximal and distal upright for KAFO

L4080 Replace metal bands KAFO, proximal thigh

L4090 Replace metal bands KAFO-AFO, calf or distal thigh

L4100 Replace leather cuff KAFO, proximal thigh

L4110 Replace leather cuff KAFO-AFO, calf or distal thigh

L4130 Replace pretibial shell

REPAIRS

L4205 Repair of orthotic device; labor component, per 15 minutes
MCM: 2100.4

L4210 repair or replace minor parts
MCM: 2133, 2100.4, 2130D

ANCILLARY ORTHOTIC SERVICES

▲**L4350** Ankle control orthosis, stirrup style, rigid, includes any type interface (e.g., pneumatic, gel), prefabricated, off-the-shelf

▲**L4360** Walking boot, pneumatic and/or vacuum, with or without joints, with or without interface material, prefabricated item that has been trimmed, bent, molded, assembled, or otherwise customized to fit a specific patient by an individual with expertise

●**L4361** Walking boot, pneumatic and/or vacuum, with or without joints, with or without interface material, prefabricated, off-the-shelf

▲**L4370** Pneumatic full leg splint, prefabricated, off-the-shelf

(L4380) Code deleted December 31, 2011

▲**L4386** Walking boot, non-pneumatic, with or without joints, with or without interface material, prefabricated item that has been trimmed, bent, molded, assembled, or otherwise customized to fit a specific patient by an individual with expertise

●**L4387** Walking boot, non-pneumatic, with or without joints, with or without interface material, prefabricated, off-the-shelf

L4392 Replacement, soft interface material; static AFO

L4394 foot drop splint

▲**L4396** Static or dynamic ankle foot orthosis, including soft interface material, adjustable for fit, for positioning, may be used for minimal ambulation, prefabricated item that has been trimmed, bent, molded, assembled, or otherwise customized to fit a specific patient by an individual with expertise

●**L4397** Static or dynamic ankle foot orthosis, including soft interface material, adjustable for fit, for positioning, may be used for minimal ambulation, prefabricated, off-the-shelf

▲**L4398** Foot drop splint, recumbent positioning device, prefabricated, off-the-shelf

L4631 Ankle foot orthosis, walking boot type, varus/valgus correction, rocker bottom, anterior tibial shell, soft interface, custom arch support, plastic or other material, includes straps and closures, custom fabricated

This page intentionally left blank

PROSTHETIC PROCEDURES

Guidelines

In addition to the information presented in the INTRODUCTION, several other items unique to this section are defined or identified here:

1. PROSTHETIC DEVICES: Prosthetic devices (other than dental) which replace all or part of an internal body organ (including contiguous tissue), or replace all or part of the function of a permanently inoperative or malfunctioning internal body organ, are covered when furnished upon a physician's order. This does not require a determination that there is no possibility that the patient's condition may improve in the future. If the medical record and the judgement of the attending physician indicate that the condition is of long and indefinite duration, the test of permanence is met. The device(s) may also be covered as a supply item when furnished incident to a physician's service.

2. SUBSECTION INFORMATION: Some of the listed subheadings or subsections have special needs or instructions unique to that section. Where these are indicated, special "notes" will be presented preceding or following the listings. Those subsections within the PROSTHETIC PROCEDURES section that have "notes" are as follows:

Subsection	Code Numbers
Prosthetic procedures-lower limb	L5000-L5999
Upper limb	L6000-L6590
Additions-upper limb	L6600-L6999

3. UNLISTED SERVICE OR PROCEDURE: A service or procedure may be provided that is not listed in this edition of HCPCS. When reporting such a service, the appropriate "unlisted procedure" code may be used to indicate the service, identifying it by "special report" as defined below. HCPCS terminology is inconsistent in defining unlisted procedures. The procedure definition may include the term(s) "unlisted", "not otherwise classified", "unspecified", "unclassified", "other" and "miscellaneous". Prior to using these codes, try to determine if a Local Level III code or CPT code is available. The "unlisted procedures" and accompanying codes for PROSTHETIC PROCEDURES are as follows:

L5999	Lower extremity prosthesis, not otherwise specified
L7499	Upper extremity prosthesis, not otherwise specified
L8039	Breast prosthesis, not otherwise specified
L8239	Gradient compression stocking, not otherwise specified
L8499	Unlisted procedure for miscellaneous prosthetic services
L8699	Prosthetic implant, not otherwise specified

4. SPECIAL REPORT: A service, material or supply that is rarely provided, unusual, variable or new may require a special report in determining medical appropriateness for reimbursement purposes. Pertinent information should include an adequate definition or description of the nature, extent, and need for the service, material or supply.

5. MODIFIERS: Listed services may be modified under certain circumstances. When appropriate, the modifying circumstance is identified by adding a modifier to the basic procedure code. CPT and HCPCS National Level II modifiers may be used with CPT and HCPCS National Level II procedure codes. Modifiers commonly used with PROSTHETIC PROCEDURES are as follows:

   -CC Procedure code change (use “CC” when the procedure code submitted was changed either for administrative reasons or because an incorrect code was filed)

   -LT Left side (used to identify procedures performed on the left side of the body)

   -RT Right side (used to identify procedures performed on the right side of the body)

   -TC Technical component. Under certain circumstances, a charge may be made for the technical component alone. Under those circumstances, the technical component charge is identified by adding modifier -TC to the usual procedure number. Technical component charges are institutional charges and are not billed separately by physicians. However, portable x-ray suppliers bill only for the technical component and should use modifier -TC. The charge data from portable x-ray suppliers will then be used to build customary and prevailing profiles.

6. CPT CODE CROSS-REFERENCE: Unless otherwise specified, the equivalent CPT code for all listings in this section is 99070.

7. DURABLE MEDICAL EQUIPMENT REGIONAL CARRIERS (DMERCS): Effective October 1, 1993 claims for prosthetics must be billed to one of four regional carriers depending upon the

residence of the beneficiary. The transition dates for DMERC claims is from November 1, 1993 to March 1, 1994, depending upon the state you practice in. See the Introduction for a complete discussion of DMERCs.

Prosthetic Procedures

LOWER LIMB

NOTE: The procedures in this section are considered as "base" or "basic" procedures, and they may be modified by listing items, procedures or special materials from the "additions" section, and adding them to the base procedure.

LOWER LIMB-PARTIAL FOOT

L5000 Partial foot; shoe insert with longitudinal arch, toe filler
MCM: 2323

L5010 molded socket, ankle height, with toe filler
MCM: 2323

L5020 molded socket, tibial tubercle height, with toe filler
MCM: 2323

LOWER LIMB-ANKLE

L5050 Ankle, symes; molded socket, SACH foot

L5060 metal frame, molded leather socket, articulated ankle/foot

LOWER LIMB-BELOW KNEE

L5100 Below knee; molded socket, shin, SACH foot

L5105 plastic socket, joints and thigh lacer, SACH foot

LOWER LIMB-KNEE DISARTICULATION

L5150 Knee disarticulation (or through knee), molded socket; external knee joints, shin, SACH foot

L5160 bent knee configuration, external knee joints, shin, SACH foot

LOWER LIMB-ABOVE KNEE

L5200 Above knee; molded socket, single axis constant friction knee, shin, SACH foot

L5210 short prosthesis, no knee joint ("stubbies"), with foot blocks, no ankle joints, each

L5220 short prosthesis, no knee joint ("stubbies"), with articulated ankle/foot, dynamically aligned, each

L5230 for proximal femoral focal deficiency, constant friction knee, shin, each foot

LOWER LIMB-HIP DISARTICULATION

L5250 Hip disarticulation; Canadian type, molded socket, hip joint, single axis constant friction knee, shin, SACH foot

L5270 tilt table type; molded socket, locking hip joint, single axis constant friction knee, shin, SACH foot

LOWER LIMB-HEMIPELVECTOMY

L5280 Hemipelvectomy, canadian type; molded socket, hip joint, single axis constant friction knee, shin, SACH foot

LOWER LIMB-ENDOSKELETAL-BELOW KNEE

L5301 Below knee, molded socket, shin, each foot, endoskeletal system

LOWER LIMB-ENDOSKELETAL-KNEE DISARTICULATION

(L5311) Code deleted December 31, 2011

L5312 Knee disarticulation (or through knee), molded socket, single axis knee, pylon, SACH foot, endoskeletal system

LOWER LIMB-ENDOSKELETAL-ABOVE KNEE

L5321 Above knee, molded socket, open end, sach foot, endoskeletal system, single axis knee

LOWER LIMB-ENDOSKELETAL-HIP DISARTICULATION

L5331 Hip disarticulation, Canadian type, molded socket, endoskeletal system, hip joint, single axis knee, sach foot

LOWER LIMB-ENDOSKELETAL-HEMIPELVECTOMY

L5341 Hemipelvectomy, Canadian type, molded socket, endoskeletal system, hip joint, single axis knee, sach foot

IMMEDIATE POST SURGICAL OR EARLY FITTING PROCEDURES

L5400 Immediate post surgical or early fitting; application of initial rigid dressing, including fitting, alignment, suspension, and one cast change, below knee

L5410 application of initial rigid dressing, including fitting, alignment and suspension, below knee, each additional cast change and realignment

L5420 application of initial rigid dressing, including fitting, alignment and suspension and one cast change "AK" or knee disarticulation

L5430 application of initial rigid dressing, including fitting, alignment and suspension, "AK" or knee disarticulation, each additional cast change and realignment

L5450 application of non-weight bearing rigid dressing, below knee

L5460 application of non-weight bearing rigid dressing, above knee

INITIAL PROSTHESIS

L5500 Initial, below knee "PTB" type socket, non-alignable system, pylon, no cover, SACH foot, plaster socket, direct formed

L5505 Initial, above knee - knee disarticulation, ischial level socket non-alignable system, pylon, no cover, SACH foot plaster socket, direct formed

PREPARATORY PROSTHESIS

L5510 Preparatory, below knee "PTB" type socket, non-alignable system, pylon, no cover, SACH foot; plaster socket, molded to model

L5520 thermoplastic or equal, direct formed

L5530 thermoplastic or equal, molded to model

L5535 Preparatory, below knee "PTB" type socket, non-alignable system, no cover, SACH foot, prefabricated, adjustable open end socket

L5540 Preparatory, below knee "PTB" type socket, non-alignable system, pylon, no cover, SACH foot, laminated socket, molded to model

L5560 Preparatory, above knee - knee disarticulation, ischial level socket, non-alignable system, pylon, no cover, SACH foot; plaster socket, molded to model

L5570 thermoplastic or equal, direct formed

L5580 thermoplastic or equal, molded to model

L5585 prefabricated adjustable open end socket

L5590 laminated socket, molded to model

L5595 Preparatory, hip disarticulation-hemipelvectomy, pylon, no cover, SACH foot; thermoplastic or equal, molded to patient model

L5600 laminated socket, molded to patient model

ADDITIONS TO LOWER EXTREMITY

L5610 Addition to lower extremity, endoskeletal system; above knee, hydracadence system

L5611 above knee - knee disarticulation, 4-bar linkage, with friction swing phase control

L5613 above knee-knee disarticulation, 4-bar linkage, with hydraulic swing phase control

L5614 above knee-knee disarticulation, 4-bar linkage, with pneumatic swing phase control

L5616 above knee, universal multiplex system, friction swing phase control

L5617 Addition to lower extremity, quick change self-aligning unit, above knee or below knee, each

ADDITIONS - TEST SOCKETS

L5618 Addition to lower extremity, test socket; Symes

L5620 below knee

L5622 knee disarticulation

L5624 above knee

L5626 hip disarticulation

L5628 hemipelvectomy

L5629 Addition to lower extremity, below knee, acrylic socket

ADDITIONS - SOCKET VARIATIONS

L5630 Addition to lower extremity, Symes type, expandable wall socket

L5631 Addition to lower extremity, above knee or knee disarticulation, acrylic socket

L5632 Addition to lower extremity, Symes type; "PTB" brim design socket

L5634 posterior opening (Canadian) socket

L5636 medial opening socket

L5637 Addition to lower extremity, below knee; total contact

L5638 leather socket

L5639 wood socket

L5640 Addition to lower extremity, knee disarticulation, leather socket

L5642 Addition to lower extremity, above knee, leather socket

L5643 Addition to lower extremity, hip disarticulation, flexible inner socket, external frame

L5644 Addition to lower extremity, above knee, wood socket

L5645 Addition to lower extremity, below knee; flexible inner socket, external frame

L5646 air, fluid, gel or equal, cushion socket

L5647 suction socket

L5648 Addition to lower extremity, above knee, air, fluid, gel or equal, cushion socket

L5649 Addition to lower extremity, ischial containment/narrow M-L socket

L5650 Addition to lower extremity, total contact, above knee or knee disarticulation socket

L5651 Addition to lower extremity, above knee, flexible inner socket, external frame

L5652 Addition to lower extremity, suction suspension, above knee or knee disarticulation socket

L5653 Addition to lower extremity, knee disarticulation, expandable wall socket

ADDITIONS - SOCKET INSERT AND SUSPENSION

L5654 Addition to lower extremity, socket insert; Symes, (Kemblo, Pelite, Aliplast, Plastazote or equal)

L5655 below knee (Kemblo, Pelite, Aliplast, Plastazote or equal)

L5656 knee disarticulation, (Kemblo, Pelite, Aliplast, Plastazote or equal)

L5658 above knee (Kemblo, Pelite, Aliplast, Plastazote or equal)

L5661 multi-durometer Symes

L5665 multi-durometer, below knee

L5666 Addition to lower extremity; below knee, cuff suspension

L5668 Addition to lower extremity; below knee, molded distal cushion

L5670 Addition to lower extremity; below knee, molded supracondylar suspension ("PTS" or similar)

L5671 Addition to lower extremity; below knee/above knee suspension locking mechanism (shuttle, lanyard or equal), excludes socket insert

L5672 below knee, removable medial brim suspension

L5673 below knee/above knee, custom fabricated from existing mold or prefabricated, socket insert, silicone gel, elastomeric or equal, for use with locking mechanism

L5676 below knee, knee joints, single axis, pair

L5677 below knee, knee joints, polycentric, pair

L5678 below knee, joint covers, pair

L5679 below knee/above knee, custom fabricated from existing mold or prefabricated, socket insert, silicone gel, elastomeric or equal, not for use with locking mechanism

L5680 below knee, thigh lacer, non-molded

L5681 below knee/above knee, custom fabricated socket insert for congenital or atypical traumatic amputee, silicone gel, elastomeric or equal, for use with or without locking mechanism, initial only (for other than initial, use code L5673 or L5679)

L5682 below knee, thigh lacer, gluteal/ischial, molded

L5683 below knee/above knee, custom fabricated socket insert for other than congenital or atypical traumatic amputee, silicone gel elastomeric or equal, for use with or without locking mechanism, initial only (for other than initial, use code L5673 or L5679)

L5684 below knee, fork strap

L5685 Addition to lower extremity prosthesis, below knee, suspension/sealing sleeve, with or without valve, any material, each

L5686 below knee, back check (extension control)

L5688 below knee, waist belt, webbing

L5690 below knee, waist belt, padded and lined

L5692 Addition to lower extremity, above knee; pelvic control belt, light

L5694 pelvic control belt, padded and lined

L5695 pelvic control, sleeve suspension, neoprene or equal, each

L5696 Addition to lower extremity, above knee or knee disarticulation; pelvic joint

L5697 pelvic band

L5698 silesian bandage

L5699 All lower extremity protheses, shoulder harness

L5700 Replacement, socket; below knee, molded to patient model

L5701 above knee/knee disarticulation, including attachment plate, molded to patient model

L5702 hip disarticulation, including hip joint, molded to patient model

L5703 Ankle, symes, molded to patient model, socket without solid ankle cushion heel (Sach) foot, replacement only

L5704 Custom shaped protective cover, below knee

L5705 Custom shaped protective cover, above knee

L5706 Custom shaped protective cover, knee disarticulation

L5707 Custom shaped protective cover, hip disarticulation

ADDITIONS - KNEE-SHIN SYSTEM

EXOSKELETAL

L5710 Addition, exoskeletal knee-shin system, single axis; manual lock

L5711 manual lock, ultra-light material

L5712 friction swing and stance phase control (safety knee)

L5714 variable friction swing phase control

L5716 Addition, exoskeletal knee-shin system, polycentric; mechanical stance phase lock

L5718 friction swing and stance phase control

L5722 Addition, exoskeletal knee-shin system, single axis; pneumatic swing, friction stance phase control

L5724 fluid swing phase control

L5726 external joints fluid swing phase control

L5728 fluid swing and stance phase control

L5780 pneumatic/hydrapneumatic swing phase control

L5781 Addition to lower limb prosthesis, vacuum pump, residual limb volume management and moisture evacuation system

L5782 Addition to lower limb prosthesis, vacuum pump, residual limb volume management and moisture evacuation system, heavy duty

L5785 Addition, exoskeletal system, below knee, ultra-light material (titanium, carbon fiber or equal)

L5790 Addition, exoskeletal system, above knee, ultra-light material (titanium, carbon fiber or equal)

L5795 Addition, exoskeletal system, hip disarticulation, ultra-light material (titanium, carbon fiber or equal)

ENDOSKELETAL

L5810 Addition, endoskeletal knee-shin system, single axis; manual lock

L5811 manual lock, ultra-light material

L5812 friction swing and stance phase control (safety knee)

L5814 Addition, endoskeletal knee-shin system, polycentric; hydraulic swing phase control, mechanical stance phase lock

L5816 mechanical stance phase lock

L5818 friction swing and stance phase control

L5822 Addition, endoskeletal knee-shin system, single axis; pneumatic swing, friction stance phase control

L5824 fluid swing phase control

L5826 hydraulic swing phase control, with miniature high activity frame

L5828 fluid swing and stance phase control

L5830 pneumatic swing phase control

L5840 Addition, endoskeletal knee-shin system, 4-bar linkage or multiaxial, pneumatic swing phase control

L5845 Addition, endoskeletal, knee-shin system; stance flexion feature, adjustable

L5848 Addition to endoskeletal, knee-shin system, fluid stance extension, dampening feature, with or without adjustability

L5850 Addition, endoskeletal system; above knee or hip disarticulation, knee extension assist

L5855 hip disarticulation, mechanical hip extension assist

L5856 Addition to lower extremity prosthesis, endoskeletal knee-shin system, microprocessor control feature, swing and stance phase, includes electronic sensor(s), any type

L5857 Addition to lower extremity prosthesis, endoskeletal knee-shin system, microprocessor control feature, swing phase only, includes electronic sensor(s), any type

L5858 Addition to lower extremity prosthesis, endoskeletal knee shin system, microprocessor control feature, stance phase only, includes electronic sensor(s), any type

L5859 Addition to lower extremity prosthesis, endoskeletal knee-shin system, powered and programmable flexion/extension assist control, includes any type motor(s)

L5910 Addition, endoskeletalsystem; below knee, alignable system

L5920 above knee or hip disarticulation, alignable system

L5925 above knee, knee disarticulation or hip disarticulation, manual lock

L5930 Addition, endoskeletal system; high activity knee control frame

L5940 below knee, ultra-light material (titanium, carbon fiber or equal)

L5950 above knee, ultra-light material (titanium, carbon fiber or equal)

L5960 hip disarticulation, ultra-light material (titanium, carbon fiber or equal)

L5961 polycentric hip joint, pneumatic or hydraulic control, rotation control, with or without flexion and/or extension control

L5962 below knee, flexible protective outer surface covering system

L5964 above knee, flexible protective outer surface covering system

L5966 hip disarticulation, flexible protective outer surface covering system

L5968 Addition to lower limb prosthesis, multiaxial ankle with swing phase active dorsiflexion feature

● **L5969** Addition, endoskeletal ankle-foot or ankle system, power assist, includes any type motor(s)

L5970 All lower extremity prostheses; foot, external keel, each foot

L5971 All lower extremity prosthesis, solid ankle cushion heel (sach) foot, replacement only

L5972 flexible keel foot (Safe, Sten, Bock Dynamic or equal)

L5973 Endoskeletal ankle foot system, microprocessor controlled feature, dorsiflexion and/or plantar flexion control, includes power source

L5974 All lower extremity prosthesis, foot, single axis ankle/foot

L5975 All lower extremity prosthesis; combination single axis ankle and flexible keel foot

L5976 energy storing foot (Seattle Carbon Copy II or equal)

L5978 foot, multiaxial ankle/foot

L5979 multiaxial ankle, dynamic response foot, one piece system

L5980 flex foot system

L5981 flex-walk system or equal

L5982 All exoskeletal lower extremity prostheses, axial rotation unit

L5984 All endoskeletal lower extremity prostheses, axial rotation unit, with or without adjustability

L5985 All endoskeletal lower extremity prostheses, dynamic prosthetic pylon

L5986 All lower extremity prostheses, multi-axial rotation unit ("MCP" or equal)

L5987 All lower extremity prosthesis, shank foot system with vertical loading pylon

L5988 Addition to lower limb prosthesis, vertical shock reducing pylon feature

L5990 Addition to lower extremity prothesis; user adjustable heel height

L5999 Lower extremity prosthesis, not otherwise specified

UPPER LIMB

NOTE: The procedures in L6000-L6599 are considered as "base" or "basic" procedures and may be modified by listing procedures from the "additions" sections. The base procedures include only standard friction wrist and control cable system unless otherwise specified.

UPPER LIMB-PARTIAL HAND

L6000 Partial hand; thumb remaining

L6010 little and/or ring ringer remaining

L6020 no finger remaining

L6025 Transcarpal/metacarpal or partial hand disarticulation prosthesis, external power, self-suspended, inner socket with removable forearm section, electrodes and cables, two batteries, charger, myoelectric control of terminal device

UPPER LIMB-WRIST DISARTICULATION

L6050 Wrist disarticulation, molded socket, flexible elbow hinges, triceps pad

UPPER LIMB-BELOW ELBOW

L6055 Wrist disarticulation, molded socket with expandable interface, flexible elbow hinges, triceps pad

L6100 Below elbow, molded socket; flexible elbow hinge, triceps pad

L6110 (Muenster or Northwestern Suspension types)

L6120 Below elbow, molded double wall split socket; step-up hinges, half cuff

L6130 stump activated locking hinge, half cuff

UPPER LIMB-ELBOW DISARTICULATION

L6200 Elbow disarticulation, molded socket, outside locking hinge, forearm

UPPER LIMB-ABOVE ELBOW

L6205 Elbow disarticulation, molded socket with expandable interface, outside locking hinges, forearm

L6250 Above elbow, molded double wall socket, internal locking elbow, forearm

UPPER LIMB-SHOULDER DISARTICULATION

L6300 Shoulder disarticulation, molded socket, shoulder bulkhead, humeral section, internal locking elbow, forearm

L6310 Shoulder disarticulation, passive restoration; (complete prosthesis)

L6320 (shoulder cap only)

UPPER LIMB-INTERSCAPULAR THORACIC

L6350 Interscapular thoracic; molded socket, shoulder bulkhead, humeral section, internal locking elbow, forearm

L6360 passive restoration (complete prosthesis)

L6370 passive restoration (shoulder cap only)

UPPER LIMB-IMMEDIATE AND EARLY POST SURGICAL PROCEDURES

L6380 Immediate post surgical or early fitting, application of initial rigid dressing, including fitting alignment and suspension of components, and one cast change; wrist disarticulation or below elbow

L6382 elbow disarticulation or above elbow

L6384 shoulder disarticulation or interscapular thoracic

L6386 Immediate post surgical or early fitting; each additional cast change and realignment

L6388 application of rigid dressing only

UPPER LIMB-ENDOSKELETAL-BELOW ELBOW

L6400 Below elbow, molded socket endoskeletal system, including soft prosthetic tissue shaping

UPPER LIMB-ENDOSKELETAL-ELBOW DISARTICULATION

L6450 Elbow disarticulation, molded socket, endoskeletal system, including soft prosthetic tissue shaping

UPPER LIMB-ENDOSKELETAL-ABOVE ELBOW

L6500 Above elbow, molded socket, endoskeletal system, including soft prosthetic tissue shaping

UPPER LIMB-ENDOSKELETAL-SHOULDER DISARTICULATION

L6550 Shoulder disarticulation, molded socket, endoskeletal system, including soft prosthetic tissue shaping

UPPER LIMB-ENDOSKELETAL-INTERSCAPULAR THORACIC

L6570 Interscapular thoracic, molded socket, endoskeletal system, including soft prosthetic tissue shaping

L6580 Preparatory, wrist disarticulation or below elbow, single wall plastic socket, friction wrist, flexible elbow hinges, figure of eight harness, humeral cuff, Bowden cable control, USMC or equal pylon, no cover, molded to patient model

L6582 Preparatory, wrist disarticulation or below elbow, single wall socket, friction wrist, flexible elbow hinges, figure of eight harness, humeral cuff, bowden cable control, USMC or equal pylon, no cover, direct formed

L6584 Preparatory, elbow disarticulation or above elbow; single wall plastic socket, friction wrist, locking elbow, figure of eight harness, fair lead cable control, USMC or equal pylon, no cover, molded to patient model

L6586 single wall socket, friction wrist, locking elbow, figure of eight harness, fair lead cable control, USMC or equal pylon, no cover, direct formed

L6588 Preparatory shoulder disarticulation or interscapular thoracic; single wall plastic socket, shoulder joint, locking elbow, friction wrist, chest strap, fair lead cable control, USMC or equal pylon, no cover, molded to patient model

L6590 single wall socket, shoulder joint, locking elbow, friction wrist, chest strap, fair lead cable control, USMC or equal pylon, no cover, direct formed

ADDITIONS - UPPER LIMB

NOTE: The following procedures, modifications and/or components may be added to other base procedures. The items in this section should reflect the additional complexity of each modification procedure, in addition to base procedure, at the time of the original order.

L6600 Upper extremity additions; polycentric hinge, pair

L6605 single pivot hinge, pair

L6610 flexible metal hinge, pair

L6611 Addition to upper extremity prosthesis, external powered, additional switch, any type

L6615 Upper extremity addition; disconnect locking wrist unit

L6616 additional disconnect insert for locking wrist unit, each

L6620 flexion/extension wrist unit, with or without friction

L6621 flexion/extension wrist with or without friction, for use with external powered terminal device

L6623 spring assisted rotational wrist unit with latch release

L6624 flexion/extension and rotation wrist unit

L6625 rotation wrist unit with cable lock

L6628 quick disconnect hook adapter, Otto Bock or equal

L6629 quick disconnect lamination collar with coupling piece, Otto Bock or equal

L6630 stainless steel, any wrist

L6632 latex suspension sleeve, each

L6635 lift assist for elbow

L6637 nudge control elbow lock

L6638 Upper extremity addition to prosthesis, electric locking feature, only for use with manually powered elbow

L6640 Upper extremity addition; shoulder abduction joint, pair

L6641 excursion amplifier, pulley type

L6642 excursion amplifier, lever type

L6645 shoulder flexion - abduction joint, each

L6646 Upper extremity addition, shoulder joint, multipositional locking, flexion, adjustable abduction friction control, for use with body powered or external powered system

L6647 Upper extremity addition, shoulder lock mechanism, body powered actuator

L6648 Upper extremity addition; shoulder lock mechanism, external powered actuator

L6650 shoulder universal joint, each

L6655 standard control cable, extra

L6660 heavy duty control cable

L6665 teflon, or equal, cable lining

L6670 hook to hand, cable adapter

L6672 harness, chest or shoulder, saddle type

L6675 harness, (eg., figure of eight type), single cable design

L6676 harness, (eg., figure of eight type), dual cable design

L6677 harness, triple control, simultaneous operation of terminal device and elbow

L6680 test socket, wrist disarticulation or below elbow

L6682 test socket, elbow disarticulation or above elbow

L6684 test socket, shoulder disarticulation or interscapular thoracic

L6686 suction socket

L6687 frame type socket, below elbow or wrist disarticulation

L6688 frame type socket, above elbow or elbow disarticulation

L6689 frame type socket, shoulder disarticulation

L6690 frame type socket, interscapular-thoracic

L6691 removable insert, each

L6692 silicone gel insert or equal, each

L6693 locking elbow, forearm counterbalance

L6694 Addition to upper extremity prosthesis, below elbow/above elbow, custom fabricated from existing mold or prefabricated, socket insert, silicone gel, elastomeric or equal, for use with locking mechanism

L6695 Addition to upper extremity prosthesis, below elbow/above elbow, custom fabricated from existing mold or prefabricated, socket insert, silicone gel, elastomeric or equal, not for use with locking mechanism

L6696 Addition to upper extremity prosthesis, below elbow/above elbow, custom fabricated socket insert for congenital or atypical traumatic amputee, silicone gel, elastomeric or equal, for use with or without locking mechanism, initial only (for other than initial, use code L6694 or L6695)

L6697 Addition to upper extremity prosthesis, below elbow/above elbow, custom fabricated socket insert for other than congenital or atypical traumatic amputee, silicone gel, elastomeric or equal, for use with or without locking mechanism, initial only (for other than initial, use code L6694 or L6695)

L6698 Addition to upper extremity prosthesis, below elbow/above elbow, lock mechanism, excludes socket insert

TERMINAL DEVICES

HOOKS

L6703 Terminal device, passive hand/mitt, any material, any size

L6704 Terminal device, sport/recreational/work attachment, any material, any size

L6706 Terminal device, hook, mechanical, voluntary opening, any material, any size, lined or unlined

L6707 Terminal device, hook, mechanical, voluntary closing, any material, any size, lined or unlined

L6708 Terminal device, hand, mechanical, voluntary opening, any material, any size

L6709 Terminal device, hand, mechanical, voluntary closing, any material, any size

L6711 Terminal device, hook, mechanical, voluntary opening, any material, any size, lined or unlined, pediatric

L6712 Terminal device, hook, mechanical, voluntary closing, any material, any size, lined or unlined, pediatric

L6713 Terminal device, hand, mechanical, voluntary opening, any material, any size, pediatric

L6714 Terminal device, hand, mechanical, voluntary closing, any material, any size, pediatric

L6715 Terminal device, multiple articulating digit, includes motor(s), initial issue or replacement

L6721 Terminal device, hook or hand, heavy duty, mechanical, voluntary opening, any material, any size, lined or unlined

L6722 Terminal device, hook or hand, heavy duty, mechanical, voluntary closing, any material, any size, lined or unlined

L6805 Addition to terminal device; modifier wrist unit
MCM: 2133

L6810 Addition to terminal device; precision pinch device
MCM: 2133

HANDS

L6880 Electric hand, switch or myoelectric controlled, independently articulating digits, any grasp pattern or combination of grasp patterns, includes motor(s)

L6881 Automatic grasp feature, addition to upper limb electric prosthetic terminal device

L6882 Microprocessor control feature, addition to upper limb prosthetic terminal device
MCM: 2133

L6883 Replacement socket, below elbow/wrist disarticulation, molded to patient model, for use with or without external power

L6884 Replacement socket, above elbow/elbow disarticulation, molded to patient model, for use with or without external power

L6885 Replacement socket, shoulder disarticulation/interscapular thoracic, molded to patient model, for use with or without external power

GLOVES FOR ABOVE HANDS

L6890 Addition to upper extremity prosthesis, glove for terminal device, any material, prefabricated, includes fitting and adjustment

L6895 Addition to upper extremity prosthesis, glove for terminal device, any material, custom fabricated

HAND RESTORATION

L6900 Hand restoration (casts, shading and measurements included), partial hand; with glove, thumb or one finger remaining

L6905 with glove, multiple fingers remaining

L6910 with glove, no fingers remaining

L6915 Hand restoration (shading, and measurements included), replacement glove for above

EXTERNAL POWER - BASE DEVICES

L6920 Wrist disarticulation, external power, self-suspended inner socket, removable forearm shell, Otto Bock or equal; switch, cables, two batteries and one charger, switch control of terminal device

L6925 electrodes, cables, two batteries and one charger, myoelectronic control of terminal device

L6930 Below elbow, external power, self-suspended inner socket, removable forearm shell; Otto Bock or equal switch, cables, two batteries and one charger, switch control of terminal device

L6935 Otto Bock or equal electrodes, cables, two batteries and one charger, myoelectronic control of terminal device

L6940 Elbow disarticulation, external power, molded inner socket, removable humeral shell, outside locking hinges, forearm; Otto Bock or equal switch, cables, two batteries and one charger, switch control of terminal device

L6945 Otto Bock or equal electrodes, cables, two batteries and one charger, myoelectronic control of terminal device

L6950 Above elbow, external power, molded inner socket, removable humeral shell, internal locking elbow, forearm; Otto Bock or equal switch, cables two batteries and one charger, switch control of terminal device

L6955 Otto Bock or equal electrodes, cables, two batteries and one charger, myoelectronic control of terminal device

L6960 Shoulder disarticulation, external power, molded inner socket, removable shoulder shell, shoulder bulkhead, humeral section, mechanical elbow, forearm; Otto Bock or equal switch, cables, two batteries and one charger, switch control of terminal device

L6965 Otto Bock or equal electrodes, cables, two batteries and one charger, myoelectronic control of terminal device

L6970 Interscapular-thoracic, external power, molded inner socket removable shoulder shell, shoulder bulkhead, humeral section, mechanical elbow, forearm; Otto Bock or equal switch, cables, two batteries and one charger, switch control of terminal device

L6975 Otto Bock or equal electrodes cables, two batteries and one charger, myoelectronic control of terminal device

EXTERNAL POWER - TERMINAL DEVICES

L7007 Electric hand, switch or myoelectric controlled; adult

L7008 pediatric

L7009 Electric hook, switch or myoelectric controlled, adult

L7040 Prehensile actuator, switch controlled

L7045 Electronic hook, switch or myoelectric controlled, pediatric

EXTERNAL POWER - ELBOW

L7170 Electronic elbow; hosmer or equal, switch controlled

L7180 microprocessor sequential control of elbow and terminal device

L7181 Electronic elbow, microprocessor simultaneous control of elbow and terminal device

L7185 adolescent, Variety Village or equal, switch controlled

L7186 child, Variety Village or equal, switch controlled

L7190 adolescent, Variety Village or equal, myoelectronically controlled

L7191 child, Variety Village or equal, myoelectronically controlled

EXTERNAL POWER - CONTROL MODULES

L7260 Electronic wrist rotator; Otto Bock or equal

L7261 for Utah arm

(L7266) Code deleted December 31, 2011

(L7272) Code deleted December 31, 2011

(L7274 Code deleted December 31, 2011

EXTERNAL POWER - BATTERY COMPONENTS

L7360 Six volt battery, each

L7362 Battery charger, six volt, each

L7364 Twelve volt battery, each

L7366 Battery charger, twelve volt, each

L7367 Lithium ion battery, replacement

L7368 Lithium ion battery charger, replacement only

L7400 Addition to upper extremity prosthesis; below elbow/wrist disarticulation, ultralight material (titanium, carbon fiber or equal)

L7401 above elbow disarticulation, ultralight material (titanium, carbon fiber or equal)

L7402 shoulder disarticulation/interscapular thoracic, ultralight material (titanium, carbon fiber or equal)

L7403 below elbow/wrist disarticulation, acrylic material

L7404 above elbow disarticulation, acrylic material

L7405 shoulder disarticulation/interscapular thoracic, acrylic material

L7499 Upper extremity prosthesis, not otherwise specified

REPAIRS

(L7500) Code deleted December 31, 2011

L7510 Repair of prosthetic device, repair or replace minor parts
MCM: 2100.4, 2130D, 2133

L7520 Repair prosthetic device, labor component, per 15 minutes

L7600 Prosthetic donning sleeve, any material, each

L7900 Male vacuum erection system

L7902 Tension ring, for vacuum erection device, any type, replacement only, each

GENERAL - BREAST PROSTHESES

L8000 Breast prosthesis; mastectomy bra
MCM: 2130.A

L8001 Breast prosthesis, mastectomy bra, with integrated breast prosthesis form, unilateral
MCM: 2130.A

L8002 Breast prosthesis, mastectomy bra, with integrated breast prosthesis form, bilateral
MCM: 2130.A

L8010 mastectomy sleeve
MCM: 2130.A

L8015 External breast prosthesis garment, with mastectomy form, post mastectomy
MCM: 2130

L8020 Breast prosthesis; mastectomy form
MCM: 2130.A

L8030 silicone or equal, without integral adhesive
MCM: 2130.A

L8031 Breast prosthesis; silicone or equal, with integral adhesive
MCM 2130A

L8032 Nipple prosthesis, reusable, any type, each

L8035 Custom breast prosthesis, post mastectomy, molded to patient model
MCM: 2130

L8039 Breast prosthesis, not otherwise specified

L8040 Nasal prosthesis, provided by a non-physician

L8041 Midfacial prosthesis, provided by a non-physician

L8042 Orbital prosthesis, provided by a non-physician

L8043 Upper facial prosthesis, provided by a non-physician

L8044 Hemi-facial prosthesis, provided by a non-physician

L8045 Auricular prosthesis, provided by a non-physician

L8046 Partial facial prosthesis, provided by a non-physician

L8047 Nasal septal prosthesis, provided by a non-physician

L8048 Unspecified maxillofacial prosthesis, by report, provided by a non-physician

L8049 Repair or modification of maxillofacial prosthesis, labor component, 15 minute increments, provided by a non-physician

GENERAL - TRUSSES

L8300 Truss; single with standard pad
CIM: 70-1, 70-2 MCM: 2133

L8310 double with standard pads
CIM: 70-1, 70-2 MCM: 2133

L8320 addition to standard pad, water pad
CIM: 70-1, 70-2 MCM: 2133

L8330 addition to standard pad, scrotal pad
CIM: 70-1, 70-2 MCM: 2133

PROSTHETIC SOCKS

L8400 Prosthetic sheath; below knee, each
MCM: 2133

L8410 above knee, each
MCM: 2133

L8415 upper limb, each
MCM: 2133

L8417 Prosthetic sheath/sock, including a gel cushion layer, below knee or above knee, each

L8420 Prosthetic sock, multiple ply; below knee, each
MCM: 2133

L8430 above knee, each
MCM: 2133

L8435 upper limb, each
MCM: 2133

L8440 Prosthetic shrinker; below knee, each
MCM: 2133

L8460 above knee, each
MCM: 2133

L8465 upper limb, each
MCM: 2133

L8470 Prosthetic sock, single ply, fitting; below knee, each
MCM: 2133

L8480 above knee, each
MCM: 2133

L8485 upper limb, each
MCM: 2133

L8499 Unlisted procedure for miscellaneous prosthetic services

PROSTHETIC IMPLANTS

L8500 Artificial larynx, any type
CIM: 65-5 MCM: 2130

L8501 Tracheostomy speaking valve
CIM: 65-16

L8505 Artificial larynx replacement battery/accessory, any type

L8507 Tracheo-esophageal voice prosthesis, patient inserted, any type, each

L8509 Tracheo-esophageal voice prosthesis, inserted by a licensed health care provider, any type

L8510 Voice amplifier
CIM: 65-5

L8511 Insert for indwelling tracheoesophageal prosthesis, with or without valve, replacement only, each

L8512 Gelatin capsules or equivalent, for use with tracheo-esophageal voice prosthesis, replacement only, per 10

L8513 Cleaning device used with tracheoesophageal voice prosthesis, pipet, brush, or equal, replacement only, each

L8514 Tracheoesophageal puncture dilator, replacement only, each

L8515 Gelatin capsule, application device for use with tracheoesophageal voice prosthesis, each

INTEGUMENTARY SYSTEM

L8600 Implantable breast prosthesis, silicone or equal
CIM: 35-47 MCM: 2130

L8603 Injectable bulking agent, collagen implant, urinary tract, 2.5 ml syringe, includes shipping and necessary supplies
CIM: 65.9

L8604 Injectable bulking agent, dextranomer/hyaluronic acid copolymer implant, urinary tract, 1 ml, includes shipping and necessary supplies

L8605 Injectable bulking agent, dextranomer/hyaluronic acid copolymer implant, anal canal, 1 ml, includes shipping and necessary supplies

L8606 Injectable bulking agent, synthetic implant, urinary tract, 1 ml syringe, includes shipping and necessary supplies
CIM: 65.9

HEAD (SKULL, FACIAL BONES, AND TEMPOROMANDIBULAR JOINT)

L8609 Artificial cornea

L8610 Ocular implant
MCM: 2130

L8612 Aqueous shunt
MCM: 2130

L8613 Ossicula implant
MCM: 2130

L8614 Cochlear device, includes all internal and external components
CIM: 65-14 MCM: 2130

L8615 Headset/headpiece for use with cochlear implant device, replacement
CIM: 65-14

L8616 Microphone for use with cochlear implant device, replacement
CIM: 65-14

L8617 Transmitting coil for use with cochlear implant device, replacement
CIM: 65-14

L8618 Transmitter cable for use with cochlear implant device, replacement
CIM: 65-14

L8619 Cochlear implant, external speech processor and controller, integrated system, replacement
CIM: 65-14

L8621 Zinc air battery for use with cochlear implant device, replacement, each

L8622 Alkaline battery for use with cochlear implant device, any size, replacement, each

L8623 Lithium ion battery for use with cochlear implant device speech processor; other than ear level, replacement, each

L8624 ear level, replacement, each

L8627 Cochlear implant; external speech processor, component, replacement
CIM: 65-14

L8628 external controller component, replacement
CIM: 65-14

L8629 Transmitting coil and cable, integrated, for use with cochlear implant device, replacement
CIM: 65-14

UPPER EXTREMITY

L8630 Metacarpophalangeal joint implant
MCM: 2130

L8631 Metacarpal phalangeal joint replacement, two or more pieces, metal (eg., stainless steel or cobalt chrome), ceramic-like material (eg., pyrocarbon), for surgical implantation (all sizes, includes entire system)
MCM: 2130

LOWER EXTREMITY (JOINT: KNEE, ANKLE, TOE)

L8641 Metatarsal joint implant
MCM: 2130

L8642 Hallux implant
MCM: 2130

MISCELLANEOUS MUSCULAR - SKELETAL

L8658 Interphalangeal joint spacer, silicone or equal, each
MCM: 2130

L8659 Interphalangeal finger joint replacement, 2 or more pieces, metal (eg., stainless steel or cobalt chrome), ceramic-like material (eg., pyrocarbon) for surgical implantation, any size
MCM: 2130

CARDIOVASCULAR SYSTEM

L8670 Vascular graft material, synthetic, implant
MCM: 2130

● **L8679** Implantable neurostimulator, pulse generator, any type
CIM: 65-8

L8680 Implantable neurostimulator electrode, each

L8681 Patient programmer (external) for use with implantable programmable neurostimulator pulse generator, replacement only
CIM: 65-8

L8682 Implantable neurostimulator radiofrequency receiver

L8683 Radiofrequency transmitter (external) for use with implantable neurostimulator radiofrequency receiver

L8684 Radiofrequency transmitter (external) for use with implantable sacral root neurostimulator receiver for bowel and bladder management, replacement

L8685 Implantable neurostimulator pulse generator, single array, rechargeable, includes extension

L8686 Implantable neurostimulator pulse generator, single array, non-rechargeable, includes extension

L8687 Implantable neurostimulator pulse generator, dual array, rechargeable, includes extension

L8688 Implantable neurostimulator pulse generator, dual array, non-rechargeable, includes extension

L8689 External recharging system for battery (internal) for use with implantable neurostimulator, replacement only
CIM: 65-8

L8690 Auditory osseointegrated device, includes all internal and external components

L8691 Auditory osseointegrated device, external sound processor, replacement

L8692 Auditory osseointegrated device, external sound processor, used without osseointegration, body worn, includes headband or other means of external attachment

L8693 Auditory osseointegrated device abutment, any length, replacement only

L8695 External recharging system for battery (external) for use with implantable neurostimulator, replacement only
CIM: 65-8

OTHER

L8699 Prosthetic implant, not otherwise specified

L9900 Orthotic and prosthetic supply, accessory, and/or service component of another HCPCS "L" code

This page intentionally left blank.

MEDICAL SERVICES

Guidelines

In addition to the information presented in the INTRODUCTION, several other items unique to this section are defined or identified here:

1. SUBSECTION INFORMATION: Some of the listed subheadings or subsections have special needs or instructions unique to that section. Where these are indicated, special "notes" will be presented preceding or following the listings. Those subsections within the MEDICAL SERVICES section that have "notes" are as follows:

Subsection	Code Numbers
Office services	M0000-M0009
End-stage renal disease services	M0900-M0999

2. SPECIAL REPORT: A service, material or supply that is rarely provided, unusual, variable or new may require a special report in determining medical appropriateness for reimbursement purposes. Pertinent information should include an adequate definition or description of the nature, extent, and need for the service, material or supply.

3. MODIFIERS: Listed services may be modified under certain circumstances. When appropriate, the modifying circumstance is identified by adding a modifier to the basic procedure code. CPT and HCPCS National Level II modifiers may be used with CPT and HCPCS National Level II procedure codes. Modifiers commonly used with MEDICAL SERVICES are as follows:

   -AH Clinical psychologist

   -AJ Clinical social worker

   -CC Procedure code change (use "CC" when the procedure code submitted was changed either for administrative reasons or because an incorrect code was filed)

   -EJ Subsequent claims for a defined course of therapy (eg., EPO, sodium hyaluronate, infliximab)

   -EM Emergency reserve supply (for ESRD benefit only)

-EP Service provided as part of Medicaid early periodic screening diagnosis and treatment (EPSDT) program

-FP Service provided as part of Medicaid family planning program

-Q5 Service furnished by a substitute physician under a reciprocal billing arrangement

-Q6 Service furnished by a locum tenens physician

-QC Single channel monitoring

-QD Recording and storage in solid state memory by a digital recorder

-QT Recording and storage on tape by an analog tape recorder

-SF Second opinion ordered by a professional review organization (PRO) per section 9401, P.L. 99-272 (100 percent reimbursement; no Medicare deductible or coinsurance)

-TC Technical component. Under certain circumstances, a charge may be made for the technical component alone. Under those circumstances, the technical component charge is identified by adding modifier -TC to the usual procedure number. Technical component charges are institutional charges and are not billed separately by physicians. However, portable x-ray suppliers bill only for the technical component and should use modifier -TC. The charge data from portable x-ray suppliers will then be used to build customary and prevailing profiles.

4. CPT CODE CROSS-REFERENCE: See sections for equivalent CPT code(s) for listings in this section.

Medical Services

ASC SERVICES

M0064 Brief office visit for the sole purpose of monitoring or changing drug prescriptions used in the treatment of mental psychoneurotic and personality disorders
MCM: 2476.3

OTHER MEDICAL SERVICES

M0075 Cellular therapy
CIM: 35-5

M0076 Prolotherapy
CIM: 35-13

M0100 Intragastric hypothermia using gastric freezing
CIM: 35-65

CARDIOVASCULAR SERVICES

M0300 IV chelation therapy (chemical endarterectomy)
CIM: 35-64

M0301 Fabric wrapping of abdominal aneurysm
CIM: 35-34

PHYSICAL MEDICINE SERVICES

OSTEOPATHIC MANIPULATION THERAPY (OMT)

NOTE: All OMT codes have been deleted; use CPT.

ESRD SERVICES

NOTE: For DME items for ESRD, see procedure codes E1500-E1699. For supplies for ESRD, see procedure codes A4650-A4999

This page intentionally left blank

PATHOLOGY AND LABORATORY

Guidelines

In addition to the information presented in the INTRODUCTION, several other items unique to this section are defined or identified here:

1. SPECIAL REPORT: A service, material or supply that is rarely provided, unusual, variable or new may require a special report in determining medical appropriateness for reimbursement purposes. Pertinent information should include an adequate definition or description of the nature, extent, and need for the service, material or supply.

2. MODIFIERS: Listed services may be modified under certain circumstances. When appropriate, the modifying circumstance is identified by adding a modifier to the basic procedure code. CPT and HCPCS National Level II modifiers may be used with CPT and HCPCS National Level II procedure codes. Modifiers commonly used with PATHOLOGY AND LABORATORY SERVICES are as follows:

   -CC Procedure code change (use "CC" when the procedure code submitted was changed either for administrative reasons or because an incorrect code was filed)

   -LR Laboratory round trip

   -TC Technical component. Under certain circumstances, a charge may be made for the technical component alone. Under these circumstances, the technical component charge is identified by adding the modifier -TC to the usual procedure code. Technical component charges are institutional charges and are not billed separately by physicians. Portable x-ray suppliers bill only for the technical component however, and should use modifier -TC. The charge data from portable x-ray suppliers will then be used to build customary and prevailing profiles.

3. CPT CODE CROSS-REFERENCE: See sections for equivalent CPT code(s) for all listings in this section.

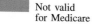

Pathology and Laboratory

CHEMISTRY AND TOXICOLOGY TESTS

P2028 Cephalin flocculation, blood
CIM: 50-34

P2029 Congo red, blood
CIM: 50-34

P2031 Hair analysis (excluding arsenic)
CIM: 50-24

P2033 Thymol turbidity, blood
CIM: 50-34

P2038 Mucoprotein, blood (seromucoid) (medical necessity procedure)
CIM: 50-34

PATHOLOGY SCREENING TESTS

P3000 Screening papanicolaou smear, cervical or vaginal, up to three smears; by technician under physician supervision
CIM: 50-20

P3001 requiring interpretation by physician
CIM: 50-20

MICROBIOLOGY TESTS

P7001 Culture, bacterial, urine; quantitative, sensitivity study

MISCELLANEOUS PATHOLOGY AND LABORATORY TESTS

P9010 Blood (whole), for transfusion, per unit
MCM: 2455.A

P9011 Blood, split unit
MCM: 2455.A

P9012 Cryoprecipitate, each unit
MCM: 2455.B

P9016 Red blood cells, leukocytes reduced, each unit
MCM: 2455.B

P9017 Fresh frozen plasma (single donor), frozen within eight hours of collection, each unit
MCM: 2455.B

P9019 Platelets, each unit
MCM: 2455.B

P9020 Platelet rich plasma, each unit
MCM: 2455.B

P9021 Red blood cells, each unit
MCM: 2455.A

P9022 Red blood cells, washed, each unit
MCM: 2455.A

P9023 Plasma, pooled multiple donor, solvent/detergent treated, frozen, each unit
MCM: 2455.B

P9031 Platelets, leukocytes reduced, each unit
MCM: 2455

P9032 Platelets, irradiated, each unit
MCM: 2455

P9033 Platelets, leukocytes reduced, irradiated, each unit
MCM: 2455

P9034 Platelets, pheresis, each unit
MCM: 2455

P9035 Platelets, pheresis, leukocytes reduced, each unit
MCM: 2455

P9036 Platelets, pheresis, irradiated, each unit
MCM: 2455

P9037 Platelets, pheresis, leukocytes reduced, irradiated, each unit
MCM: 2455

P9038 Red blood cells, irradiated, each unit
MCM: 2455

P9039 Red blood cells, deglycerolized, each unit
MCM: 2455

P9040 Red blood cells, leukocytes reduced, irradiated, each unit
MCM: 2455

P9041 Infusion, albumin (human), 5%, 50 ml

P9043 Infusion, plasma protein fraction (human), 5%, 50 ml
MCM: 2455.B

P9044 Plasma, cryoprecipitate reduced, each unit
MCM: 2455.B

P9045 Infusion, albumin (human), 5%, 250 ml

P9046 Infusion, albumin (human), 25%, 20 ml

P9047 Infusion, albumin (human), 25%, 50 ml

P9048 Infusion, plasma protein fraction (human), 5%, 250 ml

P9050 Granulocytes, pheresis, each unit

P9051 Whole blood or red blood cells, leukocytes reduced, CMV-negative, each unit

P9052 Platelets, HLA-matched leukocytes reduced, apheresis/pheresis, each unit

P9053 Platelets, pheresis, leukocytes reduced, CMV-negative, irradiated, each unit

P9054 Whole blood or red blood cells, leukocytes reduced, frozen, deglycerol, washed, each unit

P9055 Platelets, leukocytes reduced, CMV-negative, apheresis/pheresis, each unit

P9056 Whole blood, leukocytes reduced, irradiated, each unit

P9057 Red blood cells, frozen/deglycerolized/washed, leukocytes reduced, irradiated, each unit

P9058 Red blood cells, leukocytes reduced, CMV-negative, irradiated, each unit

P9059 Fresh frozen plasma between 8-24 hours of collection, each unit

P9060 Fresh frozen plasma, donor retested, each unit

P9603 Travel allowance one way in connection with medically necessary laboratory specimen collection drawn from home bound or nursing home bound patient; prorated miles actually travelled
MCM: 5114.1K

P9604 prorated trip charge
MCM: 5114.1K

P9612 Catheterization for collection of specimen; single patient, all places of service
MCM: 5114.1D

P9615 multiple patients
MCM: 5114.1D

This page intentionally left blank

TEMPORARY CODES

Guidelines

In addition to the information presented in the INTRODUCTION, several other items unique to this section are defined or identified here:

1. SUBSECTION INFORMATION: Some of the listed subheadings or subsections have special needs or instructions unique to that section. Where these are indicated, special "notes" will be presented preceding or following the listings. Those subsections within the TEMPORARY CODES section that have "notes" are as follows:

Subsection	Code Numbers
Temporary codes	Q0000-Q9999

2. SPECIAL REPORT: A service, material or supply that is rarely provided, unusual, variable or new may require a special report in determining medical appropriateness for reimbursement purposes. Pertinent information should include an adequate definition or description of the nature, extent, and need for the service, material or supply.

3. MODIFIERS: Listed services may be modified under certain circumstances. When appropriate, the modifying circumstance is identified by adding a modifier to the basic procedure code. CPT and HCPCS National Level II modifiers may be used with CPT and HCPCS National Level II procedure codes. Modifiers commonly used with TEMPORARY CODES are as follows:

   -CC Procedure code change (use "CC" when the procedure code submitted was changed either for administrative reasons or because an incorrect code was filed)

   -LL Lease/rental (used when DME equipment rental is to be applied against the purchase price)

   -LR Laboratory round trip

   -QC Single channel monitoring

   -QD Recording and storage in solid state memory by a digital recorder

-QE Prescribed amount of oxygen is less than 1 liter per minute (LPM)

-QF Prescribed amount of oxygen exceeds 4 liters per minute (LPM) and portable oxygen is prescribed

-QG Prescribed amount of oxygen is greater than 4 liters per minute (LPM)

-QH Oxygen conserving device is being used with an oxygen delivery system

-QT Recording and storage on tape by an analog tape recorder

-RP Replacement and repair (may be used to indicate replacement of DME, orthotic and prosthetic devices that have been in use for some time. The claim shows the code for the part, followed by the "RP" modifier and the charge for the part.)

-RR Rental (used when DME is to be rented)

-TC Technical component. Under certain circumstances, a charge may be made for the technical component alone. Under these circumstances, the technical component charge is identified by adding the modifier -TC to the usual procedure code. Technical component charges are institutional charges and are not billed separately by physicians. Portable x-ray suppliers bill only for the technical component however, and should use modifier -TC. The charge data from portable x-ray suppliers will then be used to build customary and prevailing profiles.

-UE Used durable medical equipment

4. CPT CODE CROSS-REFERENCE: See sections for equivalent CPT code(s) for all listings in this section.

Temporary Codes

NOTE: Temporary codes are national codes given by CMS on a temporary basis. The list contains current codes, as well as those which have been superseded by permanent alphanumeric codes as indicated by the cross-reference.

Q0035 Cardiokymography
CIM: 50-50

Q0081 Infusion therapy, using other than chemotherapeutic drugs, per visit
CIM: 60-14

Q0083 Chemotherapy administration by other than infusion technique only (e.g., subcutaneous, intramuscular, push), per visit

Q0084 Chemotherapy administration by infusion technique only, per visit
CIM: 60-14

Q0085 Chemotherapy administration by both infusion technique and other technique(s) (e.g., subcutaneous, intramuscular, push), per visit

(Q0090) Code deleted December 31, 2013.. Use J7301

Q0091 Screening papanicolaou smear; obtaining, preparing and conveyance of cervical or vaginal smear to laboratory
CIM: 50-20

Q0092 Set-up portable x-ray equipment
MCM: 2070.4

Q0111 Wet mounts, including preparations of vaginal, cervical or skin specimens

Q0112 All potassium hydroxide (koh) preparations

Q0113 Pinworm examinations

Q0114 Fern test

Q0115 Post-coital direct, qualitative examinations of vaginal or cervical mucous

Q0138 Injection, ferumoxytol, for treatment of iron deficiency anemia, 1 mg (non-ESRD use)

Q0139 Injection, ferumoxytol, for treatment of iron deficiency anemia, 1 mg (for ESRD on dialysis)

Q0144 Azithromycin dihydrate, oral, capsules/powder, 1 gram

● **Q0161** Chlorpromazine hydrochloride, 5 mg, oral, fad approved prescription anti-emetic, for use as a complete therapeutic substitute for an iv anti-emetic at the time of chemotherapy treatment, not to exceed a 48 hour dosage regimen

Q0162 Ondansetron 1 mg, oral, FDA approved prescription anti-emetic, for use as a complete therapeutic substitute for an IV anti-emetic at the time of chemotherapy treatment, not to exceed a 48 hour dosage regimen

Q0163 Diphenhydramine HCl, 50 mg, oral, FDA approved prescription anti-emetic, for use as a complete therapeutic substitute for an IV anti-emetic at time of chemotherapy treatment not to exceed a 48 hour dosage regimen

Q0164 Prochlorperazine maleate, 5 mg, oral, FDA approved prescription anti-emetic, for use as a complete therapeutic substitute for an IV anti-emetic at the time of chemotherapy treatment, not to exceed a 48 hour dosage regimen

(Q0165) Code deleted December 31, 2013

Q0166 Granisetron HCl, 1 mg, oral, FDA approved prescription anti-emetic, for use as a complete therapeutic substitute for an IV anti-emetic at the time of chemotherapy treatment, not to exceed a 24 hour dosage regimen

Q0167 Dronabinol, 2.5 mg, oral, FDA approved prescription anti-emetic, for use as a complete therapeutic substitute for an IV anti-emetic at the time of chemotherapy treatment, not to exceed a 48 hour dosage regimen

(Q0168) Code deleted December 31, 2013

Q0169 Promethazine HCl, 12.5 mg, oral, FDA approved prescription anti-emetic, for use as a complete therapeutic substitute for an IV anti-emetic at the time of chemotherapy treatment, not to exceed a 48 hour dosage regimen

(Q0170) Code deleted December 31, 2013

(Q0171) Code deleted December 31, 2013

(Q0172) Code deleted December 31, 2013

Q0173 Trimethobenzamide HCl, 250 mg, oral, FDA approved prescription anti-emetic, for use as a complete therapeutic substitute for an IV anti-emetic at the time of chemotherapy treatment, not to exceed a 48 hour dosage regimen

Q0174 Thiethylperazine maleate, 10 mg, oral, FDA approved prescription anti-emetic, for use as a complete therapeutic substitute for an IV anti-emetic at the time of chemotherapy treatment, not to exceed a 48 hour dosage regimen

Q0175 Perphenzaine, 4 mg, oral, FDA approved prescription anti-emetic, for use as a complete therapeutic substitute for an IV anti-emetic at the time of chemotherapy treatment, not to exceed a 48 hour dosage regimen

(Q0176) Code deleted December 31, 2013

Q0177 Hydroxyzine pamoate, 25 mg, oral, FDA approved prescription anti-emetic, for use as a complete therapeutic substitute for an IV anti-emetic at the time of chemotherapy treatment, not to exceed a 48 hour dosage regimen

(Q0178) Code deleted December 31, 2013

(Q0179) Code deleted December 31, 2011

Q0180 Dolasetron mesylate, 100 mg, oral, FDA approved prescription anti-emetic, for use as a complete therapeutic substitute for an IV anti-emetic at the time of chemotherapy treatment, not to exceed a 24 hour dosage regimen

Q0181 Unspecified oral dosage form, FDA approved prescription anti-emetic, for use as a complete therapeutic substitute for an IV anti-emetic at the time of chemotherapy treatment, not to exceed a 48 hour dosage regimen

Q0478 Power adapter for use with electric or electric/pneumatic ventricular assist device, vehicle type

Q0479 Power module for use with electric or electric/pneumatic ventricular assist device, replacement only

Q0480 Driver for use with pneumatic ventricular assist device, replacement only

Q0481 Microprocessor control unit for use with electric ventricular assist device, replacement only

Q0482 Microprocessor control unit for use with electric/pneumatic combination ventricular assist device, replacement only

Q0483 Monitor/display module for use with electric ventricular assist device, replacement only

Q0484 Monitor/display module for use with electric or electric/pneumatic ventricular assist device, replacement only

Q0485 Monitor control cable for use with electric ventricular assist device, replacement only

Q0486 Monitor control cable for use with electric/pneumatic ventricular assist device, replacement only

Q0487 Leads (pneumatic/electrical) for use with any type electric/pneumatic ventricular assist device, replacement only

Q0488 Power pack base for use with electric ventricular assist device, replacement only

Q0489 Power pack base for use with electric/pneumatic ventricular assist device, replacement only

Q0490 Emergency power source for use with electric ventricular assist device, replacement only

Q0491 Emergency power source for use with electric/pneumatic ventricular assist device, replacement only

Q0492 Emergency power supply cable for use with electric ventricular assist device, replacement only

Q0493 Emergency power supply cable for use with electric/pneumatic ventricular assist device, replacement only

Q0494 Emergency hand pump for use with electric or electric/pneumatic ventricular assist device, replacement only

Q0495 Battery/power pack charger for use with electric or electric/pneumatic ventricular assist device, replacement only

Q0496 Battery, other than lithium-ion, for use with electric or electric/pneumatic ventricular assist device, replacement only

Q0497 Battery clips for use with electric or electric/pneumatic ventricular assist device, replacement only

Q0498 Holster for use with electric or electric/pneumatic ventricular assist device, replacement only

Q0499 Belt/vest/bag for use to carry external peripheral components of any type ventricular assist device, replacement only

Q0500 Filters for use with electric or electric/pneumatic ventricular assist device, replacement only

Q0501 Shower cover for use with electric or electric/pneumatic ventricular assist device, replacement only

Q0502 Mobility cart for pneumatic ventricular assist device, replacement only

Q0503 Battery for pneumatic ventricular assist device, replacement only, each

Q0504 Power adapter for pneumatic ventricular assist device, replacement only, vehicle type

(Q0505) Code deleted 3/31/2013

Q0506 Battery, lithium-ion, for use with electric or electric/pneumatic ventricular assist device, replacement only

● **Q0507** Miscellaneous supply or accessory for use with an external ventricular assist device

● **Q0508** Miscellaneous supply or accessory for use with an implanted ventricular assist device

● **Q0509** Miscellaneous supply or accessory for use with ayn implanted ventricular assist device for which payment was not made under Medicare Part A

Q0510 Pharmacy supply fee for initial immunosuppressive drug(s), first month following transplant

Q0511 Pharmacy supply fee for oral anti-cancer, oral anti-emetic or immunosuppressive drug(s); for the first prescription in a 30-day period

Q0512 for a subsequent prescription in a 30-day period

Q0513 Pharmacy dispensing fee for inhalation drug(s); per 30 days

Q0514 per 90 days

Q0515 Injection, sermorelin acetate, 1 microgram
MCM: 2049

(Q1003) Code deleted March 31, 2011.

Q1004 New technology intraocular lens category 4 as defined in Federal Register notice

Q1005 New technology intraocular lens category 5 as defined in Federal Register notice

Q2004 Irrigation solution for treatment of bladder calculi, for example Renacidin, per 500 ml
MCM: 2049

Q2009 Injection, fosphenytoin, 50 mg phenytoin equivalent
MCM: 2049

Q2017 Injection, teniposide, 50 mg
MCM: 2049

Q2026 Injection, radiesse, 0.1 ml

(Q2027) Code deleted December 31, 2013..

● **Q2028** Injection, Sculptra, 0.5 mg

● **Q2033** Influenza vaccine, recombinant hemagglutinin antigens, for intramuscular use (Flublok)
MCM: 2049.4

Q2034 Influenza virus vaccine, split virus, for intramuscular use (Agriflu)

Q2035 Influenza virus vaccine, split virus, when administered to individuals 3 years of age and older, for intramuscular use (Afluria)
MCM: 2049.4

Q2036 Influenza virus vaccine, split virus, when administered to individuals 3 years of age and older, for intramuscular use (Flulaval)
MCM: 2049.4

Q2037 Influenza virus vaccine, split virus, when administered to individuals 3 years of age and older, for intramuscular use (Fluvirin)
MCM: 2049.4

Q2038 Influenza virus vaccine, split virus, when administered to individuals 3 years of age and older, for intramuscular use (Fluzone)
MCM: 2049.4

Q2039 Influenza virus vaccine, split virus, when administered to individuals 3 years of age and older, for intramuscular use (not otherwise specified)
MCM: 2049.4

(Q2040) Code deleted December 31, 2011; see J0588

(Q2041) Code deleted December 31, 2011; see J7183

(Q2042) Code deleted December 31, 2011; see J1725

Q2043 Sipuleucel-T-t, minimum of 50 million autologous CD54+ cells activated with pap-gm-csf, including leukapheresis and all other preparatory procedures, per infusion

(Q2044) Code deleted December 31, 2011; see J0490

(Q2045) Code deleted December 31, 2012. Use J7178

(Q2046) Code deleted December 31, 2012. Use J0178

(Q2047) Code deleted December 31, 2012. Use J0890

(Q2048) Code deleted December 31, 2012. Use J9002

Q2049 Injection, doxorubicin hydrochloride, liposomal, imported lipodox, 10 mg

● **Q2050** Injection, doxorubicin hydrochloride, liposomal, Doxil, 10 mg
MCM: 2049.4

(Q2051) Code deleted December 31, 2013.

● **Q2052** Services, supplies and accessories used in the home under the medicare intravenous immune globulin (IVIG) demonstration

Q3001 Radioelements for brachytherapy, any type, each
MCM: 15022

Q3014 Telehealth originating site facility fee

(Q3025) Code deleted December 31, 2013.

(Q3026) Code deleted December 31, 2013.

● **Q3027** Injection, interferon beta-1a, 1 mcg for intramuscular use
MCM: 2049

● **Q3028** Injection, interferon beta-1a, 1 mcg for subcutaneous use

Q3031 Collagen skin test
CIM: 65-9

Q4001 Cast supplies, body cast adult, with or without head, plaster

Q4002 Cast supplies, body cast adult, with or without head, fiberglass

Q4003 Cast supplies, shoulder cast, adult (11 years +), plaster

Q4004 Cast supplies, shoulder cast, adult (11 years +), fiberglass

Q4005 Cast supplies, long arm cast, adult (11 years +), plaster

Q4006 Cast supplies, long arm cast, adult (11 years +), fiberglass

Q4007 Cast supplies, long arm cast, pediatric (0-10 years), plaster

Q4008 Cast supplies, long arm cast, pediatric (0-10 years), fiberglass

Q4009 Cast supplies, short arm cast, adult (11 years +), plaster

Q4010 Cast supplies, short arm cast, adult (11 years +), fiberglass

Q4011 Cast supplies, short arm cast, pediatric (0-10 years), plaster

Q4012 Cast supplies, short arm cast, pediatric (0-10 years), fiberglass

Q4013 Cast supplies, gauntlet cast (includes lower forearm and hand), adult (11 years +), plaster

Q4014 Cast supplies, gauntlet cast (includes lower forearm and hand), adult (11 years +), fiberglass

Q4015 Cast supplies, gauntlet cast (includes lower forearm and hand), pediatric (0-10 years), plaster

Q4016 Cast supplies, gauntlet cast (includes lower forearm and hand), pediatric (0-10 years), fiberglass

Q4017 Cast supplies, long arm splint, adult (11 years +), plaster

Q4018 Cast supplies, long arm splint, adult (11 years +), fiberglass

Q4019 Cast supplies, long arm splint, pediatric (0-10 years), plaster

Q4020 Cast supplies, long arm splint, pediatric (0-10 years), fiberglass

Q4021 Cast supplies, short arm splint, adult (11 years +), plaster

Q4022 Cast supplies, short arm splint, adult (11 years +), fiberglass

Q4023 Cast supplies, short arm splint, pediatric (0-10 years), plaster

Q4024 Cast supplies, short arm splint, pediatric (0-10 years), fiberglass

Q4025 Cast supplies, hip spica (one or both legs), adult (11 years +), plaster

Q4026 Cast supplies, hip spica (one or both legs), adult (11 years +), fiberglass

Q4027 Cast supplies, hip spica (one or both legs), pediatric (0-10 years), plaster

Q4028 Cast supplies, hip spica (one or both legs), pediatric (0-10 years), fiberglass

Q4029 Cast supplies, long leg cast, adult (11 years +), plaster

Q4030 Cast supplies, long leg cast, adult (11 years +), fiberglass

Q4031 Cast supplies, long leg cast, pediatric (0-10 years), plaster

Q4032 Cast supplies, long leg cast, pediatric (0-10 years), fiberglass

Q4033 Cast supplies, long leg cylinder cast, adult (11 years +), plaster

Q4034 Cast supplies, long leg cylinder cast, adult (11 years +), fiberglass

Q4035 Cast supplies, long leg cylinder cast, pediatric (0-10 years), plaster

Q4036 Cast supplies, long leg cylinder cast, pediatric (0-10 years), fiberglass

Q4037 Cast supplies, short leg cast, adult (11 years +), plaster

Q4038 Cast supplies, short leg cast, adult (11 years +), fiberglass

Q4039 Cast supplies, short leg cast, pediatric (0-10 years), plaster

Q4040 Cast supplies, short leg cast, pediatric (0-10 years), fiberglass

Q4041 Cast supplies, long leg splint, adult (11 years +), plaster

Q4042 Cast supplies, long leg splint, adult (11 years +), fiberglass

Q4043 Cast supplies, long leg splint, pediatric (0-10 years), plaster

Q4044 Cast supplies, long leg splint, pediatric (0-10 years), fiberglass

Q4045 Cast supplies, short leg splint, adult (11 years +), plaster

Q4046 Cast supplies, short leg splint, adult (11 years +), fiberglass

Q4047 Cast supplies, short leg splint, pediatric (0-10 years), plaster

Q4048 Cast supplies, short leg splint, pediatric (0-10 years), fiberglass

Q4049 Finger splint, static

Q4050 Cast supplies, for unlisted types and materials of casts

Q4051 Splint supplies, miscellaneous (includes thermoplastics, strapping, fasteners, padding and other supplies)

Q4074 Iloprost, inhalation solution, FDA-approved final product, non-compounded, administered through DME, unit dose form, up to 20 micrograms

INJECTION CODES FOR EPO

Q4081 Injection, epoetin alfa, 100 units (for ESRD on dialysis)
MCM: 4273.1

Q4082 Drug or biological, not otherwise classified, Part B drug competitive acquisition program (CAP)

Q4100 Skin substitute, not otherwise specified

Q4101 Apligraf, per square centimeter

Q4102 Oasis wound matrix, per square centimeter

Q4103 Oasis burn matrix, per square centimeter

Q4104 Integra bilayer matrix wound dressing (bmwd), per square centimeter

Q4105 Integra dermal regeneration template (drt), per square centimeter

Q4106 Dermagraft, per square centimeter

Q4107 Graftjacket, per square centimeter

Q4108 Integra matrix, per square centimeter

Q4110 Primatrix, per square centimeter

Q4111 Gammagraft, per square centimeter

Q4112 Cymetra, injectable, 1cc

Q4113 Graftjacket xpress, injectable, 1cc

Q4114 Integra flowable wound matrix, injectable, 1cc

Q4115 Alloskin, per square centimeter

Q4116 Alloderm, per square centimeter

Q4117 Hyalomatrix, per square centimeter

Q4118 Matristem micromatrix, 1 mg

Q4119 Matristem wound matrix, per square centimeter

Q4120 Matristem burn matrix, per square centimeter

Q4121 Theraskin, per square centimeter

Q4122 Dermicel, per square centimeter

Q4123 Alloskin RT, per square centimeter

Q4124 Oasis ultra tri-layer wound matrix, per square centimeter

Q4125 Arthroflex, per square centimeter

Q4126 Memoderm, per square centimeter

Q4127 Talymed, per square centimeter

Q4128 Flexhd or allopatch hd, per square centimeter

Q4129 Unite Biomatrix, per square centimeter

Q4130 Strattice tm, per square centimeter

Q4131 Epifix, per square centimeter

Q4132 Grafix core, per square centimeter

Q4133 Grafix prime, per square centimeter

Q4134 Hmatrix, per square centimeter

Q4135 Mediskin, per square centimeter

Q4136 Ez-derm, per square centimeter

● **Q4137** Amnioexcel or biodexcel, per square centimeter

● **Q4138** Biodefense dry flex, per square centimeter

● **Q4139** Amniomatrix or Biomatrix, injectable, 1 cc

● **Q4140** Biodefense, per square centimeter

● **Q4141** Alloskin ac, per square centimeter

● **Q4142** Xcm biologic tissue matrix, per square centimeter

● **Q4143** Repriza, per square centimeter

● **Q4145** Epifix, injectable, 1 mg

● **Q4146** Tensix, per square centimeter

● **Q4147** Architect extracellular matrix, per square centimeter

● **Q4148** Neox 1k, per square centimeter

● **Q4149** Excellagen, 0.1 cc

▲ **Q5001** Hospice or home health care provided in patient's home/residence

▲ **Q5002** Hospice or home health care provided in assisted living facility

Q5003 Hospice care provided in nursing long term care facility (LTC) or non-skilled nursing facility (NF)

Q5004 Hospice care provided in skilled nursing facility (SNF)

Q5005 Hospice care provided in inpatient hospital

Q5006 Hospice care provided in inpatient hospice facility

Q5007 Hospice care provided in long term care facility (LTC)

Q5008 Hospice care provided in inpatient psychiatric facility

▲**Q5009** Hospice or home health care provided in place not otherwise specified (NOS)

Q5010 Hospice home care provided in a hospice facility

Q9951 Low osmolar contrast material, 400 or greater mg/ml iodine concentration, per ml
MCM: 15022

Q9953 Injection, iron-based magnetic resonance contrast agent, per ml
MCM: 15022

Q9954 Oral magnetic resonance contrast agent, per 100 ml
MCM: 15022

Q9955 Injection, perflexane lipid microspheres, per ml

Q9956 Injection, octafluoropropane microspheres, per ml

Q9957 Injection, perflutren lipid microspheres, per ml

Q9958 High osmolar contrast material, up to 149 mg/ml iodine concentration, per ml
MCM: 15022

Q9959 High osmolar contrast material, 150-199 mg/ml iodine concentration, per ml
MCM: 15022

Q9960 High osmolar contrast material, 200-249 mg/ml iodine concentration, per ml
MCM: 15022

Q9961 High osmolar contrast material, 250-299 mg/ml iodine concentration, per ml
MCM: 15022

Q9962 High osmolar contrast material, 300-349 mg/ml iodine concentration, per ml
MCM: 15022

Q9963 High osmolar contrast material, 350-399 mg/ml iodine concentration, per ml
MCM: 15022

Q9964 High osmolar contrast material, 400 or greater mg/ml iodine concentration, per ml
MCM: 15022

Q9965 Low osmolar contrast material, 100-199 mg/ml iodine concentration, per ml
MCM: 15022

Q9966 Low osmolar contrast material, 200-299 mg/ml iodine concentration, per ml
MCM: 15022

Q9967 Low osmolar contrast material, 300-399 mg/ml iodine concentration, per ml
MCM: 15022

Q9968 Injection, non-radioactive, non-contrast, visualization adjunct (eg., methylene blue, isosulfan blue), 1 mg

Q9969 Tc-99m from non-highly enriched uranium source, full cost recovery add-on, per study dose

This page intentionally left blank

DIAGNOSTIC RADIOLOGY SERVICES

Guidelines

In addition to the information presented in the INTRODUCTION, several other items unique to this section are defined or identified here:

1. SPECIAL REPORT: A service, material or supply that is rarely provided, unusual, variable or new may require a special report in determining medical appropriateness for reimbursement purposes. Pertinent information should include an adequate definition or description of the nature, extent, and need for the service, material or supply.

2. MODIFIERS: Listed services may be modified under certain circumstances. When appropriate, the modifying circumstance is identified by adding a modifier to the basic procedure code. CPT and HCPCS National Level II modifiers may be used with CPT and HCPCS National Level II procedure codes. Modifiers commonly used with DIAGNOSTIC RADIOLOGY SERVICES are as follows:

   -CC Procedure code change (use "CC" when the procedure code submitted was changed either for administrative reasons or because an incorrect code was filed)

   -LT Left side (used to identify procedures performed on the left side of the body)

   -RT Right side (used to identify procedures performed on the right side of the body)

   -TC Technical component. Under certain circumstances, a charge may be made for the technical component alone. Under those circumstances, the technical component charge is identified by adding modifier -TC to the usual procedure number. Technical component charges are institutional charges and are not billed separately by physicians. However, portable x-ray suppliers bill only for the technical component and should use modifier -TC. The charge data from portable x-ray suppliers will then be used to build customary and prevailing profiles.

3. CPT CODE CROSS-REFERENCE: There are no equivalent CPT codes for procedures listed in this section.

Diagnostic Radiology Services

R0070 Transportation of portable x-ray equipment and personnel to home or nursing home, per trip to facility or location; one patient seen
MCM: 2070.4, 5244.B

R0075 more than one patient seen, per patient
MCM: 2070.4, 5244.B

R0076 Transportation of portable EKG to facility or location, per patient
CIM: 50-15 MCM: 2070.1, 2070.4

PRIVATE PAYER CODES

Guidelines

HCPCS "S" codes are temporary national codes established by the private payers for private payer use. Prior to using "S" codes on insurance claims to private payers, you should consult with the payer to confirm that the "S" codes are acceptable. "S" codes are not valid for Medicare use.

In addition to the information presented in the INTRODUCTION, several other items unique to this section are defined or identified here.

1. SPECIAL REPORT: A service, material or supply that is rarely provided, unusual, variable or new may require a special report in determining medical appropriateness for reimbursement purposes. Pertinent information should include an adequate definition or description of the nature, extent, and need for the service, material or supply.

2. MODIFIERS: Listed services may be modified under certain circumstances. When appropriate, the modifying circumstance is identified by adding a modifier to the basic procedure code. CPT and HCPCS National Level II modifiers may be used with CPT and HCPCS National Level II procedure codes.

Private Payer Codes

S0012 Butorphanol tartrate, nasal spray, 25 mg

S0014 Tacrine HCl, 10 mg

S0017 Injection, aminocaproic acid, 5 gram

S0020 Injection, bupivicaine HCl, 30 ml

S0021 Injection, ceftoperazone sodium, 1 gram

S0023 Injection, cimetidine HCl, 300 mg

S0028 Injection, fanotidine, 20 mg

S0030 Injection, metronidazole, 500 mg

Not valid for Medicare | Non-covered by Medicare | Special coverage instructions | Carrier discretion

S0032 Injection, nafcillin sodium, 2 grams

S0034 Injection, ofloxacin, 400 mg

S0039 Injection, sulfamethoxazole and trimethoprim, 10 ml

S0040 Injection, ticarcillin disodium and clavulanate potassium, 3.1 grams

S0073 Injection, aztreonam, 500 mg

S0074 Injection, cefotetan disodium, 500 mg

S0077 Injection, clindamycin phosphate, 300 mg

S0078 Injection, fosphenytoin sodium, 750 mg

S0080 Injection, pentamidine isethionate, 300 mg

S0081 Injection, piperacillin sodium, 500 mg

S0088 Imatinib, 100 mg

S0090 Sildenafil citrate, 25 mg

S0091 Granisetron hydrochloride, 1mg (for circumstances falling under the Medicare statute, use Q0166)

S0092 Injection, hydromorphone hydrochloride, 250 mg (loading dose for infusion pump)

S0093 Injection, morphine sulfate, 500 mg (loading dose for infusion pump)

S0104 Zidovudine, oral, 100 mg

S0106 Bupropion HCl sustained release tablet, 150 mg, per bottle of 60 tablets

S0108 Mercaptopurine, oral, 50 mg

S0109 Methadone, oral, 5 mg

S0117 Tretinoin, topical, 5 grams

S0119	Ondansetron, oral, 4 mg (for circumstances falling under the Medicare statute, use HCPCS Q code)
S0122	Injection, menotropins, 75 IU
S0126	Injection, follitropin alfa, 75 IU
S0128	Injection, follitropin beta, 75 IU
S0132	Injection, ganirelix acetate, 250 mcg
S0136	Clozapine, 25 mg
S0137	Didanosine (DDI), 25 mg
S0138	Finasteride, 5 mg
S0139	Minoxidil, 10 mg
S0140	Saquinavir, 200 mg
S0142	Colistimethate sodium, inhalation solution administered through DME, concentrated form, per mg
S0145	Injection, pegylated interferon alfa-2a, 180 mcg per ml
S0148	Injection, pegylated interferon alfa-2b, 10 mcg
S0155	Sterile dilutant for epoprostenol, 50 ml
S0156	Exemestane, 25 mg
S0157	Becaplermin gel 0.01%, 0.5 gram
S0160	Dextroamphetamine sulfate, 5 mg
S0164	Injection, pantoprazole sodium, 40 mg
S0166	Injection, olanzapine, 2.5 mg
S0169	Calcitrol, 0.25 microgram
S0170	Anastrozole, oral, 1 mg
S0171	Injection, bumetanide, 0.5 mg

S0172 Chlorambucil, oral, 2 mg

S0174 Dolasetron mesylate, oral 50 mg (for circumstances falling under the medicare statute, use Q0180)

S0175 Flutamide, oral, 125 mg

S0176 Hydroxyurea, oral, 500 mg

S0177 Levamisole hydrochloride, oral, 50 mg

S0178 Lomustine, oral, 10 mg

S0179 Megestrol acetate, oral, 20 mg

(S0181) Code deleted December 31, 2011

S0182 Procarbazine hydrochloride, oral, 50 mg

S0183 Prochlorperazine maleate, oral, 5 mg (for circumstances falling under the medicare statute, use Q0164 - Q0165)

S0187 Tamoxifen citrate, oral, 10 mg

S0189 Testosterone pellet, 75 mg

S0190 Mifepristone, oral, 200 mg

S0191 Misoprostol, oral, 200 mcg

S0194 Dialysis/stress vitamin supplement, oral, 100 capsules

S0195 Pneumococcal conjugate vaccine, polyvalent, intramuscular, for children from five years to nine years of age who have not previously received the vaccine

S0197 Prenatal vitamins, 30-day supply

S0199 Medically induced abortion by oral ingestion of medication including all associated services and supplies (e.g., patient counseling, office visits, confirmation of pregnancy by HCG, ultrasound to confirm duration of pregnancy, ultrasound to confirm completion of abortion) except drugs

S0201 Partial hospitalization services, less than 24 hours, per diem

S0207 Paramedic intercept, non-hospital-based ALS service (non-voluntary), non-transport

S0208 Paramedic intercept, hospital-based ALS service (non-voluntary), non-transport

S0209 Wheelchair van, mileage, per mile

S0215 Non-emergency transportation; mileage, per mile

S0220 Medical conference by a physician with interdisciplinary team of health professionals or representatives of community agencies to coordinate activities of patient care (patient is present); approximately 30 minutes

S0221 Medical conference by a physician with interdisciplinary team of health professionals or representatives of community agencies to coordinate activities of patient care (patient is present); approximately 60 minutes

S0250 Comprehensive geriatric assessment and treatment planning performed by assessment team

S0255 Hospice referral visit (advising patient and family of care options) performed by nurse, social worker, or other designated staff

S0257 Counseling and discussion regarding advance directives or end of life care planning and decisions, with patient and/or surrogate (list separately in addition to code for appropriate evaluation and management service)

S0260 History and physical (outpatient or office) related to surgical procedure (list separately in addition to code for appropriate evaluation and management service)

S0265 Genetic counseling, under physician supervision, each 15 minutes

S0270 Physician management of patient home care, standard monthly case rate (per 30 days)

S0271 Physician management of patient home care, hospice monthly case rate (per 30 days)

S0272 Physician management of patient home care, episodic care monthly case rate (per 30 days)

S0273 Physician visit at member's home, outside of a capitation arrangement

S0274 Nurse practitioner visit at member's home, outside of a capitation arrangement

S0280 Medical home program, comprehensive care coordination and planning, initial plan

S0281 Medical home program, comprehensive care coordination and planning, maintenance of plan

S0302 Completed early periodic screening diagnosis and treatment (EPSDT) service (list in addition to code for appropriate evaluation and management service)

S0310 Hospitalist services (list separately in addition to code for appropriate evaluation and management service)

S0315 Disease management program; initial assessment and initiation of the program

S0316 follow-up/reassessment

S0317 Disease management program; per diem

S0320 Telephone calls by a registered nurse to a disease management program member for monitoring purposes; per month

S0340 Lifestyle modification program for management of coronary artery disease, including all supportive services; first quarter/stage

S0341 Lifestyle modification program for management of coronary artery disease, including all supportive services; second or third quarter/stage

S0342 Lifestyle modification program for management of coronary artery disease, including all supportive services; fourth quarter/stage

S0353 Treatment planning and care coordination management for cancer initial treatment

S0354 Treatment planning and care coordination management for cancer established patient with a change of regimen

S0390 Routine foot care; removal and/or trimming of corns, calluses and/or nails and preventive maintenance, per visit

S0395 Impression casting of a foot performed by a practitioner other than the manufacturer of the orthotic

S0400 Global fee for extracorporeal shock wave lithotripsy treatment of kidney stone(s)

S0500 Disposable contact lens, per lens

S0504 Single vision prescription lens (safety, athletic or sunglass), per lens

S0506 Bifocal vision prescription lens (safety, athletic or sunglass), per lens

S0508 Trifocal vision prescription lens (safety, athletic or sunglass), per lens

S0510 Non-prescription lens (safety, athletic or sunglass), per lens

S0512 Daily wear specialty contact lens, per lens

S0514 Color contact lens, per lens

S0515 Scleral lens, liquid bandage device, per lens

S0516 Safety eyeglass frames

S0518 Sunglasses frames

S0580 Polycarbonate lens (List this code in addition to the basic code for the lens)

S0581 Nonstandard lens (List this code in addition to the basic code for the lens)

S0590 Integral lens service, miscellaneous services reported separately

S0592 Comprehensive contact lens evaluation

S0595 Dispensing new spectacle lenses for patient supplied frame

S0596 Phakic intraocular lens for correction of refractive error

S0601 Screening proctoscopy

S0610 Annual gynecological examination; new patient

S0612 established patient

S0613 clinical breast examination without pelvic evaluation

S0618 Audiometry for hearing aid evaluation to determine the level and degree of hearing loss

S0620 Routine ophthalmological examination including refraction; new patient

S0621 established patient

S0622 Physical exam for college, new or established patient (list separately in addition to appropriate evaluation and management code)

(S0625) Code deleted December 31, 2011

S0630 Removal of sutures by a physician other than the physician who originally closed the wound

S0800 Laser in situ keratomileusis (LASIK)

S0810 Photorefractive keratectomy (PRK)

S0812 Phototherapeutic keratectomy (PTK)

S1001 Deluxe item, patient aware (List in addition to code for basic item)

S1002 Customized item (List in addition to code for basic item)

S1015 IV tubing extension set

S1016 Non-PVC (polyvinyl chloride) intravenous administration set, for use with drugs that are not stable in PVC, e.g., paclitaxel

S1030 Continuous noninvasive glucose monitoring device, purchase (for physician interpretation of data, use CPT code)

S1031 Continuous noninvasive glucose monitoring device, rental, including sensor, sensor replacement, and download to monitor (for physician interpretation of data, use CPT code)

S1040 Cranial remolding orthosis, pediatric, rigid, with soft interface material, custom fabricated, includes fitting and adjustment(s)

S1090 Mometasone furoate sinus implant, 370 micrograms

S2053 Transplantation of small intestine and liver allografts

S2054 Transplantation of multivisceral organs

S2055 Harvesting of donor multivisceral organs, with preparation and maintenance of allografts; from cadaver donor

S2060 Lobar lung transplantation

S2061 Donor lobectomy (lung) for transplantation, living donor

S2065 Simultaneous pancreas kidney transplantation

S2066 Breast reconstruction with gluteal artery perforator (GAP) flap, including harvesting of the flap, microvascular transfer, closure of donor site and shaping the flap into a breast, unilateral

S2067 Breast reconstruction of a single breast with "stacked" deep inferior epigastric perforator (DIEP) flap(s) and/or gluteal artery perforator (GAP) flap(s), including harvesting of the flap(s), microvascular transfer, closure of donor site(s) and shaping the flap into a breast, unilateral

S2068 Breast reconstruction with deep inferior epigastric perforator (DIEP) flap or superficial inferior epigastric artery (SIEA) flap, including harvesting of the flap, microvascular transfer, closure of donor site and shaping the flap into a breast, unilateral

S2070 Cystourethroscopy, with ureteroscopy and/or pyeloscopy; with endoscopic laser treatment of ureteral calculi (includes ureteral catheterization)

S2079 Laparoscopic esophagomyotomy (heller type)

S2080 Laser-assisted uvulopalatoplasty (laup)

S2083 Adjustment of gastric band diameter via subcutaneous port by injection or aspiration of saline

S2095 Transcatheter occlusion or embolization for tumor destruction, percutaneous, any method, using yttrium-90 microspheres

S2102 Islet cell tissue transplant from pancreas; allogenic

S2103 Adrenal tissue transplant to brain

S2107 Adoptive immunotherapy i.e., development of specific anti-tumor reactivity (e.g. tumor-infiltrating lymphocyte therapy) per course of treatment

S2112 Arthroscopy, knee, surgical for harvesting cartilage (chondrocyte cells)

S2115 Osteotomy, periacetabular, with internal fixation

S2117 Arthroereisis, subtalar

S2118 Metal-on-metal total hip resurfacing, including acetabular and femoral components

S2120 Low density lipoprotein (LDL) apheresis using heparin-induced extracorporeal LDL precipitation

S2140 Cord blood harvesting for transplantation, allogenic

S2142 Cord blood-derived stem cell transplantation, allogenic

S2150 Bone marrow or blood-derived stem cells (peripheral or umbilical), allogeneic or autologous, harvesting, transplantation, and related complications; including: pheresis and cell preparation/storage; marrow ablative therapy; drugs, supplies, hospitalization with outpatient follow-up; medical/surgical, diagnostic, emergency, and rehabilitative services; and the number of days of pre- and post-transplant care in the global definition

S2152 Solid organ(s), complete or segmental, single organ or combination of organs; deceased or living donor(s), procurement, transplantation, and related complications; including: drugs; supplies; hospitalization with outpatient follow-up; medical/surgical, diagnostic, emergency, and rehabilitative services, and the number of days of pre- and post-transplant care in the global definition

S2202 Echosclerotherapy

S2205 Minimally invasive direct coronary artery bypass surgery involving mini-thoracotomy or mini-sternotomy surgery, performed under direct vision; using arterial graft(s), single coronary arterial graft

S2206 using arterial graft(s), two coronary arterial grafts

S2207 using venous graft only, single coronary venous graft

S2208 using single arterial and venous graft(s), single venous graft

S2209 using two arterial grafts and single venous graft

S2225 Myringotomy, laser-assisted

S2230 Implantation of magnetic component of semi-implantable hearing device on ossicles in middle ear

S2235 Implantation of auditory brain stem implant

S2260 Induced abortion, 17 to 24 weeks

S2265 Induced abortion, 25-28 weeks

S2266 Induced abortion, 29-31 weeks

S2267 Induced abortion, 32 weeks or greater

(S2270) Code deleted March 31, 2011

S2300 Arthroscopy, shoulder, surgical; with thermally-induced capsulorrhaphy

S2325 Hip core decompression

S2340 Chemodenervation of abductor muscle(s) of vocal cord

S2341 Chemodenervation of adductor muscle(s) of vocal cord

S2342 Nasal endoscopy for post-operative debridement following functional endoscopic sinus surgery, nasal and/or sinus cavity(s), unilateral or bilateral

(S2344) Code deleted March 31, 2011

S2348 Decompression procedure, percutaneous, of nucleus pulposus of intervertebral disc, using radiofrequency energy, single or multiple levels, lumbar

S2350 Diskectomy, anterior, with decompression of spinal cord and/or nerve root(s), including osteophytectomy; lumbar, single interspace

S2351 Diskectomy, anterior, with decompression of spinal cord and/or nerve root(s), including osteophytectomy; lumbar, each additional interspace (list separately in addition to code for primary procedure)

S2360 Percutaneous vertebroplasty, one vertebral body, unilateral or bilateral injection; cervical

S2361 Each additional cervical vertebral body (list separately in addition to code for primary procedure)

S2400 Repair, congenital diaphragmatic hernia in the fetus using temporary tracheal occlusion, procedure performed in utero

S2401 Repair, urinary tract obstruction in the fetus, procedure performed in utero

S2402 Repair, congenital cystic adenomatoid malformation in the fetus, procedure performed in utero

S2403 Repair, extralobar pulmonary sequestration in the fetus, procedure performed in utero

S2404 Repair, myelomeningocele in the fetus, procedure performed in utero

S2405 Repair of sacrococcygeal teratoma in the fetus, procedure performed in utero

S2409 Repair, congenital malformation of fetus, procedure performed in utero, not otherwise classified

S2411 Fetoscopic laser therapy for treatment of twin-to-twin transfusion syndrome

S2900 Surgical techniques requiring use of robotic surgical system (list separately in addition to code for primary procedure)

S3000 Diabetic indicator; retinal eye exam, dilated, bilateral

S3005 Performance measurement, evaluation of patient self assessment, depression

S3600 Stat laboratory request (situations other than S3601)

S3601 Emergency stat laboratory charge for patient who is homebound or residing in a nursing facility

S3620 Newborn metabolic screening panel, includes test kit, postage and the following tests: hemoglobin; electrophoresis; hydroxyprogesterone; 17-D; phenalanine (PKU); and thyroxine, total

(S3625) Code deleted December 31, 2013

(S3626) Code deleted December 31, 2013

(S3628) Code deleted June 30, 2011

S3630 Eosinophil count, blood, direct

S3645 HIV-1 antibody testing of oral mucosal transudate

S3650 Saliva test, hormone level; during menopause

S3652 to assess preterm labor risk

S3655 Antisperm antibodies test (immunobead)

S3708 Gastrointestinal fat absorption study

(S3711) Code deleted March 31, 2012

(S3713) Code deleted March 31, 2012

S3721 Prostate cancer antigen 3 (PCa3) testing

S3722 Dose optimization by area under the curve (AUC) analysis, for infusional 5-fluorouracil

S3800 Genetic testing for amyotrophic lateral sclerosis (ALS)

(S3818) Code deleted March 31, 2012

(S3819) Code deleted March 31, 2012

(S3820) Code deleted March 31, 2012

(S3822) Code deleted March 31, 2012

(S3823) Code deleted March 31, 2012

(S3828) Code deleted March 31, 2012

(S3829) Code deleted March 31, 2012

(S3830) Code deleted March 31, 2012

(S3831) Code deleted March 31, 2012

(S3833) Code deleted December 31, 2013

(S3834) Code deleted December 31, 2013

(S3835) Code deleted March 31, 2012

(S3837) Code deleted March 31, 2012

S3840 DNA analysis for germline mutations of the RET proto-oncogene for susceptibility to multiple endocrine neoplasia type 2

S3841 Genetic testing for retinoblastoma

S3842 Genetic testing for von Hippel-Lindau disease

(S3843) Code deleted March 31, 2012

S3844 DNA analysis of the connexin 26 gene (GJB2) for susceptibility to congenital, profound deafness

S3845 Genetic testing for alpha-thalassemia

S3846 Genetic testing for hemoglobin E beta-thalassemia

(S3847) Code deleted March 31, 2012

(S3848) Code deleted March 31, 2012

S3849 Genetic testing for Niemann-Pick disease

S3850 Genetic testing for sickle cell anemia

(S3851) Code deleted March 31, 2012

S3852 DNA analysis for APOE epsilon 4 allele for susceptibility to Alzheimer's disease

S3853 Genetic testing for myotonic muscular dystrophy

S3854 Gene expression profiling panel for use in the management of breast cancer treatment

S3855 Genetic testing for detection of mutations in the presenilin, 1 gene

(S3860) Code deleted March 31, 2012

S3861 Genetic testing, sodium channel, voltage-gated, type V, alpha subunit (scn5a) and variants for suspected Brugada syndrome

(S3862) Code deleted March 31, 2012

S3865 Comprehensive gene sequence analysis for hypertrophic cardiomyopathy

S3866 Genetic analysis for a specific gene mutation for hypertrophic cardiomyopathy (HCM) in an individual with a known mutation in the family

▲**S3870** Comparative genomic hybridization (CGH) microarray testing for developmental delay, autism spectrum disorder and/or intellectual disability

S3890 DNA analysis, fecal, for colorectal cancer screening

S3900 Surface electromyography (EMG)

S3902 Ballistocardiogram

S3904 Masters two step

(S3905) Code deleted March 31, 2011

S4005 Interim labor facility global (labor occurring but not resulting in delivery)

S4011 In vitro fertilization; including but not limited to identification and incubation of mature oocytes, fertilization with sperm, incubation of embryo(s), and subsequent visualization for determination of development

S4013 Complete cycle, gamete intrafallopian transfer (GIFT), case rate

S4014 Complete cycle, zygote intrafallopian transfer (ZIFT), case rate

S4015 Complete in vitro fertilization cycle, case rate not otherwise specified

S4016 Frozen in vitro fertilization cycle, case rate

S4017 Incomplete cycle, treatment canceled prior to stimulation, case rate

S4018 Frozen embryo transfer procedure canceled before transfer, case rate

S4020 In vitro fertilization procedure canceled before aspiration, case rate

S4021 In vitro fertilization procedure canceled after aspiration, case rate

S4022 Assisted oocyte fertilization, case rate

S4023 Donor egg cycle, incomplete, case rate

S4025 Donor services for in vitro fertilization (sperm or embryo), case rate

S4026 Procurement of donor sperm from sperm bank

S4027 Storage of previously frozen embryos

S4028 Microsurgical epididymal sperm aspiration (mesa)

S4030 Sperm procurement and cryopreservation services; initial visit

S4031 Sperm procurement and cryopreservation services; subsequent visit

S4035 Stimulated intrauterine insemination (IU), case rate

S4037 Cryopreserved embryo transfer, case rate

S4040 Monitoring and storage of cryopreserved embryos, per 30 days

S4042 Management of ovulation induction (interpretation of diagnostic tests and studies, non-face-to-face medical management of the patient), per cycle

S4981 Insertion of levonorgestrel-releasing intrauterine system

S4989 Contraceptive intrauterine device (e.g., progestacert IUD), including implants and supplies

S4990 Nicotine patches, legend

S4991 Nicotine patches, non-legend

S4993 Contraceptive pills for birth control

S4995 Smoking cessation gum

S5000 Prescription drug, generic

S5001 Prescription drug, brand name

S5010 5% dextrose and 0.45% normal saline, 1000 ml

S5011 5% dextrose in lactated ringer's, 1000 ml

S5012 5% dextrose with potassium chloride, 1000 ml

S5013 5% dextrose/0..45% normal saline with potassium chloride and magnesium sulfate, 1000 ml

S5014 5% dextrose/0.45% normal saline with potassium chloride and magnesium sulfate, 1500 ml

S5035 Home infusion therapy, routine service of infusion device (e.g., pump maintenance)

S5036 Home infusion therapy, repair of infusion device (e.g., pump repair)

S5100 Day care services, adult; per 15 minutes

S5101 per half day

S5102 per diem

S5105 Day care services, center-based; services not included in program fee, per diem

S5108 Home care training to home care client; per 15 minutes

S5109 per session

S5110 Home care training, family; per 15 minutes

S5111 per session

S5115 Home care training, non-family; per 15 minutes

S5116 per session

S5120 Chore services; per 15 minutes

S5121 per diem

S5125 Attendant care services; per 15 minutes

S5126 per diem

S5130 Homemaker service, NOS; per 15 minutes

S5131 per diem

S5135 Companion care, adult (e.g., IADL/ADL); per 15 minutes

S5136 per diem

S5140 Foster care, adult, per diem

S5141 per month

S5145 Foster care, therapeutic, child; per diem

S5146 per month

S5150 Unskilled respite care, not hospice; per 15 minutes

S5151 per diem

S5160 Emergency response system; installation and testing

S5161 service fee, per month (excludes installation and testing)

S5162 purchase only

S5165 Home modifications; per service

S5170 Home delivered meals, including preparation; per meal

S5175 Laundry service, external, professional; per order

S5180 Home health respiratory therapy, initial evaluation

S5181 Home health respiratory therapy NOS, per diem

S5185 Medication reminder service, non-face-to-face; per month

S5190 Wellness assessment, performed by non-physician

S5199 Personal care item, NOS, each

S5497 Home infusion therapy, catheter care/maintenance, not otherwise classified; includes administrative services, professional pharmacy services, care coordination, and all necessary supplies and equipment (drugs and nursing visits coded separately), per diem

S5498 Home infusion therapy, catheter care/maintenance, simple (single lumen), includes administrative services, professional pharmacy services, care coordination and all necessary supplies and equipment, (drugs and nursing visits coded separately), per diem

S5501 Home infusion therapy, catheter care/maintenance, complex (more than one lumen), includes administrative services, professional pharmacy services, care coordination, and all necessary supplies and equipment (drugs and nursing visits coded separately), per diem

S5502 Home infusion therapy, catheter care/maintenance, implanted access device, includes administrative services, professional pharmacy services, care coordination and all necessary supplies and equipment, (drugs and nursing visits coded separately), per diem (use this code for interim maintenance of vascular access not currently in use)

S5517 Home infusion therapy, all supplies necessary for restoration of catheter patency or declotting

S5518 Home infusion therapy, all supplies necessary for catheter repair

S5520 Home infusion therapy, all supplies (including catheter) necessary for a peripherally inserted central venous catheter (PICC) line insertion

S5521 Home infusion therapy, all supplies (including catheter) necessary for a midline catheter insertion

S5522 Home infusion therapy, insertion of peripherally inserted central venous catheter (PICC), nursing services only (no supplies or catheter included)

S5523 Home infusion therapy, insertion of midline venous catheter, nursing services only (no supplies or catheter included)

S5550 Insulin, rapid onset; 5 units

S5551 Insulin, most rapid onset (lispro or aspart); 5 units

S5552 Insulin, intermediate acting (NPH or lente); 5 units

S5553 Insulin, long acting; 5 units

S5560 Insulin delivery device, reusable pen; 1.5 ml size

S5561 Insulin delivery device, reusable pen; 3 ml size

S5565 Insulin cartridge for use in insulin delivery device other than pump; 150 units

S5566 Insulin cartridge for use in insulin delivery device other than pump; 300 units

S5570 Insulin delivery device, disposable pen (including insulin); 1.5 ml size

S5571 Insulin delivery device, disposable pen (including insulin); 3 ml size

S8030 Scleral application of tantalum ring(s) for localization of lesions for proton beam therapy

S8035 Magnetic source imaging

S8037 Magnetic resonance cholangiopancreatography (MRCP)

S8040 Topographic brain mapping

S8042 Magnetic resonance imaging (MRI), low-field

(S8049) Code deleted March 31, 2012

S8055 Ultrasound guidance for multifetal pregnancy reduction(s), technical component (only to be used when the physician doing the reduction procedure does not perform the ultrasound, guidance is included in the CPT code for multifetal pregnancy reduction - 59866)

S8080 Scintimammography (radioimmunoscintigraphy of the breast), unilateral, including supply of radiopharmaceutical

S8085 Fluorine-18 fluorodeoxyglucose (F-18 FDG) imaging using dual-head coincidence detection system (non-dedicated PET scan)

S8092 Electron beam computed tomography (also known as ultrafast CT, cine CT)

S8096 Portable peak flow meter

S8097 Asthma kit (including but not limited to portable peak expiratory flow meter, instructional video, brochure, and/or spacer)

S8100 Holding chamber or spacer for use with an inhaler or nebulizer; without mask

S8101 with mask

S8110 Peak expiratory flow rate (physician services)

S8120 Oxygen contents, gaseous, 1 unit equals 1 cubic foot

S8121 Oxygen contents, liquid, 1 unit equals 1 pound

S8130 Interferential current stimulator, 2 channel

S8131 Interferential current stimulator, 4 channel

S8185 Flutter device

S8186 Swivel adaptor

S8189 Tracheostomy supply, not otherwise classified

S8210 Mucus trap

S8262 Mandibular orthopedic repositioning device, each

S8265 Haberman feeder for cleft lip/palate

S8270 Enuresis alarm, using auditory buzzer and/or vibration device

S8301 Infection control supplies, not otherwise specified

S8415 Supplies for home delivery of infant

S8420 Gradient pressure aid (sleeve and glove combination), custom made

S8421 Gradient pressure aid (sleeve and glove combination), ready made

S8422 Gradient pressure aid (sleeve), custom made, medium weight

S8423 Gradient pressure aid (sleeve), custom made, heavy weight

S8424 Gradient pressure aid (sleeve), ready made

S8425 Gradient pressure aid (glove), custom made, medium weight

S8426 Gradient pressure aid (glove), custom made, heavy weight

S8427 Gradient pressure aid (glove), ready made

S8428 Gradient pressure aid (gauntlet), ready made

S8429 Gradient pressure exterior wrap

S8430 Padding for compression bandage, roll

S8431 Compression bandage, roll

S8450 Splint, prefabricated, digit (specify digit by use of modifier)

S8451 Splint, prefabricated, wrist or ankle

S8452 Splint, prefabricated, elbow

S8460 Camisole, post mastectomy

S8490 Insulin syringes (100 syringes, any size)

S9830 Electrical stimulation of auricular acupuncture points; each 15 minutes of personal one-on-one contact with the patient

S8940 Equestrian/hippotherapy, per session

S8948 Application of a modality (requiring constant provider attendance) to one or more areas, low-level laser, each 15 minutes

S8950 Complex lymphedema therapy, each 15 min

S8990 Physical or manipulative therapy performed for maintenance rather than restoration

S8999 Resuscitation bag (for use by patient on artificial respiration during power failure or other catastrophic event)

S9001 Home uterine monitor with or without associated nursing services

S9007 Ultrafiltration monitor

S9015 Automated EEG monitoring

S9024 Paranasal sinus ultrasound

S9025 Omnicardiogram/cardiointegram

S9034 Extracorporeal shockwave lithotripsy for gall stones (if performed with ERCP, use 43265)

S9055 Procuren or other growth factor preparation to promote wound healing

S9056 Coma stimulation per diem

S9061 Home administration of aerosolized drug therapy (e.g., pentamidine); administative services, professional pharmacy services, care coordination, all necesary supplies and equipment (drugs and nursing visits coded separately), per diem

(S9075) Code deleted June 30, 2011

S9083 Global fee urgent care centers

S9088 Services provided in an urgent care center (list in addition to code for service)

S9090 Vertebral axial decompression, per session

S9097 Home visit for wound care

S9098 Home visit, phototherapy services (e.g., Bili-lite), including equipment rental, nursing services, blood draw, supplies, and other services, per diem

(S9109) Code deleted December 31, 2012.

S9110 Telemonitoring of patient in their home, including all necessary equipment; computer system, connections, and software; maintenance; patient education and support; per month

S9117 Back school, per visit

S9122 Home health aide or certified nurse assistant, providing care in the home; per hour

S9123 Nursing care, in the home; by registered nurse, per hour (use for general nursing care only, not to be used when CPT codes 99500-99602 can be used)

S9124 by licensed practical nurse, per hour

S9125 Respite care, in the home, per diem

S9126 Hospice care, in the home, per diem

S9127 Social work visit, in the home, per diem

S9128 Speech therapy, in the home, per diem

S9129 Occupational therapy, in the home, per diem

S9131 Physical therapy; in the home, per diem

S9140 Diabetic management program; follow-up visit to non-MD provider

S9141 follow-up visit to MD provider

S9145 Insulin pump initiation, instruction in initial use of pump (pump not included)

S9150 Evaluation by ocularist

S9152 Speech therapy, re-evaluation

S9208 Home management of pre-term labor, including administrative services, professional pharmacy services, care coordination, and all necessary supplies or equipment (drugs and nursing visits coded separately), per diem (do not use this code with any home infusion per diem code)

S9209 Home management of pre-term premature rupture of membranes (PPROM), including administrative services, professional pharmacy services, care coordination, and all necessary supplies or equipment (drugs and nursing visits coded separately), per diem (do not use this code with any home infusion per diem code)

S9211 Home management of gestational hypertension, includes administrative services, professional pharmacy services, care coordination and all necessary supplies and equipment (drugs and nursing visits coded separately); per diem (do not use this code with any home infusion per diem code)

S9212 Home management of postpartum hypertension, includes administrative services, professional pharmacy services, care coordination, and all necessary supplies and equipment (drugs and nursing visits coded separately), per diem (do not use this code with any home infusion per diem code)

S9213 Home management of preeclampsia, includes administrative services, professional pharmacy services, care coordination, and all necessary supplies and equipment (drugs and nursing services coded separately); per diem (do not use this code with any home infusion per diem code)

S9214 Home management of gestational diabetes, includes administrative services, professional pharmacy services, care coordination, and all necessary supplies and equipment (drugs and nursing visits coded separately); per diem (do not use this code with any home infusion per diem code)

S9325 Home infusion therapy, pain management infusion; administrative services, professional pharmacy services, care coordination, and all necessary supplies and equipment, (drugs and nursing visits coded separately), per diem (do not use this code with S9326, S9327 or S9328)

S9326 Home infusion therapy, continuous (twenty-four hours or more) pain management infusion; administrative services, professional pharmacy services, care coordination and all necessary supplies and equipment (drugs and nursing visits coded separately), per diem

S9327 Home infusion therapy, intermittent (less than twenty-four hours) pain management infusion; administrative services, professional pharmacy services, care coordination, and all necessary supplies and equipment (drugs and nursing visits coded separately), per diem

S9328 Home infusion therapy, implanted pump pain management infusion; administrative services, professional pharmacy services, care coordination, and all necessary supplies and equipment (drugs and nursing visits coded separately), per diem

S9329 Home infusion therapy, chemotherapy infusion; administrative services, professional pharmacy services, care coordination, and all necessary supplies and equipment (drugs and nursing visits coded separately), per diem (do not use this code with S9330 or S9331)

S9330 Home infusion therapy, continuous (twenty-four hours or more) chemotherapy infusion; administrative services, professional pharmacy services, care coordination, and all necessary supplies and equipment (drugs and nursing visits coded separately), per diem

S9331 Home infusion therapy, intermittent (less than twenty-four hours) chemotherapy infusion; administrative services, professional pharmacy services, care coordination, and all necessary supplies and equipment (drugs and nursing visits coded separately), per diem

S9335 Home therapy, hemodialysis; administrative services, professional pharmacy services, care coordination, and all necessary supplies and equipment (drugs and nursing services coded separately), per diem

S9336 Home infusion therapy, continuous anticoagulant infusion therapy (e.g., Heparin), administrative services, professional pharmacy services, care coordination and all necessary supplies and equipment (drugs and nursing visits coded separately), per diem

S9338 Home infusion therapy, immunotherapy (e.g., intravenous immunoglobulin, interferon); administrative services, professional pharmacy services, care coordination, and all necessary supplies and equipment (drugs and nursing visits coded separately), per diem

S9339 Home therapy; peritoneal dialysis, administrative services, professional pharmacy services, care coordination and all necessary supplies and equipment (drugs and nursing visits coded separately), per diem

S9340 Home therapy; enteral nutrition; administrative services, professional pharmacy services, care coordination, and all necessary supplies and equipment (enteral formula and nursing visits coded separately), per diem

S9341 Home therapy; enteral nutrition via gravity; administrative services, professional pharmacy services, care coordination, and all necessary supplies and equipment (enteral formula and nursing visits coded separately), per diem

S9342 Home therapy; enteral nutrition via pump; administrative services, professional pharmacy services, care coordination, and all necessary supplies and equipment (enteral formula and nursing visits coded separately), per diem

S9343 Home therapy; enteral nutrition via bolus; administrative services, professional pharmacy services, care coordination, and all necessary supplies and equipment (enteral formula and nursing visits coded separately), per diem

S9345 Home infusion therapy, anti-hemophilic agent infusion therapy (e.g., Factor VIII); administrative services, professional pharmacy services, care coordination, and all necessary supplies and equipment (drugs and nursing visits coded separately), per diem

S9346 Home infusion therapy, alpha-1-proteinase inhibitor (e.g., Prolastin); administrative services, professional pharmacy services, care coordination, and all necessary supplies and equipment (drugs and nursing visits coded separately), per diem

S9347 Home infusion therapy, uninterrupted, long-term, controlled rate intravenous or subcutaneous infusion therapy (e.g. epoprostenol); administrative services, professional pharmacy services, care coordination, and all necessary supplies and equipment (drugs and nursing visits coded separately), per diem

S9348 Home infusion therapy, sympathomimetic/inotropic agent infusion therapy (e.g., Dobutamine); administrative services, professional pharmacy services, care coordination, all necessary supplies and equipment (drugs and nursing visits coded separately), per diem

S9349 Home infusion therapy, tocolytic infusion therapy; administrative services, professional pharmacy services, care coordination, and all necessary supplies and equipment (drugs and nursing visits coded separately), per diem

S9351 Home infusion therapy, continuous or intermittent anti-emetic infusion therapy; administrative services, professional pharmacy services, care coordination, and all necessary supplies and equipment (drugs and visits coded separately), per diem

S9353 Home infusion therapy, continuous insulin infusion therapy; administrative services, professional pharmacy services, care coordination, and all necessary supplies and equipment (drugs and nursing visits coded separately), per diem

S9355 Home infusion therapy, chelation therapy; administrative services, professional pharmacy services, care coordination, and all necessary supplies and equipment (drugs and nursing visits coded separately), per diem

S9357 Home infusion therapy, enzyme replacement intravenous therapy; (e.g., Imiglucerase); administrative services, professional pharmacy services, care coordination, and all necessary supplies and equipment (drugs and nursing visits coded separately), per diem

S9359 Home infusion therapy, anti-tumor necrosis factor intravenous therapy; (e.g., Infliximab); administrative services, professional pharmacy services, care coordination, and all necessary supplies and equipment (drugs and nursing visits coded separately), per diem

S9361 Home infusion therapy, diuretic intravenous therapy; administrative services, professional pharmacy services, care coordination, and all necessary supplies and equipment (drugs and nursing visits coded separately), per diem

S9363 Home infusion therapy, anti-spasmotic intravenous therapy; administrative services, professional pharmacy services, care coordination, and all necessary supplies and equipment (drugs and nursing visits coded separately), per diem

S9364 Home infusion therapy, total parenteral nutrition (TPN); administrative services, professional pharmacy services, care coordination, and all necessary supplies and equipment, including standard TPN formula (lipids, specialty amino acid formulas, drugs other than in standard formula, and nursing visits coded separately) per diem (Do not use with home infusion codes S9365-S9368 using daily volume scales)

S9365 Home infusion therapy, total parenteral nutrition (TPN); one liter per day, administrative services, professional pharmacy services, care coordination, and all necessary supplies and equipment, including standard TPN formula (lipids, specialty amino acid formulas, drugs other than in standard formula, and nursing visits coded separately), per diem

S9366 Home infusion therapy, total parenteral nutrition (TPN); more than one liter but no more than two liters per day, administrative services, professional pharmacy services, care coordination, and all necessary supplies and equipment, including standard TPN formula (lipids, specialty amino acid formulas, drugs other than in standard formula, and nursing visits coded separately), per diem

S9367 Home infusion therapy, total parenteral nutrition (TPN); more than two liters but no more than three liters per day, administrative services, professional pharmacy services, care coordination, and all necessary supplies and equipment, including standard TPN formula (lipids, specialty amino acid formulas, drugs other than in standard formula, and nursing visits coded separately), per diem

S9368 Home infusion therapy, total parenteral nutrition (TPN); more than three liters per day, administrative services, professional pharmacy services, care coordination, and all necessary supplies and equipment, including standard TPN formula (lipids, specialty amino acid formulas, drugs other than in standard formula, and nursing visits coded separately), per diem

S9370 Home therapy, intermittent anti-emetic injection therapy; administrative services, professional pharmacy services, care coordination, and all necessary supplies and equipment (drugs and nursing visits coded separately), per diem

S9372 Home therapy; intermittent anticoagulant injection therapy (e.g., heparin); administrative services, professional pharmacy services, care coordination, and all necessary supplies and equipment (drugs and nursing visits coded separately), per diem (do not use this code for flushing of infusion devices with heparin to maintain patency)

S9373 Home infusion therapy, hydration therapy; administrative services, professional pharmacy services, care coordination, and all necessary supplies and equipment (drugs and nursing visits coded separately), per diem (do not use with hydration therapy codes S9374-S9377 using daily volume scales)

S9374 Home infusion therapy, hydration therapy; one liter per day, administrative services, professional pharmacy services, care coordination, and all necessary supplies and equipment (drugs and nursing visits coded separately), per diem

S9375 Home infusion therapy, hydration therapy; more than one liter but no more than two liters per day, administrative services, professional pharmacy services, care coordination, and all necessary supplies and equipment (drugs and nursing visits coded separately), per diem

S9376 Home infusion therapy, hydration therapy; more than two liters but no more than three liters per day, administrative services, professional pharmacy services, care coordination, and all necessary supplies and equipment (drugs and nursing visits coded separately), per diem

S9377 Home infusion therapy, hydration therapy; more than three liters per day, administrative services, professional pharmacy services, care coordination, and all necessary supplies (drugs and nursing visits coded separately), per diem

S9379 Home infusion therapy, infusion therapy, not otherwise classified; administrative services, professional pharmacy services, care coordination, and all necessary supplies and equipment (drugs and nursing visits coded separately), per diem

S9381 Delivery or service to high risk areas requiring escort or extra protection, per visit

S9401 Anticoagulation clinic, inclusive of all services except laboratory tests, per session

S9430 Pharmacy compounding and dispensing services

S9433 Medical food nutritionally complete, administered orally, providing 100% of nutritional intake

S9434 Modified solid food supplements for inborn errors of metabolism

S9435 Medical foods for inborn errors of metabolism

S9436 Childbirth preparation/Lamaze classes, non-physician provider, per session

S9437 Childbirth refresher classes, non-physician provider, per session

S9438 Cesarean birth classes, non-physician provider, per session

S9439 VBAC (vaginal birth after cesarean) classes, non-physician provider, per session

S9441 Asthma education, non-physician provider, per session

S9442 Birthing classes, non-physician provider, per session

S9443 Lactation classes, non-physician provider, per session

S9444 Parenting classes, non-physician provider, per session

S9445 Patient education, not otherwise classified, non-physician provider, individual, per session

S9446 Patient education, not otherwise classified, non-physician provider, group, per session

S9447 Infant safety (including CPR) classes, non-physician provider, per session

S9449 Weight management classes, non-physician provider, per session

S9451 Exercise classes, non-physician provider, per session

S9452 Nutrition classes, non-physician provider, per session

S9453 Smoking cessation classes, non-physician provider, per session

S9454 Stress management classes, non-physician provider, per session

S9455 Diabetic management program; group session

S9460 nurse visit

S9465 dietician visit

S9470 Nutritional counseling, dietitian visit

S9472 Cardiac rehabilitation program, non-physician provider, per diem

S9473 Pulmonary rehabilitation program, non-physician provider, per diem

S9474 Enterostomal therapy by a registered nurse certified in enterostomal therapy, per diem

S9475 Ambulatory setting substance abuse treatment or detoxification services, per diem

S9476 Vestibular rehabilitation program, non-physician provider, per diem

S9480 Intensive outpatient psychiatric services, per diem

S9482 Family stabilization services, per 15 minutes

S9484 Crisis intervention mental health services, per hour

S9485 Crisis intervention mental health services, per diem

S9490 Home infusion therapy, corticosteroid infusion; administrative services, professional pharmacy services, care coordination, and all necessary supplies and equipment (drugs and nursing visits coded separately), per diem

S9494 Home infusion therapy, antibiotic, antiviral, or antifungal therapy; administrative services, professional pharmacy services, care coordination, and all necessary supplies and equipment (drugs and nursing visits coded separately), per diem (do not use with home infusion codes for hourly dosing schedules S9497-S9504)

S9497 Home infusion therapy, antibiotic, antiviral, or antifungal therapy; once every 3 hours; administrative services, professional pharmacy services, care coordination, and all necessary supplies and equipment (drugs and nursing visits coded separately), per diem

S9500 Home infusion therapy, antibiotic, antiviral, or antifungal therapy; once every 24 hours; administrative services, professional pharmacy services, care coordination, and all necessary supplies and equipment (drugs and nursing visits coded separately), per diem

S9501 Home infusion therapy, antibiotic, antiviral, or antifungal therapy; once every 12 hours; administrative services, professional pharmacy services, care coordination, and all necessary supplies and equipment (drugs and nursing visits coded separately), per diem

S9502 Home infusion therapy, antibiotic, antiviral, or antifungal therapy; once every 8 hours, administrative services, professional pharmacy services, care coordination, and all necessary supplies and equipment (drugs and nursing visits coded separately), per diem

S9503 Home infusion therapy, antibiotic, antiviral, or antifungal; once every 6 hours; administrative services, professional pharmacy services, care coordination, and all necessary supplies and equipment (drugs and nursing visits coded separately), per diem

S9504 Home infusion therapy, antibiotic, antiviral, or antifungal; once every 4 hours; administrative services, professional pharmacy services, care coordination, and all necessary supplies and equipment (drugs and nursing visits coded separately), per diem

S9529 Routine venipuncture for collection of specimen(s), single home bound, nursing home, or skilled nursing facility patient

S9537 Home therapy, hematopoietic hormone injection therapy (e.g., erythropoietin, G-CSF, GM-CSF); administrative services, professional pharmacy services, care coordination, and all necessary supplies and equipment (drugs and nursing visits coded separately), per diem

S9538 Home transfusion of blood product(s); administrative services, professional pharmacy services, care coordination and all necessary supplies and equipment (blood products, drugs, and nursing visits coded separately), per diem

S9542 Home injectable therapy; not otherwise classified, including administrative services, professional pharmacy services, care coordination, and all necessary supplies and equipment (drugs and nursing visits coded separately), per diem

S9558 Home injectable therapy; growth hormone, including administrative services, professional pharmacy services, care coordination, and all necessary supplies and equipment (drugs and nursing visits coded separately), per diem

S9559 Home injectable therapy; interferon, including administrative services, professional pharmacy services, care coordination, and all necessary supplies and equipment (drugs and nursing visits coded separately), per diem

S9560 Home injectable therapy; hormonal therapy (e.g., leuprolide, goserelin), including administrative services, professional pharmacy services, care coordination, and all necessary supplies and equipment (drugs and nursing visits coded separately), per diem

S9562 Home injectable therapy, palivizumab, including administrative services, professional pharmacy services, care coordination, and all necessary supplies and equipment (drugs and nursing visits coded separately), per diem

S9590 Home therapy, irrigation therapy (e.g. Sterile irrigation of an organ or anatomical cavity); including administrative services, professional pharmacy services, care coordination, and all necessary supplies and equipment (drugs and nursing visits coded separately), per diem

S9810 Home therapy; professional pharmacy services for provision of infusion, specialty drug administration, and/or disease state management, not otherwise classified, per hour (do not use this code with any per diem code)

S9900 Services by authorized Christian Science Practitioner for the process of healing, per diem. Not to be used for rest or study. Excludes in-patient services.

● **S9960** Ambulance service, conventional air services, nonemergency transport, one way (fixed wing)

● **S9961** Ambulance service, conventional air service, nonemergency transport, one way (rotary

S9970 Health club membership, annual

S9975 Transplant related lodging, meals, and transportation, per diem

S9976 Lodging, per diem, not otherwise classified

S9977 Meals, per diem, not otherwise specified

S9981 Medical records copying fee, administrative

S9982 Medical records copying fee, per page

S9986 Not medically necessary service (patient is aware that service not medically necessary)

S9988 Services provided as part of a phase I clinical trial

S9989 Services provided outside of the United States of America (list in addition to code(s) for services(s))

S9990 Services provided as part of a phase II clinical trial

S9991 Services provided as part of a phase III clinical trial

S9992 Transportation costs to and from trial location and local transportation costs (e.g., fares for taxicab or bus) for clinical trial participant and one caregiver/companion

S9994 Lodging costs (e.g., hotel charges) for clinical trial participant and one caregiver/companion

S9996 Meals for clinical trial participant and one caregiver/companion

S9999 Sales tax

This page intentionally left blank.

STATE MEDICAID AGENCY CODES

Guidelines

"T" codes were added to HCPCS in 2002. These codes are exclusively for the use of state Medicaid agencies. Prior to using "T" codes on health insurance claims to your state Medicaid processor, you should verify that these codes are acceptable. "T" codes are not valid for Medicare use.

In addition to the information presented in the INTRODUCTION, several other items unique to this section are defined or identified here.

1. SPECIAL REPORT: A service, material or supply that is rarely provided, unusual, variable or new may require a special report in determining medical appropriateness for reimbursement purposes. Pertinent information should include an adequate definition or description of the nature, extent, and need for the service, material or supply.

2. MODIFIERS: Listed services may be modified under certain circumstances. When appropriate, the modifying circumstance is identified by adding a modifier to the basic procedure code. CPT and HCPCS National Level II modifiers may be used with CPT and HCPCS National Level II procedure codes.

State Medicaid Agency Codes

T1000 Private duty/independent nursing service(s), licensed, up to 15 minutes

T1001 Nursing assessment/evaluation

T1002 RN services, up to 15 minutes

T1003 LPN/LVN services, up to 15 minutes

T1004 Services of a qualified nursing aide, up to 15 minutes

T1005 Respite care services, up to 15 minutes

T1006 Alcohol and/or substance abuse services, family/couple counseling

T1007 Alcohol and/or substance abuse services, treatment plan development and/or modification

T1009 Child sitting services for children of the individual receiving alcohol and/or substance abuse services

T1010 Meals for individuals receiving alcohol and/or substance abuse services (when meals are not included in the program)

T1012 Alcohol and/or substance abuse services, skills development

T1013 Sign language or oral interpreter services, per 15 minutes

T1014 Telehealth transmission, per minute, professional services bill separately

T1015 Clinic visit/encounter, all-inclusive

T1016 Case management, each 15 mintues

T1017 Targeted case management, each 15 minutes

T1018 School-based individualized education program (IEP) services, bundled

T1019 Personal care services, per 15 minutes, not for an inpatient or resident of a hospital, nursing facility, ICF/MR or IMD, part of the individualized plan of treatment (code may not be used to identify services provided by home health aide or certified nurse assistant)

T1020 Personal care services, per diem, not for an inpatient or resident of a hospital, nursing facility, ICF/MR or IMD, part of the individualized plan of treatment (code may not be used to identify services provided by home health aide or certified nurse assistant)

T1021 Home health aide or certified nurse assistant, per visit

T1022 Contracted home health agency services, all services provided under contract, per day

T1023 Screening to determine the appropriateness of consideration of an individual for participation in a specified program, project or treatment protocol, per encounter

T1024 Evaluation and treatment by an integrated, specialty team contracted to provide coordinated care to multiple or severely handicapped children, per encounter

T1025 Intensive, extended multidisciplinary services provided in a clinic setting to children with complex medical, physical, medical and psychosocial impairments, per diem

T1026 Intensive, extended multidisciplinary services provided in a clinic setting to children with complex medical, physical, medical and psychosocial impairments, per hour

T1027 Family training and counseling for child development, per 15 mintues

T1028 Assessment of home, physical and family environment, to determine suitability to meet patient's medical needs

T1029 Comprehensive environmental lead investigation, not including laboratory analysis, per dwelling

T1030 Nursing care, in the home, by registered nurse, per diem

T1031 Nursing care, in the home, by licensed practical nurse, per diem

T1502 Administration of oral, intramuscular and/or subcutaneous medication by health care agency/professional, per visit

T1503 Administration of medication, other than oral and/or injectable, by a health care agency/professional, per visit

T1505 Electronic medication compliance management device, includes all components and accessories, not otherwise classified

T1999 Miscellaneous therapeutic items and supplies, retail purchases, not otherwise classified. Identify product in "remarks."

T2001 Non-emergency transportation; patient attendant/escort

Not valid for Medicare | Non-covered by Medicare | Special coverage instructions | Carrier discretion

T2002 Non-emergency tranportation; per diem

T2003 Non-emergency transportation; encounter/trip

T2004 Non-emergency transportation; commercial carrier, multi-pass

T2005 Non-emergency transportation; stretcher van

T2007 Transportation waiting time, air ambulance, and non-emergency vehicle, one-half (1/2) hour increments

T2010 Preadmission screening and resident review (PASRR) Level I Identification Screening, per screen

T2011 Preadmission screening and resident review (PASRR) Level II Evaluation, per evaluation

T2012 Habilitation, educational, waiver; per diem

T2013 Habilitation, educational, waiver; per hour

T2014 Habilitation, prevocational, waiver; per diem

T2015 Habilitation, prevocational, waiver; per hour

T2016 Habilitation, residential, waiver; per diem

T2017 Habilitation, residential, waiver; per hour

T2018 Habilitation, supported employment, waiver; per diem

T2019 Habilitation, supported employment, wiaver; per 15 minutes

T2020 Day habilitation, waiver; per diem

T2021 Day habilitation, waiver; per 15 minutes

T2022 Case management; per month

T2023 Targeted case management; per month

T2024 Service assessment/plan of care development, waiver

T2025 Waiver services; not otherwise specified (NOS)

T2026 Specialized childcare, waiver; per diem

T2027 Specialized childcare, waiver; per 15 minutes

T2028 Specialized supply, not otherwise specified, waiver

T2029 Specialized medical equipment, not otherwise specified, waiver

T2030 Assisted living, waiver; per month

T2031 Assisted living, waiver; per diem

T2032 Residential care, not otherwise specified (NOS), waiver; per month

T2033 Residential care, not otherwise specified (NOS), waiver; per diem

T2034 Crisis intervention waiver; per diem

T2035 Utility services to support medical equipment and assistive technology/devices, waiver

T2036 Therapeutic camping, overnight, waiver; each session

T2037 Therapeutic camping, day, waiver; each session

T2038 Community transition, waiver; per service

T2039 Vehicle modifications, waiver; per service

T2040 Financial management, self-directed, waiver; per 15 minutes

T2041 Supports brokerage, self-directed, waiver; per 15 minutes

T2042 Hospice routine home care; per diem

T2043 Hospice continuous home care; per hour

T2044 Hospice inpatient respite care; per diem

T2045 Hospice general inpatient care; per diem

T2046 Hospice long term care, room and board only; per diem

T2048 Behavioral health; long-term care residential (non-acute care in a residential treatment program where stay is typically longer than 30 days), with room and board, per diem

T2049 Non-emergency transportation; stretcher van, mileage; per mile

T2101 Human breast milk processing, storage and distribution only

T4521 Adult sized disposable incontinence product, brief/diaper, small, each
CIM: 60-9

T4522 Adult sized disposable incontinence product, brief/diaper, medium, each
CIM: 60-9

T4523 Adult sized disposable incontinence product, brief/diaper, large, each
CIM: 60-9

T4524 Adult sized disposable incontinence product, brief/diaper, extra large, each
CIM: 60-9

T4525 Adult sized disposable incontinence product, protective underwear/pull-on, small size, each
CIM: 60-9

T4526 Adult sized disposable incontinence product, protective underwear/pull-on, medium size, each
CIM: 60-9

T4527 Adult sized disposable incontinence product, protective underwear/pull-on, large size, each
CIM: 60-9

T4528 Adult sized disposable incontinence product, protective underwear/pull-on, extra large size, each
CIM: 60-9

T4529 Pediatric sized disposable incontinence product, brief/diaper, small/medium size, each
CIM: 60-9

T4530 Pediatric sized disposable incontinence product, brief/diaper, large size, each
CIM: 60-9

T4531 Pediatric sized disposable incontinence product, protective underwear/pull-on, small/medium size, each
CIM: 60-9

T4532 Pediatric sized disposable incontinence product, protective underwear/pull-on, large size, each
CIM: 60-9

T4533 Youth sized disposable incontinence product, brief/diaper, each
CIM: 60-9

T4534 Youth sized disposable incontinence product, protective underwear/pull-on, each
CIM: 60-9

T4535 Disposable liner/shield/guard/pad/undergarment, for incontinence, each
CIM: 60-9

T4536 Incontinence product, protective underwear/pull-on, reusable, any size, each
CIM: 60-9

T4537 Incontinence product, protective underpad, reusable, bed size, each
CIM: 60-9

T4538 Diaper service, reusable diaper, each diaper
CIM: 60-9

T4539 Incontinence product, diaper/brief, reusable, any size, each
CIM: 60-9

T4540 Incontinence product, protective underpad, reusable, chair size, each
CIM: 60-9

T4541 Incontinence product, disposable underpad, large, each

T4542 Incontinence product, disposable underpad, small size, each

▲**T4543** Adult sized disposable incontinence product, protective brief/diaper, above extra large, each
CIM: 60-9

●**T4544** Adult sized disposable incontinence product, protective underwear/pull-on, above extra large, each
CIM: 60-9

T5001 Positioning seat for persons with special orthopedic needs

T5999 Supply, not otherwise specified

VISION SERVICES

Guidelines

In addition to the information presented in the INTRODUCTION, several other items unique to this section are defined or identified here:

1. SUBSECTION INFORMATION: Some of the listed subheadings or subsections have special needs or instructions unique to that section. Where these are indicated, special "notes" will be presented preceding or following the listings. Those subsections within the VISION SERVICES section that have "notes" are as follows:

Subsection	Code Numbers
Spectacle lenses	V2100-V2499
Contact lenses	V2500-V2599
Low vision aids	V2600-V2615

2. UNLISTED SERVICE OR PROCEDURE: A service or procedure may be provided that is not listed in this edition of HCPCS. When reporting such a service, the appropriate "unlisted procedure" code may be used to indicate the service, identifying it by "special report" as defined below. HCPCS terminology is inconsistent in defining unlisted procedures. The procedure definition may include the term(s) "unlisted", "not otherwise classified", "unspecified", "unclassified", "other" and "miscellaneous". Prior to using these codes, try to determine if a Local Level III code or CPT code is available. The "unlisted procedures" and accompanying codes for VISION SERVICES are as follows:

V2199	Not otherwise classified, single vision lens, bifocal, glass or plastic
V2499	Variable sphericity lens, other type
V2599	Not otherwise classified, contact lens
V2629	Prosthetic eye, other type
V2799	Vision service, miscellaneous

3. SPECIAL REPORT: A service, material or supply that is rarely provided, unusual, variable or new may require a special report in determining medical appropriateness for reimbursement purposes. Pertinent information should include an adequate definition or description of the nature, extent, and need for the service, material or supply.

Q-R-S CODES

4. MODIFIERS: Listed services may be modified under certain circumstances. When appropriate, the modifying circumstance is identified by adding a modifier to the basic procedure code. CPT and HCPCS National Level II modifiers may be used with CPT and HCPCS National Level II procedure codes. Modifiers commonly used with VISION SERVICES are as follows:

    -AP Determination of refractive state was not performed in the course of diagnostic ophthalmological examination

    -CC Procedure code change (use "CC" when the procedure code submitted was changed either for administrative reasons or because an incorrect code was filed)

    -LS FDA-monitored intraocular lens implant

    -LT Left side (used to identify procedures performed on the left side of the body)

    -PL Progressive addition lenses

    -RT Right side (used to identify procedures performed on the right side of the body)

    -SF Second opinion ordered by a professional review organization (PRO) per section 9401, P.L. 99-272. (100 percent reimbursement; no Medicare deductible or coinsurance)

    -TC Technical component. Under certain circumstances, a charge may be made for the technical component alone. Under those circumstances, the technical component charge is identified by adding modifier -TC to the usual procedure number. Technical component charges are institutional charges and are not billed separately by physicians. However, portable x-ray suppliers bill only for the technical component and should use modifier -TC. The charge data from portable x-ray suppliers will then be used to build customary and prevailing profiles.

    -VP Aphakic patient

5. CPT CODE CROSS-REFERENCE: See sections for equivalent CPT code(s) for all listings in this section.

Vision Services

FRAMES

V2020 Frames, purchases
MCM: 2130

V2025 Deluxe frame
MCM: 3045.4

SPECTACLE LENSES

NOTE: If CPT code 92390 or 92395 is reported, recode with the specific lens type listed below. For aphakic temporary spectacle correction, see CPT code 92358.

SINGLE VISION, GLASS OR PLASTIC

V2100 Sphere, single vision; plano to plus or minus 4.00, per lens

V2101 plus or minus 4.12 to plus or minus 7.00d, per lens

V2102 plus or minus 7.12 to plus or minus 20.00d, per lens

V2103 Spherocylinder, single vision, plano to plus or minus 4.00d sphere; .12 to 2.00d cylinder, per lens

V2104 2.12 to 4.00d cylinder, per lens

V2105 4.25 to 6.00d cylinder, per lens

V2106 over 6.00d cylinder, per lens

V2107 Spherocylinder, single vision, plus or minus 4.25d to plus or minus 7.00d sphere; .12 to 2.00d cylinder, per lens

V2108 2.12 To 4.00d cylinder, per lens

V2109 4.25 to 6.00d cylinder, per lens

V2110 over 6.00d cylinder, per lens

V2111 Spherocylinder, single vision, plus or minus 7.25 to plus or minus 12.00d sphere; .25 to 2.25d cylinder, per lens

V2112 2.25d to 4.00d cylinder, per lens

V2113 4.25 to 6.00d cylinder, per lens

V2114 Spherocylinder, single vision, sphere over plus or minus 12.00d per lens

V2115 Lenticular, (myodisc), per lens, single vision

V2118 Aniseikonic lens, single vision

V2121 Lenticular lens, per lens, single
MCM: 2130.B

V2199 Not otherwise classified, single vision lens

BIFOCAL, GLASS OR PLASTIC

(Up to and including 28mm seg width, add power up to and including 3.25d)

V2200 Sphere, bifocal, plano to plus or minus 4.00d, per lens

V2201 Sphere, bifocal, plus or minus 4.12 to plus or minus 7.00d, per lens

V2202 Sphere, bifocal, plus or minus 7.12 to plus or minus 20.00d, per lens

V2203 Spherocylinder, bifocal, plano to plus or minus 4.00d sphere; .12 to 2.00d cylinder, per lens

V2204 2.12 to 4.00d cylinder, per lens

V2205 4.25 to 6.00d cylinder, per lens

V2206 over 6.00d cylinder, per lens

V2207 Spherocylinder, bifocal, plus or minus 4.25 to plus or minus 7.00d sphere; .12 to 2.00d cylinder, per lens

V2208 2.12 to 4.00d cylinder, per lens

V2209 4.25 to 6.00d cylinder, per lens

V2210 over 6.00d cylinder, per lens

V2211 Spherocylinder, bifocal, plus or minus 7.25 to plus or minus 12.00d sphere; .25 to 2.25d cylinder, per lens

V2212 2.25 to 4.00d cylinder, per lens

V2213 4.25 to 6.00d cylinder, per lens

V2214 Spherocylinder, bifocal, sphere over plus or minus 12.00d, per lens

V2215 Lenticular (myodisc), per lens, bifocal

V2218 Aniseikonic, per lens, bifocal

V2219 Bifocal seg width over 28mm

V2220 Bifocal add over 3.25d

V2221 Lenticular lens, per lens, bifocal
MCM: 2130.B

V2299 Specialty bifocal (by report)

TRIFOCAL, GLASS OR PLASTIC

(Up to and including 28mm seg width, add power up to and including 3.25d)

V2300 Sphere, trifocal, plano to plus or minus 4.00d, per lens

V2301 Sphere, trifocal, plus or minus 4.12 to plus or minus 7.00d, per lens

V2302 Sphere, trifocal, plus or minus 7.12 to plus or minus 20.00, per lens

V2303 Spherocylinder, trifocal, plano to plus or minus 4.00d sphere; .12 to 2.00d cylinder, per lens

V2304 2.25 to 4.00d cylinder, per lens

V2305 4.25 to 6.00d cylinder, per lens

V2306 over 6.00d cylinder, per lens

V2307 Spherocylinder, trifocal, plus or minus 4.25 to plus or minus 7.00d sphere; .12 to 2.00d cylinder, per lens

V2308 2.12 to 4.00d cylinder, per lens

V2309 4.25 to 6.00d cylinder, per lens

V2310 over 6.00d cylinder, per lens

V2311 Spherocylinder, trifocal, plus or minus 7.25 to plus or minus 12.00d sphere; .25 to 2.25d cylinder, per lens

V2312 2.25 to 4.00d cylinder, per lens

V2313 4.25 to 6.00d cylinder, per lens

V2314 Spherocylinder, trifocal, sphere over plus or minus 12.00d, per lens

V2315 Lenticular, (myodisc), per lens, trifocal

V2318 Aniseikonic lens, trifocal

V2319 Trifocal seg width over 28mm

V2320 Trifocal add over 3.25d

V2321 Lenticular lens, per lens, trifocal
MCM: 2130.B

V2399 Specialty trifocal (by report)

VARIABLE ASPHERICITY

(Welsh 4-drop, hyperaspheric, double drop, etc.)

V2410 Variable asphericity lens; single vision, full field, glass or plastic, per lens

V2430 bifocal, full field, glass or plastic, per lens

V2499 other type

CONTACT LENSES (CPT 92391 OR 92396)

NOTE: If CPT code 92391 or 92396 is reported, recode with specific lens type listed below, per lens.

V2500 Contact lens, PMMA; spherical, per lens

V2501 toric or prism ballast, per lens

V2502 bifocal, per lens

V2503 color vision deficiency, per lens

V2510 Contact lens, gas permeable; spherical, per lens

V2511 toric, prism ballast, per lens

V2512 bifocal, per lens

V2513 extended wear, per lens

V2520 Contact lens hydrophilic; spherical, per lens
CIM: 45-7, 65-1

V2521 toric, or prism ballast, per lens
CIM: 45-7, 65-1

V2522 bifocal, per lens
CIM: 45-7, 65-1

V2523 extended wear, per lens
CIM: 45-7, 65-1

V2530 Contact lens, scleral, gas impermeable, per lens (for contact lens modification, see 92325)

V2531 Contact lens, scleral, gas permeable, per lens (for contact lens modification, see 92325)
CIM: 65-3

V2599 Contact lens, other type

LOW VISION AIDS (CPT 92392)

NOTE: If CPT code 92392 is reported, record with specific systems listed below.

V2600 Hand held low vision aids and other nonspectacle mounted aids

V2610 Single lens spectacle mounted low vision aids

V2615 Telescopic and other compound lens system, including distance vision telescopic, near vision telescopes and compound microscopic lens system

EYE PROSTHESIS

PROSTHETIC EYE (CPT 92330 OR 92393)

V2623 Prosthetic, eye; plastic, custom
MCM: 2133

V2624 Polishing/resurfacing or ocular prosthesis

V2625 Enlargement of ocular prosthesis

V2626 Reduction of ocular prosthesis

V2627 Scleral cover shell
CIM: 65-3

V2628 Fabrication and fitting of ocular conformer

V2629 Prosthetic eye, other type

INTRAOCULAR LENSES

V2630 Anterior chamber intraocular lens
MCM: 2130

V2631 Iris supported intraocular lens
MCM: 2130

V2632 Posterior chamber intraocular lens
MCM: 2130

MISCELLANEOUS

V2700 Balance lens, per lens

V2702 Deluxe lens feature
MCM: 2130.B

V2710 Slab off prism, glass or plastic, per lens

V2715 Prism, per lens

V2718 Press-on lens, fresnell prism, per lens

V2730 Special base curve, glass or plastic, per lens

V2744 Tint, photochromatic, per lens
MCM: 2130.B

V2745 Addition to lens; tint, any color, solid, gradient or equal, excludes photochromatic, any lens material, per lens
MCM: 2130.B

V2750 Anti-reflective coating, per lens
MCM: 2130.B

V2755 U-V lens, per lens
MCM: 2130.B

V2756 Eye glass case

V2760 Scratch resistant coating, per lens

V2761 Mirror coating, any type, solid, gradient or equal, any lens material, per lens
MCM: 2130.B

V2762 Polarization, any lens material, per lens
MCM: 2130.B

V2770 Occluder lens, per lens

V2780 Oversize lens, per lens

V2781 Progressive lens, per lens

V2782 Lens, index 1.54 to 1.65 plastic or 1.60 to 1.79 glass, excluding polycarbonate, per lens
MCM: 2130.B

V2783 Lens, index greater than or equal to 1.66 plastic or greater than or equal to 1.80 glass, excludes polycarbonate, per lens
MCM: 2130.B

V2784 Lens, polycarbonate or equal, any index, per lens
MCM: 2130.B

V2785 Processing, preserving and transporting corneal tissue

V2786 Specialty occupational multifocal lens, per lens
MCM: 2130.B

V2787 Astigmatism correcting function of intraocular lens

V2788 Presbyopia correcting function of intraocular lens

V2790 Amniotic membrane for surgical reconstruction, per procedure

V2797 Vision supply, accessory and/or service component of another HCPCS vision code

V2799 Vision service, miscellaneous

HEARING SERVICES

Guidelines

In addition to the information presented in the INTRODUCTION, several other items unique to this section are defined or identified here:

1. PROSTHETIC DEVICES: Prosthetic devices that replace all or part of an internal body organ or the function of a permanently inoperative or malfunctioning internal body organ are covered when furnished on a physician's order. If the medical record and attending physician indicate the condition will be indefinite, the test of permanence is met.

2. SPEECH PATHOLOGY: Services necessary for diagnosing and treating speech disorders that result in communication disabilities, and swallowing disorders, regardless of the presence of a disability, are covered Medicare services if reasonable and necessary. The services must be considered to be an effective treatment for the patient's condition, and the patient's condition must be at a level of severity that requires the service of a qualified speech pathologist.

3. UNLISTED SERVICE OR PROCEDURE: A service or procedure may be provided that is not listed in this edition of HCPCS. When reporting such a service, the appropriate "unlisted procedure" code may be used to indicate the service, identifying it by "special report" as defined below. HCPCS terminology is inconsistent in defining unlisted procedures. The procedure definition may include the term(s) "unlisted", "not otherwise classified", "unspecified", "unclassified", "other" and "miscellaneous". Prior to using these codes, try to determine if a Local Level III code or CPT code is available. The "unlisted procedures" and accompanying codes for HEARING SERVICES are as follows:

   V5299 Hearing service, miscellaneous

4. SPECIAL REPORT: A service, material or supply that is rarely provided, unusual, variable or new may require a special report in determining medical appropriateness for reimbursement purposes. Pertinent information should include an adequate definition or description of the nature, extent, and need for the service, material or supply.

5. MODIFIERS: Listed services may be modified under certain circumstances. When appropriate, the modifying circumstance is identified by adding a modifier to the basic procedure code. CPT and

HCPCS National Level II modifiers may be used with CPT and HCPCS National Level II procedure codes. Modifiers commonly used with HEARING SERVICES are as follows:

-CC Procedure code change (use "CC" when the procedure code submitted was changed either for administrative reasons or because an incorrect code was filed)

-LT Left side (used to identify procedures performed on the left side of the body)

-RT Right side (used to identify procedures performed on the right side of the body)

-SF Second opinion ordered by a professional review organization (PRO) per sectoin 9401, P.L. 99-272 (100 percent reimbursement; no Medicare deductible or coinsurance)

-TC Technical component. Under certain circumstances, a charge may be made for the technical component alone. Under those circumstances, the technical component charge is identified by adding modifier -TC to the usual procedure number. Technical component charges are institutional charges and are not billed separately by physicians. However, portable x-ray suppliers bill only for the technical component and should use modifier -TC. The charge data from portable x-ray suppliers will then be used to build customary and prevailing profiles.

6. CPT CODE CROSS-REFERENCE: See sections for equivalent CPT code(s) for all listings in this section.

Hearing Services

V5008 Hearing screening
MCM: 2320

V5010 Assessment for hearing aid

V5011 Fitting/orientation/checking of hearing aid

V5014 Repair/modification of a hearing aid

V5020 Conformity evaluation

V5030 Hearing aid, monaural; body worn, air conduction

V5040 body worn, bone conduction

V5050 in the ear

V5060 behind the ear

V5070 Glasses; air conduction

V5080 bone conduction

V5090 Dispensing fee, unspecified hearing aid

V5095 Semi-implantable middle ear hearing prosthesis

V5100 Hearing aid, bilateral, body worn

V5110 Dispensing fee, bilateral

V5120 Binaural; body

V5130 in the ear

V5140 behind the ear

V5150 glasses

V5160 Dispensing fee, binaural

V5170 Hearing aid, CROS; in the ear

V5180 behind the ear

V5190 glasses

V5200 Dispensing fee, CROS

V5210 Hearing aid, bicros; in the ear

V5220 behind the ear

V5230 glasses

V5240 Dispensing fee, bicros

V5241 Dispensing fee, monaural hearing aid, any type

V5242 Hearing aid, analog, monaural, cic (completely in the ear canal)

V5243 Hearing aid, analog, monaural, itc (in the canal)

V5244 Hearing aid, digitally programmable analog, monaural, cic

V5245 Hearing aid, digitally programmable, analog, monaural, itc

V5246 Hearing aid, digitally programmable analog, monaural, ite (in the ear)

V5247 Hearing aid, digitally programmable analog, monaural, bte (behind the ear)

V5248 Hearing aid, analog, binaural, cic

V5249 Hearing aid, analog, binaural, itc

V5250 Hearing aid, digitally programmable analog, binaural, cic

V5251 Hearing aid, digitally programmable analog, binaural, itc

V5252 Hearing aid, digitally programmable, binaural, ite

V5253 Hearing aid, digitally programmable, binaural, bte

V5254 Hearing aid, digital, monaural, cic

V5255 Hearing aid, digital, monaural, itc

V5256 Hearing aid, digital, monaural, ite

V5257 Hearing aid, digital, monaural, bte

V5258 Hearing aid, digital, binaural, cic

V5259 Hearing aid, digital, binaural, itc

V5260 Hearing aid, digital, binaural, ite

V5261 Hearing aid, digital, binaural, bte

V5262 Hearing aid, disposable, any type, monaural

V5263 Hearing aid, disposable, any type, binaural

V5264 Ear mold/insert, not disposable, any type

V5265 Ear mold/insert, disposable, any type

V5266 Battery for use in hearing device

V5267 Hearing aid supplies/accessories

V5268 Assistive listening device, telephone amplifier, any type

V5269 Assistive listening device, alerting, any type

V5270 Assistive listening device, television amplifier, any type

V5271 Assistive listening device, television caption decoder

V5272 Assistive listening device, TDD

V5273 Assistive listening device, for use with cochlear implant

V5274 Assistive learning device, not otherwise specified

V5275 Ear impression, each

V5281 Assistive listening device, personal fm/dm system, monaural, (1 receiver, transmitter, microphone), any type

V5282 Assistive listening device, personal fm/dm system, binaural, (2 receivers, transmitter, microphone), any type

V5283 Assistive listening device, personal fm/dm neck, loop induction receiver

V5284 Assistive listening device, personal fm/dm, ear level receiver

V5285 Assistive listening device, personal fm/dm, direct audio input receiver

V5286 Assistive listening device, personal blue tooth fm/dm receiver

V5287 Assistive listening device, personal fm/dm receiver, not otherwise specified

V5288 Assistive listening device, personal fm/dm transmitter assistive listening device

V5289 Assistive listening device, personal fm/dm adapter/boot coupling device for receiver, any type

V5290 Assistive listening device, transmitter microphone, any type

V5298 Hearing aid, not otherwise classified

V5299 Hearing service, miscellaneous
MCM: 2320

SPEECH-LANGUAGE PATHOLOGY SERVICES

V5336 Repair/modification of augmentative communicative system or device (excludes adaptive hearing aid)

V5362 Speech screening

V5363 Language screening

V5364 Dysphagia screening

APPENDIX A: MODIFIERS

HCPCS National Level II Modifiers

The following list is the complete list of HCPCS National Level II modifiers and descriptions.

-A1 Dressing for one wound

-A2 Dressing for two wounds

-A3 Dressing for three wounds

-A4 Dressing for four wounds

-A5 Dressing for five wounds

-A6 Dressing for six wounds

-A7 Dressing for seven wounds

-A8 Dressing for eight wounds

-A9 Dressing for nine or more wounds

-AA Anesthesia services performed personally by anesthesiologist
MCM: 3350.5

-AD Medical supervision by a physician; more than four concurrent anesthesia procedures
MCM: 3350.5

-AE Registered dietician

-AF Specialty physician

-AG Primary physician

-AH Clinical psychologist
MCM: 2150, 5112

-AI Principal physician of record

-AJ Clinical social worker
MCM: 2152, 5113

-AK Non-participating physician

-AM Physician, team member service
MCM: 4105.7

● **-AO** Alternate payment method declined by provider of service

-AP Determination of refractive state was not performed in the course of diagnostic ophthalmological examination

-AQ Physician providing a service in an unlisted health professional shortage area (HPSA)

-AR Physician provider services in a physician scarcity area

-AS Physician assistant, nurse practitioner or clinical nurse specialist services for assistant at surgery

-AT Acute treatment (this modifier should be used when reporting service 98940, 98941, 98942)

-AU Item furnished in conjunction with a urological, ostomy, or tracheostomy supply

-AV Item furnished in conjunction with a prosthetic device, prosthetic or orthotic

-AW Item furnished in conjunction with a surgical dressing

-AX Item furnished in conjunction with dialysis services

-AY Item or service furnished to an ESRD patient that is not for the treatment of ESRD

-AZ Physician providing a service in a dental health professional shortage area for the purpose of an electronic health record incentive payment

-BA Item furnished in conjunction with parenteral enteral nutrition (PEN) services

-BL Special acquisition of blood and blood products

-BO Orally administered nutrition, not by feeding tube

-BP The beneficiary has been informed of the purchase and rental options and has elected to purchase the item

-BR The beneficiary has been informed of the purchase and rental options and has elected to rent the item

-BU The beneficiary has been informed of the purchase and rental options and after 30 days has not informed the supplier of his/her decision

-CA Procedure payable only in the inpatient setting when performed emergently on an outpatient who expires prior to admission

-CB Service ordered by a renal dialysis facility (RDF) physician as part of the ESRD beneficiary's dialysis benefit, is not part of the composite rate, and is separately reimbursable

-CC Procedure code change (use -CC when the procedure code submitted was changed either for administrative reasons or because an incorrect code was filed)

-CD AMCC test has been ordered by an ESRD facility or MCP physician that is part of the composite rate and is not separately billable
MCM: 4270.2

-CE AMCC test has been ordered by an ESRD facility or MCP physician that is a composite rate test but is beyond the normal frequency covered under the rate and is separately reimbursable based on medical necessity
MCM: 4270.2

-CF AMCC test has been ordered by an ESRD facility or MCP physician that is not part of the composite rate and is separately billable
MCM: 4270.2

-CG Policy criteria applied

-CH 0 percent impaired, limited or restricted

-CI At least 1 percent but less than 20 percent impaired, limited or restricted

-CJ At least 20 percent but less than 40 percent impaired, limited or restricted

-CK At least 40 percent but less than 60 percent impaired, limited or restricted

-CL At least 60 percent but less than 80 percent impaired, limited or restricted

-CM At least 80 percent but less than 100 percent impaired, limited or restricted

-CM 100 percent impaired, limited or restricted

-CR Catastrophe/disaster related

-CS Item or service related, in whole or in part, to an illness, injury, or condition that was caused by or exacerbated by the effects, direct or indirect, of the 2010 oil spill in the Gulf Of Mexico, including but not limited to subsequent clean-up activities

-DA Oral health assessment by a licensed health professional other than a dentist

-E1 Upper left, eyelid

-E2 Lower left, eyelid

-E3 Upper right, eyelid

-E4 Lower right, eyelid

-EA Erythropoetic stimulating agent (ESA) administered to treat anemia due to anti-cancer chemotherapy

-EB Erythropoetic stimulating agent (ESA) administered to treat anemia due to anti-cancer radiotherapy

-EC Erythropoetic stimulating agent (ESA) administered to treat anemia not due to anti-cancer radiotherapy or anti-cancer chemotherapy

-ED Hematocrit level has exceeded 39% (or hemoglobin level has exceeded 13.0 g/dl) for 3 or more consecutive billing cycles immediately prior to and including the current cycle

-EE Hematocrit level has not exceeded 39% (or hemoglobin level has not exceeded 13.0 g/dl) for 3 or more consecutive billing cycles immediately prior to and including the current cycle

-EJ Subsequent claims for a defined course of therapy, e.g., EPO, sodium hyaluronate, infliximab
MCM: 4273.2

-EM Emergency reserve supply (for ESRD benefit only)
MCM: 3045.7

-EP Service provided as part of Medicaid early periodic screening, diagnosis, and treatment (EPSDT) program

-ET Emergency services

-EY No physician or other licensed health care provider order for this item or service

-F1 Left hand, second digit

-F2 Left hand, third digit

-F3 Left hand, fourth digit

-F4 Left hand, fifth digit

-F5 Right hand, thumb

-F6 Right hand, second digit

-F7 Right hand, third digit

-F8 Right hand, fourth digit

-F9 Right hand, fifth digit

-FA Left hand, thumb

-FB Item provided without cost to provider, supplier or practitioner, or full credit received for replaced device (examples, but not limited to: covered under warranty, replaced due to defect, free samples)

-FC Partial credit received for replaced device

-FP Service provided as part of family planning program

-G1 Most recent URR reading of less than 60

-G2 Most recent URR reading of 60 to 64.9

-G3 Most recent URR reading of 65 to 69.9

-G4 Most recent URR reading of 70 to 74.9

-G5 Most recent URR reading of 75 or greater

-G6 ESRD patient for whom less than six dialysis sessions have been provided in a month

-G7 Pregnancy resulted from rape or incest or pregnancy certified by physician as life threatening
CIM: 35-99 MCM: 2005.1

-G8 Monitored anesthesia care (MAC) for deep complex, complicated, or markedly invasive surgical procedure

-G9 Monitored anesthesia care for patient who has history of severe cardio-pulmonary condition

-GA Waiver of liability statement issued as required by payer policy, individual case

-GB Claim being re-submitted for payment because it is no longer covered under a global payment demonstration

-GC This service has been performed in part by a resident under the direction of a teaching physician
MCM: 3350.5, 4116

-GD Units of service exceeds medically unlikely edit value and represents reasonable and necessary services

-GE This service has been performed by a resident without the presence of a teaching physician under the primary care exception
MCM: 4116

-GF Non-physician (eg., nurse practitioner (NP), certified registered nurse anesthetist (CRNA), certified registered nurse (CRN), clinical nurse specialist (CNS), physician assistant (PA)) services in a critical access hospital

-GG Performance and payment of a screening mammogram and diagnostic mammogram on the same patient, same day

-GH Diagnostic mammogram converted from screening mammogram on same day

-GJ "Opt Out" physician or practitioner emergency or urgent service

-GK Reasonable and necessary item/service associated with a -GA or -GZ modifier

-GL Medically unnecessary upgrade provided instead of non-upgraded item, no charge, no advance beneficiary notice (ABN)

-GM Multiple patients on one ambulance trip

-GN Services delivered under an outpatient speech language pathology plan of care

-GO Services delivered under an outpatient occupational therapy plan of care

-GP Services delivered under an outpatient physical therapy plan of care

-GQ Via asynchronous telecommunications system

-GR This service was performed in whole or in part by a resident in a department of veterans affairs medical center or clinic, supervised in accordance with VA policy

-GS Dosage of EPO or darbepoetin alfa has been reduced and maintained in response to hematocrit or hemoglobin level
MCM: 4273.1

-GT Via interactive audio and video telecommunication systems

-GU Waiver of liability statement issued as required by payer policy, routine notice

-GV Attending physician not employed or paid under arrangement by the patient's hospice provider
MCM: 4175-5

-GW Service not related to the hospice patient's terminal condition
MCM: 4175-5

-GX Notice of liability issued, voluntary under payer policy

-GY Item or service statutorily excluded, does not meet the definition of any Medicare benefit or, for non-Medicare insurers, is not a contract benefit

-GZ Item or service expected to be denied as not reasonable and necessary
MCM: 2000

-H9 Court-ordered

-HA Child/adolescent program

-HB Adult program, non geriatric

-HC Adult program, geriatric

-HD Pregnant/parenting women's program

-HE Mental health program

-HF Substance abuse program

-HG Opioid addiction treatment program

-HH Integrated mental health/substance abuse program

▲**-HI** Integrated mental health and intellectual disability/developmental disabilities program

-HJ Employee assistance program

-HK Specialized mental health programs for high-risk populations

-HL Intern

-HM Less than bachelor degree level

-HN Bachelors degree level

-HO Masters degree level

-HP Doctoral level

-HQ Group setting

-HR Family/couple with client present

-HS Family/couple without client present

-HT Multi-disciplinary team

-HU Funded by child welfare agency

-HV Funded state addictions agency

-HW Funded by state mental health agency

-HX Funded by county/local agency

-HY Funded by juvenile justice agency

-HZ Funded by criminal justice agency

-J1 Competitive acquisition program no-pay submission for a prescription number

-J2 Competitive acquisition program, restocking of emergency drugs after emergency administration

-J3 Competitive acquisition program (CAP), drug not available through CAP as written, reimbursed under average sales price methodology

-J4 DMEPOS item subject to DMEPOS competitive bidding program that is furnished by a hospital upon discharge

-JA Administered intravenously

-JB Administered subcutaneously

-JC Skin substitute used as a graft

-JD Skin substitute not used as a graft

● **-JE** Administered via dialysate

-JW Drug amount discarded/not administered to any patient

-K0 Lower extremity prosthesis functional level 0: Does not have the ability or potential to ambulate or transfer safely with or without assistance and a prosthesis does not enhance their quality of life or mobility

-K1 Lower extremity prosthesis functional level 1: Has the ability or potential to use a prosthesis for transfers or ambulation on level surfaces at fixed cadence. Typical of the limited and unlimited household ambulator.

-K2 Lower extremity prosthesis functional level 2: Has the ability or potential for ambulation with the ability to traverse low-level environmental barriers such as curbs, stairs or uneven surfaces. Typical of the limited community ambulator.

-K3 Lower extremity prosthesis functional level 3: Has the ability or potential for ambulation with variable cadence. Typical of the community ambulator who has the ability to traverse most environmental barriers and may have vocational, therapeutic or exercise activity that demands prosthetic utilization beyond simple locomotion.

-K4 Lower extremoty prosthesis functional level 4: Has the ability or potential for prosthetic ambulation that exceeds the basic ambulation skills, exhibiting high impact, stress or energy levels, typical of the prosthetic demands of the child, active adult, or athlete.

-KA Add on option/accessory for wheelchair

-KB Beneficiary requested upgrade for ABN, more than 4 modifiers identified on claim

-KC Replacement of special power wheelchair interface

-KD Drug or biological infused through DME

-KE Bid under round one of the DMEPOS competitive bidding program for use with non-competitive bid base equipment

-KF Item designated by FDA as class III device

-KG Dmepos item subject to dmepos competitive bidding program number 1

-KH DMEPOS item, initial claim, purchase or first month rental

-KI DMEPOS item, second or third month rental

-KJ DMEPOS item, parenteral enteral nutrition (PEN) pump or capped rental, months four to fifteen

-KK Dmepos item subject to dmepos competitive bidding program number 2

-KL Dmepos item delivered via mail

-KM Replacement of facial prosthesis including new impression/moulage

-KN Replacement of facial prosthesis using previous master model

-KO Single drug unit dose formulation

-KP First drug of a multiple drug unit dose formulation

-KQ Second or subsequent drug of a multiple drug unit dose formulation

-KR Rental item, billing for partial month

-KS Glucose monitor supply for diabetic beneficiary not treated with insulin

-KT Beneficiary resides in a competitive bidding area and travels outside that competitive bidding area and receives a competitive bid item

-KU Dmepos item subject to dmepos competitive bidding program number 3

-KV Dmepos item subject to dmepos competitive bidding program that is furnished as part of a professional service

-KW Dmepos item subject to dmepos competitive bidding program number 4

-KX Requirements specified in the medical policy have been met

-KY Dmepos item subject to dmepos competitive bidding program number 5

-KZ New coverage not implemented by managed care

-LC Left circumflex coronary artery

-LD Left anterior descending coronary artery

-LL Lease/rental (use the -LL modifier when DME equipment rental is to be applied against the purchase price)

-LM Left main coronary artery

-LR Laboratory round trip

-LS FDA-monitored intraocular lens implant
CIM: 65-7

-LT Left side (used to identify procedures performed on the left side of the body)

-M2 Medicare secondary payer (MSP)

-MS Six-month maintenance and servicing fee for reasonable and necessary parts and labor which are not covered under any manufacturer or supplier warranty

-NB Nebulizer system, any type, FDA-cleared for use with specific drug

-NR New when rented (use the -NR modifier when DME which was new at the time of rental is subsequently purchased)

-NU New equipment

-P1 A normal healthy patient

-P2 A patient with mild systemic disease

-P3 A patient with severe systemic disease

-P4 A patient with severe systemic disease that is a constant threat to life

-P5 A moribund patient who is not expected to survive without the operation

-P6 A declared brain-dead patient whose organs are being removed for donor purposes

-PA Surgical or other invasive procedure on wrong body party

-PB Surgical or other invasive procedure on wrong patient

-PC Wrong surgery or other invasive procedure on patient

-PD Diagnostic or related non diagnostic item or service provided in a wholly owned or operated entity to a patient who is admitted as an inpatient within 3 days

-PI Positron emission tomography (PET) or PET/Computed Tomography (CT) to inform the initial treatment strategy of tumors that are biopsy proven or strongly suspected of being cancerous based on other diagnostic testing

-PL Progressive addition lenses

-PS Positron emission tomography (PET) or PET/Computed Tomography (CT) to inform the subsequent treatment strategy of cancerous tumors when the beneficiary's treating physician determines that the PET study is needed to inform subsequent anti-tumor strategy

-PT Colorectal cancer screening test; converted to diagnostic test or other procedure

-Q0 Investigational clinical service provided in a clinical research study that is in an approved clinical research study

-Q1 Routine clinical service provided in a clinical research study that is in an approved clinical research study

-Q2 HCFA/ORD demonstration project procedure/service

-Q3 Live kidney donor surgery and related services

-Q4 Service for ordering/referring physician qualifies as a service exemption

-Q5 Service furnished by a substitute physician under a reciprocal billing arrangement
MCM: 3060.6

-Q6 Service furnished by a locum tenens physician
MCM: 3060.7

-Q7 One class A finding

-Q8 Two class B findings

-Q9 One class B and two class C findings

-QC Single channel monitoring

-QD Recording and storage in solid state memory by a digital recorder

-QE Prescribed amount of oxygen is less than one liter per minute (LPM)

-QF Prescribed amount of oxygen exceeds 4 liters per minute (LPM) and portable oxygen is prescribed

-QG Prescribed amount of oxygen is greater than four liters per minute (LPM)

-QH Oxygen conserving device is being used with an oxygen delivery system

-QJ Services/items provided to a prisoner or patient in state or local custody, however the state or local government, as applicable, meets the requirements in 42 CFR 411.4 (B)

-QK Medical direction of two, three or four concurrent anesthesia procedures involving qualified individuals
MCM: 3350.5

-QL Patient pronounced dead after ambulance called

-QM Ambulance service provided under arrangement by a provider of services

-QN Ambulance service furnished directly by a provider of services

-QP Documentation is on file showing that the laboratory test(s) was ordered individually or ordered as a CPT-recognized panel other than automated profile codes 80002-80019, G0058, G0059, and G0060.
MCM: 7517.1

-QS Monitored anesthesia care service
CIM: 15018I

-QT Recording and storage on tape by an analog tape recorder

-QW CLIA waived test

-QX CRNA service: with medical direction by a physician

-QY Medical direction of one certified registered nurse anesthetist (CRNA) by an anesthesiologist
MCM: 3350.5

-QZ CRNA service: without medical direction by a physician

-RA Replacement of a DME, orthotic or prosthetic item

-RB Replacement of a part of a DME, orthotic or prosthetic item furnished as part of a repair

-RC Right coronary artery

-RD Drug provided to beneficiary, but not administered incident-to

-RE Furnished in full compliance with FDA-mandated risk evaluation and mitigation strategy (REMS)

-RI Ramus intermedius coronary artery

-RR Rental (use the -RR modifier when DME is to be rented)

-RT Right side (used to identify procedures performed on the right side of the body)

-SA Nurse practitioner rendering service in collaboration with a physician

-SB Nurse midwife

-SC Medically necessary service or supply

-SD Services provided by registered nurse with specialized, highly technical home infusion training

-SE State and/or federally funded programs/services

-SF Second opinion ordered by a professional review organization (PRO) per section 9401, P.L. 99-272 (100% reimbursement — no Medicare deductible or coinsurance)

-SG Ambulatory surgical center (ASC) facility service

-SH Second concurrently administered infusion therapy

-SJ Third or more concurrently administered infusion therapy

-SK Member of high-risk population (use only with codes for immunization)

-SL State supplied vaccine

-SM Second surgical opinion

-SN Third surgical opinion

-SQ Item ordered by home health

-SS Home infusion services provided in the infusion suite of the IV therapy provider

-ST Related to trauma or injury

-SU Procedure performed in physician's office (to denote use of facility and equipment)

-SV Pharmaceuticals delivered to patient's home but not utilized

-SW Services provided by a certified diabetic educator

-SY Persons who are in close contact with member of high-risk population (use only with codes for immunization)

-T1 Left foot, second digit

-T2 Left foot, third digit

-T3 Left foot, fourth digit

-T4 Left foot, fifth digit

-T5 Right foot, great toe

-T6 Right foot, second digit

-T7 Right foot, third digit

-T8 Right foot, fourth digit

-T9 Right foot, fifth digit

-TA Left foot, great toe

-TC Technical component. Under certain circumstances, a charge may be made for the technical component alone. Under those circumstances the technical component charge is identified by adding modifier -TC to the usual procedure number. Technical component charges are institutional charges and not billed separately by physicians. However, portable x-ray suppliers only bill for technical component and should utilize modifier -TC. The charge data from portable x-ray suppliers will then be used to build customary and prevailing profiles.

-TD RN

-TE LPN/LVN

-TF Intermediate level of care

-TG Complex/high tech level of care

-TH Obstetrical treatment/services, prenatal or postpartum

-TJ Program group, child and/or adolescent

-TK Extra patient or passenger, non-ambulance
(Note: use modifier "-GM: Multiple patients on one ambulance trip" for ambulance claims)

-TL Early intervention/individualized family services plan (IFSP)

-TM Individualized education program (IEP)

-TN Rural/outside providers customary service area

-TP Medical transport, unloaded vehicle

-TQ Basice life support (BLS) transport by a volunteer ambulance provider

-TR School-based individualized education program (IEP) services provided outside the public school district responsible for the student

-TS Follow-up service

-TT Individualized service provided to more than one patient in same setting

-TU Special payment rate, overtime

-TV Special payment rates, holidays/weekends

-TW Back-up equipment

-U1 Medicaid level of care 1, as defined by each state

-U2 Medicaid level of care 2, as defined by each state

-U3 Medicaid level of care 3, as defined by each state

-U4 Medicaid level of care 4, as defined by each state

-U5 Medicaid level of care 5, as defined by each state

-U6 Medicaid level of care 6, as defined by each state

-U7 Medicaid level of care 7, as defined by each state

-U8 Medicaid level of care 8, as defined by each state

-U9 Medicaid level of care 9, as defined by each state

-UA Medicaid level of care 10, as defined by each state

-UB Medicaid level of care 11, as defined by each state

-UC Medicaid level of care 12, as defined by each state

-UD Medicaid level of care 13, as defined by each state

-UE Used durable medical equipment

-UF Services provided in the morning

-UG Services provided in the afternoon

-UH Services provided in the evening

-UJ Services provided at night

-UK Services provided on behalf of the client to someone other than the client (collateral relationship)

-UN Two patients served

-UP Three patients served

-UQ Four patients served

-UR Five patients served

-US Six or more patients served

-V5 Vascular catheter (alone or with any other vascular access)

-V6 Arteriovenous graft (or other vascular access not including a vascular catheter)

-V7 Arteriovenous fistula only (in use with two needles)

(-V8) Code deleted March 31, 2012

(-V9) Code deleted March 31, 2012

-VP Aphakic patient

AMBULANCE SERVICE MODIFIERS

For ambulance service, one-digit modifiers are combined to form a two-digit modifier that identifies the ambulance's place of origin with the first digit, and ambulance's destination with the second digit. They are used in items 12 and 13 on the CMS Form 1491.

One digit modifiers:

-D Diagnostic or therapeutic site other than -P or -H when these are used as origin codes

-E Residential, domiciliary, custodial facility (other than an 1819 facility)

-G Hospital-based dialysis facility (hospital or hospital related)

-H Hospital

-I Site of transfer (for example, airport or helicopter pad) between types of ambulance

-J Non-hospital-based dialysis facility

-N Skilled nursing facility (SNF) (1819 facility)

-P Physician's office (includes HMO non-hospital facility, clinic, etc.)

-R Residence

-S Scene of accident or acute event

-X (Destination code only) Intermediate stop at physician's office on the way to the hospital (includes HMO non-hospital facility, clinic, etc.)

PET SCAN MODIFIERS

Use these single-digit alpha characters in combination as two-character modifiers to indicate the results of a current PET scan and a previous test.

-N Negative

-E Equivocal

-P Positive, but not suggestive of extensive ischemia

-S Positive and suggestive of extensive ischemia (>20 percent of the left ventricle)

APPENDIX B: SUMMARY OF CHANGES

Summary of Official HCPCS Additions, Changes, and Deletions for 2014

-AO Alternate payment method declined by provider of services
New modifier

-HI Integrated mental health and intellectual disability/developmental disabilities program
Revised modifier

-JE Administered via dialysate
New modifier

A4555 Electrode/transducer for use with electrical stimulation device used for cancer treatment, replacement only
New code

A5081 Stoma plug or seal, any type
Revised code

A7047 Oral interface used with respiratory suction pump, each
New code

A9272 Wound suction, disposable, includes dressing, all accessories and components, any type, each
Revised code

A9520 Technetium tc-99m, tilmanocept, diagnostic, up to 0.5 millicuries
New code

A9575 Injection, gadoterate meglumine, 0.1 ml
New code

A9599 Radiopharmaceutical, diagnostic, for beta-amyloid positron emission tomography (pet) imaging, per study dose
New code

C1204 Code deleted December 31, 2013. Use A9520.

C1841 Retinal prosthesis, includes all internal and external components

New code

C2618 Probe/needle, cryoablation
Revised code

C5271 Application of low cost skin substitute graft to trunk, arms, legs, total wound surface area up to 100 sq cm; first 25 sq cm or less wound surface area
New code

C5272 Application of low cost skin substitute graft to trunk, arms, legs, total wound surface area up to 100 sq cm; each additional 25 sq cm wound surface area, or part thereof (list separately in addition to code for primary procedure)
New code

C5273 Application of low cost skin substitute graft to trunk, arms, legs, total wound surface area greater than or equal to 100 sq cm; first 100 sq cm wound surface area, or 1% of body area of infants and children
New code

C5274 Application of low cost skin substitute graft to trunk, arms, legs, total wound surface area greater than or equal to 100 sq cm; each additional 100 sq cm wound surface area, or part thereof, or each additional 1% of body area of infants and children, or part thereof (list separately in addition to code for primary procedure)
New code

C5275 Application of low cost skin substitute graft to face, scalp, eyelids, mouth, neck, ears, orbits, genitalia, hands, feet, and/or multiple digits, total wound surface area up to 100 sq cm; first 25 sq cm or less wound surface area
New code

C5276 Application of low cost skin substitute graft to face, scalp, eyelids, mouth, neck, ears, orbits, genitalia, hands, feet, and/or multiple digits, total wound surface area up to 100 sq cm; each additional 25 sq cm wound surface area, or part thereof (list separately in addition to code for primary procedure)
New code

C5277 Application of low cost skin substitute graft to face, scalp, eyelids, mouth, neck, ears, orbits, genitalia, hands, feet, and/or multiple digits, total wound surface area greater than or equal to 100 sq cm; first 100 sq cm wound surface area, or 1% of body area of infants and children
New code

C5278 Application of low cost skin substitute graft to face, scalp, eyelids, mouth, neck, ears, orbits, genitalia, hands, feet, and/or multiple digits, total wound surface area greater than or equal to 100 sq cm; each additional 100 sq cm wound surface area, or part thereof, or each additional 1% of body area of infants and children, or part thereof (list separately in addition to code for primary procedure)
New code

C9130 Code deleted December 31, 2013. Use J1556.

C9131 Code deleted December 31, 2013. Use J9354.

C9132 Prothrombin complex concentrate (human), centra, per i.u. of factor ix activity
New code

C9133 Factor ix (antihemophilic factor, recombinant), rixibus, per i.u.
New code

C9292 Code deleted December 31, 2013. Use J9306.

C9294 Code deleted December 31, 2013. Use J3060.

C9295 Code deleted December 31, 2013. Use J9047.

C9296 Code deleted December 31, 2013. Use J9400.

C9297 Code deleted December 31, 2013. Use J9262.

C9298 Code deleted December 31, 2013. Use J7316.

C9441 Injection, ferric carboxymaltose, 1 mg
New code

C9497 Loxapine, inhalation powder, 10 mg
New code

C9734 Focused ultrasound ablation/therapeutic intervention, other than uterine leiomyomata, with magnetic resonance (mr) guidance
Revised code

C9735 Anoscopy; with directed submucosal injection(s), any substance
New code

C9736 Code deleted December 31, 2013.

C9737 Laparoscopy, surgical, esophageal sphincter augmentation with device (eg, magnetic band)
New code

E0601 Continuous positive airway pressure (CPAP) device
Revised code

E0766 Electrical stimulation device used for cancer treatment, includes all accessories, any type
New code

E1352 Oxygen accessory, flow regulator capable of positive inspiratory pressure
New code

E2300 Wheelchair accessory, power seat elevation system, any type
Revised code

E2301 Wheelchair accessory, power standing system, any type
Revised code

G0275 Code deleted December 31, 2013.

G0416 Surgical pathology, gross and microscopic examinations, for prostate needle biopsy, any method, 10-20 specimens
Revised code

G0417 Surgical pathology, gross and microscopic examination, for prostate needle biopsy, any method, 21-40 specimens
Revised code

G0418 Surgical pathology, gross and microscopic examination, for prostate needle biopsy, any method, 41-60 specimens
Revised code

G0419 Surgical pathology, gross and microscopic examination, for prostate needle biopsy, any method, 60 specimens
Revised code

G0461 Immunohistochemistry or immunocytochemistry, per specimen; first single or multiplex antibody stain
New code

G0462 Immunohistochemistry or immunocytochemistry, per specimen; each additional single or multiplex antibody stain (list separately in addition to code for primary procedure)
New code

G0463 Hospital outpatient clinic visit for assessment and management of a patient
New code

G8126 Patient with a diagnosis of major depression documented as being treated with antidepressant medication during the entire 84 day (12 week) acute treatment phase
Revised code

G8127 Patient with a diagnosis of major depression not documented as being treated with antidepressant medication during the entire 84 day (12 week) acute treatment phase
Revised code

G8417 BME is documented above normal parameters and a follow- up plan is documented
Revised code

G8418 BME is documented below normal parameters and a follow- up plan is documented
Revised code

G8419 BME documented outside normal parameters, no follow-up plan documented, no reason given
Revised code

G8420 BME is documented within normal parameters and no follow-up plan is required
Revised code

G8421 BME not documented and no reason is given
Revised code

G8422 BME not documented, documentation the patient is not eligible for bei calculation
Revised code

G8427 Eligible professional attests to documenting in the medical record they obtained, updated, or reviewed the patient's current medications
Revised code

G8428 Current list of medications not documented as obtained, updated, or reviewed by the eligible professional, reason not given
Revised code

G8430 Eligible professional attests to documenting in the medical record the patient is not eligible for a current list of medications being obtained, updated, or reviewed by the eligible professional
Revised code

G8431 Screening for clinical depression is documented as being positive and a follow-up plan is documented
Revised code

G8433 Screening for clinical depression not documented, documentation stating the patient is not eligible
Revised code

G8442 Pain assessment not documented as being performed, documentation the patient is not eligible for a pain assessment using a standardized tool
Revised code

G8451 Beta-blocker therapy for LVEF 40% not prescribed for reasons documented by the clinician (e.g., low blood pressure, fluid overload, asthma, patients recently treated with an intravenous positive inotropic agent, allergy, intolerance, other medical reasons, patient declined, other patient reasons, or other reasons attributable to the healthcare system)
Revised code

G8459 Code deleted December 31, 2013.

G8462 Code deleted December 31, 2013.

G8463 Code deleted December 31, 2013.

G8509 Pain assessment documented as positive using a standardized tool, follow-up plan not documented, reason not given
Revised code

G8510 Screening for clinical depression is documented as negative, a follow-up plan is not required
Revised code

G8511 Screening for clinical depression documented as positive, follow up plan not documented, reason not given
Revised code

G8535 Elder maltreatment screen not documented; documentation that patient not eligible for the elder maltreatment screen
Revised code

G8539 Functional outcome assessment documented as positive using a standardized tool and a care plan based on identified deficiencies on the date of functional outcome assessment, is documented
Revised code

G8540 Functional outcome assessment not documented as being performed, documentation the patient is not eligible for a functional outcome assessment using a standardized tool
Revised code

G8542 Functional outcome assessment using a standardized tool is documented; no functional deficiencies identified, care plan not required
Revised code

G8543 Documentation of a positive functional outcome assessment using a standardized tool; care plan not documented, reason not given
Revised code

G8553 Code deleted December 31, 2013.

G8556 Code deleted December 31, 2013.

G8557 Code deleted December 31, 2013.

G8558 Code deleted December 31, 2013.

G8569 Prolonged postoperative intubation (24 hrs) required
Revised code

G8570 Prolonged postoperative intubation (24 hrs) not required
Revised code

G8588 Code deleted December 31, 2013.

G8589 Code deleted December 31, 2013.

G8590 Code deleted December 31, 2013.

G8591 Code deleted December 31, 2013.

G8592 Code deleted December 31, 2013.

G8596 Code deleted December 31, 2013.

G8603 Code deleted December 31, 2013.

G8604 Code deleted December 31, 2013.

G8605 Code deleted December 31, 2013.

G8606 Code deleted December 31, 2013.

G8607 Code deleted December 31, 2013.

G8608 Code deleted December 31, 2013.

G8609 Code deleted December 31, 2013.

G8610 Code deleted December 31, 2013.

G8611 Code deleted December 31, 2013.

G8612 Code deleted December 31, 2013.

G8613 Code deleted December 31, 2013.

G8614 Code deleted December 31, 2013.

G8615 Code deleted December 31, 2013.

G8616 Code deleted December 31, 2013.

G8617 Code deleted December 31, 2013.

G8618 Code deleted December 31, 2013.

G8619 Code deleted December 31, 2013.

G8620 Code deleted December 31, 2013.

G8621 Code deleted December 31, 2013.

G8622 Code deleted December 31, 2013.

G8623 Code deleted December 31, 2013.

G8624 Code deleted December 31, 2013.

G8625 Code deleted December 31, 2013.

G8626 Code deleted December 31, 2013.

G8642 Code deleted December 31, 2013.

G8643 Code deleted December 31, 2013.

G8644 Code deleted December 31, 2013.

G8682 LVF testing documented as being performed prior to discharge or in the previous 12 months
Revised code

G8683 LVF testing not performed prior to discharge or in the previous 12 months for a medical or patient documented reason
Revised code

G8685 LVF testing not documented as being performed prior to discharge or in the previous 12 months, reason not given
Revised code

G8709 Patient prescribed or dispensed antibiotic for documented medical reason(s) (e.g. intestinal infection, pertussis, bacterial infection, lyme disease, otitis media, acute sinusitis, acute pharyngitis, acute tonsillitis, chronic sinusitis, infection of the pharynx/larynx/tonsils/adenoids, prostatitis, cellulitis, mastoiditis, or bone infections, acute lymphadenitis, impetigo, skin staph infections, pneumonia/gonococcal infections, venereal disease (syphilis, chlamydia, inflammatory diseases (female reproductive organs)), infections of the kidney, cystitis or UTI, and acne)
Revised code

G8722 Documentation of medical reason(s) for not including the pt category, the PN category or the histologic grade in the pathology report (e.g., re-excision without residual tumor; non-carcinomas anal canal)
Revised code

G8730 Pain assessment documented as positive using a standardized tool and a follow-up plan is documented
Revised code

G8731 Pain assessment using a standardized tool is documented as negative, no follow-up plan required
Revised code

G8733 Elder maltreatment screen documented as positive and a follow-up plan is documented
Revised code

G8741 Code deleted December 31, 2013.

G8742 Code deleted December 31, 2013.

G8743 Code deleted December 31, 2013.

G8744 Code deleted December 31, 2013.

G8745 Code deleted December 31, 2013.

G8746 Code deleted December 31, 2013.

G8747 Code deleted December 31, 2013.

G8748 Code deleted December 31, 2013.

G8768 Documentation of medical reason(s) for not performing lipid profile (e.g., patients with palliative goals or for whom treatment of hypertension with standard treatment goals is not clinically appropriate)
Revised code

G8772 Documentation of medical reason(s) for not performing urine protein test (e.g., patients with palliative goals or for whom treatment of hypertension with standard treatment goals is not clinically appropriate)
Revised code

G8775 Documentation of medical reason(s) for not performing serum creatinine test (e.g., patients with palliative goals or for whom treatment of hypertension with standard treatment goals is not clinically appropriate)
Revised code

G8778 Documentation of medical reason(s) for not performing diabetes screening test (e.g., patients with a diagnosis of diabetes, or with palliative goals or for whom treatment of hypertension with standard treatment goals is not clinically appropriate)
Revised code

G8781 Documentation of medical reason(s) for patient not receiving counseling for diet and physical activity (e.g., patients with palliative goals or for whom treatment of hypertension with standard treatment goals is not clinically appropriate)
Revised code

G8784 Blood pressure reading not documented, documentation the patient is not eligible
Revised code

G8790 Code deleted December 31, 2013.

G8791 Code deleted December 31, 2013.

G8792 Code deleted December 31, 2013.

G8793 Code deleted December 31, 2013.

G8794 Code deleted December 31, 2013.

G8795 Code deleted December 31, 2013.

G8796 Code deleted December 31, 2013.

G8799 Code deleted December 31, 2013.

G8800 Code deleted December 31, 2013.

G8801 Code deleted December 31, 2013.

G8808 Performance of trans-abdominal or trans-vaginal ultrasound not ordered, reason not given (e.g., patient has visited the ed multiple times with no documentation of a trans-abdominal or trans-vaginal ultrasound within ed or from referring eligible professional)
Revised code

G8810 Rh-immunoglobulin (RhoGAM) not ordered for reasons documented by clinician (e.g., patient had prior documented receipt of RhoGAM within 12 weeks, patient refusal)
Revised code

G8812 Code deleted December 31, 2013.

G8813 Code deleted December 31, 2013.

G8814 Code deleted December 31, 2013.

G8827 Code deleted December 31, 2013.

G8835 Code deleted December 31, 2013.

G8880 Documentation of reason(s) sentinel lymph node biopsy not performed (e.g., reasons could include but not limited to; non-invasive cancer, incidental discovery of breast cancer on prophylactic mastectomy, incidental discovery of breast cancer on reduction mammoplasty, pre-operative biopsy proven lymph node (ln) metastases, inflammatory carcinoma, stage 3 locally advanced cancer, recurrent invasive breast cancer, patient refusal after informed consent)
Revised code

G8882 Sentinel lymph node biopsy procedure not performed, reason not given
Revised code

G8887 Documentation of medical reason(s) for most recent blood pressure not being under control (e.g., patients with palliative goals or for whom treatment of hypertension with standard treatment goals is not clinically appropriate)
Revised code

G8891 Documentation of medical reason(s) for most recent LDL-c not under control (e.g., patients with palliative goals for whom treatment of hypertension with standard treatment goals is not clinically appropriate)
Revised code

G8892 Documentation of medical reason(s) for not performing LDL-c test (e.g. patients with palliative goals or for whom treatment of hypertension with standard treatment goals is not clinically appropriate)
Revised code

G8919 Code deleted December 31, 2013.

G8920 Code deleted December 31, 2013.

G8921 Code deleted December 31, 2013.

G8922 Code deleted December 31, 2013.

G8928 Adjuvant chemotherapy not prescribed or previously received for documented reasons (e.g., medical co-morbidities, diagnosis date more than 5 years prior to the current visit date, patient's cancer has metastasized, medical contraindication/allergy, poor performance status, other medical reasons, patient refusal, other patient reasons, patient is currently enrolled in a clinical trial that precludes prescription of chemotherapy, other system reasons)
Revised code

G8929 Adjuvant chemotherapy not prescribed or previously received, reason not specified
Revised code

G8938 BME is documented as being outside of normal limits, follow-up plan is not documented, documentation the patient is not eligible
Revised code

G8939 Pain assessment documented as positive, follow-up plan not documented, documentation the patient is not eligible
Revised code

G8940 Screening for clinical depression documented as positive, a follow-up plan not documented, documentation stating the patient is not eligible
Revised code

G8941 Elder maltreatment screen documented as positive, follow-up plan not documented, documentation the patient is not eligible
Revised code

G8942 Functional outcomes assessment using a standardized tool is documented within the previous 30 days and care plan, based on identified deficiencies on the date of the functional outcome assessment, is documented
Revised code

G8945 Code deleted December 31, 2013.

G8946 Minimally invasive biopsy method attempted but not diagnostic of breast cancer (e.g., high risk lesion of breast such as atypical ductal hyperplasia, lobular neoplasia, atypical lobular hyperplasia, lobular carcinoma in situ, atypical columnar hyperplastica, flat epithelial atypia, radial scar, complex sclerosing lesion, papillary lesion, or any lesion with spindle cells)
Revised code

G8950 Pre-hypertensive or hypertensive blood pressure reading documented, and the indicated follow-up is documented
Revised code

G8951 Pre-hypertensive or hypertensive blood pressure reading documented, indicated follow-up not documented, documentation the patient is not eligible
Revised code

G8954 Code deleted December 31, 2013.

G8968 Documentation of medical reason(s) for not prescribing warfarin or another oral anticoagulant that is fad approved for the prevention of thromboembolism (e.g. patients with mitral stenosis or prosthetic heart valves, patients with transient or reversible causes of af (e.g., pneumonia or hyperthyroidism), postoperative patients, patients who are pregnant, allergy, risk of bleeding, other medical reasons)
Revised code

G8969 Documentation of patient reason(s) for not prescribing warfarin or another oral anticoagulant that is fad approved (e.g., economic, social, and/or religious impediments, noncompliance patient refusal, other patient reasons)
Revised code

G8985 Carrying, moving and handling objects, projected goal status, at therapy episode outset, at reporting intervals, and at discharge or to end reporting
Revised code

G8990 Other physical or occupational therapy primary functional limitation, current status, at therapy episode outset and at reporting intervals
Revised code

G8991 Other physical or occupational therapy primary functional limitation, projected goal status, at therapy episode outset, at reporting intervals, and at discharge or to end reporting
Revised code

G8992 Other physical or occupational therapy primary functional limitation, discharge status, at discharge from therapy or to end reporting
Revised code

G8993 Other physical or occupational therapy subsequent functional limitation, current status, at therapy episode outset and at reporting intervals
Revised code

G8994 Other physical or occupational therapy subsequent functional limitation, projected goal status, at therapy episode outset, at reporting intervals, and at discharge or to end reporting
Revised code

G8995 Other physical or occupational therapy subsequent functional limitation, discharge status, at discharge from therapy or to end reporting
Revised code

G8996 Swallowing functional limitation, current status at therapy episode outset and at reporting intervals
Revised code

G8997 Swallowing functional limitation, projected goal status, at therapy episode outset, at reporting intervals, and at discharge or to end reporting
Revised code

G8998 Swallowing functional limitation, discharge status, at discharge from therapy or to end reporting
Revised code

G8999 Motor speech functional limitation, current status at therapy episode outset and at reporting intervals
Revised code

G9158 Motor speech functional limitation, discharge status, at discharge from therapy or to end reporting
Revised code

G9159 Spoken language comprehension functional limitation, current status at therapy episode outset and at reporting intervals
Revised code

G9160 Spoken language comprehension functional limitation, projected goal status at therapy episode outset, at reporting intervals, and at discharge from or to end reporting
Revised code

G9161 Spoken language comprehension functional limitation, discharge status, at discharge from therapy or to end reporting
Revised code

G9162 Spoken language expression functional limitation, current status at therapy episode outset and at reporting intervals
Revised code

G9163 Spoken language expression functional limitation, projected goal status at therapy episode outset, at reporting intervals, and at discharge from or to end reporting
Revised code

G9164 Spoken language expression functional limitation, discharge status at discharge from therapy or to end reporting
Revised code

G9165 Attention functional limitation, current status at therapy episode outset and at reporting intervals
Revised code

G9166 Attention functional limitation, projected goal status at therapy episode outset, at reporting intervals, and at discharge from or to end reporting
Revised code

G9167 Attention functional limitation, discharge status at discharge from therapy or to end reporting
Revised code

G9168 Memory functional limitation, current status at therapy episode outset and at reporting intervals
Revised code

G9169 Memory functional limitation, projected goal status at therapy episode outset, at reporting intervals, and at discharge from or to end reporting
Revised code

G9170 Memory functional limitation, discharge status at discharge from therapy or to end reporting
Revised code

G9171 Voice functional limitation, current status at therapy episode outset and at reporting intervals
Revised code

G9172 Voice functional limitation, projected goal status at therapy episode outset, at reporting intervals, and at discharge from or to end reporting
Revised code

G9173 Voice functional limitation, discharge status at discharge from therapy or to end reporting
Revised code

G9174 Other speech language pathology functional limitation, current status at therapy episode outset and at reporting intervals
Revised code

G9175 Other speech language pathology functional limitation, projected goal status at therapy episode outset, at reporting intervals, and at discharge from or to end reporting
Revised code

G9176 Other speech language pathology functional limitation, discharge status at discharge from therapy or to end reporting
Revised code

G9186 Motor speech functional limitation, projected goal status at therapy episode outset, at reporting intervals, and at discharge from or to end reporting
Revised code

G9187 Bundled payments for care improvement initiative home visit for patient assessment performed by a qualified health care professional for individuals not considered homebound including, but not limited to, assessment of safety, falls, clinical status, fluid status, medication reconciliation/management, patient compliance with orders/plan of care, performance of activities of daily living, appropriateness of care setting; (for use only in the Medicare-approved bundled payments for care improvement initiative); may not be billed for a 30-day period covered by a transitional care management code
New code

G9188 Beta-blocker therapy not prescribed, reason not given
New code

G9189 Beta-blocker therapy prescribed or currently being taken
New code

G9190 Documentation of medical reason(s) for not prescribing beta-blocker therapy (eg, allergy, intolerance, other medical reasons)
New code

G9191 Documentation of patient reason(s) for not prescribing beta-blocker therapy (eg, patient declined, other patient reasons)
New code

G9192 Documentation of system reason(s) for not prescribing beta-blocker therapy (eg, other reasons attributable to the health care system)
New code

G9193 Clinician documented that patient with a diagnosis of major depression was not an eligible candidate for antidepressant medication treatment or patient did not have a diagnosis of major depression
New code

G9194 Patient with a diagnosis of major depression documented as being treated with antidepressant medication during the entire 180 day (6 month) continuation treatment phase
New code

G9195 Patient with a diagnosis of major depression not documented as being treated with antidepressant medication during the entire 180 day (6 months) continuation treatment phase
New code

G9196 Documentation of medical reason(s) for not ordering first or second generation cephalosporin for antimicrobial prophylaxis
New code

G9197 Documentation of order for first or second generation cephalosporin for antimicrobial prophylaxis
New code

G9198 Order for first or second generation cephalosporin for antimicrobial prophylaxis was not documented, reason not given

New code

G9199 Venous thromboembolism (vote) prophylaxis not administered the day of or the day after hospital admission for documented reasons (eg, patient is ambulatory, patient expired during inpatient stay, patient already on warfarin or another anticoagulant, other medical reason(s) or eg, patient left against medical advice, other patient reason(s))
New code

G9200 Venous thromboembolism (vote) prophylaxis was not administered the day of or the day after hospital admission, reason not given
New code

G9201 Venous thromboembolism (vote) prophylaxis administered the day of or the day after hospital admission
New code

G9202 Patients with a positive hepatitis C antibody test
New code

G9203 RNA testing for hepatitis C documented as performed within 12 months prior to initiation of antiviral treatment for hepatitis C
New code

G9204 RNA testing for hepatitis C was not documented as performed within 12 months prior to initiation of antiviral treatment for hepatitis C, reason not given
New code

G9205 Patient starting antiviral treatment for hepatitis C during the measurement period
New code

G9206 Patient starting antiviral treatment for hepatitis C during the measurement period
New code

G9207 Hepatitis c genotype testing documented as performed within 12 months prior to initiation of antiviral treatment for hepatitis C
New code

G9208 Hepatitis C genotype testing was not documented as performed within 12 months prior to initiation of antiviral treatment for hepatitis C, reason not given
New code

G9209 Hepatitis c quantitative rna testing documented as performed between 4-12 weeks after the initiation of antiviral treatment
New code

G9210 Hepatitis c quantitative rna testing not performed between 4- 12 weeks after the initiation of antiviral treatment for reasons documented by clinician (eg, patients whose treatment was deleted during the testing period prior to testing, other medical reasons, patient declined, other patient reasons)
New code

G9211 Hepatitis c quantitative rna testing was not documented as performed between 4-12 weeks after the initiation of antiviral treatment, reason not given
New code

G9212 DSM-IV criteria for major depressive disorder documented at the initial evaluation
New code

G9213 DSMT-iv-TR criteria for major depressive disorder not documented at the initial evaluation, reason not otherwise specified
New code

G9214 Cd4+ cell count or cd4+ cell percentage results documented
New code

G9215 Cd4+ cell count or percentage not documented as performed, reason not given
New code

G9216 (No Suggestions) prophylaxis was not prescribed at time of diagnosis of hiv, reason not given
New code

G9217 (No Suggestions) prophylaxis was not prescribed within 3 months of low cd4+ cell count below 200 cells/mm3, reason not given
New code

G9218 (No Suggestions) prophylaxis was not prescribed within 3 months of low cd4+ cell count below 500 cells/mm3 or a cd4 percentage below 15%, reason not given
New code

G9219 Pneumocystis jiroveci pneumonia prophylaxis not prescribed within 3 months of low cd4+ cell count below 200 cells/mm3 for medical reason (i.e., patient's cd4+ cell count above threshold within 3 months after cd4+ cell count below threshold, indicating that the patient's cd4+ levels are within an acceptable range and the patient does not require pcx prophylaxis)
New code

G9220 Pneumocystis jiroveci pneumonia prophylaxis not prescribed within 3 months of low cd4+ cell count below 500 cells/mm3 or a cd4 percentage below 15% for medical reason (i.e., patient's cd4+ cell count above threshold within 3 months after cd4+ cell count below threshold, indicating that the patient's cd4+ levels are within an acceptable range and the patient does not require pcx prophylaxis)
New code

G9221 Pneumocystis jiroveci pneumonia prophylaxis prescribed
New code

G9222 Pneumocystis jiroveci pneumonia prophylaxis prescribed within 3 months of low cd4+ cell count below 200 cells/mm3
New code

G9223 Pneumocystis jiroveci pneumonia prophylaxis prescribed within 3 months of low cd4+ cell count below 500 cells/mm3 or a cd4 percentage below 15%
New code

G9224 Documentation of medical reason for not performing foot exam (e.g., patient with bilateral foot/leg amputation)
New code

G9225 Foot exam was not performed, reason not given
New code

G9226 Foot examination performed (includes examination through visual inspection, sensory exam with monofilament, and pulse exam - report when all of the 3 components are completed)
New code

G9227 Functional outcome assessment documented, care plan not documented, documentation the patient is not eligible for a care plan
New code

G9228 Chlamydia, gonorrhea and syphilis screening results documented (report when results are present for all of the 3 screenings)
New code

G9229 Chlamydia, gonorrhea, and syphilis not screened, due to documented reason (patient refusal is the only allowed exclusion)
New code

G9230 Chlamydia, gonorrhea, and syphilis not screened, reason not given
New code

G9231 Documentation of end stage renal disease (esrd), dialysis, renal transplant or pregnancy
New code

G9232 Clinician treating major depressive disorder did not communicate to clinician treating comorbid condition for specified patient reason
New code

G9233 All quality actions for the applicable measures in the total knee replacement measures group have been performed for this patient
New code

G9234 I intend to report the total knee replacement measures group
New code

G9235 All quality actions for the applicable measures in the general surgery measures group have been performed for this patient
New code

G9236 All quality actions for the applicable measures in the optimizing patient exposure to ionizing radiation measures group have been performed for this patient
New code

G9237 I intend to report the general surgery measures group
New code

G9238 I intend to report the optimizing patient exposure to ionizing radiation measures group
New code

G9239 Documentation of reasons for patient initiating maintenance hemodialysis with a catheter as the mode of vascular access (eg, patient has a maturing aVF/avg, time-limited trial of hemodialysis, patients undergoing palliative dialysis, other medical reasons, patient declined aVF/avg, other patient reasons, patient followed by reporting nephrologist for fewer than 90 days, other system reasons)
New code

G9240 Patient whose mode of vascular access is a catheter at the time maintenance hemodialysis is initiated
New code

G9241 Patient whose mode of vascular access is not a catheter at the time maintenance hemodialysis is initiated
New code

G9242 Documentation of viral load equal to or greater than 200 copies/ml
New code

G9243 Documentation of viral load less than 200 copies/ml
New code

G9244 Antiretroviral therapy not prescribed
New code

G9245 Antiretroviral therapy prescribed
New code

G9246 Patient did not have at least one medical visit in each 6 month period of the 24 month measurement period, with a minimum of 60 days between medical visits
New code

G9247 Patient had at least one medical visit in each 6 month period of the 24 month measurement period, with a minimum of 60 days between medical visits
New code

G9248 Patient did not have a medical visit in the last 6 months
New code

G9249 Patient had a medical visit in the last 6 months
New code

G9250 Documentation of patient pain brought to a comfortable level within 48 hours from initial assessment
New code

G9251 Documentation of patient with pain not brought to a comfortable level within 48 hours from initial assessment
New code

G9252 Adenoma(s) or other neoplasm detected during screening colonoscopy
New code

G9253 Adenoma(s) or other neoplasm not detected during screening colonoscopy
New code

G9254 Documentation of patient discharged to home later than post-operative day 2 following cas
New code

G9255 Documentation of patient discharged to home no later than post operative day 2 following cas
New code

G9256 Documentation of patient death following cas
New code

G9257 Documentation of patient stroke following cas
New code

G9258 Documentation of patient stroke following CEA
New code

G9259 Documentation of patient survival and absence of stroke following CAS
New code

G9260 Documentation of patient death following CEA
New code

G9261 Documentation of patient survival and absence of stroke following CEA
New code

G9262 Documentation of patient death in the hospital following endovascular aaa repair
New code

G9263 Documentation of patient survival in the hospital following endovascular aaa repair
New code

G9264 Documentation of patient receiving maintenance hemodialysis for greater than or equal to 90 days with a catheter for documented reasons (eg, patient is undergoing palliative dialysis with a catheter, patient approved by a qualified transplant program and scheduled to receive a living donor kidney transplant, other medical reasons, patient declined aVF/avg, other patient reasons)
New code

G9265 Patient receiving maintenance hemodialysis for greater than or equal to 90 days with a catheter as the mode of vascular access
New code

G9266 Patient receiving maintenance hemodialysis for greater than or equal to 90 days without a catheter as the mode of vascular access
New code

G9267 Documentation of patient with one or more complications or mortality within 30 days
New code

G9268 Documentation of patient with one or more complications within 90 days
New code

G9269 Documentation of patient without one or more complications and without mortality within 30 days
New code

G9270 Documentation of patient without one or more complications within 90 days
New code

G9271 LDL value 100
New code

G9272 LDL value = 100
New code

G9273 Blood pressure has a systolic value of 140 and a diastolic value of 90
New code

G9274 Blood pressure has a systolic value of =140 and a diastolic value of = 90 or systolic value 140 and diastolic value = 90 or systolic value = 140 and diastolic value 90
New code

G9275 Documentation that patient is a current non-tobacco user
New code

G9276 Documentation that patient is a current tobacco user
New code

G9277 Documentation that the patient is on daily aspirin or has documentation of a valid contraindication to aspirin automatic contraindications include anti-coagulant use, allergy, and history of gastrointestinal bleed; additionally, any reason documented by the physician as a reason for not taking daily aspirin is acceptable (examples include non-steroidal anti-inflammatory agents, risk for drug interaction, or uncontrolled hypertension defined as 180 systolic or 110 diastolic)
New code

G9278 Documentation that the patient is not on daily aspirin regimen
New code

G9279 Pneumococcal screening performed and documentation of vaccination received prior to discharge
New code

G9280 Pneumococcal vaccination not administered prior to discharge, reason not specified
New code

G9281 Screening performed and documentation that vaccination not indicated/patient refusal
New code

G9282 Documentation of medical reason(s) for not reporting the histological type or NSCLC-nos classification with an explanation (e.g., biopsy taken for other purposes in a patient with a history of non- small cell lung cancer or other documented medical reasons)
New code

G9283 Non small cell lung cancer biopsy and cytology specimen report documents classification into specific histologic type or classified as NSCLC-nos with an explanation
New code

G9284 Non small cell lung cancer biopsy and cytology specimen report does not document classification into specific histologic type or classified as NSCLC-nos with an explanation
New code

G9285 Specimen site other than anatomic location of lung or is not classified as non small cell lung cancer
New code

G9286 Documentation of antibiotic regimen prescribed within 7 days of diagnosis or within 10 days after onset of symptoms
New code

G9287 No antibiotic regimen prescribed within 7 days of diagnosis or within 10 days after onset of symptoms
New code

G9288 Documentation of medical reason(s) for not reporting the histological type or NSCLC-nos classification with an explanation (e.g., a solitary fibrous tumor in a person with a history of non-small cell carcinoma or other documented medical reasons)
New code

G9289 Non small cell lung cancer biopsy and cytology specimen report documents classification into specific histologic type or classified as NSCLC-nos with an explanation
New code

G9290 Non small cell lung cancer biopsy and cytology specimen report does not document classification into specific histologic type or classified as NSCLC-nos with an explanation
New code

G9291 Specimen site other than anatomic location of lung, is not classified as non small cell lung cancer or classified as NSCLC-nos
New code

G9292 Documentation of medical reason(s) for not reporting pt category and a statement on thickness and ulceration and for pt1, mitotic rate (e.g., negative skin biopsies in a patient with a history of melanoma or other documented medical reasons)
New code

G9293 Pathology report does not include the pt category and a statement on thickness and ulceration and for pt1, mitotic rate
New code

G9294 Pathology report includes the pt category and a statement on thickness and ulceration and for pt1, mitotic rate
New code

G9295 Specimen site other than anatomic cutaneous location
New code

G9296 Patients with documented shared decision-making including discussion of conservative (non-surgical) therapy prior to the procedure
New code

G9297 Shared decision-making including discussion of conservative (non-surgical) therapy prior to the procedure not documented, reason not given
New code

G9298 Patients who are evaluated for venous thromboembolic and cardiovascular risk factors within 30 days prior to the procedure including history of DVT, pe, mi, arrhythmia and stroke
New code

G9299 Patients who are not evaluated for venous thromboembolic and cardiovascular risk factors within 30 days prior to the procedure including history of DVT, pe, mi, arrhythmia and stroke, reason not given
New code

G9300 Documentation of medical reason(s) for not completely infusing the prophylactic antibiotic prior to the inflation of the proximal tourniquet (e.g., a tourniquet was not used)
New code

G9301 Patients who had the prophylactic antibiotic completely infused prior to the inflation of the proximal tourniquet
New code

G9302 Prophylactic antibiotic not completely infused prior to the inflation of the proximal tourniquet, reason not given
New code

G9303 Operative report does not identify the prosthetic implant specifications including the prosthetic implant manufacturer, the brand name of the prosthetic implant and the size of the prosthetic implant, reason not given
New code

G9304 Operative report identifies the prosthetic implant specifications including the prosthetic implant manufacturer, the brand name of the prosthetic implant and the size of the prosthetic implant
New code

G9305 Intervention for presence of leak of endoluminal contents through an anastomosis not required
New code

G9306 Intervention for presence of leak of endoluminal contents through an anastomosis required
New code

G9307 No return to the operating room for a surgical procedure, for any reason, within 30 days of the principal operative procedure
New code

G9308 Unplanned return to the operating room for a surgical procedure, for any reason, within 30 days of the principal operative procedure
New code

G9309 No unplanned hospital readmission within 30 days of principal procedure
New code

G9310 Unplanned hospital readmission within 30 days of principal procedure
New code

G9311 No surgical site infection
New code

G9312 Surgical site infection
New code

G9313 Amoxicillin, with or without clavulanate, not prescribed as first line antibiotic at the time of diagnosis for documented reason (eg, cystic fibrosis, immotile cilia disorders, ciliary dyskinesia, immune deficiency, prior history of sinus surgery within the past 12 months, and anatomic abnormalities, such as deviated nasal septum, resistant organisms, allergy to medication, recurrent sinusitis, chronic sinusitis, or other reasons)
New code

G9314 Amoxicillin, with or without clavulanate, not prescribed as first line antibiotic at the time of diagnosis, reason not given
New code

G9315 Documentation amoxicillin, with or without clavulanate, prescribed as a first line antibiotic at the time of diagnosis
New code

G9316 Documentation of patient-specific risk assessment with a risk calculator based on multi-institutional clinical data, the specific risk calculator used, and communication of risk assessment from risk calculator with the patient or family
New code

G9317 Documentation of patient-specific risk assessment with a risk calculator based on multi-institutional clinical data, the specific risk calculator used, and communication of risk assessment from risk calculator with the patient or family not completed
New code

G9318 Imaging study named according to standardized nomenclature
New code

G9319 Imaging study not named according to standardized nomenclature, reason not given
New code

G9320 Documentation of medical reason(s) for not naming ct studies according to a standardized nomenclature provided (eg, ct studies performed for radiation treatment planning or image-guided radiation treatment delivery)
New code

G9321 Count of previous ct (any type of ct) and cardiac nuclear medicine (myocardial perfusion) studies documented in the 12-month period prior to the current study
New code

G9322 Count of previous ct and cardiac nuclear medicine (myocardial perfusion) studies not documented in the 12-month period prior to the current study, reason not given
New code

G9323 Documentation of medical reason(s) for not counting previous ct and cardiac nuclear medicine (myocardial perfusion) studies (eg, ct studies performed for radiation treatment planning or image-guided radiation treatment delivery)
New code

G9324 All necessary data elements not included, reason not given
New code

G9325 Ct studies not reported to a radiation dose index registry due to medical reasons (eg, ct studies performed for radiation treatment planning or image-guided radiation treatment delivery)
New code

G9326 Ct studies performed not reported to a radiation dose index registry, reason not given
New code

G9327 Ct studies performed reported to a radiation dose index registry with all necessary data elements
New code

G9328 DICOM format image data availability not documented in final report due to medical reasons (eg, ct studies performed for radiation treatment planning or image-guided radiation treatment delivery)
New code

G9329 DICOM format image data available to non-affiliated external entities on a secure, media free, reciprocally searchable basis with patient authorization for at least a 12-month period after the study not documented in final report, reason not given
New code

G9340 Final report documented that DICOM format image data available to non-affiliated external entities on a secure, media free, reciprocally searchable basis with patient authorization for at least a 12- month period after the study
New code

G9341 Search conducted for prior patient ct imaging studies completed at non-affiliated external entities within the past 12-months and are available through a secure, authorized, media-free, shared archive prior to an imaging study being performed
New code

G9342 Search conducted for prior patient imaging studies completed at non-affiliated external entities within the past 12-months and are available through a secure, authorized, media-free, shared archive prior to an imaging study being performed not completed, reason not given
New code

G9343 Search for prior patient completed DICOM format images not completed due to medical reasons (eg, ct studies performed for radiation treatment planning or image-guided radiation treatment delivery)
New code

G9344 Search for prior patient completed DICOM format images not completed due to system reasons (ie, facility does not have archival abilities through a shared archival system)
New code

G9345 Follow-up recommendations according to recommended guidelines for incidentally detected pulmonary nodules (eg, follow-up ct imaging studies needed or that no follow-up is needed) based at a minimum on nodule size and patient risk factors documented
New code

G9346 Follow-up recommendations according to recommended guidelines for incidentally detected pulmonary nodules not documented due to medical reasons (eg, patients with known malignant disease, patients with unexplained fever, ct studied performed for radiation treatment planning or image-guided radiation treatment delivery)
New code

G9347 Follow-up recommendations according to recommended guidelines for incidentally detected pulmonary nodules not documented, reason not given
New code

G9348 Ct scan of the paranasal sinuses ordered at the time of diagnosis for documented reasons (eg, persons with sinusitis symptoms lasting at least 7 to 10 days, antibiotic resistance, immunocompromised, recurrent sinusitis, acute frontal sinusitis, acute sphenoid sinusitis, periorbital cellulitis, or other medical)
New code

G9349 Documentation of a ct scan of the paranasal sinuses ordered at the time of diagnosis or received within 28 days after date of diagnosis
New code

G9350 Ct scan of the paranasal sinuses not ordered at the time of diagnosis or received within 28 days after date of diagnosis
New code

G9351 More than one ct scan of the paranasal sinuses ordered or received within 90 days after diagnosis
New code

G9352 More than one ct scan of the paranasal sinuses ordered or received within 90 days after the date of diagnosis, reason not given
New code

G9353 More than one ct scan of the paranasal sinuses ordered or received within 90 days after the date of diagnosis for documented reasons (eg, patients with complications, second ct obtained prior to surgery, other medical reasons)
New code

G9354 More than one ct scan of the paranasal sinuses not ordered within 90 days after the date of diagnosis
New code

G9355 Elective delivery or early induction not performed
New code

G9356 Elective delivery or early induction performed
New code

G9357 Post-partum screenings, evaluations and education performed
New code

G9358 Post-partum screenings, evaluations and education not performed
New code

G9359 Documentation of negative or managed positive t.b. screen with further evidence that t.b. is not active
New code

G9360 No documentation of negative or managed positive t.b. screen
New code

J0151 Injection, adenosine for diagnostic use, 1 mg (not to be used to report any adenosine phosphate compounds, instead use a9270)
New code

J0152 Code deleted December 31, 2013.

J0401 Injection, aripiprazole, extended release, 1 mg
New code

J0717 Injection, Certolizumab pegol, 1 mg (code may be used for medicare when drug administered under the direct supervision of a physician, not for use when drug is self administered)
New code

J0718 Code deleted December 31, 2013.

J1440 Code deleted December 31, 2013.

J1441 Code deleted December 31, 2013.

J1442 Injection, filgrastim (g-csf), 1 microgram
New code

J1446 Injection, to-filgrastim, 5 micrograms
New code

J1556 Injection, immune globulin (bivigam), 500 mg
New code

J1602 Injection, golimumab, 1 mg, for intravenous use
New code

J3060 Injection, taliglucerase alfa, 10 units
New code

J3487 Code deleted December 31, 2013.

J3488 Code deleted December 31, 2013.

J3489 Injection, zoledronic acid, 1 mg
New code

J7301 Levonorgestrel-releasing intrauterine contraceptive system (skylark), 13.5 mg
New code

J7316 Injection, Ocriplasmin, 0.125 mg
New code

J7507 Tacrolimus, immediate release, oral, 1 mg
Revised code

J7508 Tacrolimus, extended release, oral, 0.1 mg
New code

J9002 Code deleted December 31, 2013.

J9047 Injection, carfilzomib, 1 mg
New code

J9262 Injection, omacetaxine mepesuccinate, 0.01 mg
New code

J9306 Injection, pertuzumab, 1 mg
New code

J9354 Injection, ado-trastuzumab emtansine, 1 mg
New code

J9371 Injection, vincristine sulfate liposome, 1 mg
New code

J9400 Injection, Ziv-aflibercept, 1 mg
New code

K0008 Custom manual wheelchair/base
New code

K0013 Custom motorized/power wheelchair base
New code

K0900 Customized durable medical equipment, other than wheelchair
New code

L0120 Cervical, flexible, non-adjustable, prefabricated, off-the-shelf (foam collar)
Revised code

L0160 Cervical, semi-rigid, wire frame occipital/mandibular support, prefabricated, off-the-shelf
Revised code

L0172 Cervical, collar, semi-rigid thermoplastic foam, two-piece, prefabricated, off-the-shelf
Revised code

L0174 Cervical, collar, semi-rigid, thermoplastic foam, two piece with thoracic extension, prefabricated, off-the-shelf
Revised code

L0430 Code deleted December 31, 2013.

L0450 TLSO, flexible, provides trunk support, upper thoracic region, produces intracavitary pressure to reduce load on the intervertebral disks with rigid stays or panel(s), includes shoulder straps and closures, prefabricated, off-the-shelf
Revised code

L0454 TLSO flexible, provides trunk support, extends from sacrococcygeal junction to above t-9 vertebra, restricts gross trunk motion in the sagittal plane, produces intracavitary pressure to reduce load on the intervertebral disks with rigid stays or panel(s), includes shoulder straps and closures, prefabricated item that has been trimmed, bent, molded, assembled, or otherwise customized to fit a specific patient by an individual with expertise
Revised code

L0455 TLSO, flexible, provides trunk support, extends from sacrococcygeal junction to above t-9 vertebra, restricts gross trunk motion in the sagittal plane, produces intracavitary pressure to reduce load on the intervertebral disks with rigid stays or panel(s), includes shoulder straps and closures, prefabricated, off-the-shelf
New code

L0456 TLSO, flexible, provides trunk support, thoracic region, rigid posterior panel and soft anterior apron, extends from the sacrococcygeal junction and terminates just inferior to the scapular spine, restricts gross trunk motion in the sagittal plane, produces intracavitary pressure to reduce load on the intervertebral disks, includes straps and closures, prefabricated item that has been trimmed, bent, molded, assembled, or otherwise customized to fit a specific patient by an individual with expertise
Revised code

L0457 TLSO, flexible, provides trunk support, thoracic region, rigid posterior panel and soft anterior apron, extends from the sacrococcygeal junction and terminates just inferior to the scapular spine, restricts gross trunk motion in the sagittal plane, produces intracavitary pressure to reduce load on the intervertebral disks, includes straps and closures, prefabricated, off-the-shelf
New code

L0460 TLSO, triplanar control, modular segmented spinal system, two rigid plastic shells, posterior extends from the sacrococcygeal junction and terminates just inferior to the scapular spine, anterior extends from the symphysis pubis to the sternal notch, soft liner, restricts gross trunk motion in the sagittal, coronal, and transverse planes, lateral strength is provided by overlapping plastic and stabilizing closures, includes straps and closures, prefabricated item that has been trimmed, bent, molded, assembled, or otherwise customized to fit a specific patient by an individual with expertise
Revised code

L0466 TLSO, sagittal control, rigid posterior frame and flexible soft anterior apron with straps, closures and padding, restricts gross trunk motion in sagittal plane, produces intracavitary pressure to reduce load on intervertebral disks, prefabricated item that has been trimmed, bent, molded, assembled, or otherwise customized to fit a specific patient by an individual with expertise
Revised code

L0467 TLSO, sagittal control, rigid posterior frame and flexible soft anterior apron with straps, closures and padding, restricts gross trunk motion in sagittal plane, produces intracavitary pressure to reduce load on intervertebral disks, prefabricated, off-the-shelf
New code

L0468 TLSO, sagittal-coronal control, rigid posterior frame and flexible soft anterior apron with straps, closures and padding, extends from sacrococcygeal junction over scapulae, lateral strength provided by pelvic, thoracic, and lateral frame pieces, restricts gross trunk motion in sagittal, and coronal planes, produces intracavitary pressure to reduce load on intervertebral disks, prefabricated item that has been trimmed, bent, molded, assembled, or otherwise customized to fit a specific patient by an individual with expertise
Revised code

L0469 TLSO, sagittal-coronal control, rigid posterior frame and flexible soft anterior apron with straps, closures and padding, extends from sacrococcygeal junction over scapulae, lateral strength provided by pelvic, thoracic, and lateral frame pieces, restricts gross trunk motion in sagittal and coronal planes, produces intracavitary pressure to reduce load on intervertebral disks, prefabricated, off-the-shelf
New code

L0621 Sacroiliac orthosis, flexible, provides pelvic-sacral support, reduces motion about the sacroiliac joint, includes straps, closures, may include pendulous abdomen design, prefabricated, off-the-shelf
Revised code

L0623 Sacroiliac orthosis, provides pelvic-sacral support, with rigid or semi-rigid panels over the sacrum and abdomen, reduces motion about the sacroiliac joint, includes straps, closures, may include pendulous abdomen design, prefabricated, off-the-shelf
Revised code

L0625 Lumbar orthosis, flexible, provides lumbar support, posterior extends from l-1 to below l-5 vertebra, produces intracavitary pressure to reduce load on the intervertebral discs, includes straps, closures, may include pendulous abdomen design, shoulder straps, stays, prefabricated, off-the-shelf
Revised code

L0626 Lumbar orthosis, sagittal control, with rigid posterior panel(s), posterior extends from l-1 to below l-5 vertebra, produces intracavitary pressure to reduce load on the intervertebral discs, includes straps, closures, may include padding, stays, shoulder straps, pendulous abdomen design, prefabricated item that has been trimmed, bent, molded, assembled, or otherwise customized to fit a specific patient by an individual with expertise
Revised code

L0627 Lumbar orthosis, sagittal control, with rigid anterior and posterior panels, posterior extends from l-1 to below l-5 vertebra, produces intracavitary pressure to reduce load on the intervertebral discs, includes straps, closures, may include padding, shoulder straps, pendulous abdomen design, prefabricated item that has been trimmed, bent, molded, assembled, or otherwise customized to fit a specific patient by an individual with expertise
Revised code

L0628 Lumbar-sacral orthosis, flexible, provides lumbo-sacral support, posterior extends from sacrococcygeal junction to t-9 vertebra, produces intracavitary pressure to reduce load on the intervertebral discs, includes straps, closures, may include stays, shoulder straps, pendulous abdomen design, prefabricated, off-the-shelf
Revised code

L0630 Lumbar-sacral orthosis, sagittal control, with rigid posterior panel(s), posterior extends from sacrococcygeal junction to t-9 vertebra, produces intracavitary pressure to reduce load on the intervertebral discs, includes straps, closures, may include padding, stays, shoulder straps, pendulous abdomen design, prefabricated item that has been trimmed, bent, molded, assembled, or otherwise customized to fit a specific patient by an individual with expertise
Revised code

L0631 Lumbar-sacral orthosis, sagittal control, with rigid anterior and posterior panels, posterior extends from sacrococcygeal junction to t-9 vertebra, produces intracavitary pressure to reduce load on the intervertebral discs, includes straps, closures, may include padding, shoulder straps, pendulous abdomen design,

prefabricated item that has been trimmed, bent, molded, assembled, or otherwise customized to fit a specific patient by an individual with expertise
Revised code

L0633 Lumbar-sacral orthosis, sagittal-coronal control, with rigid posterior frame/panel(s), posterior extends from sacrococcygeal junction to t-9 vertebra, lateral strength provided by rigid lateral frame/panels, produces intracavitary pressure to reduce load on intervertebral discs, includes straps, closures, may include padding, stays, shoulder straps, pendulous abdomen design, prefabricated item that has been trimmed, bent, molded, assembled, or otherwise customized to fit a specific patient by an individual with expertise
Revised code

L0637 Lumbar-sacral orthosis, sagittal-coronal control, with rigid anterior and posterior frame/panels, posterior extends from sacrococcygeal junction to t-9 vertebra, lateral strength provided by rigid lateral frame/panels, produces intracavitary pressure to reduce load on intervertebral discs, includes straps, closures, may include padding, shoulder straps, pendulous abdomen design, prefabricated item that has been trimmed, bent, molded, assembled, or otherwise customized to fit a specific patient by an individual with expertise
Revised code

L0639 Lumbar-sacral orthosis, sagittal-coronal control, rigid shell(s)/panel(s), posterior extends from sacrococcygeal junction to t-9 vertebra, anterior extends from symphysis pubis to xyphoid, produces intracavitary pressure to reduce load on the intervertebral discs, overall strength is provided by overlapping rigid material and stabilizing closures, includes straps, closures, may include soft interface, pendulous abdomen design, prefabricated item that has been trimmed, bent, molded, assembled, or otherwise customized to fit a specific patient by an individual with expertise
Revised code

L0641 Lumbar orthosis, sagittal control, with rigid posterior panel(s), posterior extends from l-1 to below l-5 vertebra, produces intracavitary pressure to reduce load on the intervertebral discs, includes straps, closures, may include padding, stays, shoulder straps, pendulous abdomen design, prefabricated, off-the-shelf
New code

L0642 Lumbar orthosis, sagittal control, with rigid anterior and posterior panels, posterior extends from l-1 to below l-5 vertebra, produces intracavitary pressure to reduce load on the intervertebral discs, includes straps, closures, may include padding, shoulder straps, pendulous abdomen design, prefabricated, off-the-shelf
New code

L0643 Lumbar-sacral orthosis, sagittal control, with rigid posterior panel(s), posterior extends from sacrococcygeal junction to t-9 vertebra, produces intracavitary pressure to reduce load on the intervertebral discs, includes straps, closures, may include padding, stays, shoulder straps, pendulous abdomen design, prefabricated, off- the-shelf
New code

L0648 Lumbar-sacral orthosis, sagittal control, with rigid anterior and posterior panels, posterior extends from sacrococcygeal junction to t-9 vertebra, produces intracavitary pressure to reduce load on the intervertebral discs, includes straps, closures, may include padding, shoulder straps, pendulous abdomen design, prefabricated, off-the-shelf
New code

L0649 Lumbar-sacral orthosis, sagittal-coronal control, with rigid posterior frame/panel(s), posterior extends from sacrococcygeal junction to t-9 vertebra, lateral strength provided by rigid lateral frame/panels, produces intracavitary pressure to reduce load on intervertebral discs, includes straps, closures, may include padding, stays, shoulder straps, pendulous abdomen design, prefabricated, off- the-shelf
New code

L0650 Lumbar-sacral orthosis, sagittal-coronal control, with rigid anterior and posterior frame/panel(s), posterior extends from sacrococcygeal junction to t-9 vertebra, lateral strength provided by rigid lateral frame/panel(s), produces intracavitary pressure to reduce load on intervertebral discs, includes straps, closures, may include padding, shoulder straps, pendulous abdomen design, prefabricated, off-the-shelf
New code

L0651 Lumbar-sacral orthosis, sagittal-coronal control, rigid shell(s)/panel(s), posterior extends from sacrococcygeal junction to t-9 vertebra, anterior extends from symphysis pubis to xyphoid, produces intracavitary pressure to reduce load on the intervertebral discs, overall strength is provided by overlapping rigid material and stabilizing closures, includes straps, closures, may include soft interface, pendulous abdomen design, prefabricated, off-the-shelf
New code

L0980 Peroneal straps, prefabricated, off-the-shelf, pair
Revised code

L0982 Stocking supporter grips, prefabricated, off-the-shelf, set of four (4)
Revised code

L0984 Protective body sock, prefabricated, off-the-shelf, each
Revised code

L1600 Hip orthosis, abduction control of hip joints, flexible, Frejka type with cover, prefabricated item that has been trimmed, bent, molded, assembled, or otherwise customized to fit a specific patient by an individual with expertise
Revised code

L1610 Hip orthosis, abduction control of hip joints, flexible, (Frejka cover only), prefabricated item that has been trimmed, bent, molded, assembled, or otherwise customized to fit a specific patient by an individual with expertise
Revised code

L1620 Hip orthosis, abduction control of hip joints, flexible, (Pavlik harness), prefabricated item that has been trimmed, bent, molded, assembled, or otherwise customized to fit a specific patient by an individual with expertise
Revised code

L1810 Knee orthosis, elastic with joints, prefabricated item that has been trimmed, bent, molded, assembled, or otherwise customized to fit a specific patient by an individual with expertise
Revised code

L1812 Knee orthosis, elastic with joints, prefabricated, off-the-shelf
New code

L1830 Knee orthosis, immobilizer, canvas longitudinal, prefabricated, off-the-shelf
Revised code

L1832 Knee orthosis, adjustable knee joints (unicentric or polycentric), positional orthosis, rigid support, prefabricated item that has been trimmed, bent, molded, assembled, or otherwise customized to fit a specific patient by an individual with expertise
Revised code

L1833 Knee orthosis, adjustable knee joints (unicentric or polycentric), positional orthosis, rigid support, prefabricated, off-the shelf
New code

L1836 Knee orthosis, rigid, without joint(s), includes soft interface material, prefabricated, off-the-shelf
Revised code

L1843 Knee orthosis, single upright, thigh and calf, with adjustable flexion and extension joint (unicentric or polycentric), medial-lateral and rotation control, with or without varus/valgus adjustment, prefabricated item that has been trimmed, bent, molded, assembled, or otherwise customized to fit a specific patient by an individual with expertise
Revised code

L1845 Knee orthosis, double upright, thigh and calf, with adjustable flexion and extension joint (unicentric or polycentric), medial-lateral and rotation control, with or without varus/valgus

adjustment, prefabricated item that has been trimmed, bent, molded, assembled, or otherwise customized to fit a specific patient by an individual with expertise
Revised code

L1847 Knee orthosis, double upright with adjustable joint, with inflatable air support chamber(s), prefabricated item that has been trimmed, bent, molded, assembled, or otherwise customized to fit a specific patient by an individual with expertise
Revised code

L1848 Knee orthosis, double upright with adjustable joint, with inflatable air support chamber(s), prefabricated, off-the-shelf
New code

L1850 Knee orthosis, Swedish type, prefabricated, off-the-shelf
Revised code

L1902 Ankle foot orthosis, ankle gauntlet, prefabricated, off-the- shelf
Revised code

L1904 Ankle orthosis, ankle gauntlet, custom-fabricated
Revised code

L1906 Ankle foot orthosis, multiligamentous ankle support, prefabricated, off-the-shelf
Revised code

L1907 Ankle orthosis, supramalleolar with straps, with or without interface/pads, custom fabricated
Revised code

L3100 Hallus-valgus night dynamic splint, prefabricated, off-the- shelf
Revised code

L3170 Foot, plastic, silicone or equal, heel stabilizer, prefabricated, off-the-shelf, each
Revised code

L3650 Shoulder orthosis, figure of eight design abduction restrainer, prefabricated, off-the-shelf
Revised code

L3660 Shoulder orthosis, figure of eight design abduction restrainer, canvas and webbing, prefabricated, off-the-shelf
Revised code

L3670 Shoulder orthosis, acromio/clavicular (canvas and webbing type), prefabricated, off-the-shelf
Revised code

L3675 Shoulder orthosis, vest type abduction restrainer, canvas webbing type or equal, prefabricated, off-the-shelf
Revised code

L3677 Shoulder orthosis, shoulder joint design, without joints, may include soft interface, straps, prefabricated item that has been trimmed, bent, molded, assembled, or otherwise customized to fit a specific patient by an individual with expertise
Revised code

L3678 Shoulder orthosis, shoulder joint design, without joints, may include soft interface, straps, prefabricated, off-the-shelf
New code

L3710 Elbow orthosis, elastic with metal joints, prefabricated, off-the-shelf
Revised code

L3762 Elbow orthosis, rigid, without joints, includes soft interface material, prefabricated, off-the-shelf
Revised code

L3807 Wrist hand finger orthosis, without joint(s), prefabricated item that has been trimmed, bent, molded, assembled, or otherwise customized to fit a specific patient by an individual with expertise
Revised code

L3809 Wrist hand finger orthosis, without joint(s), prefabricated, off-the-shelf, any type
New code

L3908 Wrist hand orthosis, wrist extension control cock-up, non molded, prefabricated, off-the-shelf
Revised code

L3912 Hand finger orthosis (hof), flexion glove with elastic finger control, prefabricated, off-the-shelf
Revised code

L3915 Wrist hand orthosis, includes one or more non torsion joint(s), elastic bands, turnbuckles, may include soft interface, straps, prefabricated item that has been trimmed, bent, molded, assembled, or otherwise customized to fit a specific patient by an individual with expertise
Revised code

L3916 Wrist hand orthosis, includes one or more non torsion joint(s), elastic bands, turnbuckles, may include soft interface, straps, prefabricated, off-the-shelf
New code

L3917 Hand orthosis, metacarpal fracture orthosis, prefabricated item that has been trimmed, bent, molded, assembled, or otherwise customized to fit a specific patient by an individual with expertise
Revised code

L3918 Hand orthosis, metacarpal fracture orthosis, prefabricated, off-the-shelf
New code

L3923 Hand finger orthosis, without joints, may include soft interface, straps, prefabricated item that has been trimmed, bent, molded, assembled, or otherwise customized to fit a specific patient by an individual with expertise
Revised code

L3924 Hand finger orthosis, without joints, may include soft interface, straps, prefabricated, off-the-shelf
New code

L3925 Finger orthosis, proximal interphalangeal (pip)/distal interphalangeal (dip), non torsion joint/spring, extension/flexion, may include soft interface material, prefabricated, off-the-shelf
Revised code

L3927 Finger orthosis, proximal interphalangeal (pip)/distal interphalangeal (dip), without joint/spring, extension/flexion (e.g. static or ring type), may include soft interface material, prefabricated, off-the- shelf
Revised code

L3929 Hand finger orthosis, includes one or more non torsion joint(s), turnbuckles, elastic bands/springs, may include soft interface material, straps, prefabricated item that has been trimmed, bent, molded, assembled, or otherwise customized to fit a specific patient by an individual with expertise
Revised code

L3930 Hand finger orthosis, includes one or more non torsion joint(s), turnbuckles, elastic bands/springs, may include soft interface material, straps, prefabricated, off-the-shelf
New code

L4350 Ankle control orthosis, stirrup style, rigid, includes any type interface (e.g., pneumatic, gel), prefabricated, off-the-shelf
Revised code

L4360 Walking boot, pneumatic and/or vacuum, with or without joints, with or without interface material, prefabricated item that has been trimmed, bent, molded, assembled, or otherwise customized to fit a specific patient by an individual with expertise
Revised code

L4361 Walking boot, pneumatic and/or vacuum, with or without joints, with or without interface material, prefabricated, off-the-shelf
New code

L4370 Pneumatic full leg splint, prefabricated, off-the-shelf
Revised code

L4386 Walking boot, non-pneumatic, with or without joints, with or without interface material, prefabricated item that has been trimmed, bent, molded, assembled, or otherwise customized to fit a specific patient by an individual with expertise
Revised code

L4387 Walking boot, non-pneumatic, with or without joints, with or without interface material, prefabricated, off-the-shelf
New code

L4396 Static or dynamic ankle foot orthosis, including soft interface material, adjustable for fit, for positioning, may be used for minimal ambulation, prefabricated item that has been trimmed, bent, molded, assembled, or otherwise customized to fit a specific patient by an individual with expertise
Revised code

L4397 Static or dynamic ankle foot orthosis, including soft interface material, adjustable for fit, for positioning, may be used for minimal ambulation, prefabricated, off-the-shelf
New code

L4398 Foot drop splint, recumbent positioning device, prefabricated, off-the-shelf
Revised code

L5969 Addition, endoskeletal ankle-foot or ankle system, power assist, includes any type motor(s)
New code

L8679 Implantable neurostimulator, pulse generator, any type
New code

Q0090 Code deleted December 31, 2013. Use J7301.

Q0161 Chlorpromazine hydrochloride, 5 mg, oral, fad approved prescription anti-emetic, for use as a complete therapeutic substitute for an iv anti-emetic at the time of chemotherapy treatment, not to exceed a 48 hour dosage regimen
New code

Q0165 Code deleted December 31, 2013.

Q0168 Code deleted December 31, 2013.

Q0170 Code deleted December 31, 2013.

Q0171 Code deleted December 31, 2013.

Q0172 Code deleted December 31, 2013.

Q0176 Code deleted December 31, 2013.

Q0178 Code deleted December 31, 2013.

Q0507 Miscellaneous supply or accessory for use with an external ventricular assist device
New code

Q0508 Miscellaneous supply or accessory for use with an implanted ventricular assist device
New code

Q0509 Miscellaneous supply or accessory for use with any implanted ventricular assist device for which payment was not made under medicare part A
New code

Q2027 Code deleted December 31, 2013.

Q2028 Injection, Sculptra, 0.5 mg
New code

Q2050 Injection, doxorubicin hydrochloride, liposomal, not otherwise specified, 10mg
New code

Q2051 Code deleted December 31, 2013.

Q2052 Services, supplies and accessories used in the home under the medicare intravenous immune globulin (IVIG) demonstration
New code

Q3025 Code deleted December 31, 2013.

Q3026 Code deleted December 31, 2013.

Q3027 Injection, interferon beta-1a, 1 mcg for intramuscular use
New code

Q3028 Injection, interferon beta-1a, 1 mcg for subcutaneous use
New code

Q4137 Amnioexcel or biodexcel, per square centimeter
New code

Q4138 Biodefense dry flex, per square centimeter
New code

Q4139 Amniomatrix or Biomatrix, injectable, 1 cc
New code

Q4140 Biodefense, per square centimeter
New code

Q4141 Alloskin ac, per square centimeter
New code

Q4142 Xcm biologic tissue matrix, per square centimeter
New code

Q4143 Repriza, per square centimeter
New code

Q4145 Epifix, injectable, 1 mg
New code

Q4146 Tensix, per square centimeter
New code

Q4147 Architect extracellular matrix, per square centimeter
New code

Q4148 Neox 1k, per square centimeter
New code

Q4149 Excellagen, 0.1 cc
New code

Q5001 Hospice or home health care provided in patient's home/residence
Revised code

Q5002 Hospice or home health care provided in assisted living facility
Revised code

Q5009 Hospice or home health care provided in place not otherwise specified (nos)
Revised code

S3625 Code deleted December 31, 2013.

S3626 Code deleted December 31, 2013.

S3833 Code deleted December 31, 2013.

S3834 Code deleted December 31, 2013.

S3870 Comparative genomic hybridization (CGH) microarray testing for developmental delay, autism spectrum disorder and/or intellectual disability
Revised code

S9960 Ambulance service, conventional air services, nonemergency transport, one way (fixed wing)
New code

S9961 Ambulance service, conventional air service, nonemergency transport, one way (rotary wing)
New code

T4543 Adult sized disposable incontinence product, protective brief/diaper, above extra large, each
Revised code

T4544 Adult sized disposable incontinence product, protective underwear/pull-on, above extra large, each
New code

APPENDIX C: TABLE OF DRUGS

HCPCS TABLE OF DRUGS

Directions for the Use of the Table:

1. All drugs are listed in strict alphabetical order by generic drug name.
2. HCPCS code numbers for drugs are listed only under the generic drug name. Users should first look for entries under generic names of drugs. When a drug is known only by brand name, look for the brand name and you will be directed to the generic name of the drug (see "generic name".
3. Cancer chemotherapy drugs are preceded by an asterisk ().
4. In all cases except those preceded by a pound sign (#), the amount stated includes the amount as well as any amount "up to" that which is stated in the column. When a pound sign appears, it designated that the amount of the drug is only the amount listed.
5. A dash (—) appearing in a column signifies that no information is given for that particular variable for the drug listed.
6. Information which is indented and appears beneath the first line for a drug is to be considered a continuation of the line preceding it. All drug entries should be checked for indented lines beneath it as a continuation of that entry.
7. When one drug has more than one entry as a result of different routes of administration or different amounts, the drug name is not repeated. All entries for the same drug are listed beneath that drug.
8. The following abbreviations are used in the "routes of administration" column:

   amp = ampule

   DME = durable medical equipment

   EPI = epidural

g = gram

IA = intra-arterial administration

IM = intramuscular administration

INF = infusion

INH = administration by inhaled solution

INJ = injection

IO = intraocular

IT = intrathecal

IU = international unit

IV = intravenous administration

mcg = microgram

mg = milligram

ml = milliliter

ORAL= administered orally

OTH = other routes of administration

PAR = parenteral

SC = subcutaneous administration

TABS = tablets

U = units

VAR = various routes of administration

A

DESCRIPTION	DOSE	ROUTE	CODE
Abatacept	10 mg	IV	J0129
Abbokinase, see Urokinase			
Abbokinase, Open Cath, see Urokinase			
Abciximab	10 mg	IV	J0130
Abelcet, see Amphotericin B lipid complex			
ABLC, see Amphotericin B			
AbobotulinumtoxintypeA	5 units	IM	J0586
Acetaminophen	10 mg	IV	J0131
Acetazolamide sodium	up to 500 mg	IM/IV	J1120
Acetylcysteine, injection	100 mg	IV	J0132
Acetylcysteine, unit dose form	per gram	INH	J7604, J7608
Achromycin, see Tetracycline			
Actemra, see Tocilizumab			
ACTH, see Corticotropin			
Acthar, see Corticotropin			
Actimmune, see Interferon gamma 1-B			
Activase, see Alteplase recombinant			
Acyclovir	5 mg		J0133
Adalimumab	20 mg		J0135
Adcetis, *see* Brentuximab vedotin			
Adenocard, see Adenosine			
Adenoscan, see Adenosine			
Adenosine	6 mg	IV	J0150
	1 mg	IV	J0151

DESCRIPTION	DOSE	ROUTE	CODE
Ado-trastuzumab emtansine	1 mg	IV	J9354
Adrenalin Chloride, see Adrenalin, epinephrine			
Adrenalin, epinephrine	0.1 mg	SC/IM	J0171
Adriamycin PFS, see Doxorubicin HCl			
Adriamycin RDF, see Doxorubicin HCl			
Adrucil, see Fluorouracil			
Aflibercept	1 mg	OTH	J0178
Agalsidase beta	1 mg	IV	J0180
Aggrastat, see Tirofiban hydrochloride			
A-hydroCort, see Hydrocortisone sodium phosphate			
Akineton, see Biperiden			
Alatrofloxacin mesylate, injection	100 mg	IV	J0200
Albuterol	0.5 mg	INH	J7620
Albuterol, concentrated form	1 mg	INH	J7610, J7611
Albuterol, unit dose form	1 mg	INH	J7609, J7613
Aldesleukin	per single use vial	IM/IV	J9015
Aldomet, see Methyldopate HCl			
Alefacept	0.5 mg	IM/IV	J0215
Alemtuzumab	10 mg	IV	J9010
Alferon N, see Interferon alfa-n3			
Alglucerase	per 10 units	IV	J0205
Alglucosidase alfa	10 mg	IV	J0220, J0221
Alkaban-AQ, see Vinblastine sulfate			
Alkeran, see Melphalan, oral			

DESCRIPTION	DOSE	ROUTE	CODE
Alpha 1-proteinase inhibitor, human	10 mg	IV	J0256, J0257
Alphanate			J7186
Alprostadil, injection	1.25 mcg	OTH	J0270
Alprostadil, urethral suppository		OTH	J0275
Alteplase recombinant	1 mg	IV	J2997
Alupent, see Metaproterenol sulfate or Metaproterenol, compounded			
Amcort, see Triamcinolone diacetate			
A-methaPred, see Methylprednisolone sodium succinate			
Amgen, see Interferon alphacon-1			
Amifostine	500 mg	IV	J0207
Amikacin sulfate	100 mg		J0278
Aminolevalinic acid HCl	unit dose (354 mg)	OTH	J7308
Aminolevulinate	1 gram	OTH	J7309
Aminophylline/ Aminophyllin	up to 250 mg	IV	J0280
Amiodarone HCl	30 mg	IV	J0282
Amitriptyline HCl	up to 20 mg	IM	J1320
Amobarbital	up to 125 mg	IM/IV	J0300
Amphocin, see Amphotericin B			
Amphotericin B	50 mg	IV	J0285
Amphotericin B, lipid complex	10 mg	IV	J0287-J0289
Ampicillin sodium	up to 500 mg	IM/IV	J0290
Ampicillin sodium/ sulbactam sodium	per 1.5 grams	IM/IV	J0295

DESCRIPTION	DOSE	ROUTE	CODE
Amygdalin, see Laetrile, Amygdalin, vitamin B-17			
Amytal, see Amobarbital			
Anabolin LA 100, see Nandrolone decanoate			
Anadulafungin	1 mg	IV	J0348
Anascorp, see Centruroides Immune Fab			
Ancef, see Cefazolin sodium			
Andrest 90-4, see Testosterone enanthate and estradiol valerate			
Andro-Cyp, see Testosterone cypionate			
Andro-Cyp 200, see Testosterone cypionate			
Andro L.A. 200, see Testosterone enanthate			
Andro-Estro 90-4, see Testosterone enanthate and estradiol valerate			
Andro/Fem, see Testosterone cypionate and estradiol cypionate			
Androgyn L.A., see Testosterone enanthate and estradiol valerate			
Androlone-50, see Nandrolone phenpropionate			
Androlone-100, see Nandrolone decanoate			
Andronaq-50, see Testosterone suspension			
Andronaq-LA, see Testosterone cypionate			
Andronate-200, see Testosterone cypionate			

DESCRIPTION	DOSE	ROUTE	CODE
Andronate-100, see Testosterone cypionate			
Andropository 100, see Testosterone enanthate			
Andryl 200, see Testosterone enanthate			
Anectine, see Succinylcholine chloride			
Anergan 25, see Promethazine HCl			
Anergan 50, see Promethazine HCl			
Anistreplase	30 units	IV	J0350
Anti-Inhibitor	per IU	IV	J7198
Antispas, see Dicyclomine HCl			
Antithrombin III (human)	per IU	IV	J7197
Antithrombin recominant	50 IU	IV	J7196
Anzemet, see Dolasetron mesylate injection			
A.P.L., see Chorionic gonadotropin			
Apomorphine HCl	1 mg	SC	J0364
Apresoline, see Hydralazine HCl			
Aprotinin	10,000 KIU		J0365
AquaMEPHYTON, see Vitamin K			
Aralen, see Chloroquine HCl			
Aramine, see Metaraminol			
Aranesp, see Darbepoetin Alfa			
Arbutamine	1 mg	IV	J0395
Arcalyst, see Rilanocept			
Aredia, see Pamidronate disodium			

DESCRIPTION	DOSE	ROUTE	CODE
Arfonad, see Trimethaphan camsylate			
Arformoterol tartrate	15 mcg	INH	J7605
Aridol, see Mannitol			
Aripiprazole	0.25 mg	IM	J0400
Aripiprazole, extended release	1 mg	INJ	J0401
Aristocort Forte, see Triamcinolone diacetate			
Aristocort Intralesional, see Triamcinolone diacetate			
Aristospan Intra-Articular, see Triamcinolone hexacetonide			
Aristospan Intralesional, see Triamcinolone hexacetonide			
Arrestin, see Trimethobenzamide HCl			
Arsenic trioxide	1 mg	IV	J9017
Arzerra, see Ofatumumab			
Asparaginase	1,000 units	IV/IM	J9019
	10,000 units	IV/IM	J9020
Astramorph PF, see Morphine sulfate			
Atgam, see Lymphocyte immune globulin			
Ativan, see Lorazepam			
Atropine, concentrated form	per mg	INH	J7635
Atropine, unit dose form	per mg	INH	J7636
Atropine sulfate	0.01 mg	IV/IM/SC	J0461
Atrovent, see Ipratropium bromide			
Atryn, see Antithrombin recominant			
Aurothioglucose	up to 50 mg	IM	J2910

DESCRIPTION	DOSE	ROUTE	CODE
Autologous cultured chondrocytes implant		OTH	J7330
Autoplex T, see Hemophilia clotting factors			
Avonex, see Interferon beta-1a			
Azacitidine	1 mg	SC	J9025
Azathioprine	50 mg	ORAL	J7500
Azathioprine, parenteral	100 mg	IV	J7501
Azithromycin, dihydrate	1 gram	ORAL	Q0144
Azithromycin, injection	500 mg	IV	J0456

B

DESCRIPTION	DOSE	ROUTE	CODE
Baclofen	10 mg	IT	J0475
Baclofen for intrathecal trial	50 mcg	OTH	J0476
Bactocill, see Oxacillin sodium			
BAL in oil, see Dimercaprol			
Banflex, see Orphenadrine citrate			
Basiliximab	20 mg		J0480
BCG (Bacillus Calmette and Guérin), live instillation	per vial	IV	J9031
Beclomethasone inhalation solution, unit dose form	per mg	INH	J7622
Belatacept	1 mg	IV	J0485
Belimumab	10 mg	IV	J0490
Bena-D10, see Diphenhydramine HCl			
Bena-D 50, see Diphenhydramine HCl			

DESCRIPTION	DOSE	ROUTE	CODE
Benadryl, see Diphenhydramine HCl			
Benahist 10, see Diphenhydramine HCl			
Benahist 50, see Diphenhydramine HCl			
Ben-Allergin-50, see Diphenhydramine HCl			
Bendamustine HCl	1 mg	IV	J9033
BeneFIX, see Factor IX, recombinant			
Benlysta, see Belimumab			
Benoject-10, see Diphenhydramine HCl			
Benoject-50, see Diphenhydramine HCl			
Bentyl, see Dicyclomine			
Benztropine mesylate	per 1 mg	IM/IV	J0515
Berinert, see C-1 esterase inhibitor			
Berubigen, see Vitamin B-12 cyanocobalamin			
Beta amyloid	per study dose	OTH	A9599
Betalin 12, see Vitamin B-12 cyanocobalamin			
Betameth, see Betamethasone sodium phosphate			
Betamethasone acetate & betamethasone sodium phosphate	per 3 mg	IM	J0702
Betamethasone inhalation solution, unit dose form	per mg	INH	J7624
Betaseron, see Interferon beta-1b			
Bethanechol chloride	up to 5 mg	SC	J0520
Bevacizumab	10 mg	IV	J9035

DESCRIPTION	DOSE	ROUTE	CODE
Bicillin L-A, see Penicillin G benzathine			
Bicillin C-R 900/300, see Penicillin G procaine and penicillin G benzathine			
Bicillin C-R, see Penicillin G benzathine and penicillin G procaine			
BiCNU, see Carmustine			
Biperiden lactate	per 5 mg	IM/IV	J0190
Bitolterol mesylate, concentrated form	per mg	INH	J7628
Bitolterol mesylate, unit dose form	per mg	INH	J7629
Bivalirudin	1 mg	IV	J0583
Blenoxane, see Bleomycin sulfate			
Bleomycin sulfate	15 units	IM/IV/SC	J9040
Bortezomib	0.1 mg	IV	J9041
Botox, see OnabotulinumtoxinA			
Brentuximab Vedotin	1 mg	IV	J9042
Brethine, see Terbutaline sulfate or Terbutaline, compounded			
Bricanyl Subcutaneous, see Terbutaline sulfate			
Brompheniramine maleate	per 10 mg	IM/SC/IV	J0945
Bronkephrine, see Ethylnorepinephrine HCl			
Bronkosol, see Isoetharine HCl			
Budesonide inhalation solution, concentrated form	0.25 mg	INH	J7633, J7634
Budesonide inhalation solution, unit dose form	0.5 mg	INH	J7626, J7627

DESCRIPTION	DOSE	ROUTE	CODE
Buprenorphine HCl	0.1 mg	IM	J0592
Busulfan	1 mg 2 mg	IV ORAL	J0594 J8510
Butorphanol tartrate	1 mg		J0595

C

DESCRIPTION	DOSE	ROUTE	CODE
C1 esterase inhibitor	10 units		J0597, J0598
Cabazitaxel	1 mg	IV	J9043
Cabergoline	0.25 mg	ORAL	J8515
Cafcit, see Caffeine citrate			
Caffeine citrate	5 mg	IV	J0706
Caine-1, see Lidocaine HCl			
Caine-2, see Lidocaine HCl			
Calcijex, see Calcitriol			
Calcimar, see Calcitonin-salmon			
Calcitonin-salmon	up to 400 units	SC/IM	J0630
Calcitriol	0.1 mcg	IM	J0636
Calcium Disodium Versenate, see Edetate calcium disodium			
Calcium gluconate	per 10 ml	IV	J0610
Calcium glycerophosphate & calcium lactate	per 10 ml	IM/SC	J0620
Caldolor, see Ibuprofen			
Calphosan, see Calcium glycerophosphate and calcium lactate			
Camptosar, see Irinotecan			
Canakinumab	1 mg	SC	J0638
Capecitabine	150 mg 500 mg	ORAL ORAL	J8520 J8521

DESCRIPTION	DOSE	ROUTE	CODE
Capsaicin patch	per 10 sq cm	OTH	J7335
Carbocaine with Neo-Cobefrin, see Mepivacaine			
Carbocaine, see Mepivacaine			
Carboplatin	50 mg	IV	J9045
Carfilzomib	1 mg	IV	J9047
Carmustine	100 mg	IV	J9050
Carnitor, see Levocarnitine			
Carticel, see Autologous cultured chondrocytes			
Caspofungin acetate	5 mg	IV	J0637
Cayston, see Aztreonam			
Cefadyl, see Cephapirin Sodium			
Cefazolin sodium	500 mg	IV/IM	J0690
Cefepime hydrochloride	500 mg	IV	J0692
Cefizox, see Ceftizoxime sodium			
Cefotaxime sodium	per 1 gram	IV/IM	J0698
Cefoxitin sodium	1 gram	IV/IM	J0694
Ceftaroline fosamil	1 mg		J0712
Ceftazidime	per 500 mg	IV/IM	J0713
Ceftizoxime sodium	per 500 mg	IV/IM	J0715
Ceftriaxone sodium	per 250 mg	IV/IM	J0696
Cefuroxime sodium, sterile	per 750 mg	IV/IM	J0697
Celestone Soluspan, see Betamethasone acetate and betamethasone sodium phosphate			
CellCept, see Mycophenolate mofetil			
Cel-U-Jec, see Betamethasone sodium phosphate			

DESCRIPTION	DOSE	ROUTE	CODE
Centruroides Immune Fab	up to 120 mg	IV	J0716
Cephalothin sodium	up to 1 gram	IV/IM	J1890
Cephapirin sodium	up to 1 gram	IV/IM	J0710
Ceredase, see Alglucerase			
Certolizumab pegol	1 mg	SC	J0717
Cerubidine, see Daunorubicin HCl			
Cetuximab	10 mg	IV	J9055
Chealamide, see Endrate ethylenediamine-tetra-acetic acid			
Chloramphenicol sodium succinate	up to 1 gram	IV	J0720
Chlordiazepoxide HCl	up to 100 mg	IM/IV	J1990
Chloromycetin Sodium Succinate, see Chloramphenicol sodium succinate			
Chloroprocaine HCl	per 30 ml	VAR	J2400
Chlorpromazine	5 mg	ORAL	Q0161
Chloroquine HCl	up to 250 mg	IM	J0390
Chlorothiazide sodium	per 500 mg	IV	J1205
Chlorpromazine HCL	up to 50 mg	IM/IV	J3230
Chorex-5, see Chorionic gonadotropin			
Chorex-10, see Chorionic gonadotropin			
Chorignon, see Chorionic gonadotropin			
Chorionic gonadotropin	per 1,000 USP units	IM	J0725
Choron 10, see Chorionic gonadotropin			
Cidofovir	375 mg	IV	J0740
Cilastatin sodium, imipenem	per 250 mg	IV/IM	J0743
Cimzia, see Certolizumab pegol			

DESCRIPTION	DOSE	ROUTE	CODE
Cinacort Forte, see Triamcinolone diacetate			
Cinacort A-40, see Triamcinolone acetonide			
Cinryze, see C1 esterase inhibitor			
Cipro IV, see Ciprofloxacin			
Ciprofloxacin	200 mg	IV	J0744
Cisplatin, powder or solution	per 10 mg	IV	J9060
Cladribine	per mg	IV	J9065
Claforan, see Cefotaxime sodium			
Clofarabine	1 mg	IV	J9027
Clonidine Hydrochloride	1 mg	EPI	J0735
Cobex, see Vitamin B-12 cyanocobalamin			
Codeine phosphate	per 30 mg	IM/IV/SC	J0745
Codimal-A, see Brompheniramine maleate			
Cogentin, see Benztropine mesylate			
Collagenase, Clostridium histolytium	0.01 mg	OTH	J0775
Colchicine	per 1 mg	IV	J0760
Colistimethate sodium	up to 150 mg	IM/IV	J0770
Coly-Mycin M, see Colistimethate sodium			
Compa-Z, see Prochlorperazine			
Compazine, see Prochlorperazine			
Cophene-B, see Brompheniramine maleate			

DESCRIPTION	DOSE	ROUTE	CODE
Copper contraceptive, intrauterine		OTH	J7300
Cordarone, see Amiodarone HCl			
Corgonject-5, see Chorionic gonadotropin			
Corticorelin ovine triflutate	1 mcg		J0795
Corticotropin	up to 40 units	IV/IM/SC	J0800
Cortrosyn, see Cosyntropin			
Cosmegen, see Dactinomycin			
Cosyntropin	per 0.25 mg	IM/IV	J0833, J0834
Cotranzine, see Prochlorperazine			
Crofab, see Crotalidae Polyvalent Immune Fab			
Cromolyn sodium, unit dose form	per 10 mg	INH	J7631, J7632
Crotalidae Polyvalent Immune Fab	up to 1 gram	IV	J0840
Crysticillin 300 A.S., see Penicillin G procaine			
Crysticillin 600 A.S., see Penicillin G procaine			
Cyclophosphamide	100 mg	IV	J9070
Cyclophosphamide, oral	25 mg	ORAL	J8530
Cyclosporine, oral	25 mg	ORAL	J7515
	100 mg	ORAL	J7502
Cyclosporine, parenteral	250 mg	IV	J7516
Cytarabine	100 mg	SC/IV	J9100
Cytarabine liposome	10 mg		J9098
Cytomegalovirus immune globulin intravenous (human)	per vial	IV	J0850
Cytosar-U, see Cytarabine			

DESCRIPTION	DOSE	ROUTE	CODE
Cytovene, see Ganciclovir sodium			
Cytoxan, see Cyclophosphamide; cyclophosphamide, lyophilized; and cyclophosphamide, oral			

D

DESCRIPTION	DOSE	ROUTE	CODE
D-5-W, infusion	1000 cc	IV	J7070
Dacarbazine	100 mg	IV	J9130
Daclizumab	25 mg	IV	J7513
Dactinomycin	0.5 mg	IV	J9120
Dalalone, see Dexamethasone sodium phosphate			
Dalalone L.A., see Dexamethasone acetate			
Dalteparin sodium	per 2500 IU	SC	J1645
Daptomycin	1 mg	IV	J0878
Darbepoetin Alfa	1 mcg	IV/SC	J0881, J0882
Daunorubicin citrate, liposomal formulation	10 mg	IV	J9151
Daunorubicin HCl	10 mg	IV	J9150
DaunoXome, see Daunorubicin citrate			
DDAVP, see Desmopressin acetate			
Decadron Phosphate, see Dexamethasone sodium phosphate			
Decadron, see Dexamethasone sodium phosphate			
Decadron-LA, see Dexamethasone acetate			

DESCRIPTION	DOSE	ROUTE	CODE
Deca-Durabolin, see Nandrolone decanoate			
Decaject, see Dexamethasone sodium phosphate			
Decaject-L.A., see Dexamethasone acetate			
Decitabine	1 mg	IV	J0894
Decolone-50, see Nandrolone decanoate			
Decolone-100, see Nandrolone decanoate			
De-Comberol, see Testosterone cypionate and estradiol cypionate			
Deferoxamine mesylate	500 mg	IM/SC/IV	J0895
Degarelix	1 mg	SC	J9155
Dehist, see Brompheniramine maleate			
Deladumone OB, see Testosterone enanthate and estradiol valerate			
Deladumone, see Testosterone enanthate and estradiol valerate			
Delatest, see Testosterone enanthate			
Delatestadiol, see Testosterone enanthate and estradiol valerate			
Delatestryl, see Testosterone enanthate			
Delta-Cortef, see Prednisolone, oral			
Delestrogen, see Estradiol valerate			
Demadex, see Torsemide			

DESCRIPTION	DOSE	ROUTE	CODE
Demerol HCl, see Meperidine HCl			
Denileukin diftitox	300 mcg	IV	J9160
Denosumab	1 mg	SC	J0897
DepAndro 100, see Testosterone cypionate			
DepAndro 200, see Testosterone cypionate			
DepAndrogyn, see Testosterone cypionate and estradiol cypionate			
DepGynogen, see Depo-estradiol cypionate			
DepMedalone 40, see Methylprednisolone acetate			
DepMedalone 80, see Methylprednisolone acetate			
Depo-estradiol cypionate	up to 5 mg	IM	J1000
Depogen, see Depo-estradiol cypionate			
Depoject, see Methylprednisolone acetate			
Depo-Medrol, see Methylprednisolone acetate			
Depopred-40, see Methylprednisolone acetate			
Depopred-80, see Methylprednisolone acetate			
Depo-Provera, see Medroxyprogesterone acetate			
Depotest, see Testosterone cypionate			
Depo-Testadiol, see Testosterone cypionate and estradiol cypionate			

DESCRIPTION	DOSE	ROUTE	CODE
Depotestogen, see Testosterone cypionate and estradiol cypionate			
Depo-Testosterone, see Testosterone cypionate			
Desferal Mesylate, see Deferoxamine mesylate			
Desmopressin acetate	1 mcg	IV/SC	J2597
Dexacen LA-8, see Dexamethasone acetate			
Dexacen-4, see Dexamethasone sodium phosphate			
Dexamethasone, concentrated form	per mg	INH	J7637
Dexamethasone, unit form	per mg	INH	J7638
Dexamethasone, intravitreal implant	0.1 mg	OTH	J7312
Dexamethasone, oral	0.25 mg	ORAL	J8540
Dexamethasone acetate	1 mg	IM	J1094
Dexamethasone sodium phosphate	1 mg	IM/IV/OTH	J1100
Dexasone, see Dexamethasone sodium phosphate			
Dexasone L.A., see Dexamethasone acetate			
Dexferrum, see Iron Dextran			
Dexone, see Dexamethasone sodium phosphate			
Dexone LA, see Dexamethasone acetate			
Dexrazoxane HCl	250 mg	IV	J1190
Dextran 40	500 ml	IV	J7100
Dextran 75	500 ml	IV	J7110
Dextrose 5%/normal saline solution	500 ml = 1 unit	IV	J7042

DESCRIPTION	DOSE	ROUTE	CODE
Dextrose/water (5%)	500 ml = 1 unit	IV	J7060
D.H.E. 45, see Dihydroergotamine			
Diamox, see Acetazolamide sodium			
Diazepam	up to 5 mg	IM/IV	J3360
Diazoxide	up to 300 mg	IV	J1730
Dibent, see Dicyclomine HCl			
Dicyclomine HCl	up to 20 mg	IM	J0500
Didronel, see Etidronate disodium			
Diethylstilbestrol diphosphate	250 mg	IV	J9165
Diflucan, see Fluconazole			
Digoxin	up to 0.5 mg	IM/IV	J1160
Digoxin immune fab (ovine)	per vial		J1162
Dihydrex, see Diphenhydramine HCl			
Dihydroergotamine mesylate	per 1 mg	IM/IV	J1110
Dilantin, see Phenytoin sodium			
Dilaudid, see Hydromorphone HCl			
Dilocaine, see Lidocaine HCl			
Dilomine, see Dicyclomine HCl			
Dilor, see Dyphylline			
Dimenhydrinate	up to 50 mg	IM/IV	J1240
Dimercaprol	per 100 mg	IM	J0470
Dimethyl sulfoxide, see DMSO, Dimethylsulfoxide			
Dinate, see Dimenhydrinate			

DESCRIPTION	DOSE	ROUTE	CODE
Dioval, see Estradiol valerate			
Dioval 40, see Estradiol valerate			
Dioval XX, see Estradiol valerate			
Diphenacen-50, see Diphenhydramine HCl			
Diphenhydramine HCl, injection	up to 50 mg	IV/IM	J1200
Diphenhydramine HCl, oral	50 mg	ORAL	Q0163
Dipyridamole	per 10 mg	IV	J1245
Disotate, see Endrate ethylenediamine-tetra-acetic acid			
Di-Spaz, see Dicyclomine HCl			
Ditate-DS, see Testosterone enanthate and estradiol valerate			
Diuril Sodium, see Chlorothiazide sodium			
D-Med 80, see Methylprednisolone acetate			
DMSO, Dimethyl sulfoxide	50%, 50 ml	OTH	J1212
Dobutamine HCl	per 250 mg	IV	J1250
Dobutrex, see Dobutamine HCl			
Docetaxel	20 mg	IV	J9170
Dolasetron mesylate, injection	10 mg	IV	J1260
Dolasetron mesylate, tablets	100 mg	ORAL	Q0180
Dolophine HCl, see Methadone HCl			

DESCRIPTION	DOSE	ROUTE	CODE
Dommanate, see Dimenhydrinate			
Donbax, see Doripenem			
Dopamine HCl	40 mg		J1265
Doribax, see Doripenem			
Doripenem	10 mg	IV	J1267
Dornase alpha, unit dose form	per mg	INH	J7639
Doxercalciferol	1 mcg	IV	J1270
Doxil, see Doxorubicin HCl, lipid			
Doxorubicin HCl	10 mg	IV	J9000
Dramamine, see Dimenhydrinate			
Dramanate, see Dimenhydrinate			
Dramilin, see Dimenhydrinate			
Dramocen, see Dimenhydrinate			
Dramoject, see Dimenhydrinate			
Dronabinol, oral	2.5 mg	ORAL	Q0167
Droperidol	up to 5 mg	IM/IV	J1790
Drug administered through a metered dose inhaler		INH	J3535
Droperidol and fentanyl citrate	up to 2 ml amp.	IM/IV	J1810
DTIC-Dome, see Dacarbazine			
Dua-Gen L.A., see Testosterone enanthate and estradiol valerate cypionate			
Duoval P.A., see Testosterone enanthate and estradiol valerate			

DESCRIPTION	DOSE	ROUTE	CODE
Durabolin, see Nandrolone phenpropionate			
Duraclon, see Clonidine hydrochloride			
Dura-Estrin, see Depo-estradiol cypionate			
Duracillin A.S., see Penicillin G procaine			
Duragen-10, see Estradiol valerate			
Duragen-20, see Estradiol valerate			
Duragen-40, see Estradiol valerate			
Duralone-40, see Methylprednisolone acetate			
Duralone-80, see Methylprednisolone acetate			
Duralutin, see Hydroxyprogesterone Caproate			
Duramorph, see Morphine sulfate			
Duratest-100, see Testosterone cypionate			
Duratest-200, see Testosterone cypionate			
Duratestrin, see Testosterone cypionate and estradiol cypionate			
Durathate-200, see Testosterone enanthate			
Dymenate, see Dimenhydrinate			
Dyphylline	up to 500 mg	IM	J1180
Dysport, see AbobotulinumtoxintypeA			

E

DESCRIPTION	DOSE	ROUTE	CODE
Ecallantide	1 mg	SC	J1290
Eculizumab	10 mg	IV	J1300
Edetate calcium disodium	up to 1000 mg	IV/SC/IM	J0600
Edetate disodium	per 150 mg	IV	J3520
Elavil, see Amitriptyline HCl			
Ellence, see Epirubicin HCl			
Elliotts b solution	1 ml	OTH	J9175
Elspar, see Asparaginase			
Emend, see Fosaprepitant			
Emete-Con, see Benzquinamide			
Eminase, see Anistreplase			
Enbrel, see Etanercept			
Endrate ethylenediamine-tetra-acetic acid, see Edetate disodium			
Enfuvirtide	1 mg	SC	J1324
Enovil, see Amitriptyline HCl			
Enoxaparin sodium	10 mg	SC	J1650
Eovist, see Gadoxetate disodium			
Epinephrine, adrenalin	0.1 mg	SC/IM	J0171
Epirubicin hydrochloride	2 mg		J9178
Epoetin alfa	1000 units	IV/SC	Q4081
Epoprostenol	0.5 mg	IV	J1325
Eptifibatide, injection	5 mg	IM/IV	J1327
Ergonovine maleate	up to 0.2 mg	IM/IV	J1330
Eribulin mesylate	0.1 mg	IV	J9179

DESCRIPTION	DOSE	ROUTE	CODE
Ertapenem sodium	500 mg	IM/IV	J1335
Erwinase, *see* Asparaginase			
Erythromycin lactobionate	500 mg	IV	J1364
Estra-D, see Depo-estradiol cypionate			
Estra-L 20, see Estradiol valerate			
Estra-L 40, see Estradiol valerate			
Estra-Testrin, see Testosterone enanthate and estradiol valerate			
Estradiol Cypionate, see Depo-estradiol cypionate			
Estradiol L.A., see Estradiol valerate			
Estradiol L.A. 20, see Estradiol valerate			
Estradiol L.A. 40, see Estradiol valerate			
Estradiol valerate	up to 10 mg	IM	J1380
Estro-Cyp, see Depo-estradiol cypionate			
Estrogen, conjugated	per 25 mg	IV/IM	J1410
Estroject L.A., see Depo-estradiol cypionate			
Estrone	per 1 mg	IM	J1435
Estrone 5, see Estrone			
Estrone Aqueous, see Estrone			
Estronol, see Estrone			
Estronol-L.A., see Depo-estradiol cypionate			
Etanercept, injection	25 mg	IM/IV	J1438
Ethanolamine	100 mg		J1430
Ethyol, see Amifostine			
Etidronate disodium	per 300 mg	IV	J1436

DESCRIPTION	DOSE	ROUTE	CODE
Etonogestrel implant			J7307
Etopophos, see Etoposide			
Etoposide	10 mg	IV	J9181
Etoposide, oral	50 mg	ORAL	J8560
Euflexxa	per dose	OTH	J7323
Everolimus, oral	0.25 mg	ORAL	J7527
Everone, see Testosterone Enanthate			
Eylen, see Aflibercept			

F

DESCRIPTION	DOSE	ROUTE	CODE
Factor VIIa (coagulation factor, recombinant)	1 mcg	IV	J7189
Factor VIII (anti-hemophilic factor, human)	per IU	IV	J7190
Factor VIII (anti-hemophilic factor, porcine)	per IU	IV	J7191
Factor VIII (anti-hemophilic factor, recombinant)	per IU	IV	J7185, J7192
Factor IX (anti-hemophilic factor, purified, non-recombinant)	per IU	IV	J7193
Factor IX (anti-hemophilic factor, recombinant)	per IU	IV	J7195
Factor IX, complex	per IU	IV	J7194
Factors, other hemophilia clotting	per IU	IV	J7196
Factrel, see Gonadorelin HCl			
Feiba VH Immuno, see Factors, other hemophilia clotting			
Fentanyl citrate	0.1 mg	IM/IV	J3010

DESCRIPTION	DOSE	ROUTE	CODE
Feraheme, see Ferumoxytol			
Ferrlecit, see Sodium ferricgluconate complex in sucrose injection			
Ferumoxytol	1 mg		Q0138, Q0139
Filgrastim (G-CSF)	1 mcg	SC/IV	J1442
Filgrastim (TBO)	5 mcg	SC/IV	J1446
Firazyr, *see* Icatibant			
Firmagon, see Degarelix			
Flebogamma	500 mg	IV	J1572
Flexoject, see Orphenadrine citrate			
Flexon, see Orphenadrine citrate			
Flolan, see Epoprostenol			
Floxuridine	500 mg	IV	J9200
Fluconazole	200 mg	IV	J1450
Fludara, see Fludarabine phosphate			
Fludarabine phosphate	1 mg 50 mg	ORAL IV	J8562 J9185
Flunisolide inhalation solution, unit dose form	per mg	INH	J7641
Fluocinolone		OTH	J7311
Fluorouracil	500 mg	IV	J9190
Folex, see Methotrexate sodium			
Folex PFS, see Methotrexate sodium			
Follutein, see Chorionic gonadotropin			
Folotyn, see Pralatexate			
Fomepizole	15 mg		J1451
Fomivirsen sodium	1.65 mg	IO	J1452
Fondaparinux sodium	0.5 mg	SC	J1652

DESCRIPTION	DOSE	ROUTE	CODE
Formoterol	12 mcg	INH	J7640
Formoterol fumarate	20 mcg	INH	J7606
Fortaz, see Ceftazidime			
Fosaprepitant	1 mg	IV	J1453
Foscarnet sodium	per 1, 000 mg	IV	J1455
Foscavir, see Foscarnet sodium			
Fosphenytoin	50 mg	IV	Q2009
FUDR, see Floxuridine			
Fulvestrant	25 mg	IM	J9395
Fungizone Intravenous, see Amphotericin B			
Furomide M.D., see Furosemide			
Furosemide	up to 20 mg	IM/IV	J1940

G

DESCRIPTION	DOSE	ROUTE	CODE
Gadoxetate disodium	1 ml	IV	A9581
Gallium nitrate	1 mg	IV	J1457
Galsulfase	1 mg	IV	J1458
GamaSTAN, see Gamma globulin and immune globulin			
Gammagard Liquid	500 mg	IV	J1569
Gamma globulin	1 cc	IM	J1460
	over 10 cc	IM	J1560
Gammaplex	500 mg	IV	J1557
Gammar, see Gamma globulin and immune globulin			
Gammar-IV, see Immune globulin intravenous (human)			
Gamulin RH, see Rho(D) immune globulin			

DESCRIPTION	DOSE	ROUTE	CODE
Gamunex	500 mg	IV	J1561
Ganciclovir, implant	4.5 mg	OTH	J7310
Ganciclovir sodium	500 mg	IV	J1570
Garamycin, gentamicin	up to 80 mg	IM/IV	J1580
Gatifloxacin	10 mg	IV	J1590
Gefitinib	250 mg	ORAL	J8565
Gel-One	per dose	OTH	J7326
Gemcitabine HCl	200 mg	IV	J9201
Gemsar, see Gemcitabine HCl			
Gemtuzumab ozogamicin	5 mg	IV	J9300
Gentamicin Sulfate, see Garamycin, gentamicin			
Gentran, see Dextran 40			
Gentran 75, see Dextran 75			
Gesterol 50, see Progesterone			
Glassia	10 mg	IV	J0257
Glatiramer acetate	20 mg	SC	J1595
Glucagon HCl	per 1 mg	SC/IM/IV	J1610
Glukor, see Chorionic gonadotropin			
Glycopyrrolate, concentrated form	per 1 mg	INH	J7642
Glycopyrrolate, unit dose form	per 1 mg	INH	J7643
Gold sodium thiomalate	up to 50 mg	IM	J1600
Golimumab	1 mg	IV	J1602
Gonadorelin HCl	per 100 mcg	SC/IV	J1620
Gonic, see Chorionic gonadotropin			
Goserelin acetate implant	per 3.6 mg	SC	J9202
Granisetron HCl, injection	100 mcg	IV	J1626
Granisetron HCl, oral	1 mg	ORAL	Q0166

DESCRIPTION	DOSE	ROUTE	CODE
Gynogen LA, see Estradiol valerate			

H

DESCRIPTION	DOSE	ROUTE	CODE
Halaven, see Eribulin mesylate			
Haldol, see Haloperidol			
Haloperidol	up to 5 mg	IM/IV	J1630
Haloperidol decanoate	per 50 mg	IM	J1631
Hectoral, see Doxercalciferol			
Hemin	1 mg		J1640
Hemofil M, see Factor VIII			
Hemophilia clotting factors (e.g., anti-inhibitors)	per IU	IV	J7198
Hemophilia clotting factors, NOC	per IU	IV	J7199
Hepagam B	0.5 ml	IM	J1571
	0.5 ml	IV	J1573
Hep-Lock, see Heparin sodium (heparin lock flush)			
Hep-Lock U/P, see Heparin sodium (heparin lock flush)			
Heparin sodium	1,000 units	IV/SC	J1644
Heparin sodium (heparin lock flush)	10 units	IV	J1642
Herceptin, see Trastuzumab			
Hexadrol Phosphate, see Dexamethasone sodium phosphate			
Histaject, see Brompheniramine maleate			

DESCRIPTION	DOSE	ROUTE	CODE
Histerone 50, see Testosterone suspension			
Histerone 100, see Testosterone suspension			
Histrelin acetate	10 mcg		J1675
Histrelin implant	50 mg	OTH	J9225
Hizentra, see Immune globulin			
Human fibrinogen concentrate	1 mg	INJ	J7178
Hyalgan		OTH	J7321
Hyaluronidase	up to 150 units	SC/IV	J3470
Hyaluronidase, ovine	up to 999 units	VAR	J3471
	per 1,000 units	VAR	J3472
Hyaluronidase, recombinant	1 USP	SC	J3473
Hyate:C, see Factor VIII (anti-hemophilic factor (porcine))			
Hybolin Improved, see Nandrolone phenpropionate			
Hybolin Decanoate, see Nandrolone decanoate			
Hycamtin, see Topotecan			
Hydralazine HCl	up to 20 mg	IV/IM	J0360
Hydrate, see Dimenhydrinate			
Hydrocortisone acetate	up to 25 mg	IV/IM/SC	J1700
Hydrocortisone sodium phosphate	up to 50 mg	IV/IM/SC	J1710
Hydrocortisone succinate sodium	up to 100 mg	IV/IM/SC	J1720
Hydrocortone acetate, see Hydrocortisone acetate			
Hydrocortone phosphate, see Hydrocortisone sodium phosphate			

DESCRIPTION	DOSE	ROUTE	CODE
Hydromorphone HCl	up to 4 mg	SC/IM/IV	J1170
Hydroxyprogesterone caproate	1 mg	IM	J1725
Hydroxyzine HCl	up to 25 mg	IM	J3410
Hydroxyzine Pamoate	25 mg	ORAL	Q0177
Hylan G-F 20		OTH	J7322
Hyoscyamine sulfate	up to 0.25 mg	SC/IM/IV	J1980
Hyperstat IV, see Diazoxide			
Hyper-Tet, see Tetanus immune globulin, human			
HypRho-D, see Rho(D) immune globulin			
Hyrexin-50, see Diphenhydramine HCl			
Hyzine-50, see Hydroxyzine HCl			

I

DESCRIPTION	DOSE	ROUTE	CODE
Ibandronate sodium	1 mg	IV	J1740
Ibuprofen	100 mg		J1741
Ibutilide fumarate	1 mg	IV	J1742
Icatibant	1 mg	SC	J1744
Idamycin, see Idarubicin HCl			
Idarubicin HCl	5 mg	IV	J9211
Idursulfase	1 mg	IV	J1743
Ifex, see Ifosfamide			
Ifosfamide	1 gram	IV	J9208
Ilaris, see Canakinumab			
Iloprost	20 mcg	INH	Q4074
Ilotycin, see Erythromycin gluceptate			
Imferon, see Iron dextran			

DESCRIPTION	DOSE	ROUTE	CODE
Imiglucerase	10 Units	IV	J1786
Imitrex, see Sumatriptan succinate			
Immune globulin			
Bivigam	500 mg	IV	J1556
Flebogamma	500 mg	IV	J1572
Gammagard Liquid	500 mg	IV	J1569
Gammaplex	500 mg	IV	J1557
Gamunex	500 mg	IV	J1561
HepaGam B	0.5 ml	IM	J1571
HepaGam B	0.5 ml	IV	J1573
Hizentra	100 mg	SC	J1559
NOS	500 mg	IV	J1566, J1599
Octagam	500 mg	IV	J1568
Privigen	500 mg	IV	J1459
Rhophylac	100 IU	IM	J2791
Subcutaneous	100 mg	SC	J1562
Immunosuppressive drug, not otherwise classified			J7599
Imuran, see Azathioprine			
Inapsine, see Droperidol			
Incobotulinumtoxin type A	1 unit	IM	J0588
Inderal, see Propranolol HCl			
InFeD, see Iron Dextran			
Infergen, see Interferon alfa-1			
Infliximab, injection	10 mg	IM/IV	J1745
Innohep, see Tinzarparin			
Innovar, see Droperidol with fentanyl citrate			
Insulin	5 units	SC	J1815
Insulin lispro	50 units	SC	J1817

DESCRIPTION	DOSE	ROUTE	CODE
Intal, see Cromolyn sodium or Cromolyn sodium, compounded			
Integrilin, injection, see Eptifibatide			
Interferon			
alphacon-1, recombinant	1 mcg	SC	J9212
alfa-2a, recombinant	3 million units	SC/IM	J9213
alfa-2b, recombinant	1 million units	SC/IM	J9214
alfa-n3 (human leukocyte derived)	250,000 IU	IM	J9215
beta-1a	30 mcg	IM	J1826
beta-1a	1 mcg	IM	Q3027
	1 mcg	SC	Q3028
beta-1b	0.25 mg	SC	J1830
gamma-1b	3 million units	SC	J9216
Intrauterine copper contraceptive, see Copper contraceptive, intrauterine			
Invega sustenna, see Paliperidone palmitate			
Ipilimumab	1 mg	IV	J9228
Ipratropium bromide, unit dose form	per mg	INH	J7644, J7645
Irinotecan	20 mg	IV	J9206
Iron dextran	50 mg	IV	J1750
Iron sucrose	1 mg	IV	J1756
Irrigation solution for Tx of bladder calculi	per 50 ml	OTH	Q2004
Isocaine HCl, see Mepivacaine			
Isoetharine HCl, concentrated form	per mg	INH	J7647, J7648
Isoetharine HCl, unit dose form	per mg	INH	J7649, J7650

DESCRIPTION	DOSE	ROUTE	CODE
Isoproterenol HCl, concentrated form	per mg	INH	J7657, J7658
Isoproterenol HCl, unit dose form	per mg	INH	J7659, J7660
Istodax, see Romidepsin			
Isuprel, see Isoproterenol HCl			
Itraconazole	50 mg	IV	J1835
Ixabepilone	1 mg	IV	J9207
Ixempra, see Ixabepilone			

J

DESCRIPTION	DOSE	ROUTE	CODE
Jenamicin, see Garamycin, gentamicin			
Jevtana, see Cabazitaxel			

K

DESCRIPTION	DOSE	ROUTE	CODE
Kabikinase, see Streptokinase			
Kalbitor, see Ecallantide			
Kaleinate, see Calcium gluconate			
Kanamycin sulfate	up to 75 mg	IM/IV	J1850
	up to 500 mg	IM/IV	J1840
Kantrex, see Kanamycin sulfate			
Keflin, see Cephalothin sodium			
Kefurox, see Cufuroxime sodium			
Kefzol, see Cefazolin sodium			
Kenaject-40, see Triamcinolone acetonide			
Kenalog-10, see Triamcinolone acetonide			

DESCRIPTION	DOSE	ROUTE	CODE
Kenalog-40, see Triamcinolone acetonide			
Keppra, see Levetiracetam			
Kestrone 5, see Estrone			
Ketorolac tromethamine	per 15 mg	IM/IV	J1885
Key-Pred 25, see Prednisolone acetate			
Key-Pred 50, see Prednisolone acetate			
Key-Pred-SP, see Prednisolone sodium phosphate			
K-Flex, see Orphenadrine citrate			
Klebcil, see Kanamycin sulfate			
Koate-HP, see Factor VIII			
Kogenate, see Factor VIII			
Konakion, see Vitamin K, phytonadione, etc.			
Konyne-80, see Factor IX, complex			
Krystexxa, see Pegloticase			
Kytril, see Granisetron HCl			

L

DESCRIPTION	DOSE	ROUTE	CODE
L.A.E. 20, see Estradiol valerate			
Laetrile, Amygdalin, vitamin B-17			J3570
Lanoxin, see Digoxin			
Lanreotide	1 mg	SC	J1930
Largon, see Propiomazine HCl			
Laronidase	0.1 mg	IV	J1931
Lasix, see Furosemide			

DESCRIPTION	DOSE	ROUTE	CODE
L-Caine, see Lidocaine HCl			
Lepirudin	50 mg		J1945
Leucovorin calcium	per 50 mg	IM/IV	J0640
Leukine, see Sargramostim (GM-CSF)			
Leuprolide acetate (for depot suspension)	3.75 mg	IM	J1950
	7.5 mg	IM	J9217
Leuprolide acetate	per 1 mg	IM	J9218
Leuprolide acetate implant	65 mg	OTH	J9219
Leustatin, see Cladribine			
Levalbuterol HCl, concentrated form	0.5 mg	INH	J7607, J7612
Levalbuterol HCl, unit dose form	0.5 mg	INH	J7614, J7615
Levaquin I.U., see Levofloxacin			
Levetiracetam	10 mg	IV	J1953
Levocarnitine	per 1 gram	IV	J1955
Levo-Dromoran, see Levorphanol tartrate			
Levofloxacin	250 mg	IV	J1956
Levoleucovorin calcium	0.5 mg	IV	J0641
Levonorgestrel implant		OTH	J7306
Levonorgestrel releasing intrauterin contraceptive	52 mg	OTH	J7302
Levorphanol tartrate	up to 2 mg	SC/IV	J1960
Levsin, see Hyoscyamine sulfate			
Levulan Kerastick, see Aminolevulinic acid HCl			
Lexiscan, see Regadenoson			
Librium, see Chlordiazepoxide HCl			
Lidocaine HCl	10 mg	IV	J2001

DESCRIPTION	DOSE	ROUTE	CODE
Lidoject-1, see Lidocaine HCl			
Lidoject-2, see Lidocaine HCl			
Lincocin, see Lincomycin HCl			
Lincomycin HCl	up to 300 mg	IV	J2010
Linezolid	200 mg	IV	J2020
Liquaemin Sodium, see Heparin sodium			
Lioresal, see Baclofen			
LMD (10%), see Dextran 40			
Lovenox, see Enoxaparin sodium			
Lorazepam	2 mg	IM/IV	J2060
Lufyllin, see Dyphylline			
Luminal Sodium, see Phenobarbitol sodium			
Lumizyme, see Alglucoside alfa			
Lunelle, see Medroxy-progesterone acetate/ estradiol cypionate			
Lupron, see Leuprolide acetate			
Lymphocyte immune globulin, anti-thymocyte globulin,			
equine	250 mg	IV	J7504
rabbit	25 mg	IV	J7511
Lyophilized, see Cyclophosphamide, lyophilized			

M

DESCRIPTION	DOSE	ROUTE	CODE
Magnesium sulfate	500 mg		J3475
Makena, see Hydroxy-progesterone caproate			

DESCRIPTION	DOSE	ROUTE	CODE
Mannitol	25% in 50 ml	IV	J2150
	5 mg	INH	J7665
Marmine, see Dimenhydrinate			
Maxipime, see Cefepime hydrochloride			
Mecasermin	1 mg	SC	J2170
Mechlorethamine HCl (nitrogen mustard), HN2	10 mg	IV	J9230
Medralone 40, see Methylprednisolone acetate			
Medralone 80, see Methylprednisolone acetate			
Medrol, see Methylprednisolone			
Medroxyprogesterone acetate	1 mg	IM	J1050
Mefoxin, see Cefoxitin sodium			
Melphalan HCl	50 mg	IV	J9245
Melphalan, oral	2 mg	ORAL	J8600
Menoject LA, see Testosterone cypionate and estradiol cypionate			
Mepergan Injection, see Meperdine and promethazine HCl			
Meperidine HCl	per 100 mg	IM/IV/SC	J2175
Meperidine and promethazine HCl	up to 50 mg	IM/IV	J2180
Mepivacaine HCl	per 10 ml	VAR	J0670
Meropenem	100 mg	IV	J2185
Mesna	200 mg	IV	J9209
Mesnex, see Mesna			
Metaprel, see Metaproterenol sulfate			

DESCRIPTION	DOSE	ROUTE	CODE
Metaproterenol sulfate, concentrated form	per 10 mg	INH	J7667, J7668
Metaproterenol sulfate, unit dose form	per 10 mg	INH	J7669, J7670
Metaraminol bitartrate	per 10 mg	IV/IM/SC	J0380
Metastron, see Strontium-89 chloride			
Methacholine chloride	1 mg	INH	J7674
Methadone HCl	up to 10 mg	IM/SC	J1230
Methergine, see Methylergonovine maleate			
Methocarbamol	up to 10 ml	IV/IM	J2800
Methotrexate, oral	2.5 mg	ORAL	J8610
Methotrexate sodium	5 mg	IV/IM/IT/IA	J9250
	50 mg	IV/IM/IT/IA	J9260
Methotrexate LPF, see Methotrexate sodium			
Methyldopate HCl	up to 250 mg	IV	J0210
Methylnaltrexone	0.1 mg	SC	J2212
Methylprednisolone, oral	per 4 mg	ORAL	J7509
Methylprednisolone acetate	20 mg	IM	J1020
	40 mg	IM	J1030
	80 mg	IM	J1040
Methylprednisolone sodium succinate	up to 40 mg	IM/IV	J2920
	up to 125 mg	IM/IV	J2930
Metoclopramide HCl	up to 10 mg	IV	J2765
Metvixia, see Aminolevulinate			
Miacalcin, see Calcitonin-salmon			
Micafungin sodium	1 mg		J2248
Midazolam HCl	per 1 mg	IM/IV	J2250
Milrinone lactate	5 mg	IV	J2260
Minocine, see Minocycline HCL			

DESCRIPTION	DOSE	ROUTE	CODE
Minocycline HCL	1 mg	IV	J2265
Mirena, see Levonorgestrel releasing intrauterine contraceptive			
Mithracin, see Plicamycin			
Mitomycin, ophthalmic	0.2 mg	IO	J7315
Mitomycin	5 mg	IV	J9280
Mitosol, *see* Mitomycin			
Mitoxantrone HCl	per 5 mg	IV	J9293
Monocid, see Cefonicic sodium			
Monoclate-P, see Factor VIII			
Monoclonal antibodies, parenteral	5 mg	IV	J7505
Mononine, see Factor IX, purified, non-recombinant			
Morphine sulfate	up to 10 mg	IM/IV/SC	J2270
	100 mg	IM/IV/SC	J2271
Morphine sulfate, preservative-free	per 10 mg	SC/IM/IV	J2275
Moxifloxacin	100 mg	IV	J2280
Mozobil, see Plerixafor			
M-Prednisol-40, see Methylprednisolone acetate			
M-Prednisol-80, see Methylprednisolone acetate			
Mucomyst, see Acetylcysteine or Acetylcysteine, compounded			
Mucosol, see Acetylcysteine			
Muromonab-CD3	5 mg	IV	J7505
Muse, see Alprostadil			
Mustargen, see Mechlorethamine HCl			
Mutamycin, see Mitomycin			
Mycophenolic acid	180 mg	ORAL	J7518

DESCRIPTION	DOSE	ROUTE	CODE
Mycophenolate mofetil	250 mg	ORAL	J7517
Myleran, see Busulfan			
Mylotarg, see Gemtuzumab ozogamicin			
Myobloc, see RimabotulinumtoxinB			
Myochrysine, see Gold sodium thiomalate			
Myolin, see Orphenadrine citrate			

N

DESCRIPTION	DOSE	ROUTE	CODE
Nabilone	1 mg	ORAL	J8650
Nalbuphine HCl	per 10 mg	IM/IV/SC	J2300
Naloxone HCl	per 1 mg	IM/IV/SC	J2310
Naltrexone, depot form	1 mg	IM	J2315
Nandrobolic L.A., see Nandrolone decanoate			
Nandrolone decanoate	up to 50 mg	IM	J2320
Narcan, see Naloxone HCl			
Naropin, see Ropivacaine HCl			
Nasahist B, see Brompheniramine maleate			
Nasal vaccine inhalation		INH	J3530
Natalizumab	1 mg	IV	J2323
Navane, see Thiothixene			
Navelbine, see Vinorelbine tartrate			
ND Stat, see Brompheniramine maleate			
Nebcin, see Tobramycin sulfate			

DESCRIPTION	DOSE	ROUTE	CODE
NebuPent, see Pentamidine isethionate			
Nelarabine	50 mg	IV	J9261
Nembutal Sodium Solution, see Pentobarbital sodium			
Neocyten, see Orphenadrine citrate			
Neo-Durabolic, see Nandrolone decanoate			
Neoquess, see Dicyclomine HCl			
Neosar, see Cyclophosphamide			
Neostigmine methylsulfate	up to 0.5 mg	IM/IV/SC	J2710
Neo-Synephrine, see Phenylephrine HCl			
Nervocaine 1%, see Lidocaine HCl			
Nervocaine 2%, see Lidocaine HCl			
Nesacaine, see Chloroprocaine HCl			
Nesacaine-MPF, see Chloroprocaine HCl			
Nesiritide	0.1 mg	IV	J2325
Neumega, see Oprelvekin			
Neupogen, see Filgrastim (G-CSF)			
Neutrexin, see Trimetrexate glucuronate			
Nipent, see Pentostatin			
Nordryl, see Diphenhydramine HCl			
Norflex, see Orphenadrine citrate			
Norzine, see Thiethylperazine maleate			

DESCRIPTION	DOSE	ROUTE	CODE
Not otherwise classified drugs			J3490
Not otherwise classified drugs other than INH administered through DME			J7799
Not otherwise classified drugs administered through DME		INH	J7699
Not otherwise classified drugs, anti-neoplastic			J9999
Not otherwise classified drugs, chemotherapeutic		ORAL	J8999
Not otherwise classified drugs, immuno-suppressive			J7599
Not otherwise classified drugs, non-chemotherapeutic		ORAL	J8499
Novantrone, see Mitoxantrone HCl			
Novo Seven, see Factor VIIa			
NPH, see Insulin			
Nplate, see Romiplostim			
Nubain, see Nalbuphine HCl			
Nulicaine, see Lidocaine HCl			
Nulojix, *see* Belatacept			
Numorphan, see Oxymorphone HCl			
Numorphan H.P., see Oxymorphone HCl			

O

DESCRIPTION	DOSE	ROUTE	CODE
Ocriplasmin	0.125 mg	IV	J7316
Octagam	500 mg	IV	J1568

DESCRIPTION	DOSE	ROUTE	CODE
Octreotide acetate, injection	1 mg	IM	J2353
	25 mcg	IV/SC	J2354
Oculinum, see Botulinum toxin type A			
Ofatumumab	10 mg	IV	J9302
Ofirmev, see Acetaminophen			
O-Flex, see Orphenadrine citrate			
Oforta, see Fludarabine phosphate			
Olanzapine	1 mg	IM	J2358
Omalizumab	5 mg	SC	J2357
Omacetaxine mepesuccinate	0.01 mg	IV	J9262
Omnipen-N, see Ampicillin			
Omontys, *see* Peginesatide			
OnabotulinumtoxinA	1 unit	IM	J0585
Oncaspar, see Pegaspargase			
Oncovin, see Vincristine sulfate			
Ondansetron HCI	1 mg	IV	J2405
Ondansetron HCl, oral	1 mg	ORAL	Q0162
Oprelvekin	5 mg	SC	J2355
Oraminic II, see Brompheniramine maleate			
Ormazine, see Chlorpromazine HCl			
Orphenadrine citrate	up to 60 mg	IV/IM	J2360
Orphenate, see Orphenadrine citrate			
Orthovisc		OTH	J7324
Or-Tyl, see Dicyclomine			
Oxacillin sodium	up to 250 mg	IM/IV	J2700
Oxaliplatin	0.5 mg	IV	J9263

DESCRIPTION	DOSE	ROUTE	CODE
Oxymorphone HCl	up to 1 mg	IV/SC/IM	J2410
Oxytetracycline HCl	up to 50 mg	IM	J2460
Oxytocin	up to 10 units	IV/IM	J2590
Ozurdex, see Dexamethasone intravitreal implant			

P

DESCRIPTION	DOSE	ROUTE	CODE
Paclitaxel	30 mg	IV	J9265
Paclitaxel protein-bound particles	1 mg	IV	J9264
Palifermin	50 mcg	IV	J2425
Paliperidone palmitate	1 mg	IM	J2426
Palonosetron HCl	25 mcg	IV	J2469
Pamidronate disodium	per 30 mg	IV	J2430
Panitumumab	10 mg	IV	J9303
Papaverine HCl	up to 60 mg	IV/IM	J2440
Paragard T 380 A, see Copper contraceptive, intrauterine			
Paraplatin, see Carboplatin			
Paricalcitol, injection	1 mcg	IV/IM	J2501
Pegademase bovine	25 IU		J2504
Pegaptinib	0.3 mg	OTH	J2503
Pegaspargase	per single dose vial	IM/IV	J9266
Pegfilgrastim	6 mg	SC	J2505
Peginesatide	0.1 mg	IV/SC	J0890
Pegloticase	1 mg	IV	J2507
Pemetrexed	10 mg	IV	J9305
Penicillin G benzathine	100,000 units	IM	J0561
Penicillin G benzathine & penicillin G procaine	100,000 units	IM	J0558
Penicillin G potassium	up to 600,000 units	IM/IV	J2540

DESCRIPTION	DOSE	ROUTE	CODE
Penicillin G procaine, aqueous	up to 600,000 units	IM/IV	J2510
Pentamidine isethionate	per 300 mg	INH	J2545, J7676
Pentastarch, 10%	100 ml		J2513
Pentazocine HCl	30 mg	IM/SC/IV	J3070
Pentobarbital sodium	per 50 mg	IM/IV/OTH	J2515
Pentostatin	per 10 mg	IV	J9268
Peforomist, see Fomorterol fumarate			
Permapen, see Penicillin G benzathine			
Perphenazine, injection	up to 5 mg	IM/IV	J3310
Perphenazine, tablets	4 mg	ORAL	Q0175
Persantine IV, see Dipyridamole			
Pertuxumab	1 mg	IV	J9306
Pfizerpen, see Penicillin G potassium			
Pfizerpen A.S., see Penicillin G procaine			
Phenazine 25, see Promethazine HCl			
Phenazine 50, see Promethazine HCl			
Phenergan, see Promethazine HCl			
Phenobarbital sodium	up to 120 mg	IM/IV	J2560
Phentolamine mesylate	up to 5 mg	IM/IV	J2760
Phenylephrine HCl	up to 1 ml	SC/IM/IV	J2370
Phenytoin sodium	per 50 mg	IM/IV	J1165
Photofrin, see Porfimer sodium			
Phytonadione (Vitamin K)	per 1 mg	IM/SC/IV	J3430
Piperacillin/Tazobactam Sodium, injection	1.125 grams	IV	J2543

DESCRIPTION	DOSE	ROUTE	CODE
Pitocin, see Oxytocin			
Plas+SD, see Plasma, pooled multiple donor			
Plasma, cryoprecipitate reduced	each unit	IV	P9044
Plasma, pooled multiple donor, frozen	each unit	IV	P9023
Platinol, see Cisplatin			
Platinol AQ, see Cisplatin			
Plerixafor	1 mg	SC	J2562
Plicamycin	2,500 mcg	IV	J9270
Polocaine, see Mepivacaine			
Polycillin-N, see Ampicillin			
Porfimer sodium	75 mg	IV	J9600
Potassium chloride	per 2 mEq	IV	J3480
Pralatrexate	1 mg	IV	J9307
Pralidoxime chloride	up to 1 gram	IV/IM/SC	J2730
Predalone-50, see Prednisolone acetate			
Predcor-25, see Prednisolone acetate			
Predcor-50, see Prednisolone acetate			
Predicort-50, see Prednisolone acetate			
Prednisone	per 5 mg	ORAL	J7506
Prednisolone, oral	5 mg	ORAL	J7510
Prednisolone acetate	up to 1 ml	IM	J2650
Predoject-50, see Prednisolone acetate			
Pregnyl, see Chorionic gonadotropin			
Premarin Intravenous, see Estrogen, conjugated			

DESCRIPTION	DOSE	ROUTE	CODE
Prescription, chemotherapeutic, NOS		ORAL	J8999
Prescription, non-chemotherapeutic, NOS		ORAL	J8499
Primacor, see Milrinone lactate			
Primaxin I.M., see Cilastatin sodium, imipenem			
Primaxin I.V., see Cilastatin sodium, imipenem			
Priscoline HCl, see Tolazoline HCl			
Privigen	500 mg	IV	J1459
Pro-Depo, see Hydroxyprogesterone Caproate			
Procainamide HCl	up to 1 gram	IM/IV	J2690
Prochlorperazine	up to 10 mg	IM/IV	J0780
Prochlorperazine maleate, oral	5 mg	ORAL	Q0164
Profasi HP, see Chorionic gonadotropin			
Profilnine Heat-Treated, see Factor IX			
Progestaject, see Progesterone			
Progesterone	per 50 mg	IM	J2675
Prograf, see Tacrolimus, oral or parenteral			
Prokine, see Sargramostim (GM-CSF)			
Prolastin, see Alpha 1-proteinase inhibitor, human			
Proleukin, see Aldesleukin			
Prolixin Decanoate, see Fluphenazine decanoate			

DESCRIPTION	DOSE	ROUTE	CODE
Promazine HCl	up to 25 mg	IM	J2950
Promethazine HCl, injection	up to 50 mg	IM/IV	J2550
Promethazine HCl, oral	12.5 mg	ORAL	Q0169
Pronestyl, see Procainamide HCl			
Proplex T, see Factor IX			
Proplex SX-T, see Factor IX			
Propranolol HCl	up to 1 mg	IV	J1800
Prorex-25, see Promethazine HCl			
Prorex-50, see Promethazine HCl			
Prostaphlin, see Procainamide HCl			
Prostigmin, see Neostigmine methylsulfate			
Protamine sulfate	per 10 mg	IV	J2720
Protein C Concentrate	10 IU	IV	J2724
Protirelin	per 250 mcg	IV	J2725
Prothazine, see Promethazine HCl			
Protopam Chloride, see Pralidoxime chloride			
Proventil, see Albuterol sulfate, compounded			
Prozine-50, see Promazine HCl			
Pulmicort Respules, see Budesonide			
Pyridoxine HCl	100 mg		J3415

Quelicin (see Succinylcholine chloride)

DESCRIPTION	DOSE	ROUTE	CODE
Quinupristin/dalfopristin	500 mg (150/350)	IV	J2770
Qutenza, *see* Capsaicin patch			

R

DESCRIPTION	DOSE	ROUTE	CODE
Ranibizumab	0.1 mg	OTH	J2778
Ranitidine HCl, injection	25 mg	IV/IM	J2780
Rapamune, *see* Sirolimus			
Rasburicase	0.5 mg	IV	J2783
Recombinate, *see* Factor VIII			
Redisol, *see* Vitamin B-12 cyanocobalamin			
Regadenoson	0.1 mg	IV	J2785
Regitine, *see* Phentolamine mesylate			
Reglan, *see* Metoclopramide HCl			
Regular, *see* Insulin			
Relefact TRH, see Protirelin			
Relistor, *see* methylnaltrexone			
Remicade, *see* Infliximab, injection			
Reo Pro, *see* Abciximab			
Rep-Pred 40, *see* Methylprednisolone acetate			
Rep-Pred 80, *see* Methylprednisolone acetate			
RespiGam, *see* Respiratory synctial virus			
Retavase, *see* Reteplase			
Reteplase	18.8 mg	IV	J2993

DESCRIPTION	DOSE	ROUTE	CODE
Retrovir, *see* Zidovudine			
Rheomacrodex, *see* Dextran 40			
Rhesonativ, see Rho(D) immune globulin, human			
Rheumatrex Dose Pack, see Methotrexate, oral			
Rho(D) immune globulin		IM/IV	J2791
Rho(D) immune globulin, human 1 dose pkg	300 mcg	IM	J2790
Rho(D) immune globulin, human	50 mg	IM	J2788
Rho(D)immune globulin, human, solvent detergent	100 IU	IV	J2792
RhoGAM, see Rho(D) immune globulin, human			
Rhophylac	100 IU	IM/IV	J2791
RiaSTAP, see Human fibrinogen concentrate			
Rilonacept	1 mg	SC	J2793
RimabotulinumtoxinB	100 units	IM	J0587
Ringers lactate infusion	up to 1,000 cc	IV	J7120
Risperidone	0.5 mg	IM	J2794
Rituxan, see Rituximab			
Rituximab	100 mg	IV	J9310
Robaxin, see Methocarbamol			
Rocephin, see Ceftriaxone sodium			
Roferon-A, see Interferon alfa-2A, recombinant			
Romidepsin	1 mg	IV	J9315
Romiplostim	10 mcg	SC	J2796
Ropivacaine Hydrochloride	1 mg	OTH	J2795
Rubex, see Doxorubicin HCl			

DESCRIPTION	DOSE	ROUTE	CODE
Rubramin PC, see Vitamin B-12 cyanocobalamin			

S

DESCRIPTION	DOSE	ROUTE	CODE
Saline solution, 5% dextrose	500 ml	IV	J7042
Saline solution, infusion	250 cc	IV	J7050
	1,000 cc	IV	J7030
Saline solution, sterile	500 ml = 1 unit	IV/OTH	J7040
Sandimmune, see Cyclosporine			
Sandoglobulin, see Immune globulin intravenous (human)			
Sandostatin LAR Depot, see Octreotide			
Sargramostim (GM-CSF)	50 mcg	IV	J2820
Sculptra	0.5 mg	IV	Q2028
Selestoject, see Betamethasone sodium phosphate			
Sermorelin acetate	1 mcg	SC	Q0515
Sincalide	5 mcg	IV	J2805
Sinusol-B, see Brompheniramine maleate			
Sirolimus	1 mg	ORAL	J7520
Skyla	13.5 mg	OTH	J7301
Sodium ferricgluconate in sucrose	12.5 mg		J2916
Sodium hyaluronate, Euflexxa			J7323
Sodium hyaluronate,			
Hyalgan			J7321
Orthovisc			J7324
Supartz			J7321

DESCRIPTION	DOSE	ROUTE	CODE
Solganal, see Aurothioglucose			
Solu-Cortef, see Hydrocortisone sodium phosphate (J1710)			
Solu-Medrol, see Methylprednisolone sodium succinate			
Solurex, see Dexamethasone sodium phosphate			
Solurex LA, see Dexamethasone acetate			
Somatrem	1 mg	SC	J2940
Somatropin	1 mg	SC	J2941
Somatulin depot, see Lanreotide			
Sparine, see Promazine HCl			
Spasmoject, see Dicyclomine HCl			
Spectinomycin HCl	up to 2 grams	IM	J3320
Sporanox, see Itraconazole			
Staphcillin, see Methicillin sodium			
Stelara, see Ustekinumab			
Stilphostrol, see Diethylstilbestrol diphosphate			
Streptase, see Streptokinase			
Streptokinase	per 250,000 IU	IV	J2995
Streptomycin Sulfate, see Streptomycin			
Streptomycin	up to 1 gram	IM	J3000
Streptozocin	1 gram	IV	J9320
Strontium-89 chloride	per millicurie		A9600
Sublimaze, see Fentanyl citrate			

DESCRIPTION	DOSE	ROUTE	CODE
Succinylcholine chloride	up to 20 mg	IV/IM	J0330
Sumatriptan succinate	6 mg	SC	J3030
Supartz		OTH	J7321
Surostrin, see Succinycholine chloride			
Sus-Phrine, see Adrenalin, epinephrine			
Synercid, see Quinupristin/dalfopristin			
Synkavite, see Vitamin K, phytonadione, etc.			
Syntocionon, see Oxytocin			
Synvisc and Synvisc-one	1mg	OTH	J7325
Sytobex, see Vitamin B-12 cyanocobalamin			

T

DESCRIPTION	DOSE	ROUTE	CODE
Tacrolimus, oral, extended release	0.1 mg	ORAL	J7508
Tacrolimus, oral, immediate release	per 1 mg	ORAL	J7507
Tacrolimus, parenteral	5 mg	IV	J7525
Taliglucerase alfa	10 units	IV	J3060
Talwin, see Pentazocine HCl			
Taractan, see Chlorprothixene			
Taxol, see Paclitaxel			
Taxotere, see Docetaxel			
Tazidime, see Ceftazidime			
Technetium TC Sestambi	per dose		A9500
TEEV, see Testosterone enanthate and estradiol valerate			
Teflaro, see Ceftaroline fosamil			

DESCRIPTION	DOSE	ROUTE	CODE
Telavancin	10 mg	IV	J3095
Temozolmide	1 mg	IV	J9328
	5 mg	ORAL	J8700
Temsirolimus	1 mg	IV	J9330
Tenecteplase	1 mg	IV	J3101
Teniposide	50 mg		Q2017
Tequin, see Gatifloxacin			
Terbutaline sulfate	up to 1 mg	SC/IV	J3105
Terbutaline sulfate, concentrated form	per 1 mg	INH	J7680
Terbutaline sulfate, unit dose form	per 1 mg	INH	J7681
Teriparatide	10 mcg	SC	J3110
Terramycin IM, see Oxytetracycline HCl			
Testa-C, see Testosterone cypionate			
Testadiate, see Testosterone enanthate and estradiol valerate			
Testadiate-Depo, see Testosterone cypionate			
Testaject-LA, see Testosterone cypionate			
Testaqua, see Testosterone suspension			
Test-Estro Cypionates, see Testosterone cypionate and estradiol cypionate			
Test-Estro-C, see Testosterone cypionate and estradiol cypionate			
Testex, see Testosterone propionate			
Testoject-50, see Testosterone suspension			
Testone LA 200, see Testosterone enanthate			

DESCRIPTION	DOSE	ROUTE	CODE
Testone LA 100, see Testosterone enanthate			
Testosterone Aqueous, see Testosterone suspension			
Testosterone enanthate and estradiol valerate	up to 1 cc	IM	J0900
Testosterone enanthate	up to 100 mg	IM	J3120
	up to 200 mg	IM	J3130
Testosterone cypionate	up to 100 mg	IM	J1070
	1 cc, 200 mg	IM	J1080
Testosterone cypionate and estradiol cypionate	up to 1 ml	IM	J1060
Testosterone propionate	up to 100 mg	IM	J3150
Testosterone suspension	up to 50 mg	IM	J3140
Testradiol 90/4, see Testosterone enanthate and estradiol valerate			
Testrin PA, see Testosterone enanthate			
Tetanus immune globulin, human	up to 250 units	IM	J1670
Tetracycline	up to 250 mg	IM/IV	J0120
Thallous Chloride TL 201	per MCI		A9505
Theelin aqueous, see Estrone			
Theophylline	per 40 mg	IV	J2810
TheraCys, see BCG live			
Thiamine HCl	100 mg		J3411
Thiethylperazine maleate, injection	up to 10 mg	IM	J3280
Thiethylperazine maleate, oral	10 mg	ORAL	Q0174
Thiotepa	15 mg	IV	J9340
Thorazine, see Chlorpromazine HCl			
Thymoglobulin, see Immune globulin, anti-thymocyte			

DESCRIPTION	DOSE	ROUTE	CODE
Thypinone, see Protirelin			
Thyrogen, see Thyrotropin Alfa			
Thyrotropin Alfa, injection	0.9 mg	IM/SC	J3240
Tice BCG, see BCG live			
Ticon, see Trimethobenzamide HCl			
Tigan, see Trimethobenzamide HCl			
Tigecycline	1 mg	IV	J3243
Tiject-20, see Trimethobenzamide HCl			
Tinzaparin	1000 IU	SC	J1655
Tirofiban HCl, injection	0.25 mg	IM/IV	J3246
TNKase, see Tenecteplase			
TOBI, see Tobramycin, inhalation solution			
Tobramycin, inhalation solution	300 mg	INH	J7682, J7685
Tobramycin sulfate	up to 80 mg	IM/IV	J3260
Tocilizumab	1 mg	IV	J3262
Tofranil, see Imipramine HCl			
Tolazoline HCl	up to 25 mg	IV	J2670
Topotecan	0.25 mg	ORAL	J8705
	0.1 mg	IV	J9351
Toradol, see Ketorolac tromethamine			
Torecan, see Thiethylperazine maleate			
Torisel, see Temsirolimus			
Tornalate, see Bitolterol mesylate			
Torsemide	10 mg/ml	IV	J3265
Totacillin-N, see Ampicillin			

DESCRIPTION	DOSE	ROUTE	CODE
Trastuzumab	10 mg	IV	J9355
Treanda, see Bendamustine HCl			
Treprostinil	1 mg		J3285
Tri-Kort, see Triamcinolone acetonide			
Triam-A, see Triamcinolone acetonide			
Triamcinolone, concentrated form	per 1 mg	INH	J7683
Triamcinolone, unit dose	per 1 mg	INH	J7684
Triamcinolone acetonide	1 mg		J3300
	per 10 mg	IM	J3301
Triamcinolone diacetate	per 5 mg	IM	J3302
Triamcinolone hexacetonide	per 5 mg	VAR	J3303
Triesence, see Triamcinclone acetonide			
Triflupromazine HCl	up to 20 mg	IM/IV	J3400
Trilafon, see Perphenazine			
Trilog, see Triamcinolone acetonide			
Trilone, see Triamcinolone diacetate			
Trimethobenzamide HCl, injection	up to 200 mg	IM	J3250
Trimethobenzamide HCl, oral	250 mg	ORAL	Q0173
Trimetrexate glucuronate	per 25 mg	IV	J3305
Triptorelin pamoate	3.75 mg	SC	J3315
Trisenox, see Arsenic trioxide			
Trobicin, see Spectinomycin HCl			
Trovan, see Alatrofloxacin mesylate			
Tysabri, see Natalizumab			

DESCRIPTION	DOSE	ROUTE	CODE
U			
Ultrazine-10, see Prochlorperazine			
Unasyn, see Ampicillin sodium/sulbactam sodium			
Unclassified drugs (see also Not elsewhere classified)			J3490
Unspecified oral antiemetic			Q0181
Urea	up to 40 grams	IV	J3350
Ureaphil, see Urea			
Urecholine, see Bethanechol chloride			
Urofollitropin	75 IU		J3355
Urokinase	5,000 IU vial	IV	J3364
	250,000 IU vial	IV	J3365
Ustekinumab	1 mg	SC	J3357
V			
V-Gan 25, see Promethazine HCl			
V-Gan 50, see Promethazine HCl			
Valergen 10, see Estradiol valerate			
Valergen 20, see Estradiol valerate			
Valergen 40, see Estradiol valerate			
Valertest No. 1, see Testosterone enanthate and estradiol valerate			
Valertest No. 2, see Testosterone enanthate and estradiol valerate			

DESCRIPTION	DOSE	ROUTE	CODE
Valium, see Diazepam			
Valrubicin, intravesical	200 mg	OTH	J9357
Valstar, see Valrubicin			
Vancocin, see Vancomycin HCl			
Vancoled, see Vancomycin HCl			
Vancomycin HCl	500 mg	IV/IM	J3370
Vasoxyl, see Methoxamine HCl			
Velaglucerase alfa	100 Units	IV	J3385
Velban, see Vinblastine sulfate			
Velsar, see Vinblastine sulfate			
Venofer, see Iron sucrose			
Ventolin, see Albuterol sulfate			
VePesid, see Etoposide and Etoposide, oral			
Versed, see Midazolam HCl			
Verteporfin	0.1 mg	IV	J3396
Vesprin, see Triflupromazine HCl			
Viadur, see Leuprolide acetate implant			
Vibativ, see Telavancin			
Vinblastine sulfate	1 mg	IV	J9360
Vincasar PFS, see Vincristine sulfate			
Vincristine sulfate	1 mg	IV	J9370
Vincristine sulfate liposome	1 mg	IV	J9371
Vinorelbine tartrate	per 10 mg	IV	J9390
Vistaject-25, see Hydroxyzine HCl			
Vistaril, see Hydroxyzine HCl			
Vistide, see cidofovir			
Visudyne, see Verteporfin			

DESCRIPTION	DOSE	ROUTE	CODE
Vitamin K, phytonadione, menadione, menadiol sodium diphosphate	per 1 mg	IM/SC/IV	J3430
Vitamin B-12 cyanocobalamin	up to 1,000 mcg	IM/SC	J3420
Von Willebrand Factor Complex, human	per IU	IV	J7187
Von Willebrand Factor Complex (human) Wilate	per IU	IV	J7183
Voriconazole	10 mg	IV	J3465
Vpriv, see Velaglucerase alfa			

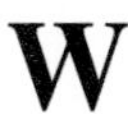

Wehamine, see Dimenhydrinate

Wehdryl, see Diphenhydramine HCl

Wellcovorin, see Leucovorin calcium

Wilate, see Von Willebrand Factor Complex (human)

Win Rho SD, see Rho(D) immuglobulin, human, solvent detergent

Wyamine Sulfate, see Mephentermine sulfate

Wycillin, see Penicillin G procaine

Wydase, see Hyaluronidase

X

Xeloda, see Capecitabine

Xeomin, see Incobotulinum toxin type A

Xgeva, see Denosumab

Xiaflex, see Collagenase

Xopenex, see Albuterol

Xylocaine HCl, see Lidocaine HCl

DESCRIPTION	DOSE	ROUTE	CODE
Xyntha, see Factor VIII (anti- hemophilic factor, recombinant)			

Y

DESCRIPTION	DOSE	ROUTE	CODE
Yervoy, see Ipilimumab			

Z

DESCRIPTION	DOSE	ROUTE	CODE
Zanosar, see Streptozocin			
Zantac, see Ranitidine HCl			
Zemplar, see Paricalcitol			
Zenapax, see Daclizumab			
Zetran, see Diazepam			
Ziconotide	1 mcg	OTH	J2278
Zidovudine	10 mg	IV	J3485
Zinacef, see Cefuroxime sodium			
Ziprasidone Mesylate	10 mg	IM	J3486
Zithromax, see Azithromycin dihydrate			
Zithromax I.V., see Azithromycin, injection			
Zofran, see Ondansetron HCl			
Zoladex, see Goserelin acetate implant			
Zoledronic Acid	1 mg	IV	J3487
Zolicef, see Cefazolin sodium			
Zortress, see Everolimus			
Zosyn, see Piperacillin			
Zyprexa relprevv, see Olanzapine			
Zyvox, see Linezolid			

APPENDIX D: MEDICARE REFERENCES

COVERAGE INSTRUCTION MANUAL (CIM) REFERENCES

The following Medicare references refer to policy issues identified in the main body of the HCPCS code section. Coverage Instruction Manual references are identified with the term CIM: followed by the reference number(s).

35-10 HYPERBARIC OXYGEN THERAPY

For purposes of coverage under Medicare, hyperbaric oxygen (HBO) therapy is a modality in which the entire body is exposed to oxygen under increased atmospheric pressure.

A. Covered Conditions.—Program reimbursement for HBO therapy will be limited to that which is administered in a chamber (including the one man unit) and is limited to the following conditions:

1. Acute carbon monoxide intoxication, (ICD-9 -CM diagnosis 986).
2. Decompression illness, (ICD-9-CM diagnosis 993.2, 993.3).
3. Gas embolism, (ICD-9-CM diagnosis 958.0, 999.1).
4. Gas gangrene, (ICD-9-CM diagnosis 0400).
5. Acute traumatic peripheral ischemia. HBO therapy is an adjunctive treatment to be used in combination with accepted standard therapeutic measures when loss of function, limb, or life is threatened. (ICD-9-CM diagnosis 902.53, 903.01, 903.1, 904.0, 904.41.)
6. Crush injuries and suturing of severed limbs. As in the previous conditions, HBO therapy would be an adjunctive treatment when loss of function, limb, or life is threatened. (ICD-9-CM diagnosis 927.00-927.03, 927.09-927.11, 927.20-927.21, 927.8-927.9, 928.00-928.01, 928.10-928.11, 928.20-928.21, 928.3, 928.8-928.9, 929.0, 929.9, 996.90-996.99.)
7. Progressive necrotizing infections (necrotizing fasciitis), (ICD-9-CM diagnosis 728.86).
8. Acute peripheral arterial insufficiency, (ICD-9-CM diagnosis 444.21, 444.22, 444.81).
9. Preparation and preservation of compromised skin grafts (not for primary management of wounds), (ICD-9CM diagnosis 996.52; excludes artificial skin graft).
10. Chronic refractory osteomyelitis, unresponsive to conventional medical and surgical management, (ICD-9-CM diagnosis 730.10-730.19).

11. Osteoradionecrosis as an adjunct to conventional treatment, (ICD-9-CM diagnosis 526.89).
12. Soft tissue radionecrosis as an adjunct to conventional treatment, (ICD-9-CM diagnosis 990).
13. Cyanide poisoning, (ICD-9-CM diagnosis 987.7, 989.0).
14. Actinomycosis, only as an adjunct to conventional therapy when the disease process is refractory to antibiotics and surgical treatment, (ICD-9-CM diagnosis 039.0-039.4, 039.8, 039.9).
15. Diabetic wounds of the lower extremities in patients who meet the following three criteria:
    a. Patient has type I or type II diabetes and has a lower extremity wound that is due to diabetes;
    b. Patient has a wound classified as Wagner grade III or higher; and
    c. Patient has failed an adequate course of standard wound therapy.

The use of HBO therapy is covered as adjunctive therapy only after there are no measurable signs of healing for at least 30-days of treatment with standard wound therapy and must be used in addition to standard wound care. Standard wound care in patients with diabetic wounds includes: assessment of a patient's vascular status and correction of any vascular problems in the affected limb if possible, optimization of nutritional status, optimization of glucose control, debridement by any means to remove devitalized tissue, maintenance of a clean, moist bed of granulation tissue with appropriate moist dressings, appropriate off-loading, and necessary treatment to resolve any infection that might be present. Failure to respond to standard wound care occurs when there are no measurable signs of healing for at least 30 consecutive days. Wounds must be evaluated at least every 30 days during administration of HBO therapy. Continued treatment with HBO therapy is not covered if measurable signs of healing have not been demonstrated within any 30-day period of treatment.

B. Noncovered Conditions.—All other indications not specified under §35-10 (A) are not covered under the Medicare program. No program payment may be made for any conditions other than those listed in §35-10(A).

No program payment may be made for HBO in the treatment of the following conditions:

1. Cutaneous, decubitus, and stasis ulcers.
2. Chronic peripheral vascular insufficiency.
3. Anaerobic septicemia and infection other than clostridial.
4. Skin burns (thermal).
5. Senility.
6. Myocardial infarction.
7. Cardiogenic shock.
8. Sickle cell anemia.
9. Acute thermal and chemical pulmonary damage, i.e., smoke inhalation with pulmonary insufficiency.
10. Acute or chronic cerebral vascular insufficiency.

11. Hepatic necrosis.
12. Aerobic septicemia.
13. Nonvascular causes of chronic brain syndrome (Pick's disease, Alzheimer's disease, Korsakoff's disease).
14. Tetanus.
15. Systemic aerobic infection.
16. Organ transplantation.
17. Organ storage.
18. Pulmonary emphysema.
19. Exceptional blood loss anemia.
20. Multiple Sclerosis.
21. Arthritic Diseases.
22. Acute cerebral edema.

C. Topical Application of Oxygen.—This method of administering oxygen does not meet the definition of HBO therapy as stated above. Also, its clinical efficacy has not been established. Therefore, no Medicare reimbursement may be made for the topical application of oxygen. (Cross reference: §35-31.)

D. Physician Supervision Requirement--For HBO therapy to be covered under the Medicare program, the physician must be in constant attendance during the entire treatment. This is a professional activity that cannot be delegated in that it requires independent medical judgement by the physician. The physician must be present, carefully monitoring the patient during the hyperbaric oxygen therapy session and be immediately available should a complication occur. This requirement applies in all settings: no payment will be made under Part A or Part B, unless the physician is in constant attendance during the HBO therapy procedure.

E. Credentials--A physician qualified in HBO therapy treatment is defined by Medicare for this purpose to be credentialed by the hospital in which HBO therapy is being performed specifically in hyperbaric medicine and the management of acute cardiopulmonary emergencies, including placement of chest tube. Credentialing includes, at a minimun, the following:

* Training, experience and privileges within the institution to manage acute cardiopulmonary emergencies, including advanced cardiac life support, and emergency myringotomy;
* Completion of a recognized hyperbaric medicine training program as established by either the American College of Hyperbaric Medicine or the Undersea and Hyperbaric Medical Society (UHMS) with a minimum of 60 hours of training and documented by a certificate of completion or an equivalent program; and
* Continuing medical education in hyperbaric medicine of a minimum of 16 hours every 2 years after initial credentialing.

An additional requirement that must be met for Medicare's payment for hyperbaric medical therapy is that cardiopulmonary resuscitation team coverage must be immediately available during the hours of the hyperbaric chamber operations.

35-13 PROLOTHERAPY, JOINT SCLEROTHERAPY, AND LIGAMENTOUS INJECTIONS WITH SCLEROSING AGENTS—NOT COVERED

The medical effectiveness of the above therapies has not been verified by scientifically controlled studies. Accordingly, reimbursement for these modalities should be denied on the ground that they are not reasonable and necessary as required by §1862(a)(1) of the law.

35-20 TREATMENT OF MOTOR FUNCTION DISORDERS WITH ELECTRIC NERVE STIMULATION—NOT COVERED

While electric nerve stimulation has been employed to control chronic intractable pain for some time, its use in the treatment of motor function disorders, such as multiple sclerosis, is a recent innovation, and the medical effectiveness of such therapy has not been verified by scientifically controlled studies. Therefore, where electric nerve stimulation is employed to treat motor function disorders, no reimbursement may be made for the stimulator or for the services related to its implantation since this treatment cannot be considered reasonable and necessary.

See §§35-27 and 65-8.

NOTE: For Medicare coverage of deep brain stimulation for essential tremor and Parkinson's disease, see §65-19.

35-27 BIOFEEDBACK THERAPY

Biofeedback therapy provides visual, auditory or other evidence of the status of certain body functions so that a person can exert voluntary control over the functions, and thereby alleviate an abnormal bodily condition. Biofeedback therapy often uses electrical devices to transform bodily signals indicative of such functions as heart rate, blood pressure, skin temperature, salivation, peripheral vasomotor activity, and gross muscle tone into a tone or light, the loudness or brightness of which shows the extent of activity in the function being measured.

Biofeedback therapy differs from electromyography, which is a diagnostic procedure used to record and study the electrical properties of skeletal muscle. An electromyography device may be used to provide feedback with certain types of biofeedback.

Biofeedback therapy is covered under Medicare only when it is reasonable and necessary for the individual patient for muscle re-education of specific muscle groups or for treating pathological muscle abnormalities of spasticity, incapacitating muscle spasm, or weakness, and more conventional treatments (heat, cold, massage, exercise, support) have not been successful. This therapy is not covered for treatment of ordinary muscle tension states or for psychosomatic conditions.

See HCFA-Pub. 14-3, §§2200ff, 2215, and 4161; HCFA-Pub. 13-3, §§3133.3, 3148, and 3149; HCFA-Pub. 10, §§242 and 242.5 for special physical therapy requirements. See also §35-20 and 65-8.)

35-34 FABRIC WRAPPING OF ABDOMINAL ANEURYSMS—NOT COVERED

Fabric wrapping of abdominal aneurysms is not a covered Medicare procedure. This is a treatment for abdominal aneurysms which involves wrapping aneurysms with cellophane or fascia lata. This procedure has not been shown to prevent eventual rupture. In extremely rare instances, external wall reinforcement may be indicated when the current accepted treatment (excision of the aneurysm and reconstruction with synthetic materials) is not a viable alternative, but external wall reinforcement is not fabric wrapping. Accordingly, fabric wrapping of abdominal aneurysms is not considered reasonable and necessary within the meaning of §1862(a)(1) of the Act.

35-46 ASSESSING PATIENT'S SUITABILITY FOR ELECTRICAL NERVE STIMULATION THERAPY

Electrical nerve stimulation is an accepted modality for assessing a patient's suitability for ongoing treatment with a transcutaneous or an implanted nerve stimulator. Accordingly, program payment may be made for the following techniques when used to determine the potential therapeutic usefulness of an electrical nerve stimulator:

A. Transcutaneous Electrical Nerve Stimulation (TENS).--This technique involves attachment of a transcutaneous nerve stimulator to the surface of the skin over the peripheral nerve to be stimulated. It is used by the patient on a trial basis and its effectiveness in modulating pain is monitored by the physician, or physical therapist. Generally, the physician or physical therapist is able to determine whether the patient is likely to derive a significant therapeutic benefit from continuous use of a transcutaneous stimulator within a trial period of 1 month; in a few cases this determination may take longer to make. Document the medical necessity for such services which are furnished beyond the first month. (See §45-25 for an explanation of coverage of medically necessary supplies for the effective use of TENS.)

If TENS significantly alleviates pain, it may be considered as primary treatment; if it produces no relief or greater discomfort than the original pain electrical nerve stimulation therapy is ruled out. However, where TENS produces incomplete relief, further evaluation with percutaneous electrical nerve stimulation may be considered to determine whether an implanted peripheral nerve stimulator would provide significant relief from pain. (See §35-46B.)

Usually, the physician or physical therapist providing the services will furnish the equipment necessary for assessment. Where the physician or physical therapist advises the patient to rent the TENS from a supplier during the trial period rather than supplying it himself/herself, program payment may be made for rental of the TENS as well as for the services of the physician or physical therapist who is evaluating its use. However, the combined program payment which is made for the physician's or physical therapist's services and the rental of the stimulator from a supplier should not exceed the amount which would be payable for the total service, including the stimulator, furnished by the physician or physical therapist alone.

B. Percutaneous Electrical Nerve Stimulation (PENS).--This diagnostic procedure which involves stimulation of peripheral nerves by a needle electrode inserted through the skin is performed only in a physician's office, clinic, or hospital outpatient department. Therefore, it is covered only when performed by a physician or incident to physician's service. If pain is effectively controlled by percutaneous stimulation, implantation of electrodes is warranted.

As in the case of TENS (described in subsection A), generally the physician should be able to determine whether the patient is likely to derive a significant therapeutic benefit from continuing use of an implanted nerve stimulator within a trial period of 1 month. In a few cases, this determination may take longer to make. The medical necessity for such diagnostic services which are furnished beyond the first month must be documented.

NOTE: Electrical nerve stimulators do not prevent pain but only alleviate pain as it occurs. A patient can be taught how to employ the stimulator, and once this is done, can use it safely and effectively without direct physician supervision. Consequently, it is inappropriate for a patient to visit his/her physician, physical therapist, or an outpatient clinic on a continuing basis for treatment of pain with electrical nerve stimulation. Once it is determined that electrical nerve stimulation should be continued as therapy and the patient has been trained to use the stimulator, it is expected that a stimulator will be implanted or the patient will employ the TENS on a continual basis in his/her home. Electrical nerve stimulation treatments furnished by a physician in his/her office, by a physical therapist or outpatient clinic are excluded from coverage by §1862(a)(1) of the Act. (See §65-8 for an explanation of coverage of the therapeutic use of implanted peripheral nerve stimulators under the prosthetic devices benefit. See §60-20 for an explanation of coverage of the therapeutic use of TENS under the durable medical equipment benefit.)

35-47 BREAST RECONSTRUCTION FOLLOWING MASTECTOMY (Effective for services performed on and after May 15, 1980.)

During recent years, there has been a considerable change in the treatment of diseases of the breast such as fibrocystic disease and cancer. While extirpation of the disease remains of primary importance, the quality of life following initial treatment is increasingly recognized as of great concern. The increased use of breast reconstruction procedures is due to several factors:

* A change in epidemiology of breast cancer, including an apparent increase in incidence;
* Improved surgical skills and techniques;
* he continuing development of better prostheses; and
* Increasing awareness by physicians of the importance of postsurgical psychological adjustment.

Reconstruction of the affected and the contralateral unaffected breast following a medically necessary mastectomy is considered a relatively safe and effective noncosmetic procedure. Accordingly, program payment may be made for breast reconstruction surgery following removal of a breast for any medical reason.

Program payment may not be made for breast reconstruction for cosmetic reasons. (Cosmetic surgery is excluded from coverage under §1862(a)(10) of the Social Security Act.)

35-48 OSTEOGENIC STIMULATION

Electrical stimulation to augment bone repair can be attained either invasively or noninvasively. Invasive devices provide electrical stimulation directly at the fracture site either through percutaneously placed cathodes or by implantation of a coiled cathode wire into the fracture site. The power pack for the latter device is implanted into soft tissue near the fracture site and subcutaneously connected to the cathode, creating a self-contained system with no external components. The power supply for the former device is externally placed and the leads connected to the inserted cathodes. With the noninvasive device, opposing pads, wired to an external power supply, are placed over the cast. An electromagnetic field is created between the pads at the fracture site.

1. Noninvasive Stimulator.—The noninvasive stimulator device is covered only for the following indications:

    * Nonunion of long bone fractures;
    * Failed fusion, where a minimum of nine months has elapsed since the last surgery;
    * Congenital pseudarthroses; and
    * As an adjunct to spinal fusion surgery for patients at high risk of pseudarthrosis due to previously failed spinal fusion at the same site or for those undergoing multiple level fusion. A multiple level fusion involves 3 or more vertebrae (e.g., L3-L5, L4-S1, etc).

2. Invasive (Implantable) Stimulator.—The invasive stimulator device is covered only for the following indications:

    * Nonunion of long bone fractures; and
    * As an adjunct to spinal fusion surgery for patients at high risk of pseudarthrosis due to previously failed spinal fusion at the same site or for those undergoing multiple level fusion.

A multiple level fusion involves 3 or more vertebrae (e.g., L3-L5, L4-S1, etc).

Effective for services performed on or after September 15, 1980, nonunion of long bone fractures, for both noninvasive and invasive devices, is considered to exist only after 6 or more months have elapsed without healing of the fracture.

Effective for services performed on or after April 1, 2000, nonunion of long bone fractures, for both noninvasive and invasive devices, is considered to exist only when serial radiographs have confirmed that fracture healing has ceased for three or more months prior to starting treatment with the electrical osteogenic stimulator. Serial radiographs must include a minimum of two sets of radiographs, each including multiple views of the fracture site, separated by a minimum of 90 days.

B. Ultrasonic Osteogenic Stimulators.—An ultrasonic osteogenic stimulator is a non-invasive device that emits low intensity, pulsed ultrasound. The ultrasound signal is applied to the skin surface at the fracture location via ultrasound, conductive gel in order to stimulate fracture healing.

Effective for services performed on or after January 1, 2001, ultrasonic osteogenic stimulators are covered as medically reasonable and necessary for the treatment of non-union fractures. In demonstrating nonunion of fractures, we would expect:

1 A minimum of two sets of radiographs obtained prior to starting treatment with the osteogenic stimulator, separated by a minimum of 90 days. Each radiograph must include multiple views of the fracture site accompanied with a written interpretation by a physician stating that there has been no clinically significant evidence of fracture healing between the two sets of radiographs.

2. Indications that the patient failed at least one surgical intervention for the treatment of the fracture.

Non-unions of the skull, vertebrae, and those that are tumor-related are excluded from coverage. The ultrasonic osteogenic stimulator may not be used concurrently with other non-invasive osteogenic devices. The national non-coverage policy related to ultrasonic osteogenic stimulators for fresh fractures and delayed unions remains in place. This policy relates only to non-union as defined above.

35-50 COCHLEOSTOMY WITH NEUROVASCULAR TRANSPLANT FOR MENIERE'S DISEASE—NOT COVERED

Ménière's disease (or syndrome) is a common cause of paroxysmal vertigo. Ménière's syndrome is usually treated medically. When medical treatment fails, surgical treatment may be required.

While there are two recognized surgical procedures used in treating Ménière's disease (decompression of the endolymphatic hydrops and labyrinthectomy), there is no scientific evidence supporting the safety and effectiveness of cochleostomy with neurovascular transplant in treatment of Ménière's syndrome. Accordingly, Medicare does not cover cochleostomy with neurovascular transplant for treatment of Ménière's disease.

35-64 CHELATION THERAPY FOR TREATMENT OF ATHEROSCLEROSIS

Chelation therapy is the application of chelation techniques for the therapeutic or preventive effects of removing unwanted metal ions from the body. The application of chelation therapy using ethylenediamine-tetra-acetic acid (EDTA) for the treatment and prevention of atherosclerosis is controversial. There is no widely accepted rationale to explain the beneficial effects attributed to this therapy. Its safety is questioned and its clinical effectiveness has never been established by well designed, controlled clinical trials. It is not widely accepted and practiced by American physicians. EDTA chelation therapy for atherosclerosis is considered experimental. For these reasons, EDTA chelation therapy for the treatment or prevention of atherosclerosis is not covered.

Some practitioners refer to this therapy as chemoendarterectomy and may also show a diagnosis other than atherosclerosis, such as arteriosclerosis or calcinosis. Claims employing such variant terms should also be denied under this section.

Cross-reference: §45-20

35-65 GASTRIC FREEZING

Gastric freezing for chronic peptic ulcer disease is a non-surgical treatment which was popular about 20 years ago but now is seldom done. It has been abandoned due to a high complication rate, only temporary improvement experienced by patients, and lack of effectiveness when tested by double- blind, controlled clinical trials. Since the procedure is now considered obsolete, it is not covered.

35-74 EXTERNAL COUNTERPULSATION (ECP) FOR SEVERE ANGINA—COVERED

External counterpulsation (ECP), commonly referred to as enhanced external counterpulsation, is a non-invasive outpatient treatment for coronary artery disease refractory to medical and/or surgical therapy. Although ECP devices are cleared by the Food and Drug Administration (FDA) for use in treating a variety of cardiac conditions, including stable or unstable angina pectoris, acute myocardial infarction and cardiogenic shock, the use of this device to treat cardiac conditions other than stable angina pectoris is not covered, since only that use has developed sufficient evidence to demonstrate its medical effectiveness. Non-coverage of hydraulic versions of these types of devices remains in force.

Coverage is provided for the use of ECP for patients who have been diagnosed with disabling angina (Class III or Class IV, Canadian Cardiovascular Society Classification or equivalent classification) who, in the opinion of a cardiologist or cardiothoracic surgeon, are not readily amenable to surgical intervention, such as PTCA or cardiac bypass because: (1) their condition is inoperable, or at high risk of operative complications or post-operative failure; (2) their coronary anatomy is not readily amenable to such procedures; or (3) they have co-morbid states which create excessive risk.

A full course of therapy usually consists of 35 one-hour treatments, which may be offered once or twice daily, usually 5 days per week. The patient is placed on a treatment table where their lower trunk and lower extremities are wrapped in a series of three compressive air cuffs which inflate and deflate in synchronization with the patient's cardiac cycle.

During diastole the three sets of air cuffs are inflated sequentially (distal to proximal) compressing the vascular beds within the muscles of the calves, lower thighs and upper thighs. This action results in an increase in diastolic pressure, generation of retrograde arterial blood flow and an increase in venous return. The cuffs are deflated simultaneously just prior to systole, which produces a rapid drop in vascular impedance, a decrease in ventricular workload and an increase in cardiac output.

The augmented diastolic pressure and retrograde aortic flow appear to improve myocardial perfusion, while systolic unloading appears to reduce cardiac workload and oxygen requirements. The increased venous return coupled with enhanced systolic flow appears to increase cardiac output. As a result of this treatment, most patients experience increased time until onset of ischemia, increased exercise tolerance, and a reduction in the number and severity of anginal episodes. Evidence was presented that this effect lasted well beyond the immediate post-treatment phase, with patients symptom-free for several months to two years.

This procedure must be done under direct supervision of a physician.

35-77 NEUROMUSCULAR ELECTRICAL STIMULATION (NMES)

Neuromuscular electrical stimulation (NMES) involves the use of a device that transmits an electrical impulse to activate muscle groups by way of electrodes. There are two broad categories of NMES. One type of device stimulates the muscle when the patient is in a resting state to treat muscle atrophy. The second type is used to enhance functional activity of neurologically impaired patients.

Treatment of Muscle Atrophy

Coverage of NMES to treat muscle atrophy is limited to the treatment of patients with disuse atrophy where the nerve supply to the muscle is intact, including brain, spinal cord and peripheral nerves and other non-neurological reasons for disuse atrophy. Examples include casting or splinting of a limb, contracture due to scarring of soft tissue as in burn lesions, and hip orthotic training begins). (See CIM 45-25 for an explanation of coverage of medically necessary supplies for the effective use of NMES).

Use for Walking in Patients with Spinal Cord Injury (SCI)

The type of NMES that is used to enhance the ability to walk of SCI patients is commonly referred to as functional electrical stimulation (FES). These devices are surface units that use electrical impulses to activate paralyzed or weak muscles in precise sequence. Coverage for the use of NMES/FES is limited to SCI patients, for walking, who have completed a training program, which consists of at least 32 physical therapy sessions with the device over a period of 3 months. The trial period of physical therapy will enable the physician treating the patient for his or her spinal cord injury to properly evaluate the person's ability to use these devices frequently and for the long term. Physical therapy sessions are only covered in the inpatient hospital, outpatient hospital, comprehensive outpatient rehabilitation facilities, and outpatient rehabilitation facilities. The physical therapy necessary to perform this training must be directly performed by the physical therapist as part of a one-on-one training program; this service cannot be done unattended.

The goal of physical therapy must be to train SCI patients on the use of NMES/FES devices to achieve walking, not to reverse or retard muscle atrophy.

Coverage for NMES/FES for walking will be limited to SCI patients with all of the following characteristics:

1) persons with intact lower motor units (L1 and below) (both muscle and peripheral nerve);
2) persons with muscle and joint stability for weight bearing at upper and lower extremities that can demonstrate balance and control to maintain an upright support posture independently;
3) persons that demonstrate brisk muscle contraction to NMES and have sensory perception of electrical stimulation sufficient for muscle contraction;
4) persons that possess high motivation, commitment and cognitive ability to use such devices for walking;
5) persons that can transfer independently and can demonstrate independent standing tolerance for at least 3 minutes;
6) persons that can demonstrate hand and finger function to manipulate controls;
7) persons with at least 6-month post recovery spinal cord injury and restorative surgery;
8) persons without hip and knee degenerative disease and no history of long bone fracture secondary to osteoporosis; and
9) persons who have demonstrated a willingness to use the device long-term.

NMES/FES for walking will not be covered in SCI patients with any of the following:

1) persons with cardiac pacemakers;
2) severe scoliosis or severe osteoporosis;
3) skin disease or cancer at area of stimulation;
4) irreversible contracture; or
5) autonomic dysreflexia.

The only settings where therapists with the sufficient skills to provide these services are employed, are inpatient hospitals, outpatient hospitals, comprehensive outpatient rehabilitation facilities and outpatient rehabilitation facilities. The physical therapy necessary to perform this training must be part of a one-on-one training program.

Additional therapy after the purchase of the DME would be limited by our general policies on coverage of skilled physical therapy.

All other uses of NMES remain non-covered.

(*Also reference Medicare Carriers' Manual, Part 3, Claims-§2210 and Medicare Intermediary Manual, Part 3, Claims-§3653 - See - Maintenance Program 271.1*)

35-82 PANCREAS TRANSPLANTS

Pancreas transplantation is performed to induce an insulin independent, euglycemic state in diabetic patients. The procedure is generally limited to those patients with severe secondary complications of diabetes, including kidney failure. However, pancreas transplantation is sometimes performed on patients with labile diabetes and hypoglycemic unawareness.

Medicare has had a policy of not covering pancreas transplantation for many years as the safety and effectiveness of the procedure had not been demonstrated. The Office of Health Technology Assessment performed an assessment on pancreas-kidney transplantation in 1994. They found reasonable graft survival outcomes for patients receiving either simultaneous pancreas-kidney transplantation and pancreas after kidney transplantation.

Effective July 1, 1999, Medicare will cover whole organ pancreas transplantation (ICD-9-CM code 52.80, or 52.82, CPT code 48554) only when it is performed simultaneous with or after a kidney transplant (ICD-9-CM code 55.69, CPT code 50360, or 50365). If the pancreas transplant occurs after the kidney transplant, immunosuppressive therapy will begin with the date of discharge from the inpatient stay for the pancreas transplant.

35-98 ELECTRICAL STIMULATION FOR THE TREATMENT OF WOUNDS

Electrical stimulation (ES) has been used or studied for many different applications, one of which is accelerating wound healing. The types of ES used for healing chronic venous and arterial wound and pressure ulcers are direct current (DC), alternating current (AC), pulsed current (PC), pulsed electromagnetic induction (PEMI), and spinal cord stimulation (SCS). An example of AC is transcutaneous electrical stimulation (TENS). The PEMI includes Pulsed Electromagnetic Field (PEMF) and Pulsed Electromagnetic Energy (PEE) using pulsed radio frequency energy, both of which are nonthermal i.e., they do not produce heat. Some ES use generators to create energy in the means such as coils, rather than by leads or surface electrodes.

There is insufficient evidence to determine any clinically significant differences in healing rates. Therefore, ES cannot be covered by Medicare because its effectiveness has not been adequately demonstrated.

35-99 ABORTION

Abortions are not covered Medicare procedures except

1. if the pregnancy is the result of an act of rape or incest; or
2. in the case where a woman suffers from a physical disorder, physical injury, or physical illness, including a life-endangering physical condition caused by or arising from the pregnancy itself, that would, as certified by a physician, place the woman in danger of death unless an abortion is performed.

This restricted coverage applies to CPT codes 59840, 59841, 59850, 59851, 59852, 59855, 59856, 59857, and 59866.

35-102 ELECTRICAL STIMULATION FOR THE TREATMENT OF WOUNDS (Effective for services on and after April 1, 2003)

Electrical stimulation (ES) has been used or studied for many different applications, one of which is accelerating wound healing. Electrical stimulation for the treatment of wounds is the application of electrical current through electrodes placed directly on the skin in close proximity to the wound. Electrical stimulation for the treatment of wounds will only be covered for chronic Stage III or Stage IV pressure ulcers, arterial ulcers, diabetic ulcers and venous stasis ulcers. All other uses of electrical stimulation for the treatment of wounds are noncovered. Chronic ulcers are defined as ulcers that have not healed within 30 days of occurrence. Electrical stimulation will not be covered as an initial treatment modality.

The use of electrical stimulation for the treatment of wounds is considered an adjunctive therapy. Electrical stimulation will be covered only after appropriate standard wound therapy has been tried for at least 30-days and there are no measurable signs of healing. This 30-day period can begin while the wound is acute. Measurable signs of improved healing include a decrease in wound size, either surface area or volume, decrease in amount of exudates and decrease in amount of necrotic tissue. Standard wound care includes: optimization of nutritional status; debridement by any means to remove devitalized tissue; maintenance of a clean, moist bed of granulation tissue with appropriate moist dressings; and necessary treatment to resolve any infection that may be present. Standard wound care based on the specific type of wound includes: frequent repositioning of a patient with pressure ulcers (usually every 2 hours); off-loading of pressure and good glucose control for diabetic ulcers; establishment of adequate circulation for arterial ulcers; and the use of a compression system for patients with venous ulcers. Continued treatment with electrical stimulation is not covered if measurable signs of healing have not been demonstrated within any 30-day period of treatment. Electrical stimulation must be discontinued when the wound demonstrates 100 per-cent epithelialized wound bed. Any form of electromagnetic therapy for the treatment of chronic wounds will not be covered.

This service can only be covered when performed by a physician, physical therapist, or incident to a physician service. Evaluation of the wound is an integral part of wound therapy. When a physician, physical therapist, or a clinician incident to a physician, performs electrical stimulation, that practitioner must evaluate the wound and contact the treating physician if the wound worsens. If electrical stimulation is being used, wounds must be evaluated at least monthly by the treating physician.

Unsupervised use of electrical stimulation for wound therapy will not be covered, as this use has not been found to be medically reasonable and necessary.

45-4 VITAMIN B12 INJECTIONS TO STRENGTHEN TENDONS, LIGAMENTS, ETC., OF THE FOOT--NOT COVERED

Vitamin B12 injections to strengthen tendons, ligaments, etc., of the foot are not covered under Medicare because (1) there is no evidence that vitamin B12 injections are effective for the purpose of strengthening weakened tendons and ligaments, and (2) this is nonsurgical treatment under the subluxation exclusion. Accordingly, vitamin B12 injections are not considered reasonable and necessary within the meaning of §1862(a)(1) of the Act.

See Intermediary Manual, §§3101.3 and 3158 and Carriers Manual, §§2050.5 and 2323.

45-7 HYDROPHILIC CONTACT LENS FOR CORNEAL BANDAGE

Some hydrophilic contact lenses are used as moist corneal bandages for the treatment of acute or chronic corneal pathology, such as bullous keratopathy, dry eyes, corneal ulcers and erosion, keratitis, corneal edema, descemetocele, corneal ectasis, Mooren.s ulcer, anterior corneal dystrophy, neurotrophic keratoconjunctivitis, and for other therapeutic reasons.

Payment may be made under §1861(s)(2) of the Act for a hydrophilic contact lens approved by the Food and Drug Administration (FDA) and used as a supply incident to a physician's service.

Payment for the lens is included in the payment for the physician.s service to which the lens is incident. Contractors are authorized to accept an FDA letter of approval or other FDA published material as evidence of FDA approval. *(See §65-1 for coverage of a hydrophilic contact lens as a prosthetic device.)*

See Intermediary Manual, §3112.4 and Carriers Manual, §§2050.1 and 15010.

45-10 LAETRILE AND RELATED SUBSTANCES—NOT COVERED

Laetrile (and the other drugs called by the various terms mentioned below) have been used primarily in the treatment or control of cancer. Although the terms "Laetrile," "laetrile," "amygdaline," "Sarcarcinase," "vitamin B-17," and "nitriloside" have been used interchangeably, the chemical identity of the substances to which these terms refer has varied.

The FDA has determined that neither Laetrile nor any other drug called by the various terms mentioned above, nor any other product which might be characterized as a "nitriloside" is generally recognized (by experts qualified by scientific training and experience to evaluate the safety and effectiveness of drugs) to be safe and effective for any therapeutic use. Therefore, use of this drug cannot be considered to be reasonable and necessary within the meaning of §1862(a)(1) of the Act and program payment may not be made for its use or any services furnished in connection with its administration.

A hospital stay only for the purpose of having laetrile (or any other drug called by the terms mentioned above) administered is not covered. Also, program payment may not be made for laetrile (or other drug noted above) when it is used during the course of an otherwise covered hospital stay, since the FDA has found such drugs to not be safe and effective for any therapeutic purpose.

45-16 CERTAIN DRUGS DISTRIBUTED BY THE NATIONAL CANCER INSTITUTE (Effective for services furnished on or after October 1, 1980.)

Under its Cancer Therapy Evaluation, the Division of Cancer Treatment of the National Cancer Institute (NCI), in cooperation with the Food and Drug Administration, approves and distributes certain drugs for use in treating terminally ill cancer patients. One group of these drugs, designated as Group C drugs, unlike other drugs distributed by the NCI, are not limited to use in clinical trials for the purpose of testing their efficacy. Drugs are classified as Group C drugs only if there is sufficient evidence demonstrating their efficacy within a tumor type and that they can be safely administered.

A physician is eligible to receive Group C drugs from the Division of Cancer Treatment only if the following requirements are met:

* A physician must be registered with the NCI as an investigator by having completed an FD-Form 1573;
* A written request for the drug, indicating the disease to be treated, must be submitted to the NCI;
* The use of the drug must be limited to indications outlined in the NCI's guidelines; and
* All adverse reactions must be reported to the Investigational Drug Branch of the Division of Cancer Treatment.

In view of these NCI controls on distribution and use of Group C drugs, intermediaries may assume, in the absence of evidence to the contrary, that a Group C drug and the related hospital stay are covered if all other applicable coverage requirements are satisfied.

If there is reason to question coverage in a particular case, the matter should be resolved with the assistance of the local PSRO, or if there is none, the assistance of your medical consultants.

Information regarding those drugs which are classified as Group C drugs may be obtained from:

Office of the Chief, Investigational Drug Branch
Division of Cancer Treatment, CTEP, Landow Building
Room 4C09, National Cancer Institute
Bethesda, Maryland 20205

45-20 ETHYLENEDIAMINE-TETRA-ACETIC (EDTA) CHELATION THERAPY FOR TREATMENT OF ATHEROSCLEROSIS

The use of EDTA as a chelating agent to treat atherosclerosis, arteriosclerosis, calcinosis, or similar generalized condition not listed by the FDA as an approved use is not covered. Any such use of EDTA is considered experimental.

See §35-64 for an explanation of this conclusion.

45-22 LYMPHOCYTE IMMUNE GLOBULIN, ANTI-THYMOCYTE GLOBULIN (EQUINE)

The lymphocyte immune globulin preparations are biologic drugs not previously approved or licensed for use in the management of renal allograft rejection. A number of other lymphocyte immune globulin products of equine, lapine, and murine origin are currently under investigation for their potential usefulness in controlling allograft rejections in human transplantation. These biologic drugs are viewed as adjunctive to traditional immunosuppressive products such as steroids and anti- metabolic drugs. At present, lymphocyte immune globulin preparations are not recommended to replace conventional immunosuppressive drugs, but to supplement them and to be used as alternatives to elevated or accelerated dosing with conventional immunosuppressive agents.

The FDA has approved one lymphocyte immune globulin preparation for marketing, lymphocyte immune globulin, anti-thymocyte globulin (equine). This drug is indicated for the management of allograft rejection episodes in renal transplantation. It is covered under Medicare when used for this purpose. Other forms of lymphocyte globulin preparation which the FDA approves for this indication in the future may be covered under Medicare.

45-23 DIMETHYL SULFOXIDE (DMSO)

DMSO is an industrial solvent produced as a chemical byproduct of paper production from wood pulp. The Food and Drug Administration has determined that the only purpose for which DMSO is safe and effective for humans is in the treatment of the bladder condition, interstitial cystitis. Therefore, the use of DMSO for all other indications is not considered to be reasonable and necessary. Payment may be made for its use only when reasonable and necessary for a patient in the treatment of interstitial cystitis.

45-24 ANTI-INHIBITOR COAGULANT COMPLEX (AICC)

Anti-inhibitor coagulant complex, AICC, is a drug used to treat hemophilia in patients with factor VIII inhibitor antibodies. AICC has been shown to be safe and effective and has Medicare coverage when furnished to patients with hemophilia A and inhibitor antibodies to factor VIII who have major bleeding episodes and who fail to respond to other, less expensive therapies.

45-25 SUPPLIES USED IN THE DELIVERY OF TRANSCUTANEOUS ELECTRICAL NERVE STIMULATION (TENS) AND NEURO-MUSCULAR ELECTRICAL STIMULATION (NMES)—(Effective for services rendered (i.e., items rented or purchased) on or after July 14, 1988.)

Transcutaneous Electrical Nerve Stimulation (TENS) and/or Neuromuscular Electrical Stimulation (NMES) can ordinarily be delivered to patients through the use of conventional electrodes, adhesive tapes and lead wires. There may be times, however, where it might be medically necessary for certain patients receiving TENS or NMES treatment to use, as an alternative to conventional electrodes, adhesive tapes and lead wires, a form-fitting conductive garment (i.e., a garment with conductive fibers which are separated from the patients' skin by layers of fabric).

A form-fitting conductive garment (and medically necessary related supplies) may be covered under the program only when:

1. It has received permission or approval for marketing by the Food and Drug Administration;
2. It has been prescribed by a physician for use in delivering covered TENS or NMES treatment; and
3. One of the medical indications outlined below is met:

   * The patient cannot manage without the conductive garment because there is such a large area or so many sites to be stimulated and the stimulation would have to be delivered so frequently that it is not feasible to use conventional electrodes, adhesive tapes and lead wires;
   * The patient cannot manage without the conductive garment for the treatment of chronic intractable pain because the areas or sites to be stimulated are inaccessible with the use of conventional electrodes, adhesive tapes and lead wires;
   * The patient has a documented medical condition such as skin problems that preclude the application of conventional electrodes, adhesive tapes and lead wires;
   * The patient requires electrical stimulation beneath a cast either to treat disuse atrophy, where the nerve supply to the muscle is intact, or to treat chronic intractable pain; or
   * The patient has a medical need for rehabilitation strengthening (pursuant to a written plan of rehabilitation) following an injury where the nerve supply to the muscle is intact.

A conductive garment is not covered for use with a TENS device during the trial period specified in §35-46 unless:

4. The patient has a documented skin problem prior to the start of the trial period; and
5. The carrier's medical consultants are satisfied that use of such an item is medically necessary for the patient.

(See conditions for coverage of the use of TENS in the diagnosis and treatment of chronic intractable pain in §§35-46 and 60-20 and the use of NMES in the treatment of disuse atrophy in §35-77.)

50-1 CARDIAC PACEMAKER EVALUATION SERVICES (Effective for services rendered on or after October 1, 1984.)

Medicare covers a variety of services for the post-implant follow-up and evaluation of implanted cardiac pacemakers. The following guidelines are designed to assist contractors in identifying and processing claims for such services.

NOTE: These new guidelines are limited to lithium battery-powered pacemakers, because mercury-zinc battery-powered pacemakers are no longer being manufactured and virtually all have been replaced by lithium units. Contractors still receiving claims for monitoring such units should continue to apply the guidelines published in 1980 to those units until they are replaced.

There are two general types of pacemakers in current use--single-chamber pacemakers, which sense and pace the ventricles of the heart, and dual-chamber pacemakers which sense and pace both the atria and the ventricles. These differences require different monitoring patterns over the expected life of the units involved. One fact of which contractors should be aware is that many dual-chamber units may be programmed to pace only the ventricles; this may be done either at the time the pacemaker is implanted or at some time afterward. In such cases, a dual-chamber unit, when programmed or reprogrammed for ventricular pacing, should be treated as a single-chamber pacemaker in applying screening guidelines.

The decision as to how often any patient's pacemaker should be monitored is the responsibility of the patient's physician who is best able to take into account the condition and circumstances of the individual patient. These may vary over time, requiring modifications of the frequency with which the patient should be monitored. In cases where monitoring is done by some entity other than the patient's physician, such as a commercial monitoring service or hospital outpatient department, the physician's prescription for monitoring is required and should be periodically renewed (at least annually) to assure that the frequency of monitoring is proper for the patient. Where a patient is monitored both during clinic visits and transtelephonically, the contractor should be sure to include frequency data on both types of monitoring in evaluating the reasonableness of the frequency of monitoring services received by the patient.

Since there are over 200 pacemaker models in service at any given point, and a variety of patient conditions that give rise to the need for pacemakers, the question of the appropriate frequency of monitoring is a complex one. Nevertheless, it is possible to develop guidelines within which the vast majority of pacemaker monitoring will fall and contractors should do this, using their own data and experience, as well as the frequency guidelines which follow, in order to limit extensive claims development to those cases requiring special attention.

Guidelines for Transtelephonic Monitoring of Cardiac Pacemakers

A. General.—Transtelephonic monitoring of pacemakers is coming into increasingly widespread use, with the services being furnished by commercial suppliers, hospital outpatient departments and physicians' offices.

Telephone monitoring of cardiac pacemakers as described below is medically efficacious in identifying early signs of possible pacemaker failure, thus reducing the number of sudden pacemaker failures requiring emergency replacement. All systems which monitor the pacemaker rate (bpm) in both the free-running and/or magnetic mode are effective in detecting subclinical pacemaker failure due to battery depletion. More sophisticated systems are also capable of detecting internal electronic problems within the pulse generator itself and other potential problems. In the case of dual chamber pacemakers in particular, such monitoring may detect failure of synchronization of the atria and ventricles, and the need for adjustment and reprogramming of the device.

NOTE: The transmitting device furnished to the patient is simply one component of the diagnostic system, and is not covered as durable medical equipment. Those engaged in transtelephonic pacemaker monitoring should reflect the costs of the transmitters in setting their charges for monitoring.

B. Definition of Transtelephonic Monitoring.—In order for transtelephonic monitoring services to be covered, the services must consist of the following elements:

1. A minimum 30-second readable strip of the pacemaker in the free-running mode;
2. Unless contraindicated, a minimum 30-second readable strip of the pacemaker in the magnetic mode; and
3. A minimum 30 seconds of readable ECG strip.

C. Frequency Guidelines for Transtelephonic Monitoring.—The guidelines below constitute a system which contractors should use, in conjunction with their knowledge of local medical practices, to screen claims for transtelephonic monitoring prior to payment. It is important to note that they are not recommendations with respect to a minimum frequency for such monitoring, but rather a maximum frequency (within which payment may be made without further claims development). As with previous guidelines, more frequent monitoring may be covered in cases where contractors are satisfied that such monitoring are medically necessary; e.g., based on the condition of the patient, or with respect to pacemakers exhibiting unexpected defects or premature failure. Contractors should seek written justification for more frequent monitoring from the patient's physician and/or any monitoring service involved.

These guidelines are divided into two broad categories—Guideline I, which will apply to the majority of pacemakers now in use, and Guideline II, which will apply only to pacemaker systems (pacemaker and leads) for which sufficient long-term clinical information exists to assure that they meet the standards of the Inter-Society Commission for Heart Disease Resources (ICHD) for longevity and end-of-life decay. (The ICHD standards are: (1) 90 percent cumulative survival at 5 years following implant; and (2) an end-of-life decay of less than a

50 percent drop of output voltage and less than 20 percent deviation of magnet rate, or a drop of 5 beats per minute or less, over a period of 3 months or more.) Contractors should consult with their medical advisers and other appropriate individuals and organizations (such as the North American Society of Pacing and Electrophysiology, which publishes product reliability information) should questions arise over whether a pacemaker system meets the ICHD standards.

The two groups of guidelines are then further broken down into two general categories--single chamber and dual-chamber pacemakers. Contractors should be aware that the frequency with which a patient is monitored may be changed from time to time for a number of reasons, such as a change in the patient's overall condition, a reprogramming of the patient's pacemaker, the development of better information on the pacemaker's longevity or failure mode, etc. Consequently, changes in the proper set of guidelines may be required. Contractors should inform physicians and monitoring services to alert contractors to any changes in the patient's monitoring prescription that might necessitate changes in the screening guidelines applied to that patient. (Of particular importance is the reprogramming of a dual-chamber pacemaker to a single-chamber mode of operation. Such reprogramming would shift the patient from the appropriate dual-chamber guideline to the appropriate single-chamber guideline.)

Guideline I

1. Single-chamber pacemakers:

   1st month—every 2 weeks.
   2nd through 36th month—every 8 weeks.
   37th month to failure—every 4 weeks.

2. Dual-chamber pacemaker:

   1st month—every 2 weeks.
   2nd through 6th month—every 4 weeks.
   7th through 36th month—every 8 weeks.
   37th month to failure—every 4 weeks.

Guideline II

1. Single-chamber pacemakers:

   1st month—every 2 weeks.
   2nd through 48th month—every 12 weeks.
   49th through 72nd month—every 8 weeks.
   Thereafter—every 4 weeks.

2. Dual-chamber pacemaker:

   1st month—every 2 weeks.
   2nd through 30th month—every 12 weeks.
   31st through 48th month—every 8 weeks.
   Thereafter—every 4 weeks.

D. Pacemaker Clinic Services

1. General.—Pacemaker monitoring is also covered when done by pacemaker clinics. Clinic visits may be done in conjunction with transtelephonic monitoring or as a separate service; however, the services rendered by a pacemaker clinic are more extensive than those currently possible by telephone. They include, for example, physical examination of patients and reprogramming of pacemakers. Thus, the use of one of these types of monitoring does not preclude concurrent use of the other.

2. Frequency Guidelines—As with transtelephonic pacemaker monitoring, the frequency of clinic visits is the decision of the patient's physician, taking into account, among other things, the medical condition of the patient. However, contractors can develop monitoring guidelines that will prove useful in screening claims. The following are recommendations for monitoring guidelines on lithium-battery pacemakers:

   a. For single-chamber pacemakers - twice in the first 6 months following implant, then once every 12 months.
   b. For dual-chamber pacemakers - twice in the first 6 months, then once every 6 months.

50-4 GRAVLEE JET WASHER

The Gravlee Jet Washer is a sterile, disposable, diagnostic device for detecting endometrial cancer. The use of this device is indicated where the patient exhibits clinical symptoms or signs suggestive of endometrial disease, such as irregular or heavy vaginal bleeding.

Program payment cannot be made for the washer or the related diagnostic services when furnished in connection with the examination of an asymptomatic patient. Payment for routine physical checkups is precluded under the statute.

(See §1862(a)(7) of the Act.) (See Intermediary Manual, §3157 and Carriers Manual, §2320.)

50-8.1 SERVICES PROVIDED FOR THE DIAGNOSIS AND TREATMENT OF DIABETIC SENSORY NEUROPATHY WITH LOSS OF PROTECTIVE SENSATION (AKA DIABETIC PERIPHERAL NEUROPATHY)

Presently, peripheral neuropathy, or diabetic sensory neuropathy, is the most common factor leading to amputation in people with diabetes. In diabetes, sensory neuropathy is an anatomically diffuse process primarily affecting sensory and autonomic fibers; however, distal motor findings may be present in advanced cases. Long nerves are affected first, with symptoms typically beginning insidiously in the toes and then advancing proximally. This leads to loss of protective sensation (LOPS), whereby a person is unable to feel minor trauma from mechanical, thermal, or chemical sources. When foot lesions are present, the reduction in autonomic nerve functions may also inhibit wound healing.

Diabetic sensory neuropathy with LOPS is a localized illness of the feet and falls within the regulation's exception to the general exclusionary rule [see 42 C.F.R. § 411.15 (l)(1)(i)]. Foot exams for people with diabetic sensory neuropathy with LOPS are reasonable and necessary to allow for early intervention in serious complications that typically afflict diabetics with the disease.

Effective for services furnished on or after July 1, 2002, Medicare covers, as a physician service, an evaluation (examination and treatment) of the feet no more often than every six months for individuals with a documented diagnosis of diabetic sensory neuropathy and LOPS, as long as the beneficiary has not seen a foot care specialist for some other reason in the interim. LOPS shall be diagnosed through sensory testing with the 5.07 monofilament using established guidelines, such as those developed by the National Institute of Diabetes and Digestive and Kidney Diseases guidelines. Five sites should be tested on the plantar surface of each foot, according to the National Institute of Diabetes and Digestive and Kidney Diseases guidelines. The areas must be tested randomly since the loss of protective sensation may be patchy in distribution, and the patient may get clues if the test is done rhythmically. Heavily callused areas should be avoided. As suggested by the American Podiatric Medicine Association, an absence of sensation at two or more sites out of 5 tested on either foot when tested with the 5.07 Semmes-Weinstein monofilament must be present and documented to diagnose peripheral neuropathy with loss of protective sensation.

The examination includes:

1) a patient history, and
2) a physical examination that must consist of at least the following elements:
   a. visual inspection of forefoot and hindfoot (including toe web spaces);
   b. evaluation of protective sensation;
   c. evaluation of foot structure and biomechanics;
   d. evaluation of vascular status and skin integrity;
   e. evaluation of the need for special footwear; and
3) patient education.

Treatment includes, but is not limited to:

1) local care of superficial wounds;
2) debridement of corns and calluses; and
3) trimming and debridement of nails.

The diagnosis of diabetic sensory neuropathy with LOPS should be established and documented prior to coverage of foot care. Other causes of peripheral neuropathy should be considered and investigated by the primary care physician prior to initiating or referring for foot care for persons with LOPS.

50-10 VABRA ASPIRATOR

The VABRA aspirator is a sterile, disposable, vacuum aspirator which is used to collect uterine tissue for study to detect endometrial carcinoma. The use of this device is indicated where the patient exhibits clinical symptoms or signs suggestive of endometrial disease, such as irregular or heavy vaginal bleeding.

Program payment cannot be made for the aspirator or the related diagnostic services when furnished in connection with the examination of an asymptomatic patient. Payment for routine physical checkups is precluded under the statute (§1862(a)(7) of the Act).

Cross-reference: Intermediary Manual, §3157; Carriers Manual §2320; §50-4

50-15 ELECTROCARDIOGRAPHIC SERVICES

Reimbursement may be made under Part B for electrocardiographic (EKG) services rendered by a physician or incident to his/her services or by an approved laboratory or an approved supplier of portable X-ray services. Since there is no coverage for EKG services of any type rendered on a screening basis or as part of a routine examination, the claim must indicate the signs and symptoms or other clinical reason necessitating the services.

A separate charge by an attending or consulting physician for EKG interpretation is allowed only when it is the normal practice to make such charge in addition to the regular office visit charge. No payment is made for EKG interpretations by individuals other than physicians.

On a claim involving EKG services furnished by a laboratory or a portable X-ray supplier, identify the physician ordering the service and, when the charge includes both the taking of the tracing and its interpretation, include the identity of the physician making the interpretation. No separate bill for the services of a physician is paid unless it is clear that he/she was the patient's attending physician or was acting as a consulting physician. The taking of an EKG in an emergency, i.e., when the patient is or may be experiencing what is commonly referred to as a heart attack, is covered as a laboratory service or a diagnostic service by a portable X-ray supplier only when the evidence shows that a physician was in attendance at the time the service was performed or immediately thereafter.

Where EKG services are rendered in the patient's home and the laboratory's or portable X-ray supplier's charge is higher than that imposed for the same service when performed in the laboratory or portable X-ray supplier's office, the medical need for home service should be documented. In the absence of such justification, reimbursement for the service if otherwise medically necessary should be based on the reasonable charge applicable when performed in the laboratory or X-ray supplier's office.

The documentation required in the various situations mentioned above must be furnished not only when the laboratory or portable X-ray supplier bills the patient or carrier for its service, but also when such a facility bills the attending physician who, in turn, bills the patient or carrier for the EKG services. (In addition to the evidence required to document the claim, the laboratory or portable X-ray supplier must maintain in its records the referring physician's written order and the identity of the employee taking the tracing.)

Long Term EKG Monitoring, also referred to as long-term EKG recording, Holter recording, or dynamic electrocardiography, is a diagnostic procedure which provides a continuous record of the electrocardiographic activity of a patient's heart while he is engaged in his daily activities.

The basic components of the long-term EKG monitoring systems are a sensing element, the design of which may provide either for the recording of electrocardiographic information on magnetic tape or for detecting significant variations in rate or rhythm as they occur, and a component for either graphically recording the electrocardiographic data or for visual or computer assisted analysis of the information recorded on magnetic tape. The long-term EKG permits the examination in the ambulant or potentially ambulant patient of as many as 70,000 heartbeats in a 12-hour recording while the standard EKG which is obtained in the recumbent position, yields information on only 50 to 60 cardiac cycles and provides only a limited data base on which diagnostic judgments may be made.

Many patients with cardiac arrhythmias are unaware of the presence of an irregularity in heart rhythm. Due to the transient nature of many arrhythmias and the short intervals in which the rhythm of the heart is observed by conventional standard EKG techniques, the offending arrhythmias can go undetected. With the extended examination provided by the long-term EKG, the physician is able not only to detect but also to classify various types of rhythm disturbances and waveform abnormalities and note the frequency of their occurrence. The knowledge of the reaction of the heart to daily activities with respect to rhythm, rate, conduction disturbances, and changes are of great assistance in directing proper therapy and this modality is valuable in both inpatient and outpatient diagnosis and therapy. Long-term monitoring of ambulant or potentially ambulant inpatients provides significant potential for reducing the length of stay for post-coronary infarct patients in the intensive care setting and may result in earlier discharge from the hospital with greater assurance of safety to the patients. The indications for the use of this technique, noted below, are similar for both inpatients and outpatients.

The long-term EKG has proven effective in detecting transient episodes of cardiac dysrhythmia and in permitting the correlation of these episodes with cardiovascular symptomatology. It is also useful for patients who have symptoms of obscure etiology suggestive of cardiac arrhythmia. Examples of such symptoms include palpitations, chest pain, dizziness, light-headedness, near syncope, syncope, transient ischemic episodes, dyspnea, and shortness of breath.

This technique would also be appropriate at the time of institution of any arrhythmic drug therapy and may be performed during the course of therapy to evaluate response. It is also appropriate for evaluating a change of dosage and may be indicated shortly before and after the discontinuation of anti-arrhythmic medication. The therapeutic response to a drug whose duration of action and peak of effectiveness is defined in hours cannot be properly assessed by examining 30-40 cycles on a standard EKG rhythm strip. The knowledge that all patients placed on anti-arrhythmic medication do not respond to therapy and the known toxicity of anti-arrhythmic agents clearly indicate that proper assessment should be made on an individual basis to determine whether medication should be continued and at what dosage level.

The long-term EKG is also valuable in the assessment of patients with coronary artery disease. It enables the documentation of etiology of such symptoms as chest pain and shortness of breath. Since the standard EKG is often normal during the intervals between the episodes of precordial pain, it is essential to obtain EKG information while the symptoms are occurring. The long-term EKG has enabled the correlation of chest symptoms with the objective evidence of ST-segment abnormalities. It is appropriate for patients who are recovering from an acute myocardial infarction or coronary insufficiency before and after discharge from the hospital, since it is impossible to predict which of these patients is subject to ventricular arrhythmias on the basis of the presence or absence of rhythm disturbances during the period of initial coronary care. The long-term EKG enables the physician to identify patients who are at a higher risk of dying suddenly in the period following an acute myocardial infarction. It may also be reasonable and necessary where the high-risk patient with known cardiovascular disease advances to a substantially higher level of activity which might trigger increased or new types of arrhythmias necessitating treatment. Such a high-risk case would be one in which there is documentation that acute phase arrhythmias have not totally disappeared during the period of convalescence.

In view of recent developments in cardiac pacemaker monitoring techniques (see CIA 50-1), the use of the long-term EKG for routine assessment of pacemaker function can no longer be justified. Its use for the patient with an internal pacemaker would be covered only when he has symptoms suggestive of arrhythmia not revealed by the standard EKG or rhythm strip.

These guidelines are intended as a general outline of the circumstances under which the use of this diagnostic procedure would be warranted. Each patient receiving a long-term EKG should be evaluated completely, prior to performance of this diagnostic study. A complete history and physical examination should be obtained and the indications for use of the long-term EKG should be reviewed by the referring physician.

The performance of a long-term EKG does not necessarily require the prior performance of a standard EKG. Nor does the demonstration of a normal standard EKG preclude the need for a long- term EKG. Finally, the demonstration of an abnormal standard EKG does not obviate the need for a long-term EKG if there is suspicion that the dysrhythmia is transient in nature.

A period of recording of up to 24 hours would normally be adequate to detect most transient arrhythmias and provide essential diagnostic information. The medical necessity for longer periods of monitoring must be documented.

Medical documentation for adjudicating claims for the use of the long-term EKG should be similar to other EKG services, X-ray services, and laboratory procedures. Generally, a statement of the diagnostic impression of the referring physician with an indication of the patient's relevant signs and symptoms should be sufficient for purposes of making a determination regarding the reasonableness and medical necessity for the use of this procedure. However, the intermediaries or carriers should require whatever additional documentation their medical consultants deem necessary to properly adjudicate the individual claim where the information submitted is not adequate.

It should be noted that the recording device furnished to the patient is simply one component of the diagnostic system and a separate charge for it will not be recognized under the durable medical equipment benefit.

Patient-Activated EKG Recorders, distributed under a variety of brand names, permit the patient to record an EKG upon manifestation of symptoms, or in response to a physician's order (e.g., immediately following strong exertion).Most such devices also permit the patient to simultaneously voice-record in order to describe symptoms and/or activity. In addition, some of these devices permit transtelephonic transmission of the recording to a physician's office, clinic, hospital, etc., having a decoder/recorder for review and analysis, thus eliminating the need to physically transport the tape. Some of these devices also permit a "time sampling" mode of operation. However, the "time sampling" mode is not covered—only the patient-activated mode of operation, when used for the indications described below, is covered at this time.

Services in connection with patient-activated EKG recorders are covered when used as an alternative to the long-term EKG monitoring (described above) for similar indications--detecting and characterizing symptomatic arrhythmias, regulation of anti-arrhythmic drug therapy, etc. Like long- term EKG monitoring, use of these devices is covered for evaluating patients with symptoms of obscure etiology suggestive of cardiac arrhythmia such as palpitations, chest pain, dizziness, lightheadedness, near syncope, syncope, transient ischemic episodes, dyspnea and shortness of breath.

As with long-term EKG monitors, patient-activated EKG recorders may be useful for both inpatient and outpatient diagnosis and therapy. While useful for assessing some post-coronary infarct patients in the hospital setting, these devices should not, however, be covered for outpatient monitoring of recently discharged post-infarct patients.

Computer Analyzed Electrocardiograms.—Computer interpretation of EKG's is recognized as a valid and effective technique which will improve the quality and availability of cardiology services. Reimbursement may be made for such computer service when furnished in the setting and under the circumstances required for coverage of other electrocardiographic services. Where either a laboratory's or a portable x-ray supplier's charge for EKG services includes the physician review and certification of the printout as well as the computer interpretation, the certifying physician must be identified on the HCFA-1490 before the entire charge can be considered a reimbursable charge. Where the laboratory's (or portable x-ray supplier's) reviewing physician is not identified, the carrier should conclude that no professional component is involved and make its charge determination accordingly. If the supplying laboratory (or portable x-ray supplier when supplied by such a facility) does not include professional review and certification of the hard copy, a charge by the patient's physician may be recognized for the service. In any case the charge for the physician component should be substantially less than that for physician interpretation of the conventional EKG tracing in view of markedly reduced demand on the physician's time where computer interpretation is involved.

Considering the unit cost reduction expected of this innovation, the total charge for the complete EKG service (taking of tracing and interpretation) when computer interpretation is employed should never exceed that considered reasonable for the service when physician interpretation is involved.

Transtelephonic Electrocardiographic Transmissions (Formerly Referred to as EKG Telephone Reporter Systems).—Effective for services furnished on and after March 1, 1980, coverage is extended to include the use of transtelephonic electrocardiographic (EKG) transmissions as a diagnostic service for the indications described below, when performed with equipment meeting the standards described below, subject to the limitations and conditions specified below. Coverage is further limited to the amounts payable with respect to the physician's service in interpreting the results of such transmissions, including charges for rental of the equipment. The device used by the beneficiary is part of a total diagnostic system and is not considered durable medical equipment.

1. Covered Uses.—The use of transtelephonic EKGs is covered for the following uses:

    a. To detect, characterize, and document symptomatic transient arrhythmias;
    b. To overcome problems in regulating antiarrhythmic drug dosage;
    c. To carry out early posthospital monitoring of patients discharged after myocardial infarction; (only if 24-hour coverage is provided, see 4. below).

Since cardiology is a rapidly changing field, some uses other than those specified above may be covered if, in the judgment of the contractor's medical consultants, such a use was justifiable in the particular case. The enumerated uses above represent uses for which a firm coverage determination has been made, and for which contractors may make payment without extensive claims development or review.

2. Specifications for Devices—The devices used by the patient are highly portable (usually pocket-sized) and detect and convert the normal EKG signal so that it can be transmitted via ordinary telephone apparatus to a receiving station. At the receiving end, the signal is decoded and transcribed into a conventional EKG. There are numerous devices available which transmit EKG readings in this fashion. For purposes of Medicare coverage, however, the transmitting devices must meet at least the following criteria:

    a. They must be capable of transmitting EKG Leads, I, II, or III;
    b. These lead transmissions must be sufficiently comparable to readings obtained by a conventional EKG to permit proper interpretation of abnormal cardiac rhythms.

3. Potential for Abuse - Need for Screening Guidelines.--While the use of these devices may often compare favorably with more costly alternatives, this is the case only where the information they contribute is actively utilized by a knowledgeable practitioner as part of overall medical management of the patient. Consequently, it is vital that contractors be aware of the potential for abuse of these devices, and adopt necessary screening and physician education policies to detect and halt potentially abusive situations. For example, use of these devices to diagnose and treat suspected arrhythmias as a routine substitute for more conventional methods of diagnosis, such as a careful history, physical examination, and standard EKG and rhythm strip

would not be appropriate. Moreover, contractors should require written justification for use of such devices in excess of 30 consecutive days in cases involving detection of transient arrhythmias.

Contractors may find it useful to review claims for these devices with a view toward detecting patterns of practice which may be useful in developing schedules which may be adopted for screening such claims in the future.

4. Twenty-four Hour Coverage.—No payment may be made for the use of these devices to carry out early posthospital monitoring of patients discharged after myocardial infarction unless provision is made for 24 hour coverage in the manner described below.

Twenty-four hour coverage means that there must be, at the monitoring site (or sites) an experienced EKG technician receiving calls; tape recording devices do not meet this requirement. Further, such technicians should have immediate access to a physician, and have been instructed in when and how to contact available facilities to assist the patient in case of emergencies.

Cross-reference: HCFA-Pub. 13-3, §§3101.5, 3110, 3112.3, HCFA-Pub. 14-3, §§2070, 2255, 2050.1

50-20 DIAGNOSTIC PAP SMEARS (Effective for services performed on and after May 15, 1978)

A diagnostic pap smear and related medically necessary services are covered under Medicare Part B when ordered by a physician under one of the following conditions:

* Previous cancer of the cervix, uterus, or vagina that has been or is presently being treated;
* Previous abnormal pap smear;
* Any abnormal findings of the vagina, cervix, uterus, ovaries, or adnexa;
* Any significant complaint by the patient referable to the female reproductive system; or
* Any signs or symptoms that might in the physician's judgment reasonably be related to a gynecologic disorder.

In respect to the last bullet, the contractor's medical staff must determine whether in a particular case a previous malignancy at another site is an indication for a diagnostic pap smear or whether the test must be considered a screening pap smear as described in §50-20.1.

Use the following CPT codes for indicating diagnostic pap smears:

* 88150 Cytopathology, smears, cervical or vaginal (e.g., Papanicolaou), up to three smears; screening by technician under physician supervision; or
* 88151 Cytopathology, smears, cervical or vaginal (e.g., Papanicolaou), up to three smears; requiring interpretation by physician.

50-24 HAIR ANALYSIS—NOT COVERED

Hair analysis to detect mineral traces as an aid in diagnosing human disease is not a covered service under Medicare.

The correlation of hair analysis to the chemical state of the whole body is not possible at this time, and therefore this diagnostic procedure cannot be considered to be reasonable and necessary under §1862(a)(1) of the law.

50-34 OBSOLETE OR UNRELIABLE DIAGNOSTIC TESTS

A. Diagnostic Tests (Effective for services performed on or after May 15, 1980).—Do not routinely pay for the following diagnostic tests because they are obsolete and have been replaced by more advanced procedures. The listed tests may be paid for only if the medical need for the procedure is satisfactorily justified by the physician who performs it. When the services are subject to PRO review, the PRO is responsible for determining that satisfactory medical justification exists. When the services are not subject to PRO review, the intermediary or carrier is responsible for determining that satisfactory medical justification exists. This includes:

* Amylase, blood isoenzymes, electrophoretic,
* Chromium, blood,
* Guanase, blood,
* Zinc sulphate turbidity, blood,
* Skin test, cat scratch fever,
* Skin test, lymphopathia venereum,
* Circulation time, one test,
* Cephalin flocculation,
* Congo red, blood,
* Hormones, adrenocorticotropin quantitative animal tests,
* Hormones, adrenocorticotropin quantitative bioassay,
* Thymol turbidity, blood,
* Skin test, actinomycosis,
* Skin test, brucellosis,
* Skin test, psittacosis,
* Skin test, trichinosis,
* Calcium, feces, 24-hour quantitative,
* Starch, feces, screening,
* Chymotrypsin, duodenal contents,
* Gastric analysis, pepsin,
* Gastric analysis, tubeless,
* Calcium saturation clotting time,
* Capillary fragility test (Rumpel-Leede),
* Colloidal gold,

* Bendien's test for cancer and tuberculosis,
* Bolen's test for cancer,
* Rehfuss test for gastric acidity, and
* Serum seromucoid assay for cancer and other diseases.

B. Cardiovascular Tests (Effective for services performed on or after January 1, 1997).--Do not pay for the following phonocardiography and vectorcardiography diagnostic tests because they have been determined to be outmoded and of little clinical value. They include:

* CPT code 93201, Phonocardiogram with or without ECG lead; with supervision during recording with interpretation and report (when equipment is supplied by the physician),
* CPT code 93202, Phonocardiogram; tracing only, without interpretation and report
* CPT code 93204, Phonocardiogram; interpretation and report,
* CPT code 93205, Phonocardiogram with ECG lead, with indirect carotid artery and/or jugular vein tracing, and/or apex cardiogram; with interpretation and report,
* CPT code 93208, Phonocardiogram; without interpretation and report,
* CPT code 93209, Phonocardiogram; interpretation and report only,
* CPT code 93210, Intracardiac,
* CPT code 93220, Vectorcardiogram (VCG), with or without ECG; with interpretation and report,
* CPT code 93221, Vectorcardiogram; tracing only, without interpretation and report, and
* CPT code 93222, Vectorcardiogram; interpretation and report only.

50-36 POSITRON EMISSION TOMOGRAPHY (PET) SCANS

I. General Description

Positron emission tomography (PET) is a noninvasive diagnostic imaging procedure that assesses the level of metabolic activity and perfusion in various organ systems of the [human] body. A positron camera (tomograph) is used to produce cross-sectional tomographic images, which are obtained from positron emitting radioactive tracer substances (radiopharmaceuticals) such as 2-[F-18] Fluoro-D-Glucose (FDG), that are administered intravenously to the patient.

The following indications may be covered for PET under certain circumstances. Details of Medicare PET coverage are discussed later in this section. Unless otherwise indicated, the clinical conditions below are covered when PET utilizes FDG as a tracer.

NOTE: This manual section lists all Medicare-covered uses of PET scans. A particular use of PET scans is not covered unless this manual specifically provides that such use is covered. Although this section lists some non-covered uses of PET scans, it does not constitute an exhaustive list of all non-covered uses.

Clinical Condition	Effective Date	Coverage
Solitary Pulmonary Nodules (SPNs)	January 1, 1998	Characterization
Lung Cancer (Non Small Cell)	January 1, 1998	Initial staging
Lung Cancer (Non Small Cell)	July 1, 2001	Diagnosis, staging and restaging
Esophageal Cancer	July 1, 2001	Diagnosis, staging and restaging
Colorectal Cancer	July 1, 1999	Determining location of tumors if rising CEA level suggests recurrence
Colorectal Cancer	July 1, 2001	Diagnosis, staging and restaging
Lymphoma	July 1, 1999	Staging and restaging only when used as an alternative to Gallium scan
Lymphoma	July 1, 2001	Diagnosis, staging and restaging
Melanoma	July 1, 1999	Evaluating recurrence prior to surgery as an alternative to a Gallium scan
Melanoma	July 1, 2001	Diagnosis, staging and restaging; Noncovered for evaluating regional nodes
Breast Cancer	October 1, 2002	As an adjunct to standard imaging modalities for staging patients with distant metastasis or restaging patients with locoregional recurrence or metastasis; as an adjunct to standard imaging modalities for monitoring tumor response to treatment for women with locally advanced and metastatic breast cancer when a change in therapy is anticipated

Head and Neck Cancers (excluding CNS and thyroid	July 1, 2001	Diagnosis, staging and restaging
Thyroid Cancer	October 1, 2003	Restaging of recurrent or residual thyroid cancers of follicular cell origin that have been previously treated by thyroidectomy and radioiodine ablation and have a serum thyroglobulin >10ng/ml and negative I-131 whole body scan performed
Myocardial Viability	July 1, 2001 toSeptember 30, 2002	Covered only following inconclusive SPECT
Myocardial Viability	October 1, 2002	Primary or initial diagnosis, or following an inconclusive SPECT prior to revascularization. SPECT may not be used following an inconclusive PET scan
Refractory Seizures	July 1, 2001	Covered for pre-surgical evaluation only
Perfusion of the heart using Rubidium 82 tracer	March 14, 1995	Covered for noninvasive imaging of the perfusion of the heart
Perfusion of the heart using ammonia N-13 tracer	October 1, 2003	Covered for noninvasive imaging of the perfusion of the heart

Not FDG-PET.

II. General Conditions of Coverage for FDG PET

A. Allowable FDG PET Systems

1. Definitions: For purposes of this section:
   a. "Any FDA approved" means all systems approved or cleared for marketing by the FDA to image radionuclides in the body.
   b. "FDA approved" means that the system indicated has been approved or cleared for marketing by the FDA to image radionuclides in the body.
   c. "Certain coincidence systems" refers to the systems that have all the following features:
      * Crystal at least 5/8-inch thick;
      * Techniques to minimize or correct for scatter and/or randoms; and
      * Digital detectors and iterative reconstruction.

Scans performed with gamma camera PET systems with crystals thinner than 5/8-inch will not be covered by Medicare. In addition, scans performed with systems with crystals greater than or equal to 5/8-inch in thickness, but that do not meet the other listed design characteristics are not covered by Medicare.

2. Allowable PET systems by covered clinical indication:

Allowable Type of FDG PET System

Covered Clinical Condition	Before 7/1/2001	7/1/ 2001 -12/31/2001	On or after 1/1/2002
Characterization of single pulmonary nodules	Effective 1/1/1998, any FDA approved	Any FDA approved	FDA approved: Full ring Partial ring Certain coincidence systems
Initial staging of lung cancer (non small cell)	Effective 1/1/1998, any FDA approved	Any FDA approved	FDA approved: Full ring Partial ring Certain coincidence systems
Determining location of colorectal tumors if rising CEA level suggests recurrence	Effective 7/1/1999, any FDA approved	Any FDA approved	FDA approved: Full ring Partial ring Certain coincidence systems
Staging or restaging of lymphoma only when used as an alternative to a gallium scan	Effective 7/1/1999, any FDA approved	Any FDA approved	FDA approved: Full ring Partial ring Certain coincidence systems
Evaluating recurrence of melanoma prior to surgery as an alternative to a gallium scan	Effective 7/1/1999, any FDA approved.	Any FDA approved	FDA approved: Full ring Partial ring Certain coincidence systems
Diagnosis, staging, and restaging of colorectal cancer	Not covered by Medicare	Full ring	FDA approved: Full ring Partial ring
Diagnosis, staging, and restaging of esophageal cancer	Not covered by Medicare	Full ring	FDA approved: Full ring Partial ring

Diagnosis, staging, and restaging of head and neck cancers (excluding CNS and thyroid)	Not covered by Medicare	Full ring	FDA approved: Full ring Partial ring

Diagnosis, staging, and restaging of lung cancer (non small cell)	Not covered by Medicare	Full ring	FDA approved: Full ring Partial ring
Diagnosis, staging, and restaging of lymphoma	Not covered by Medicare	Full ring	FDA approved: Full ring Partial ring
Diagnosis, staging, and restaging of melanoma (noncovered for evaluating regional nodes)	Not covered by Medicare	Full ring	FDA approved: Full ring Partial ring

Determination of myocardial viability only following an inconclusive SPECT	Not covered by Medicare	Full ring	FDA approved: Full ring Partial ring
Presurgical evaluation of refractory seizures	Not covered by Medicare	Full ring	FDA approved: Full ring
Breast Cancer	Not covered	Not covered	Effective October 1, 2002, full and partial ring
Thyroid Cancer	Not covered	Not covered	Effective October 1, 2003, full and partial ring
Myocardial Viability Primary or initial diagnosis prior to revascularization	Not covered	Not covered	Effective October 1, 2002, full and partial ring

B. Regardless of any other terms or conditions, all uses of FDG PET scans, in order to be covered by the Medicare program, must meet the following general conditions prior to June 30, 2001:

1. Submission of claims for payment must include any information Medicare requires to assure that the PET scans performed were: (a) medically necessary, (b) did not unnecessarily duplicate other covered diagnostic tests, and (c) did not involve investigational drugs or procedures using investigational drugs, as determined by the Food and Drug Administration (FDA).

2. The PET scan entity submitting claims for payment must keep such patient records as Medicare requires on file for each patient for whom a PET scan claim is made.

C. Regardless of any other terms or conditions, all uses of FDG PET scans, in order to be covered by the Medicare program, must meet the following general conditions as of July 1,2001:

1. The provider of the PET scan should maintain on file the doctor's referral and documentation that the procedure involved only FDA approved drugs and devices, as is normal business practice.
2. The ordering physician is responsible for documenting the medical necessity of the study and that it meets the conditions specified in the instructions. The physician should have documentation in the beneficiary's medical record to support the referral to the PET scan provider.

IV. Covered Indications for PET Scans and Limitations/Requirements for Usage

For all uses of PET relating to malignancies the following conditions apply:

1. Diagnosis: PET is covered only in clinical situations in which the PET results may assist in avoiding an invasive diagnostic procedure, or in which the PET results may assist in determining the optimal anatomical location to perform an invasive diagnostic procedure. In general, for most solid tumors, a tissue diagnosis is made prior to the performance of PET scanning. PET scans following a tissue diagnosis are performed for the purpose of staging, not diagnosis. Therefore, the use of PET in the diagnosis of lymphoma, esophageal, and colorectal cancers as well as in melanoma should be rare.

   PET is not covered for other diagnostic uses, and is not covered for screening (testing of patients without specific signs and symptoms of disease).

2. Staging and or Restaging: PET is covered in clinical situations in which 1) (a) the stage of the cancer remains in doubt after completion of a standard diagnostic workup, including conventional imaging (computed tomography, magnetic resonance imaging, or ultrasound) or (b) the use of PET would also be considered reasonable and necessary if it could potentially replace one or more conventional imaging studies when it is expected that conventional study information is insufficient for the clinical management of the patient and 2) clinical management of the patient would differ depending on the stage of the cancer identified. PET will be covered for restaging after the completion of treatment for the purpose of detecting residual disease, for detecting suspected recurrence or to determine the extent of a known recurrence. Use of PET would also be considered reasonable and necessary if it could potentially replace one or more conventional imaging studies when it is expected that conventional study information is insufficient for the clinical management of the patient.

3. Monitoring: Use of PET to monitor tumor response during the planned course of therapy (i.e., when no change in therapy is being contemplated) is not covered except for breast cancer. Restaging only occurs after a course of treatment is completed, and this is covered, subject to the conditions above.

NOTE: In the absence of national frequency limitations, contractors, should, if necessary, develop frequency requirements on any or all of the indications covered on and after July 1, 2001.

IV. Coverage of PET for Perfusion of the Heart

A. Rubidium 82

Effective for services performed on or after March 14, 1995, PET scans performed at rest or with pharmacological stress used for noninvasive imaging of the perfusion of the heart for the diagnosis and management of patients with known or suspected coronary artery disease using the FDA-approved radiopharmaceutical Rubidium 82 (Rb 82) are covered, provided the requirements below are met.

Requirements:

* The PET scan, whether at rest alone, or rest with stress, is performed in place of, but not in addition to, a single photon emission computed tomography (SPECT); or
* The PET scan, whether at rest alone or rest with stress, is used following a SPECT that was found to be inconclusive. In these cases, the PET scan must have been considered necessary in order to determine what medical or surgical intervention is required to treat the patient. (For purposes of this requirement, an inconclusive test is a test(s) whose results are equivocal, technically uninterpretable, or discordant with a patient's other clinical data and must be documented in the beneficiary's file.)
* For any PET scan for which Medicare payment is claimed for dates of services prior to July 1, 2001, the claimant must submit additional specified information on the claim form (including proper codes and/or modifiers), to indicate the results of the PET scan. The claimant must also include information on whether the PET scan was done after an inconclusive noninvasive cardiac test. The information submitted with respect to the previous noninvasive cardiac test must specify the type of test done prior to the PET scan and whether it was inconclusive or unsatisfactory. These explanations are in the form of special G codes used for billing PET scans using Rb 82. Beginning July 1, 2001, claims should be submitted with the appropriate codes.

B. Ammonia N-13

Effective for services performed on or after October 1, 2003, PET scans performed at rest or with pharmacological stress used for noninvasive imaging of the perfusion of the heart for the diagnosis and management of patients with known or suspected coronary artery disease using the FDA-approved radiopharmaceutical ammonia N-13 are covered, provided the requirements below are met.

Requirements:

* The PET scan, whether at rest alone, or rest with stress, is performed in place of, but not in addition to, a single photon emission computed tomography (SPECT); or
* The PET scan, whether at rest alone or rest with stress, is used following a SPECT that was found to be inconclusive. In these cases, the PET scan must have been considered necessary in order to determine what medical or surgical intervention is required to treat the patient. (For purposes of this requirement, an inconclusive test is a test whose results are equivocal, technically uninterpretable, or discordant with a patient's other clinical data and must be documented in the beneficiary's file.)

V. Coverage of FDG PET for Lung Cancer

The coverage for FDG PET for lung cancer, effective January 1, 1998, has been expanded. Beginning July 1, 2001, usage of FDG PET for lung cancer has been expanded to include diagnosis, staging, and restaging (see section III) of the disease.

A. Effective for services performed on or after January 1, 1998, Medicare covers regional FDG PET chest scans, on any FDA approved scanner, for the characterization of single pulmonary nodules (SPNs). The primary purpose of such characterization should be to determine the likelihood of malignancy in order to plan future management and treatment for the patient.

Beginning July 1, 2001, documentation should be maintained in the beneficiary's medical file at the referring physician's office to support the medical necessity of the procedure, as is normal business practice.

Requirements:

* There must be evidence of primary tumor. Claims for regional PET chest scans for characterizing SPNs should include evidence of the initial detection of a primary lung tumor, usually by computed tomography (CT). This should include, but is not restricted to, a report on the results of such CT or other detection method, indicating an indeterminate or possibly malignant lesion, not exceeding four centimeters (cm) in diameter.
* PET scan claims must include the results of concurrent thoracic CT (as noted above), which is necessary for anatomic information, in order to ensure that the PET scan is properly coordinated with other diagnostic modalities.
* In cases of serial evaluation of SPNs using both CT and regional PET chest scanning, such PET scans will not be covered if repeated within 90 days following a negative PET scan.

NOTE: A tissue sampling procedure (TSP) is not routinely covered in the case of a negative PET scan for characterization of SPNs, since the patient is presumed not to have a malignant lesion, based upon the PET scan results. When there has been a negative PET, the provider must submit additional information with the claim to support the necessity of a TSP, for review by the Medicare contractor.

B. Effective for services performed from January 1, 1998 through June 30, 2001, Medicare approved coverage of FDG PET for initial staging of non-small-cell lung carcinoma (NSCLC).

Limitations: This service is covered only when the primary cancerous lung tumor has been pathologically confirmed; claims for PET must include a statement or other evidence of the detection of such primary lung tumor. The evidence should include, but is not restricted to, a surgical pathology report, which documents the presence of an NSCLC. Whole body PET scan results and results of concurrent computed tomography (CT) and follow-up lymph node biopsy must be properly coordinated with other diagnostic modalities. Claims must include both:

* The results of concurrent thoracic CT, necessary for anatomic information, and
* The results of any lymph node biopsy performed to finalize whether the patient will be a surgical candidate. The ordering physician is responsible for providing this biopsy result to the PET facility.

NOTE: Where the patient is considered a surgical candidate, (given the presumed absence of metastatic NSCLC unless medical review supports a determination of medical necessity of a biopsy) a lymph node biopsy will not be covered in the case of a negative CT and negative PET. A lymph node biopsy will be covered in all other cases, i.e., positive CT + positive PET; negative CT + positive PET; positive CT + negative PET.

C. Beginning July 1, 2001, Medicare covers FDG PET for diagnosis, staging, and restaging of NSCLC. Documentation should be maintained in the beneficiary's medical file to support the medical necessity of the procedure, as is normal business practice.

Requirements: PET is covered in either/or both of the following circumstances:

* Diagnosis - PET is covered only in clinical situations in which the PET results may assist in avoiding an invasive diagnostic procedure, or in which the PET results may assist in determining the optimal anatomical location to perform an invasive diagnostic procedure. In general, for most solid tumors, a tissue diagnosis is made prior to the performance of PET scanning. PET scans following a tissue diagnosis are performed for the purpose of staging, not diagnosis. Therefore, the use of PET in the diagnosis of lymphoma, esophageal, and colorectal cancers as well as in melanoma should be rare.
* Staging and/or Restaging - PET is covered in clinical situations in which 1) (a) the stage of the cancer remains in doubt after completion of a standard diagnostic workup, including conventional imaging (computed tomography, magnetic resonance imaging, or ultrasound) or (b) the use of PET would also be considered reasonable and necessary if it could potentially replace one or more conventional imaging studies when it is expected that conventional study information is insufficient for the clinical management of the patient and 2) clinical management of the patient would differ depending on the stage of the cancer identified. PET will be covered for restaging after the completion of treatment for the

purpose of detecting residual disease, for detecting suspected recurrence or to determine the extent of a known recurrence. Use of PET would also be considered reasonable and necessary if it could potentially replace one or more conventional imaging studies when it is expected that conventional study information is insufficient for the clinical management of the patient.

Documentation should be maintained in the beneficiary's medical record at the referring physician's office to support the medical necessity of the procedure, as is normal business practice.

VI. Coverage of FDG PET for Esophageal Cancer

A. Beginning July 1, 2001, Medicare covers FDG PET for the diagnosis, staging, and restaging of esophageal cancer. Medical evidence is present to support the use of FDG PET in Presurgical staging of esophageal cancer.

Requirements: PET is covered in either/or both of the following circumstances:

* Diagnosis - PET is covered only in clinical situations in which the PET results may assist in avoiding an invasive diagnostic procedure, or in which the PET results may assist in determining the optimal anatomical location to perform an invasive diagnostic procedure. In general, for most solid tumors, a tissue diagnosis is made prior to the performance of PET scanning. PET scans following a tissue diagnosis are performed for the purpose of staging, not diagnosis. Therefore, the use of PET in the diagnosis of lymphoma, esophageal and colorectal cancers as well as in melanoma should be rare.
* Staging and/or Restaging - PET is covered in clinical situations in which 1)(a) the stage of the cancer remains in doubt after completion of a standard diagnostic workup, including conventional imaging (computed tomography, magnetic resonance imaging, or ultrasound) or (b) the use of PET would also be considered reasonable and necessary if it could potentially replace one or more conventional imaging studies when it is expected that conventional study information is insufficient for the clinical management of the patient, and 2) clinical management of the patient would differ depending on the stage of the cancer identified. PET will be covered for restaging after the completion of treatment for the purpose of detecting residual disease, for detecting suspected recurrence, or to determine the extent of a known recurrence. Use of PET would also be considered reasonable and necessary if it could potentially replace one or more conventional imaging studies when it is expected that conventional study information is insufficient for the clinical management of the patient.

Documentation should be maintained in the beneficiary's medical record at the referring physician's office to support the medical necessity of the procedure, as is normal business practice.

VII. Coverage of FDG PET for Colorectal Cancer

Medicare coverage of FDG PET for colorectal cancer where there is a rising level of carcinoembryonic antigen (CEA) was effective July 1, 1999 through June 30, 2001. Beginning July 1, 2001, usage of FDG PET for colorectal cancer has been expanded to include diagnosis, staging, and restaging of the disease (see part III).

A. Effective July 1, 1999, Medicare covers FDG PET for patients with recurrent colorectal carcinomas, which are suggested by rising levels of the biochemical tumor marker CEA.

1. Frequency Limitations: Whole body PET scans for assessment of recurrence of colorectal cancer cannot be ordered more frequently than once every 12 months unless medical necessity documentation supports a separate re-elevation of CEA within this period.
2. Limitations: Because this service is covered only in those cases in which there has been a recurrence of colorectal tumor, claims for PET should include a statement or other evidence of previous colorectal tumor, through June 30, 2001.

B. Beginning July 1, 2001, Medicare coverage has been expanded for colorectal carcinomas for diagnosis, staging and re-staging. New medical evidence supports the use of FDG PET as a useful tool in determining the presence of hepatic/extrahepatic metastases in the primary staging of colorectal carcinoma, prior to selecting a treatment regimen. Use of FDG PET is also supported in evaluating recurrent colorectal cancer beyond the limited presentation of a rising CEA level where the patient presents clinical signs or symptoms of recurrence.

Requirements: PET is covered in either/both of the following circumstances:

Diagnosis - PET is covered only in clinical situations in which the PET results may assist in avoiding an invasive diagnostic procedure, or in which the PET results may assist in determining the optimal anatomical location to perform an invasive diagnostic procedure. In general, for most solid tumors, a tissue diagnosis is made prior to the performance of PET scanning. PET scans following a tissue diagnosis are performed for the purpose of staging, not diagnosis. Therefore, the use of PET in the diagnosis of lymphoma, esophageal, and colorectal cancers as well as in melanoma should be rare.

* Staging and/or Restaging - PET is covered in clinical situations in which 1) (a) the stage of the cancer remains in doubt after completion of a standard diagnostic workup, including conventional imaging (computed tomography, magnetic resonance imaging, or ultrasound) or (b) the use of PET would also be considered reasonable and necessary if it could potentially replace one or more conventional imaging studies when it is expected that conventional study information is insufficient for the clinical management of the patient and 2) clinical management of the patient would differ depending on the stage of the cancer identified. PET will be covered for restaging after the completion of treatment for the purpose of detecting residual disease, for detecting suspected recurrence, or to determine the extent of a known recurrence. Use of PET would also be considered reasonable and necessary if it could potentially replace one

or more conventional imaging studies when it is expected that conventional study information is insufficient for the clinical management of the patient.

Documentation that these conditions are met should be maintained by the referring physician in the beneficiary's medical record, as is normal business practice.

VIII. Coverage of FDG PET for Lymphoma

Medicare coverage of FDG PET to stage and re-stage lymphoma as alternative to a Gallium scan, was effective July 1, 1999. Beginning July 1, 2001, usage of FDG PET for lymphoma has been expanded to include diagnosis, staging and restaging (see section III) of the disease.

A. Effective July 1, 1999, FDG PET is covered for the staging and restaging of lymphoma.

Requirements:

- PET is covered only for staging or follow-up restaging of lymphoma. Claims must include a statement or other evidence of previous diagnosis of lymphoma when used as an alternative to a Gallium scan
- To ensure that the PET scan is properly coordinated with other diagnostic modalities, claims must include the results of concurrent computed tomography (CT) and/or other diagnostic modalities when they are necessary for additional anatomic information.
- In order to ensure that the PET scan is covered only as an alternative to a Gallium scan, no PET scan may be covered in cases where it is done within 50 days of a Gallium scan done by the same facility where the patient has remained during the 50-day period. Gallium scans done by another facility less than 50 days prior to the PET scan will not be counted against this screen. The purpose of this screen is to assure that PET scans are covered only when done as an alternative to a Gallium scan within the same facility. We are aware that, in order to assure proper patient care, the treating physician may conclude that previously performed Gallium scans are either inconclusive or not sufficiently reliable.

Frequency Limitation for Restaging: PET scans will be allowed for restaging no sooner than 50 days following the last staging PET scan or Gallium scan, unless sufficient evidence is presented to convince the Medicare contractor that the restaging at an earlier date is medically necessary. Since PET scans for restaging are generally done following cycles of chemotherapy, and since such cycles usually take at least 8 weeks, we believe this screen will adequately prevent medically unnecessary scans while allowing some adjustments for unusual cases. In all cases, the determination of the medical necessity for a PET scan for re-staging lymphoma is the responsibility of the local Medicare contractor.

Beginning July 1, 2001, documentation should be maintained in the beneficiary's medical record at the referring physician's office to support the medical necessity of the procedure, as is normal business practice.

B. Effective for services performed on or after July 1, 2001, the Medicare program has broadened coverage of FDG PET for the diagnosis, staging and restaging of lymphoma.

Requirements: PET is covered in either/both of the following circumstances:

* Diagnosis - PET is covered only in clinical situations in which the PET results may assist in avoiding an invasive diagnostic procedure, or in which the PET results may assist in determining the optimal anatomical location to perform an invasive diagnostic procedure. In general, for most solid tumors, a tissue diagnosis is made prior to the performance of PET scanning. PET scans following a tissue diagnosis are performed for the purpose of staging, not diagnosis. Therefore, the use of PET in the diagnosis of lymphoma, esophageal, and colorectal cancers as well as in melanoma should be rare.
* Staging and/or Restaging - PET is covered in clinical situations in which 1) (a) the stage of the cancer remains in doubt after completion of a standard diagnostic workup, including conventional imaging (computed tomography, magnetic resonance imaging, or ultrasound) or (b) the use of PET would also be considered reasonable and necessary if it could potentially replace one or more conventional imaging studies when it is expected that conventional study information is insufficient for the clinical management of the patient, and 2) clinical management of the patient would differ depending on the stage of the cancer identified. PET will be covered for restaging after the completion of treatment for the purpose of detecting residual disease, for detecting suspected recurrence, or to determine the extent of a known recurrence. Use of PET would also be considered reasonable and necessary if it could potentially replace one or more conventional imaging studies when it is expected that conventional study information is insufficient for the clinical management of the patient.

Documentation that these conditions are met should be maintained by the referring physician in the beneficiary's medical record, as is normal business practice.

IX. Coverage of FDG PET for Melanoma

Medicare covered the evaluation of recurrent melanoma prior to surgery when used as an alternative to a Gallium scan, effective July 1, 1999. For services furnished on or after July 1, 2001 FDG PET is covered for the diagnosis, staging, and restaging of malignant melanoma (see part III). FDG PET is not covered for the use of evaluating regional nodes in melanoma patients.

A. Effective for services furnished July 1, 1999 through June 30, 2001, in the case of patients with recurrent melanoma prior to surgery, FDG PET (when used as an alternative to a Gallium scan) is covered for tumor evaluation.

Frequency Limitations: Whole body PET scans cannot be ordered more frequently than once every 12 months, unless medical necessity documentation, maintained in the beneficiaries medical record, supports the specific need for anatomic localization of possible recurrent tumor within this period.

Limitations: The FDG PET scan is covered only as an alternative to a Gallium scan. PET scans can not be covered in cases where it is done within 50 days of a Gallium scan done by the same PET facility where the patient has remained under the care of the same facility during the 50-day period. Gallium scans done by another facility less than 50 days prior to the PET scan will not be counted against this screen. The purpose of this screen is to assure that PET scans are covered only when done as an alternative to a Gallium scan within the same facility. We are aware that, in order to assure proper patient care, the treating physician may conclude that previously performed Gallium scans are either inconclusive or not sufficiently reliable to make the determination covered by this provision. Therefore, we will apply this 50-day rule only to PET scans done by the same facility that performed the Gallium scan.

Beginning July 1, 2001, documentation should be maintained in the beneficiary's medical file at the referring physician's office to support the medical necessity of the procedure, as is normal business practice.

B. Effective for services performed on or after July 1, 2001 FDG PET scan coverage for the diagnosis, staging and restaging of melanoma (not the evaluation regional nodes) has been broadened.

Limitations: PET scans are not covered for the evaluation of regional nodes.

Requirements: PET is covered in either/both of the following circumstances:

Diagnosis - PET is covered only in clinical situations in which the PET results may assist in avoiding an invasive diagnostic procedure, or in which the PET results may assist in determining the optimal anatomical location to perform an invasive diagnostic procedure. In general, for most solid tumors, a tissue diagnosis is made prior to the performance of PET scanning. PET scans following a tissue diagnosis are performed for the purpose of staging, not diagnosis. Therefore, the use of PET in the diagnosis of lymphoma, esophageal, and colorectal cancers as well as in melanoma should be rare.

* Staging and/or Restaging - PET is covered in clinical situations in which 1) (a) the stage of the cancer remains in doubt after completion of a standard diagnostic workup, including conventional imaging (computed tomography, magnetic resonance imaging, or ultrasound) or (b) the use of PET would also be considered reasonable and necessary if it could potentially replace one or more conventional imaging studies when it is expected that conventional study information is insufficient for the clinical management of the patient, and 2) clinical management of the patient would differ depending on the stage of the cancer identified. PET will be covered for restaging after the completion of treatment for the purpose of detecting residual disease, for detecting suspected recurrence, or to determine the extent of a known recurrence. Use of PET would also be considered reasonable and necessary if it could potentially replace one or more conventional imaging studies when it is expected that conventional study information is insufficient for the clinical management of the patient.

Documentation that these conditions are met should be maintained by the referring physician in the beneficiary's medical file, as is normal business practice.

X. Coverage of FDG PET for Head and Neck Cancers

Effective for services performed on or after July 1, 2001, Medicare will provide coverage for cancer of the head and neck, excluding the central nervous system (CNS) and thyroid. The head and neck cancers encompass a diverse set of malignancies of which the majority is squamous cell carcinomas. Patients may present with metastases to cervical lymph nodes but conventional forms of diagnostic imaging fail to identify the primary tumor. Patients that present with cancer of the head and neck are left with two options either to have a neck dissection or to have radiation of both sides of the neck with random biopsies. PET scanning attempts to reveal the site of primary tumor to prevent the adverse effects of random biopsies or unneeded radiation.

Limitations: PET scans for head and neck cancers are not covered for CNS or thyroid cancers (prior to October 1, 2003). Refer to section XIV for coverage for thyroid cancer effective October 1, 2003.

Requirements: PET is covered in either/or both of the following circumstances:

* Diagnosis - PET is covered only in clinical situations in which the PET results may assist in avoiding an invasive diagnostic procedure, or in which the PET results may assist in determining the optimal anatomical location to perform an invasive diagnostic procedure. In general, for most solid tumors, a tissue diagnosis is made prior to the performance of PET scanning. PET scans following a tissue diagnosis are performed for the purpose of staging, not diagnosis. Therefore, the use of PET in the diagnosis of lymphoma, esophageal, and colorectal cancers as well as in melanoma should be rare.

* Staging and/or Restaging - PET is covered in clinical situations in which 1) (a) the stage of the cancer remains in doubt after completion of a standard diagnostic workup, including conventional imaging (computed tomography, magnetic resonance imaging, or ultrasound) or (b) the use of PET would also be considered reasonable and necessary if it could potentially replace one or more conventional imaging studies when it is expected that conventional study information is insufficient for the clinical management of the patient, and 2) clinical management of the patient would differ depending on the stage of the cancer identified. PET will be covered for restaging after the completion of treatment for the purpose of detecting residual disease, for detecting suspected recurrence, or to determine the extent of a known recurrence. Use of PET would also be considered reasonable and necessary if it could potentially replace one or more conventional imaging studies when it is expected that conventional study information is insufficient for the clinical management of the patient.

Documentation that these conditions are met should be maintained by the referring physician in the beneficiary's medical record, as is normal business practice.

XI. Coverage of FDG PET for Myocardial Viability

The identification of patients with partial loss of heart muscle movement or hibernating myocardium is important in selecting candidates with compromised ventricular function to determine appropriateness for revascularization. Diagnostic tests such as FDG PET distinguish between dysfunctional but viable myocardial tissue and scar tissue in order to affect management decisions in patients with ischemic cardiomyopathy and left ventricular dysfunction.

FDG PET is covered for the determination of myocardial viability following an inconclusive SPECT from July 1, 2001 through September 30, 2002. Only full ring PET scanners are covered from July 1, 2001 through December 31, 2001. However, as of January 1, 2002, full and partial ring scanners are covered.

Beginning October 1, 2002, Medicare covers FDG PET for the determination of myocardial viability as a primary or initial diagnostic study prior to revascularization, or following an inconclusive SPECT. Studies performed by full and partial ring scanners are covered.

Limitations: In the event that a patient has received a single photon computed tomography test (SPECT) with inconclusive results, a PET scan may be covered. However, if a patient received a FDG PET study with inconclusive results, a follow up SPECT is not covered.

Documentation that these conditions are met should be maintained by the referring physician in the beneficiary's medical record, as is normal business practice.

(See §50-58 of the CIM for SPECT coverage.)

XII. Coverage of FDG PET for Refractory Seizures

Beginning July 1, 2001, Medicare will cover FDG-PET for pre-surgical evaluation for the purpose of localization of a focus of refractory seizure activity.

Limitations: Covered only for pre-surgical evaluation.

Documentation that these conditions are met should be maintained by the referring physician in the beneficiary's medical record, as is normal business practice.

XIII. Breast Cancer

Beginning October 1, 2002, Medicare covers FDG PET as an adjunct to other imaging modalities for staging patients with distant metastasis, or restaging patients with locoregional recurrence or metastasis. Monitoring treatment of a breast cancer tumor when a change in therapy is contemplated is also covered as an adjunct to other imaging modalities.

Limitations: Effective October 1, 2002, Medicare continues to have a national non-coverage determination for initial diagnosis of breast cancer and staging of axillary lymph nodes. Medicare coverage for staging patients with distant metastasis or restaging patients with locoregional recurrence or metastasis; and for monitoring tumor response to treatment for women with locally advanced and metastatic breast cancer when a change in therapy is anticipated, is only covered as an adjunct to other imaging modalities.

Documentation that these conditions are met should be maintained by the referring physician in the beneficiary's medical record, as is normal business practice.

XIV. Thyroid Cancer

1. Effective for services furnished on or after October 1, 2003, Medicare covers the use of FDG PET for thyroid cancer only for restaging of recurrent or residual thyroid cancers of follicular cell origin that have been previously treated by thyroidectomy and radioiodine ablation and have a serum thyroglobulin >10ng/ml and negative I-131 whole body scan performed.

2. All other uses of FDG PET in the diagnosis and treatment of thyroid cancer remain noncovered.

XV. Soft Tissue Sarcoma - NOT COVERED

Following a thorough review of the scientific literature, including a technology assessment on the topic, Medicare maintains its national noncoverage determination for all uses of FDG PET for soft tissue sarcoma.

XVI. Dementia and Neurogenerative Diseases - NOT COVERED

Following a thorough review of the scientific literature, including a technology assessment on the topic and consideration by the Medicare Coverage Advisory Committee, Medicare maintains its national noncoverage determination for all uses of FDG-PET for the diagnosis and management of dementia or other neurogenerative diseases

50-42 AMBULATORY BLOOD PRESSURE MONITORING

Ambulatory blood pressure monitoring (ABPM) involves the use of a non-invasive device which is used to measure blood pressure in 24-hour cycles. These 24-hour measurements are stored in the device and are later interpreted by the physician. ABPM must be performed for at least 24 hours to meet coverage criteria.

ABPM is only covered for those patients with suspected white coat hypertension. Suspected white coat hypertension is defined as 1) office blood pressure >140/90 mm Hg on at least three separate clinic/office visits with two separate measurements made at each visit; 2) at least two documented blood pressure measurements taken outside the office which are <140/90 mm Hg; and 3) no evidence of end-organ damage. The information obtained by ABPM is necessary in order to determine the appropriate management of the patient. ABPM is not covered for any other uses. In the rare circumstance that ABPM needs to be performed more than once in a patient, the qualifying criteria described above must be met for each subsequent ABPM test.

For those patients that undergo ABPM and have an ambulatory blood pressure of <135/85 with no evidence of end-organ damage, it is likely that their cardiovascular risk is similar to that of normotensives. They should be followed over time. Patients for which ABPM demonstrates a blood pressure of >135/85 may be at increased cardiovascular risk, and a physician may wish to consider antihypertensive therapy.

50-44 BONE (MINERAL) DENSITY STUDIES—Effective for services rendered on or after March 4, 1983.

Bone (mineral) density studies are used to evaluate diseases of bone and/or the responses of bone diseases to treatment. The studies assess bone mass or density associated with such diseases as osteoporosis, osteomalacia, and renal osteodystrophy. Various single or combined methods of measurement may be required to: (a) diagnose bone disease, (b) monitor the course of bone changes with disease progression, or (c) monitor the course of bone changes with therapy. Bone density is usually studied by using photodensitometry, single or dual photon absorptiometry, or bone biopsy.

The following bone (mineral) density studies are covered under medicare:

A. Single Photon Absorptiometry. A non-invasive radiological technique that measures absorption of a monochromatic photon beam by bone material. The device is placed directly on the patient, uses a low dose of radionuclide, and measures the mass absorption efficiency of the energy used. It provides a quantitative measurement of the bone mineral of cortical and trabecular bone, and is used in assessing an individual's treatment response at appropriate intervals.

   Single photon absorptiometry is covered under Medicare when used in assessing changes in bone density of patients with osteodystrophy or osteoporosis when performed on the same individual at intervals of 6 to 12 months.

B. Bone Biopsy. A physiologic test which is a surgical, invasive procedure. A small sample of bone (usually from the ilium) is removed, generally by a biopsy needle. The biopsy sample is then examined histologically, and provides a qualitative measurement of the bone mineral of trabecular bone. This procedure is used in ascertaining a differential diagnosis of bone disorders and is used primarily to differentiate osteomalacia from osteoporosis.

   Bone biopsy is covered under Medicare when used for the qualitative evaluation of bone no more than four times per patient, unless there is special justification given. When used more than four times on a patient, bone biopsy leaves a defect in the pelvis and may produce some patient discomfort.

C. Photodensitometry (radiographic absorptiometry). A noninvasive radiological procedure that attempts to assess bone mass by measuring the optical density of extremity radiographs with a photodensitometer, usually with a reference to a standard density wedge placed on the film at the time of exposure. This procedure provides a quantitative measurement of the bone mineral of cortical bone, and is used for monitoring gross bone change.

The following bone (mineral) density study is not covered under medicare:

Dual Photon Absorptiometry.—A noninvasive radiological technique that measures absorption of a dichromatic beam by bone material. This procedure is not covered under Medicare because it is still considered to be in the investigational stage.

50-50 DISPLACEMENT CARDIOGRAPHY

Displacement cardiography, including cardiokymography and photokymography, is a noninvasive diagnostic test used in evaluating coronary artery disease.

A. Cardiokymography.—(Effective For Services Rendered On Or After October 12, 1988).

Cardiokymography is a covered service only when it is used as an adjunct to electrocardiographic stress testing in evaluating coronary artery disease and only when the following clinical indications are present:

* For male patients, atypical angina pectoris or nonischemic chest pain; or
* For female patients, angina, either typical or atypical.

B. Photokymography.—NOT COVERED

Photokymography remains excluded from coverage.

50-55 PROSTATE CANCER SCREENING TESTS—COVERED (Effective for services furnished on or after January 1, 2000)

A. General.—Section 4103 of the Balanced Budget Act of 1997 provides for coverage of certain prostate cancer screening tests subject to certain coverage, frequency, and payment limitations. Effective for services furnished on or after January 1, 2000. Medicare will cover prostate cancer screening tests/procedures for the early detection of prostate cancer. Coverage of prostate cancer screening tests includes the following procedures furnished to an individual for the early detection of prostate cancer:

* Screening digital rectal examination; and
* Screening prostate specific antigen blood test.

B. Screening Digital Rectal Examinations. Screening digital rectal examinations (HCPCS code G0102) are covered at a frequency of once every 12 months for men who have attained age 50 (at least 11 months have passed following the month in which the last Medicare-covered screening digital rectal examination was performed). Screening digital rectal examination means a clinical examination of an individual's prostate for nodules or other abnormalities of the prostate. This screening must be performed by a doctor of medicine or osteopathy (as defined in §1861(r)(1) of the Act), or by a physician assistant, nurse practitioner, clinical nurse specialist, or certified nurse midwife (as defined in §1861(aa) and §1861(gg) of the Act) who is authorized under State law to perform the examination, fully knowledgeable about the beneficiary's medical condition, and would be responsible for using the results of any examination performed in the overall management of the beneficiary's specific medical problem.

C. Screening Prostate Specific Antigen Tests. Screening prostate specific antigen tests (code G0103) are covered at a frequency of once every 12 months for men who have attained age 50 (at least 11 months have passed following the month in which the last Medicare-covered screening prostate specific antigen test was performed). Screening prostate specific antigen tests (PSA) means a test to detect the marker for adenocarcinoma of prostate. PSA is a reliable immunocytochemical marker for primary and metastatic adenocarcinoma of prostate. This screening must be ordered by the beneficiary's physician or by the beneficiary's physician assistant, nurse practitioner, clinical nurse specialist, or certified nurse midwife (the term "attending physician" is defined in §1861(r)(1) of the Act to mean a doctor of medicine or osteopathy and the terms "physician assistant, nurse practitioner, clinical nurse specialist, or certified nurse midwife" are defined in §1861(aa) and §1861(gg) of the Act) who is fully knowledgeable about the beneficiary's medical condition, and who would be responsible for using the results of any examination (test) performed in the overall management of the beneficiary's specific medical problem.

50-57.1 CURRENT PERCEPTION THRESHOLD/SENSORY NERVE CONDUCTION THRESHOLD TEST (sNCT) NONCOVERED

The Current Perception Threshold/Sensory Nerve Conduction Threshold (sNCT) test is a diagnostic test used to diagnose sensory neuropathies. The device is a noninvasive test that uses transcutaneous electrical stimuli to evoke a sensation. There is insufficient scientific or clinical evidence to consider this device reasonable and necessary within the meaning of Section 1862(a)(1)(A) of the law and will not be covered by Medicare.

55-1 WATER PURIFICATION AND SOFTENING SYSTEMS USED IN CONJUNCTION WITH HOME DIALYSIS

A. Water Purification Systems—Water used for home dialysis should be chemically free of heavy trace metals and/or organic contaminants which could be hazardous to the patient. It should also be as free of bacteria as possible but need not be biologically sterile. Since the characteristics of natural water supplies in most areas of the country are such that some type of water purification system is needed, such a system used in conjunction with a home dialysis (either peritoneal or hemodialysis) unit is covered uner Medicare.

There are two types of water purification systems which will satisfy these requirements:

* Deionization-The removal of organic substances, mineral salts of magnesium and calcium (causing hardness), compounds of fluoride and chloride from tap water using the process of filtration and ion exchange; or
* Reverse Osmosis-The process used to remove impurities from tap water utilizing pressure to force water through a porous membrane.

Use of both a deionization unit and reverse osmosis unit in series, theoretically to provide the advantages of both systems, has been determined medically unnecessary since either system can provide water which is both chemically and bacteriologically pure enough for acceptable use in home dialysis. In addition, spare deionization tanks are not covered since they are essentially a precautionary supply rather than a current requirement for treatment of the patient. Activated carbon filters used as a component of water purification systems to remove unsafe concentrations of chlorine and chloramines are covered when prescribed by a physician.

B. Water Softening System.-Except as indicated below, a water softening system used in conjunction with home dialysis is excluded from coverage under Medicare as not being reasonable and necessary within the meaning of S1862(a)(1) of the law. Such a system, in conjunction with a home dialysis unit, does not adequately remove the hazardous heavy metal contaminants (such as arsenic) which may be present in trace amounts.

A water softening system may be covered when used to pretreat water to be purified by a reverse osmosis (RO) unit for home dialysis where:

* The manufacturer of the RO unit has set standards for the quality of water entering the RO (e.g., the water to be purified by the RO must be of a certain quality if the unit is to perform as intended);
* The patients water is demonstrated to be of a lesser quality than required; and
* The softener is used only to soften water entering the RO unit, and thus, used only for dialysis. (The softener need not actually be built into the RO unit, but must be an integral part of the dialysis system.)

C. Developing Need When a Water Softening System is Replaced with a Water Purification Unit in an Existing Home Dialysis System.-The medical necessity of water purification units must be care fully developed when they replace water softening systems in existing home dialysis systems. A purification system may be ordered under these circumstances for a number of reasons. For example, changes in the medical community's opinions regarding the quality of water necessary for safe dialysis may lead the physician to decide the quality of water previously used should be improved, or the water quality itself may have deteriorated. Patients may have dialyzed using only an existing water softener previous to Medicare ESRD coverage because of inability to pay for a purification system. On the other hand, in some cases, the installation of a purification system is not medically necessary. Thus, when such a case comes to your attention, ask the physician to furnish the reason for the changes. Supporting documentation, such as the supplier's recommendations or water analysis, may be required. All such cases should be reviewed by your medical consultants.

Cross-refer: Intermediary Manual, SS3113, 3643 (item ic); Carriers Manual, SS2100, 2100.2 2130, 2105 (item ic); Hospital Manual, S235.

60-3 WHITE CANE FOR USE BY A BLIND PERSON—NOT COVERED

A white cane for use by a blind person is more an identifying and self-help device rather than an item which makes a meaningful contribution in the treatment of an illness or injury.

60-4 HOME USE OF OXYGEN

A. General.—Medicare coverage of home oxygen and oxygen equipment under the durable medical equipment (DME) benefit (see §1861(s)(6)of the Act) is considered reasonable and necessary only for patients with significant hypoxemia who meet the medical documentation, laboratory evidence, and health conditions specified in subsections B, C, and D. This section also includes special coverage criteria for portable oxygen systems. Finally, a statement on the absence of coverage of the professional services of a respiratory therapist under the DME benefit is included in subsection F.

B. Medical documentation.—Initial claims for oxygen services must include a completed Form HCFA-484 (Certificate of Medical Necessity: Oxygen)to establish whether coverage criteria are met and to ensure that the oxygen services provided are consistent with the physician's prescription or other medical documentation. The treating physician's prescription or other medical documentation must indicate that other forms of treatment (e.g., medical and physical therapy directed at secretions, bronchospasm and infection) have been tried, have not been sufficiently successful, and oxygen therapy is still required. While there is no substitute for oxygen therapy, each patient must receive optimum therapy before long-term home oxygen therapy is ordered. Use Form HCFA-484 for recertifications. (See Medicare Carriers Manual §3312 for completion of Form HCFA-484.)

The medical and prescription information in section B of Form HCFA-484 can be completed only by the treating physician, the physician's employee, or another clinician (e.g., nurse, respiratory therapist, etc.) as long as that person is not the DME supplier. Although hospital discharge coordinators and medical social workers may assist in arranging for physician-prescribed home oxygen, they do not have the authority to prescribe the services. Suppliers may not enter this information. While this section may be completed by nonphysician clinician or a physician employee, it must be reviewed and the form HCFA-484 signed by the attending physician.

A physician's certification of medical necessity for oxygen equipment must include the results of specific testing before coverage can be determined.

Claims for oxygen must also be supported by medical documentation in the patient's record. Separate documentation is used with electronic billing. (See Medicare Carriers Manual, Part 3, §4105.5.) This documentation may be in the form of a prescription written by the patient's attending physician who has recently examined the patient (normally within a month of the start of therapy) and must specify:

* A diagnosis of the disease requiring home use of oxygen;
* The oxygen flow rate; and

An estimate of the frequency, duration of use (e.g., 2 liters per minute, 10 minutes per hour, 12 hours per day), and duration of need (e.g., 6 months or lifetime).

NOTE: A prescription for "Oxygen PRN" or "Oxygen as needed" does not meet this last requirement. Neither provides any basis for determining if the amount of oxygen is reasonable and necessary for the patient.

A member of the carrier's medical staff should review all claims with oxygen flow rates of more than 4 liters per minute before payment can be made.

The attending physician specifies the type of oxygen delivery system to be used (i.e., gas, liquid, or concentrator) by signing the completed form HCFA-484. In addition the supplier or physician may use the space in section C for written confirmation of additional details of the physician's order. The additional order information contained in section C may include the means of oxygen delivery (mask, nasal, cannula, etc.), the specifics of varying flow rates, and/or the noncontinuous use of oxygen as appropriate. The physician confirms this order information with their signature in section D.

New medical documentation written by the patient's attending physician must be submitted to the carrier in support of revised oxygen requirements when there has been a change in the patient's condition and need for oxygen therapy.

Carriers are required to conduct periodic, continuing medical necessity reviews on patients whose conditions warrant these reviews and on patients with indefinite or extended periods of necessity as described in Medicare Carriers Manual, Part 3, §4105.5. When indicated, carriers may also request documentation of the results of a repeat arterial blood gas or oximetry study.

NOTE: Section 4152 of OBRA 1990 requires earlier recertification and retesting of oxygen patients who begin coverage with an arterial blood gas result at or above a partial pressure of 55 or an arterial oxygen saturation percentage at or above 89. (See Medicare Carriers Manual §4105.5 for certification and retesting schedules.)

C. Laboratory Evidence.—Initial claims for oxygen therapy must also include the results of a blood gas study that has been ordered and evaluated by the attending physician. This is usually in the form of a measurement of the partial pressure of oxygen (PO2) in arterial blood. (See Medicare Carriers Manual, Part 3, §2070.1 for instructions on clinical laboratory tests.) A measurement of arterial oxygen saturation obtained by ear or pulse oximetry, however, is also acceptable when ordered and evaluated by the attending physician and performed under his or her supervision or when performed by a qualified provider or supplier of laboratory services. When the arterial blood gas and the oximetry studies are both used to document the need for home oxygen therapy and the results are conflicting, the arterial blood gas study is the preferred source of documenting medical need. A DME supplier is not considered a qualified provider or supplier of laboratory services for purposes of these guidelines. This prohibition does not extend to the results of blood gas test conducted by a hospital certified to do such tests. The conditions under which the laboratory tests are performed must be specified in writing and submitted with the initial claim, i.e., at rest, during exercise, or during sleep.

The preferred sources of laboratory evidence are existing physician and/or hospital records that reflect the patient's medical condition. Since it is expected that virtually all patients who qualify for home oxygen coverage for the first time under these guidelines have recently been discharged from a hospital where they submitted to arterial blood gas tests, the carrier needs to request that such test results be submitted in support of their initial claims for home oxygen. If more than one arterial blood gas test is performed during the patient's hospital stay, the test result obtained closest to, but no earlier than 2 days prior to the hospital discharge date is required as evidence of the need for home oxygen therapy.

For those patients whose initial oxygen prescription did not originate during a hospital stay, blood gas studies should be done while the patient is in the chronic stable state, i.e., not during a period of an acute illness or an exacerbation of their underlying disease."

Carriers may accept a attending physician's statement of recent hospital test results for a particular patient, when appropriate, in lieu of copies of actual hospital records.

A repeat arterial blood gas study is appropriate when evidence indicates that an oxygen recipient has undergone a major change in their condition relevant to home use of oxygen. If the carrier has reason to believe that there has been a major change in the patient's physical condition, it may ask for documentation of the results of another blood gas or oximetry study.

D. Health Conditions.—Coverage is available for patients with significant hypoxemia in the chronic stable state if: (1) the attending physician has determined that the patient has a health condition outlined in subsection D.1, (2) the patient meets the blood gas evidence requirements specified in subsection D.3, and (3) the patient has appropriately tried other alternative treatment measures without complete success. (See subsection B.)

1. Conditions for Which Oxygen Therapy May Be Covered.—

   * A severe lung disease, such as chronic obstructive pulmonary disease, diffuse interstitial lung disease, whether of known or unknown etiology; cystic fibrosis bronchiectasis; widespread pulmonary neoplasm; or
   * Hypoxia-related symptoms or findings that might be expected to improve with oxygen therapy. Examples of these symptoms and findings are pulmonary hypertension, recurring congestive heart failure due to chronic cor pulmonale, erythrocytosis, impairment of the cognitive process, nocturnal restlessness, and morning headache.

2. Conditions for Which Oxygen Therapy Is Not Covered.—

   * Angina pectoris in the absence of hypoxemia. This condition is generally not the result of a low oxygen level in the blood, and there are other preferred treatments;
   * Breathlessness without cor pulmonale or evidence of hypoxemia. Although intermittent oxygen use is sometimes prescribed to relieve this condition, it is potentially harmful and psychologically addicting;
   * Severe peripheral vascular disease resulting in clinically evident desaturation in one or more extremities. There is no evidence that increased PO2 improves the oxygenation of tissues with impaired circulation; or

* Terminal illnesses that do not affect the lungs.

3. Covered Blood Gas Values.—If the patient has a condition specified in subsection D.1, the carrier must review the medical documentation and laboratory evidence that has been submitted for a particular patient (see subsections B and C) and determine if coverage is available under one of the three group categories outlined below.

   a. Group I.—Except as modified in subsection d, coverage is provided for patients with significant hypoxemia evidenced by any of the following:

      (1) An arterial PO2 at or below 55 mm Hg, or an arterial oxygen saturation at or below 88 percent, taken at rest, breathing room air.

      (2) An arterial PO2 at or below 55 mm Hg, or an arterial oxygen saturation at or below 88 percent, taken during sleep for a patient who demonstrates an arterial PO2 at or above 56 mm Hg, or an arterial oxygen saturation at or above 89 percent, while awake; or a greater than normal fall in oxygen level during sleep (a decrease in arterial PO2 more than 10 mm Hg, or decrease in arterial oxygen saturation more than 5 percent) associated with symptoms or signs reasonably attributable to hypoxemia (e.g., impairment of cognitive processes and nocturnal restlessness or insomnia). In either of these cases, coverage is provided only for use of oxygen during sleep, and then only one type of unit will be covered. Portable oxygen, therefore, would not be covered in this situation.

      (3) An arterial PO2 at or below 55 mm Hg or an arterial oxygen saturation at or below 88 percent, taken during exercise for a patient who demonstrates an arterial PO2 at or above 56 mm Hg, or an arterial oxygen saturation at or above 89 percent, during the day while at rest. In this case, supplemental oxygen is provided for during exercise if there is evidence the use of oxygen improves the hypoxemia that was demonstrated during exercise when the patient was breathing room air.

   b. Group II.—Except as modified in subsection d, coverage is available for patients whose arterial PO2 is 56-59 mm Hg or whose arterial blood oxygen saturation is 89 percent, if there is evidence of:

      (1) Dependent edema suggesting congestive heart failure;

      (2) Pulmonary hypertension or cor pulmonale, determined by measurement of pulmonary artery pressure, gated blood pool scan, echocardiogram, or "P" pulmonale on EKG (P wave greater than 3 mm in standard leads II, III, or AVFL; or

      (3) Erythrocythemia with a hematocrit greater than 56 percent.

   c. Group III.—Except as modified in subsection d, carriers must apply a rebuttable presumption that a home program of oxygen use is not medically necessary for patients with arterial PO2 levels at or above 60 mm Hg, or arterial blood oxygen saturation at or above 90 percent. In order for claims in this category to be reimbursed, the carrier's reviewing physician needs to review any documentation submitted in rebuttal of this presumption and grant specific approval of the claims. HCFA expects few claims to be approved for coverage in this category.

d. Variable Factors That May Affect Blood Gas Values.—In reviewing the arterial PO2 levels and the arterial oxygen saturation percentages specified in subsections D. 3. a, b and c, the carrier's medical staff must take into account variations in oxygen measurements that may result from such factors as the patient's age, the altitude level, or the patient's decreased oxygen carrying capacity.

E. Portable Oxygen Systems.—A patient meeting the requirements specified below may qualify for coverage of a portable oxygen system either (1) by itself or (2) to use in addition to a stationary oxygen system. A portable oxygen system is covered for a particular patient if:

* The claim meets the requirements specified in subsections A-D, as appropriate; and
* The medical documentation indicates that the patient is mobile in the home and would benefit from the use of a portable oxygen system in the home. Portable oxygen systems are not covered for patients who qualify for oxygen solely based on blood gas studies obtained during sleep.

F. Respiratory Therapists.—Respiratory therapists' services are not covered under the provisions for coverage of oxygen services under the Part B durable medical equipment benefit as outlined above. This benefit provides for coverage of home use of oxygen and oxygen equipment, but does not include a professional component in the delivery of such services.

(See §60-9; Intermediary Manual, Part 3, §3113ff; and Medicare Carriers Manual, Part 3, §2100ff.)

60-5 POWER-OPERATED VEHICLES THAT MAY BE USED AS WHEELCHAIRS

Power-operated vehicles that may be appropriately used as wheelchairs are covered under the durable medical equipment provision.

These vehicles have been appropriately used in the home setting for vocational rehabilitation and to improve the ability of chronically disabled persons to cope with normal domestic, vocational and social activities. They may be covered if a wheelchair is medically necessary and the patient is unable to operate a wheelchair manually.

A specialist in physical medicine, orthopedic surgery, neurology, or rheumatology must provide an evaluation of the patient's medical and physical condition and a prescription for the vehicle to assure that the patient requires the vehicle and is capable of using it safely. When an intermediary determines that such a specialist is not reasonably accessible, e.g., more than 1 day's round trip from the beneficiary's home, or the patient's condition precludes such travel, a prescription from the beneficiary's physician is acceptable.

The intermediary's medical staff reviews all claims for a power-operated vehicle, including the specialists' or other physicians' prescriptions and evaluations of the patient's medical and physical conditions, to insure that all coverage requirements are met. (See §60-9 and Intermediary Manual, Part 3, §3629.)

60-6 SPECIALLY SIZED WHEELCHAIRS

Payment may be made for a specially sized wheelchair even though it is more expensive than a standard wheelchair. For example, a narrow wheelchair may be required because of the narrow doorways of a patient's home or because of a patient's slender build. Such difference in the size of the wheelchair from the standard model is not considered a deluxe feature.

A physician's certification or prescription that a special size is needed is not required where you can determine from the information in file or other sources that a specially sized wheelchair (rather than a standard one) is needed to accommodate the wheelchair to the place of use or the physical size of the patient.

To determine the reasonable charge in these cases, use the criteria set out in Carriers Manual, §§5022, 5022.1, 5200, and 5205, as necessary.

Cross-reference: Intermediary Manual, §§3113.2C, 3642.1, 3643 (item 3); Carriers Manual, §§2100.2c, 2105, 4105.2, 5107; Hospital Manual, §§235.2c, 420.1 (item 13).

60-7 SELF-CONTAINED PACEMAKER MONITORS

Self-contained pacemaker monitors are accepted devices for monitoring cardiac pacemakers. Accordingly, program payment may be made for the rental or purchase of either of the following pacemaker monitors when it is prescribed by a physician for a patient with a cardiac pacemaker:

A. Digital Electronic Pacemaker Monitor.—This device provides the patient with an instantaneous digital readout of his pacemaker pulse rate. Use of this device does not involve professional services until there has been a change of five pulses (or more) per minute above or below the initial rate of the pacemaker; when such change occurs, the patient contacts his physician.

B. Audible/Visible Signal Pacemaker Monitor.—This device produces an audible and visible signal which indicates the pacemaker rate. Use of this device does not involve professional services until a change occurs in these signals; at such time, the patient contacts his physician.

NOTE: The design of the self-contained pacemaker monitor makes it possible for the patient to monitor his pacemaker periodically and minimizes the need for regular visits to the outpatient department of the provider.

Therefore, documentation of the medical necessity for pacemaker evaluation in the outpatient department of the provider should be obtained where such evaluation is employed in addition to the self-contained pacemaker monitor used by the patient in his home.

Cross-reference: §50-1

60-8 SEAT LIFT

Reimbursement may be made for the rental or purchase of a medically necessary seat lift when prescribed by a physician for a patient with severe arthritis of the hip or knee and patients with muscular dystrophy or other neuromuscular diseases when it has been determined the patient can benefit therapeutically from use of the device. In establishing medical necessity for the seat lift, the evidence must show that the item is included in the physician's course of treatment, that it is likely to effect improvement, or arrest or retard deterioration in the patient's condition, and that the severity of the condition is such that the alternative would be chair or bed confinement.

Coverage of seat lifts is limited to those types which operate smoothly, can be controlled by the patient, and effectively assist a patient in standing up and sitting down without other assistance. Excluded from coverage is the type of lift which operates by a spring release mechanism with a sudden, catapult-like motion and jolts the patient from a seated to a standing position. Limit the payment for units which incorporate a recliner feature along with the seat lift to the amount payable for a seat lift without this feature.

Cross reference: Carriers Manual, § 5107

60-9 DURABLE MEDICAL EQUIPMENT REFERENCE LIST

The durable medical equipment (DME) list which follows is designed to facilitate your processing of DME claims. This section is designed to be used as a quick reference tool for determining the coverage status of certain pieces of DME and especially for those items which are commonly referred to by both brand and generic names. The information contained herein is applicable (where appropriate) to all DME coverage determinations discussed in the DME portion of this manual. The list is organized into two columns. The first column lists alphabetically various generic categories of equipment on which national coverage decisions have been made by HCFA; and the second column notes the coverage status of each equipment category.

In the case of equipment categories that have been determined by HCFA to be covered under the DME benefit, the list outlines the conditions of coverage that must be met if payment is to be allowed for the rental or purchase of the DME by a particular patient, or cross-refers to another section of the manual where the applicable coverage criteria are described in more detail. With respect to equipment categories that cannot be covered as DME, the list includes a brief explanation of why the equipment is not covered. This DME list will be updated periodically to reflect any additional national coverage decisions that HCFA may make with regard to other categories of equipment.

When you receive a claim for an item of equipment which does not appear to fall logically into any of the generic categories listed, you have the authority and responsibility for deciding whether those items are covered under the DME benefit. These decisions must be made by each contractor based on the advice of its medical consultants, taking into account:

* The general DME coverage instructions in the Carriers Manual, §2100ff and Intermediary Manual, §3113ff (see below for brief summary);

* Whether the item has been approved for marketing by the Food and Drug Administration (FDA) (see Carriers Manual, §2303.1 and Intermediary Manual, §3151.1) and is otherwise generally considered to be safe and effective for the purpose intended; and
* Whether the item is reasonable and necessary for the individual patient.
* As provided in the Carriers Manual, § 2100.1, and Intermediary Manual, §3113.1, the term DME is defined as equipment which
* Can withstand repeated use; i.e., could normally be rented, and used by successive patients;
* Is primarily and customarily used to serve a medical purpose;
* Generally is not useful to a person in the absence of illness or injury; and
* Is appropriate for use in a patient's home.

Durable Medical Equipment Reference List:

Item	Coverage Status
Air Cleaners	deny--environmental control equipment; not primarily medical in nature (§186l(n) of the Act)
Air Conditioners	deny--environmental control equipment; not primarily medical in nature (§l861(n) of the Act)
Air-Fluidized Bed	(See §60-19.)
Alternating Pressure Pads, and Mattresses and Lambs Wool Pads	covered if patient has, or is highly susceptible to, decubitus ulcers and patient's physician has specified that he will be supervising its use in connection with his course of treatment.
Audible/Visible Signal Pacemaker Monitor	(See Self-Contained Pacemaker Monitor.)
Augmentative Communication Device	(See Speech Generating Devices, §60-23.)
Bathtub Lifts	deny--convenience item; not primarily medical in nature (§l861(n) of the Act)
Bathtub Seats	deny--comfort or convenience item; hygienic equipment; not primarily medical in nature (§l861(n) of the Act)
Bead Bed	(See §60-19.)
Bed Baths (home type)	deny--hygienic equipment; not primarily medical in nature (§l861(n) of the Act)
Bed Lifter (bed elevator)	deny--not primarily medical in nature (§1861(n) of the Act.
Bedboards	deny--not primarily medical in nature (§1861(n) of the Act)
Bed Pans (autoclavable hospital type)	covered if patient is bed confined

Bed Side Rails	(See Hospital Beds, §60-18.)
Beds-Lounge (power or manual)	deny--not a hospital bed; comfort or convenience item; not primarily medical in nature (§1861(n) of the Act)
Beds--Oscillating	deny--institutional equipment; inappropriate for home use
Bidet Toilet Seat	(See Toilet Seats.)
Blood Glucose Analyzer Reflectance Colorimeter	deny--unsuitable for home use (See §60-11.)
Blood Glucose Monitor	covered if patient meets certain conditions (See §60-11.)
Braille Teaching Texts	deny--educational equipment; not primarily medical in nature (§1861(n) of the Act)
Canes	covered if patient's condition impairs ambulation (See §60-3.)
Carafes	deny--convenience item; not primarily medical in nature (§1861(n) of the Act)
Catheters	deny--nonreusable disposable supply (§1861(n) of the Act)

Commodes	covered if patient is confined to bed or room. NOTE: The term "room confined" means that the patient's condition is such that leaving the room is medically contraindicated. The accessibility of bathroom facilities generally would not be a factor in this determination. However, confinement of a patient to his home in a case where there are no toilet facilities in the home may be equated to room confinement. Moreover, payment may also be made if a patient's medical condition confines him to a floor of his home and there is no bathroom located on that floor (See hospital beds in §60-18 for definition of "bed confinement".)

Communicator	(See §60-23, Speech Generating Devices)

Continuous Passive Motion	Continuous passive motion devices are devices covered for patients who have received a total knee replacement. To qualify for coverage, use of the device must commence within 2 days following surgery. In addition, coverage is limited to that portion of the three week period following surgery during which the device is used in the patient's home.There is insufficient evidence to justify coverage of these devices for longer periods of time or for other applications.
Continuous Positive Airway Pressure (CPAP)	(See §60-17.)
Crutches	covered if patient's condition impairs Ambulation
Cushion Lift Power Seat	(See Seat Lifts.)
Dehumidifiers (room or central heating system type)	deny--environmental control equipment; not primarily medical in nature (§l861(n) of the Act
Diathermy Machines (standard pulses wave types)	deny--inappropriate for home use (See and §35-41.)

Digital Electronic Pacemaker Monitor	(See Self-Contained Pacemaker Monitor.)
Disposable Sheets and Bags	deny--nonreusable disposable supplies (§l861(n) of the Act)
Elastic Stockings	deny--nonreusable supply; not rental-type items (§l861(n) of the Act)
Electric Air Cleaners	deny--(See Air Cleaners.) (§l861(n) of the Act)
Electric Hospital Beds	(See Hospital Beds §60-18.)
Electrical Stimulation for Wounds	deny--inappropriate for home use
Electrostatic Machines	deny--(See Air Cleaners and Air Conditioners.) (§l861(n) of the Act)
Elevators	deny--convenience item; not primarily medical in nature (§l861(n) of the Act)
Emesis Basins	deny--convenience item; not primarily medical in nature (§l861(n) of the Act)
Esophageal Dilator	deny--physician instrument; inappropriate for patient use
Exercise Equipment	deny--not primarily medical in nature (§l861(n) of the Act)
Fabric Supports	deny--nonreusable supplies; not rental-type it (§l861(n) of the Act)
Face Masks (oxygen)	covered if oxygen is covered (See § 60-4.)

Face Masks (surgical)	deny--nonreusable disposable items (§l861(n) of the Act)
Flowmeter	(See Medical Oxygen Regulators)
Fluidic Breathing Assister	(See IPPB Machines.)
Fomentation Device	(See Heating Pads.)
Gel Flotation Pads and Mattresses	(See Alternating Pressure Pads and Mattresses.)
Grab Bars	deny--self-help device; not primarily medical in nature (§l861(n) of the Act)
Heat and Massage Foam Cushion Pad	deny--not primarily medical in nature; personal comfort item (§§ l861(n) and l862(a)(6) of the Act)
Heating and Cooling Plants	deny--environmental control equipment; not primarily medical in nature(§l861(n) of the Act)
Heating Pads	covered if the contractor's medical staff determines patient's medical condition is one for which the application of heat in the form of a heating pad is therapeutically effective.
Heat Lamps	covered if the contractor's medical staff determines patient's medical condition is one for which the application of heat in the form of a heat lamp is therapeutically effective.
Hospital Beds	(See § 60-18.)
Hot Packs	(See Heating Pads.)
Humidifiers (oxygen)	(See Oxygen Humidifiers.)
Humidifiers (room or central heating system types)	deny--environmental control equipment; not medical in nature (§l861(n) of the Act)
Hydraulic Lift	(See Patient Lifts.)
Incontinent Pads	deny--nonreusable supply; hygienic item (§ l861(n) of the Act.)
Infusion Pumps	For external and implantable pumps, see §60-14. If the pump is used with an enteral or parenteral malnutritional therapy system, see §§65-10 - 65.10.2 0.2 for special coverage rules.
Injectors (hypodermic jet devices for injection of insulin	deny-- noncovered self-administered drug supply, §1861(s)(2)(A) of the Act)
IPPB Machines	covered if patient's ability to breathe is severely impaired

Iron Lungs	(See Ventilators.)
Irrigating Kit	deny--nonreusable supply; hygienic equipment (§1861(n) of the Act)
Lambs Wool Pads	covered under same conditions as alternating pressure pads and mattresses
Leotards	deny--(See Pressure Leotards.) (§1861(n)of the Act)
Lymphedema Pumps	covered (See §60-16.)(segmental and non-segmental therapy types)
Massage Devices	deny--personal comfort items; not primarily medical in nature (§§1861(n) and 1862(a)(6) of the Act)
Mattress	covered only where hospital bed is medically necessary (Separate Charge for replacement mattresses should not be allowed where hospital bed with mattress is rented.) (See §60-18.)
Medical Oxygen Regulators	covered if patient's ability to breathe is severely impaired (See §60-4.)
Mobile Geriatric Chair	(See Rolling Chairs.)
Motorized Wheelchairs	(See Wheelchairs (power operated).)
Muscle Stimulators	Covered for certain conditions (See §35-77.)
Nebulizers	covered if patient's ability to breathe is severely impaired
Oscillating Beds	deny--institutional equipment--inappropriate for home use
Overbed Tables	deny--convenience item; not primarily medical in nature (§1861(n) of the Act)
Oxygen	covered if the oxygen has been prescribed for use in connection with medically necessary durable medical equipment (See §60-4.)
Oxygen Humidifiers	covered if a medical humidifier has been prescribed for use in connection with medically necessary durable medical equipment for purposes of moisturizing oxygen (See §60-4.)
Oxygen Regulators (Medical)	(See Medical Oxygen Regulators.)
Oxygen Tents	(See § 60-4.)
Paraffin Bath Units (Portable)	(See Portable Paraffin Bath Units.)
Paraffin Bath Units (Standard)	deny--institutional equipment; inappropriate for home use

Parallel Bars	deny--support exercise equipment; primarily for institutional use; in the home setting other devices (e.g., a walker) satisfy the patient's need
Patient Lifts	covered if contractor's medical staff determines patient's condition is such that periodic movement is necessary to effect improvement or to arrest or retard deterioration in his condition.
Percussors	covered for mobilizing respiratory tract secretions in patients with chronic obstructive lung disease, chronic bronchitis, or emphysema, when patient or operator of powered percussor has received appropriate training by a physician or therapist, and no one competent to administer manual therapy is available.
Portable Oxygen Systems	1. Regulated (adjustable --covered under conditions specified in flow rate)§60-4. Refer all claims to medical staff for this determination. 2. Preset (flow rate --deny--emergency, first-aid, or not adjustable) precautionary equipment; essentially not therapeutic in nature
Portable Paraffin Bath Units	covered when the patient has undergone a successful trial period of paraffin therapy ordered by a physician and the patient's condition is expected to be relieved by long term use of this modality.
Portable Room Heaters	deny--environmental control equipment; not primarily medical in nature (§l861(n) of the Act)
Portable Whirlpool Pumps	deny--not primarily medical in nature; personal comfort items (§§l861(n) and l862(a)(6) of the Act)
Postural Drainage Boards	covered if patient has a chronic pulmonary condition
Preset Portable Oxygen Units	deny--emergency, first-aid, or precautionary equipment; essentially not therapeutic in nature
Pressure Leotards	deny--nonreusable supply, not rental-type item (§l861(n) of the Act)

Pulse Tachometer	deny--not reasonable or necessary for monitoring pulse of homebound patient with or without a cardiac pacemaker
Quad-Canes	(See Walkers.)
Raised Toilet Seats	deny--convenience item; hygienic equipment; not primarily medical in nature (§1861(n) of the Act)
Reflectance Colorimeters	(See Blood Glucose Analyzers.)
Respirators	(See Ventilators.)
Rolling Chairs	covered if the contractor's medical staff determines that the patient's condition is such that there is a medical need for this item and it has been prescribed by the patient's physician in lieu of a wheelchair. Coverage is limited to those rollabout chairs having casters of at least 5 inches in diameter and specifically designed to meet the needs of ill, injured, or otherwise impaired individuals. Coverage is denied for the wide range of chairs with smaller casters as are found in general use in homes, offices, and institutions for many purposes not related to the care or treatment of ill or injured persons. This type is not primarily medical in nature. (§1861(n) of the Act)
Safety Roller	(See §60-15.)
Sauna Baths	deny--not primarily medical in nature; personal comfort items (§§1861(n) and (1862(a)(6) of the Act)
Seat Lift	covered under the conditions specified in §60-8. Refer all to medical staff for this determination.
Self-Contained Pacemaker Monitor	covered when prescribed by a physician for a patient with a cardiac pacemaker (See §§50-1C and 60-7.)
Sitz Bath	covered if the contractor's medical staff determines patient has an infection or injury of the perineal area and the item has been prescribed by the patient's physician as a part of his planned regimen of treatment in the patient's home.
Spare Tanks of Oxygen	deny--convenience or precautionary supply

Speech Teaching Machine	deny--education equipment; not primarily medical in nature (§1861(n) of the Act)

Stairway Elevators	deny--(See Elevators.) (§1861(n) of the Act)
Standing Table	deny--convenience item; not primarily medical in nature (§1861(n) of the Act)

Steam Packs	these packs are covered under the same condition as a heating pad (See Heating Pads.)
Suction Machine	covered if the contractor's medical staff determines that the machine specified in the claim is medically required and appropriate for home use without technical or professional supervision.
Support Hose	deny (See Fabric Supports.) (§1861(n) of the Act)
Surgical Leggings	deny--nonreusable supply; not rental-type item (§1861(n) of the Act)
Telephone Alert Systems	deny--these are emergency communications systems and do not serve a diagnostic or therapeutic purpose

Telephone Arms	deny--convenience item; not medical in nature (§1861(n) of the Act)
Toilet Seats	deny--not medical equipment (§1861(n)of the Act)
Traction Equipment	covered if patient has orthopedic impairment requiring traction equipment which prevents ambulation during the period of use (Consider covering devices usable during ambulation; e.g., cervical traction collar, under the brace provision)
Trapeze Bars	covered if patient is bed confined and the patient needs a trapeze bar to sit up because of respiratory condition, to change body position for other medical reasons, or to get in and out of bed.
Treadmill Exerciser	deny--exercise equipment; not primarily medical in nature(§1861(n) of the Act)

Ultraviolet Cabinet	covered for selected patients with generalized intractable psoriasis. Using appropriate consultation, the contractor should determine whether medical and other factors justify treatment at home rather than at alternative sites, e.g., outpatient department of a hospital.
Urinals (autoclavable hospital type)	covered if patient is bed confined
Vaporizers	covered if patient has a respiratory illness
Ventilators	covered for treatment of neuromuscular diseases, thoracic restrictive diseases, and chronic respiratory failure consequent to chronic obstructive pulmonary disease. Includes both positive and negative pressure types.
Walkers	covered if patient's condition impairs ambulation (See also §60-15.)
Water and Pressure Pads and Mattresses	(See Alternating Pressure Pads and Mattresses.)
Wheelchairs	covered if patient's condition is such that without the use of a wheelchair he would otherwise be bed or chair confined. An individual may qualify for a wheelchair and still be considered bed confined.
Wheelchairs (power operated) and wheelchairs with other special features	covered if patient's condition is such and that a wheelchair is medically necessary and the patient is unable to operate the wheelchair manually. Any claim involving a power wheelchair or a wheelchair with other special features should be referred for medical consultation since payment for the special features is limited to those which are medically required because of the patient's condition. (See §60-5 for power operated and §60-6 for specially sized wheelchairs.) NOTE: A power-operated vehicle that may appropriately be used as a wheelchair can be covered. (See §60-5 for coverage details.)

Whirlpool Bath Equipment	covered if patient is homebound and has a (standard) condition for which the whirlpool bath can be expected to provide substantial therapeutic benefit justifying its cost. Where patient is not homebound but has such a condition, payment is restricted to the cost of providing the services elsewhere; e.g., an outpatient department of a participating hospital, if that alternative is less costly. In all cases, refer claim to medical staff for a determination.
Whirlpool Pumps	deny--(See Portable Whirlpool Pumps.) (§1861(n) of the Act)

60-11 HOME BLOOD GLUCOSE MONITORS

There are several different types of blood glucose monitors that use reflectance meters to determine blood glucose levels. Medicare coverage of these devices varies, both with respect to the type of device and the medical condition of the patient for whom the device is prescribed.

Reflectance colorimeter devices used for measuring blood glucose levels in clinical settings are not covered as durable medical equipment for use in the home because their need for frequent professional re-calibration makes them unsuitable for home use. However, some types of blood glucose monitors which use a reflectance meter specifically designed for home use by diabetic patients may be covered as durable medical equipment, subject to the conditions and limitations described below.

Blood glucose monitors are meter devices that read color changes produced on specially treated reagent strips by glucose concentrations in the patient's blood. The patient, using a disposable sterile lancet, draws a drop of blood, places it on a reagent strip and, following instructions which may vary with the device used, inserts it into the device to obtain a reading. Lancets, reagent strips, and other supplies necessary for the proper functioning of the device are also covered for patients for whom the device is indicated. Home blood glucose monitors enable certain patients to better control their blood glucose levels by frequently checking and appropriately contacting their attending physician for advice and treatment. Studies indicate that the patient's ability to carefully follow proper procedures is critical to obtaining satisfactory results with these devices. In addition, the cost of the devices, with their supplies, limits economical use to patients who must make frequent checks of their blood glucose levels. Accordingly, coverage of home blood glucose monitors is limited to patients meeting the following conditions:

* The patient has been diagnosed as having diabetes;
* The patient's physician states that the patient is capable of being trained to use the particular device prescribed in an appropriate manner. In some cases, the patient may not be able to perform this function, but a responsible individual can be trained to use the equipment and monitor

the patient to assure that the intended effect is achieved. This is permissible if the record is properly documented by the patient's physician; and

* The device is designed for home rather than clinical use.

There is also a blood glucose monitoring system designed especially for use by those with visual impairments. The monitors used in such systems are identical in terms of reliability and sensitivity to the standard blood glucose monitors described above. They differ by having such features as voice synthesizers, automatic timers, and specially designed arrangements of supplies and materials to enable the visually impaired to use the equipment without assistance.

These special blood glucose monitoring systems are covered under Medicare if the following conditions are met:

* The patient and device meet the three conditions listed above for coverage of standard home blood glucose monitors; and

* The patient's physician certifies that he or she has a visual impairment severe enough to require use of this special monitoring system.

The additional features and equipment of these special systems justify a higher reimbursement amount than allowed for standard blood glucose monitors. Separately identify claims for such devices and establish a separate reimbursement amount for them. For those carriers using HCPCS, the procedure code and definition is: E0609--Blood Glucose Monitor--with special features (e.g., voice synthesizers, automatic timer).

60-14 INFUSION PUMPS

The following indications for treatment using infusion pumps are covered under medicare:

A. External Infusion Pumps.—

1. Iron Poisoning (Effective for Services Performed On or After 9/26/84).—When used in the administration of deferoxamine for the treatment of acute iron poisoning and iron overload, only external infusion pumps are covered.
2. Thromboembolic Disease (Effective for Services Performed On or After 9/26/84).—When used in the administration of heparin for the treatment of thromboembolic disease and/or pulmonary embolism, only external infusion pumps used in an institutional setting are covered.
3. Chemotherapy for Liver Cancer (Effective for Services Performed On or After 1/29/85).—The external chemotherapy infusion pump is covered when used in the treatment of primary hepatocellular carcinoma or colorectal cancer where this disease is unresectable or where the patient refuses surgical excision of the tumor.
4. Morphine for Intractable Cancer Pain (Effective for Services Performed On or After 4/22/85).—Morphine infusion via an external infusion pump is covered when used in the treatment of intractable pain caused by cancer (in either an inpatient or outpatient setting, including a hospice).

5. Continuous subcutaneous insulin infusion pumps (CSII) (Effective for Services Performed On or After 4/1/2000).—

An external infusion pump and related drugs/supplies are covered as medically necessary in the home setting in the following situation:

Treatment of Diabetes

In order to be covered, patients must meet criterion A or B:

(A)The patient has completed a comprehensive diabetes education program, and has been on a program of multiple daily injections of insulin (i.e. at least 3 injections per day), with frequent self-adjustments of insulin dose for at least 6 months prior to initiation of the insulin pump, and has documented frequency of glucose self-testing an average of at least 4 times per day during the 2 months prior to initiation of the insulin pump, and meets one or more of the following criteria while on the multiple daily injection regimen:

(1) Glycosylated hemoglobin level (HbAlc) > 7.0 percent

(2) History of recurring hypoglycemia

(3) Wide fluctuations in blood glucose before mealtime

(4) Dawn phenomenon with fasting blood sugars frequently Exceeding 200 mg/dl

(5) History of severe glycemic excursions

(B)The patient with diabetes has been on a pump prior to enrollment in Medicare and has documented frequency of glucose self-testing an average of at least 4 times per day during the month prior to Medicare enrollment.

Diabetes needs to be documented by a fasting C-peptide level that is less than or equal to 110 percent of the lower limit of normal of the laboratory's measurement method. (Effective for Services Performed on or after January 1, 2002.)

Continued coverage of the insulin pump would require that the patient has been seen and evaluated the treating physician at least every 3 months.

The pump must be ordered by and follow-up care of the patient must be managed by a physician who manages multiple patients with CSII and who works closely with a team including nurses, diabetes educators, and dietitians who are knowledgeable in the use of CSII.

6. Other uses of external infusion pumps are covered if the contractor's medical staff verifies the appropriateness of the therapy and of the prescribed pump for the individual patient.

   NOTE: Payment may also be made for drugs necessary for the effective use of an external infusion pump as long as the drug being used with the pump is itself reasonable and necessary for the patient's treatment.

B. Implantable Infusion Pumps.—

1. Chemotherapy for Liver Cancer (Effective for Services Performed On or After 9/26/84).—The implantable infusion pump is covered for intra-arterial infusion of 5-FUdR for the treatment of liver cancer for patients with primary hepatocellular carcinoma or Duke's Class D colorectal cancer, in whom the metastases are limited to the liver, and where (1) the disease is unresectable or (2) where the patient refuses surgical excision of the tumor.
2. Anti-Spasmodic Drugs for Severe Spasticity.—An implantable infusion pump is covered when used to administer anti-spasmodic drugs intrathecally (e.g., baclofen) to treat chronic intractable spasticity in patients who have proven unresponsive to less invasive medical therapy as determined by the following criteria:

   * As indicated by at least a 6-week trial, the patient cannot be maintained on noninvasive methods of spasm control, such as oral anti-spasmodic drugs, either because these methods fail to control adequately the spasticity or produce intolerable side effects, and
   * Prior to pump implantation, the patient must have responded favorably to a trial intrathecal dose of the anti-spasmodic drug.

3. Opioid Drugs for Treatment of Chronic Intractable Pain.—An implantable infusion pump is covered when used to administer opioid drugs (e.g., morphine) intrathecally or epidurally for treatment of severe chronic intractable pain of malignant or nonmalignant origin in patients who have a life expectancy of at least 3 months and who have proven unresponsive to less invasive medical therapy as determined by the following criteria:

   * The patient's history must indicate that he/she would not respond adequately to non-invasive methods of pain control, such as systemic opioids (including attempts to eliminate physical and behavioral abnormalities which may cause an exaggerated reaction to pain); and
   * A preliminary trial of intraspinal opioid drug administration must be undertaken with a temporary intrathecal/epidural catheter to substantiate adequately acceptable pain relief and degree of side effects (including effects on the activities of daily living) and patient acceptance.

4. Coverage of Other Uses of Implanted Infusion Pumps .—Determinations may be made on coverage of other uses of implanted infusion pumps if the contractor's medical staff verifies that:

   The drug is reasonable and necessary for the treatment of the individual patient;

   * It is medically necessary that the drug be administered by an implanted infusion pump; and
   * The FDA approved labeling for the pump must specify that the drug being administered and the purpose for which it is administered is an indicated use for the pump.

5. Implantation of Infusion Pump Is Contraindicated.—The implantation of an infusion pump is contraindicated in the following patients:

   * Patients with a known allergy or hypersensitivity to the drug being used (e.g., oral baclofen, morphine, etc.);
   * Patients who have an infection;
   * Patients whose body size is insufficient to support the weight and bulk of the device; and
   * Patients with other implanted programmable devices since crosstalk between devices may inadvertently change the prescription.

NOTE: Payment may also be made for drugs necessary for the effective use of an implantable infusion pump as long as the drug being used with the pump is itself reasonable and necessary for the patient's treatment.

The following indications for treatment using infusion pumps are not covered under medicare:

A. External Infusion Pumps.—

1. Vancomycin (Effective for Services Beginning On or After September 1, 1996).—Medicare coverage of vancomycin as a durable medical equipment infusion pump benefit is not covered. There is insufficient evidence to support the necessity of using an external infusion pump, instead of a disposable elastomeric pump or the gravity drip method, to administer vancomycin in a safe and appropriate manner.

B. Implantable Infusion Pump.—

1. Thromboembolic Disease (Effective for Services Performed On or After 9/26/84).—According to the Public Health Service, there is insufficient published clinical data to support the safety and effectiveness of the heparin implantable pump. Therefore, the use of an implantable infusion pump for infusion of heparin in the treatment of recurrent thromboembolic disease is not covered.
2. Diabetes—Implanted infusion pumps for the infusion of insulin to treat diabetes is not covered. The data do not demonstrate that the pump provides effective administration of insulin.

60-15 SAFETY ROLLER (Effective for Claims Adjudicated On or After 6/3/85)

"Safety roller" is the generic name applied to devices for patients who cannot use standard wheeled walkers. They may be appropriate, and therefore covered, for some patients who are obese, have severe neurological disorders, or restricted use of one hand, which makes it impossible to use a wheeled walker that does not have the sophisticated braking system found on safety rollers.

In order to assure that payment is not made for a safety roller when a less expensive standard wheeled walker would satisfy the patient's medical needs, carriers refer safety roller claims to their medical consultants. The medical consultant determines whether some or all of the features provided in a safety roller are necessary, and therefore covered and reimbursable. If it is determined that the patient could use a standard wheeled walker, the charge for the safety roller is reduced to the charge of a standard wheeled walker.

Some obese patients who could use a standard wheeled walker if their weight did not exceed the walker's strength and stability limits can have it reinforced and its wheel base expanded. Such modifications are routine mechanical adjustments and justify a moderate surcharge. In these cases the carrier reduces the charge for the safety roller to the charge for the standard wheeled walker plus the surcharge for modifications.

In the case of patients with medical documentation showing severe neurological disorders or restricted use of one hand which makes it impossible for them to use a wheeled walker that does not have a sophisticated braking system, a reasonable charge for the safety roller may be determined without relating it to the reasonable charge for a standard wheeled walker. (Such reasonable charge should be developed in accordance with the instructions in Medicare Carriers Manual §§5010 and 5205.)

Cross reference: Carriers Manual §§2100ff., §60-9.

60-16 PNEUMATIC COMPRESSION DEVICES

Pneumatic compression devices consist of an inflatable garment for the arm or leg and an electrical pneumatic pump that fills the garment with compressed air. The garment is intermittently inflated and deflated with cycle times and pressures that vary between devices. Pneumatic devices are covered for the treatment of lymphedema or for the treatment of chronic venous insufficiency with venous stasis ulcers.

Lymphedema

Lymphedema is the swelling of subcutaneous tissues due to the accumulation of excessive lymph fluid. The accumulation of lymph fluid results from impairment to the normal clearing function of the lymphatic system and/or from an excessive production of lymph. Lymphedema is divided into two broad classes according to etiology. Primary lymphedema is a relatively uncommon, chronic condition which may be due to such causes as Milroy's Disease or congenital anomalies. Secondary lymphedema, which is much more common, results from the destruction of or damage to formerly functioning lymphatic channels, such as surgical removal of lymph nodes or post radiation fibrosis, among other causes.

Pneumatic compression devices are covered in the home setting for the treatment of lymphedema if the patient has undergone a four-week trial of conservative therapy and the treating physician determines that there has been no significant improvement or if significant symptoms remain after the trial. The trial of conservative therapy must include use of an appropriate compression bandage system or compression garment, exercise, and elevation of the limb. The garment may be prefabricated or custom-fabricated but must provide adequate graduated compression.

Chronic Venous Insufficiency with Venous Stasis Ulcers

Chronic venous insufficiency (CVI) of the lower extremities is a condition caused by abnormalities of the venous wall and valves, leading to obstruction or reflux of blood flow in the veins. Signs of CVI include hyperpigmentation, stasis dermatitis, chronic edema, and venous ulcers.

Pneumatic compression devices are covered in the home setting for the treatment of CVI of the lower extremities only if the patient has one or more venous stasis ulcer(s) which have failed to heal after a 6 month trial of conservative therapy directed by the treating physician. The trial of conservative therapy must include a compression bandage system or compression garment, appropriate dressings for the wound, exercise, and elevation of the limb.

General Coverage Criteria

Pneumatic compression devices are covered only when prescribed by a physician and when they are used with appropriate physician oversight, i.e., physician evaluation of the patient's condition to determine medical necessity of the device, assuring suitable instruction in the operation of the machine, a treatment plan defining the pressure to be used and the frequency and duration of use, and ongoing monitoring of use and response to treatment.

The determination by the physician of the medical necessity of a pneumatic compression device must include (1) the patient's diagnosis and prognosis; (2) symptoms and objective findings, including measurements which establish the severity of the condition; (3) the reason the device is required, including the treatments which have been tried and failed; and (4) the clinical response to an initial treatment with the device. The clinical response includes the change in pre-treatment measurements, ability to tolerate the treatment session and parameters, and ability of the patient (or caregiver) to apply the device for continued use in the home.

The only time that a segmented, calibrated gradient pneumatic compression device (HCPCS code E0652) would be covered is when the individual has unique characteristics that prevent them from receiving satisfactory pneumatic compression treatment using a nonsegmented device in conjunction with a segmented appliance or a segmented compression device without manual control of pressure in each chamber.

Cross reference: §60-9.

60-17 CONTINUOUS POSITIVE AIRWAY PRESSURE (CPAP)

CPAP is a non-invasive technique for providing single levels of air pressure from a flow generator, via a nose mask, through the nares. The purpose is to prevent the collapse of the oropharyngeal walls and the obstruction of airflow during sleep, which occurs in obstructive sleep apnea (OSA).

Effective for services furnished between and including January 12, 1987 and March 31, 2002:

The diagnosis of OSA requires documentation of at least 30 episodes of apnea, each lasting a minimum of 10 seconds, during 6-7 hours of recorded sleep. The use of CPAP is covered under Medicare when used in adult patients with moderate or severe OSA for whom surgery is a likely alternative to CPAP.

Initial claims must be supported by medical documentation (separate documentation where electronic billing is used), such as a prescription written by the patient's attending physician, that specifies:

* a diagnosis of moderate or severe obstructive sleep apnea, and
* surgery is a likely alternative.

The claim must also certify that the documentation supporting a diagnosis of OSA (described above) is available.

Effective for services furnished on or after April 1, 2002:

The use of CPAP devices are covered under Medicare when ordered and prescribed by the licensed treating physician to be used in adult patients with OSA if either of the following criteria using the Apnea-Hypopnea Index (AHI) are met:

* AHI = 15 events per hour, or
* AHI = 5 and = 14 events per hour with documented symptoms of excessive daytime sleepiness, impaired cognition, mood disorders or insomnia, or documented hypertension, ischemic heart disease or history of stroke.

The AHI is equal to the average number of episodes of apnea and hypopnea per hour and must be based on a minimum of 2 hours of sleep recorded by polysomnography using actual recorded hours of sleep (i.e., the AHI may not be extrapolated or projected).

Apnea is defined as a cessation of airflow for at least 10 seconds. Hypopnea is defined as an abnormal respiratory event lasting at least 10 seconds with at least a 30% reduction in thoracoabdominal movement or airflow as compared to baseline, and with at least a 4% oxygen desaturation.

The polysomnography must be performed in a facility - based sleep study laboratory, and not in the home or in a mobile facility.

Initial claims for CPAP devices must be supported by information contained in the medical record indicating that the patient meets Medicare's stated coverage criteria.

Cross reference: §60-9.

60-18 HOSPITAL BEDS

A. General Requirements for Coverage of Hospital Beds.—A physician's prescription, and such additional documentation as the contractors' medical staffs may consider necessary, including medical records and physicians' reports, must establish the medical necessity for a hospital bed due to one of the following reasons:

* The patient's condition requires positioning of the body; e.g., to alleviate pain, promote good body alignment, prevent contractures, avoid respiratory infections, in ways not feasible in an ordinary bed; or
* The patient's condition requires special attachments that cannot be fixed and used on an ordinary bed.

B. Physician's Prescription.—The physician's prescription, which must accompany the initial claim, and supplementing documentation when required, must establish that a hospital bed is medically necessary. If the stated reason for the need for a hospital bed is the patient's condition requires positioning, the prescription or other documentation must describe the medical condition, e.g., cardiac disease, chronic obstructive pulmonary disease, quadriplegia or paraplegia, and also the severity and frequency of the symptoms of the condition, that necessitates a hospital bed for positioning.

If the stated reason for requiring a hospital bed is the patient's condition requires special attachments, the prescription must describe the patient's condition and specify the attachments that require a hospital bed.

C. Variable Height Feature.—In well documented cases, the contractors' medical staffs may determine that a variable height feature of a hospital bed, approved for coverage under subsection A above, is medically necessary and, therefore, covered, for one of the following conditions:

* Severe arthritis and other injuries to lower extremities; e.g., fractured hip. The condition requires the variable height feature to assist the patient to ambulate by enabling the patient to place his or her feet on the floor while sitting on the edge of the bed;
* Severe cardiac conditions. For those cardiac patients who are able to leave bed, but who must avoid the strain of "jumping" up or down;
* Spinal cord injuries, including quadriplegic and paraplegic patients, multiple limb amputee and stroke patients. For those patients who are able to transfer from bed to a wheelchair, with or without help; or
* Other severely debilitating diseases and conditions, if the variable height feature is required to assist the patient to ambulate.

D. Electric Powered Hospital Bed Adjustments.—Electric powered adjustments to lower and raise head and foot may be covered when the contractor's medical staff determines that the patient's condition requires frequent change in body position and/or there may be an immediate need for a change in body position (i.e., no delay can be tolerated) and the patient can operate the controls and cause the adjustments. Exceptions may be made to this last requirement in cases of spinal cord injury and brain damaged patients.

E. Side Rails.—If the patient's condition requires bed side rails, they can be covered when an integral part of, or an accessory to, a hospital bed.

Cross reference: Carriers Manual, §5015.4

60-19 AIR-FLUIDIZED BED (Effective for services rendered on or after: 07/30/90)

An air-fluidized bed uses warm air under pressure to set small ceramic beads in motion which simulate the movement of fluid. When the patient is placed in the bed, his body weight is evenly distributed over a large surface area which creates a sensation of "floating." Medicare payment for home use of the air-fluidized bed for treatment of pressure sores can be made if such use is reasonable and necessary for the individual patient.

A decision that use of an air-fluidized bed is reasonable and necessary requires that:

* The patient has a stage 3 (full thickness tissue loss) or stage 4 (deep tissue destruction) pressure sore;
* The patient is bedridden or chair bound as a result of severely limited mobility;
* In the absence of an air-fluidized bed, the patient would require institutionalization;
* The air-fluidized bed is ordered in writing by the patient's attending physician based upon a comprehensive assessment and evaluation of the patient after completion of a course of conservative treatment designed to optimize conditions that promote wound healing. This course of treatment must have been at least one month in duration without progression toward wound healing. This month of prerequisite conservative treatment may include some period in an institution as long as there is documentation available to verify that the necessary conservative treatment has been rendered.
* Use of wet-to-dry dressings for wound debridement, begun during the period of conservative treatment and which continue beyond 30 days, will not preclude coverage of air-fluidized bed. Should additional debridement again become necessary, while a patient is using an air-fluidized bed (after the first 30-day course of conservative treatment) that will not cause the air-fluidized bed to become non-covered. In all instances documentation verifying the continued need for the bed must be available.
* Conservative treatment must include:
    - Frequent repositioning of the patient with particular attention to relief of pressure over bony prominences (usually every 2 hours);
    - Use of a specialized support surface (Group II) designed to reduce pressure and shear forces on healing ulcers and to prevent new ulcer formation;

- Necessary treatment to resolve any wound infection;
- Optimization of nutrition status to promote wound healing;
- Debridement by any means (including wet to dry dressings-which does not require an occlusive covering) to remove devitalized tissue from the wound bed;
- Maintenance of a clean, moist bed of granulation tissue with appropriate moist dressings protected by an occlusive covering, while the wound heals.

* A trained adult caregiver is available to assist the patient with activities of daily living, fluid balance, dry skin care, repositioning, recognition and management of altered mental status, dietary needs, prescribed treatments, and management and support of the air-fluidized bed system and its problems such as leakage;
* A physician directs the home treatment regimen, and reevaluates and recertifies the need for the air-fluidized bed on a monthly basis; and
* All other alternative equipment has been considered and ruled out.

Home use of the air-fluidized bed is not covered under any of the following circumstances:

* The patient has coexisting pulmonary disease (the lack of firm back support makes coughing ineffective and dry air inhalation thickens pulmonary secretions);
* The patient requires treatment with wet soaks or moist wound dressings that are not protected with an impervious covering such as plastic wrap or other occlusive material; an air-fluidized bed;
* The caregiver is unwilling or unable to provide the type of care required by the patient on an air-fluidized bed;
* Structural support is inadequate to support the weight of the air-fluidized bed system (it generally weighs 1600 pounds or more);
* Electrical system is insufficient for the anticipated increase in energy consumption; or
* Other known contraindications exist.

Coverage of an air-fluidized bed is limited to the equipment itself. Payment for this covered item may only be made if the written order from the attending physician is furnished to the supplier prior to the delivery of the equipment. Payment is not included for the caregiver or for architectural adjustments such as electrical or structural improvement.

Cross reference: Carriers Manual, §5102.2.

60-21 INTRAPULMONARY PERCUSSIVE VENTILATOR (IPV)—NOT COVERED

IPV is a mechanized form of chest physical therapy. Instead of a therapist clapping or slapping the patient's chest wall, the IPV delivers mini-bursts (more than 200 per minute) of respiratory gasses to the lungs via a mouthpiece. Its intended purpose is to mobilize endobronchial secretions and diffuse patchy atelectasis. The patient controls variables such as inspiratory time, peak pressure and delivery rates.

Studies do not demonstrate any advantage of IPV over that achieved with good pulmonary care in the hospital environment and there are no studies in the home setting. There are no data to support the effectiveness of the device. Therefore, IPV in the home setting is not covered.

60-23 SPEECH GENERATING DEVICES

Effective January 1, 2001, augmentative and alternative communication devices or communicators, which are hereafter referred to as "speech generating devices" are now considered to fall within the DME benefit category established by §1861(n) of the Social Security Act. They may be covered if the contractor's medical staff determines that the patient suffers from a severe speech impairment and that the medical condition warrants the use of a device based on the following definitions.

Definition of Speech Generating Devices

Speech generating devices are defined as speech aids that provide an individual who has a severe speech impairment with the ability to meet his functional speaking needs. Speech generating are characterized by:

* Being a dedicated speech device, used solely by the individual who has a severe speech impairment;
* May have digitized speech output, using pre-recorded messages, less than or equal to 8 minutes recording time;
* May have digitized speech output, using pre-recorded messages, greater than 8 minutes recording time;
* May have synthesized speech output, which requires message formulation by spelling and device access by physical contact with the device-direct selection techniques;
* May have synthesized speech output, which permits multiple methods of message formulation and multiple methods of device access; or
* May be software that allows a laptop computer, desktop computer or personal digital assistant (PDA) to function as a speech generating device.

Devices that would not meet the definition of speech generating devices and therefore, do not fall within the scope of §1861(n) are characterized by:

* Devices that are not dedicated speech devices, but are devices that are capable of running software for purposes other than for speech generation, e.g., devices that can also run a word processing package, an accounting program, or perform other non-medical function.
* Laptop computers, desktop computers, or PDAs, which may be programmed to perform the same function as a speech generating device, are non-covered since they are not primarily medical in nature and do not meet the definition of DME. For this reason, they cannot be considered speech generating devices for Medicare coverage purposes.

* A device that is useful to someone without severe speech impairment is not considered a speech generating device for Medicare coverage purposes.

60-24 NON-IMPLANTABLE PELVIC FLOOR ELECTRICAL STIMULATOR

Non-implantable pelvic floor electrical stimulators provide neuromuscular electrical stimulation through the pelvic floor with the intent of strengthening and exercising pelvic floor musculature. Stimulation is generally delivered by vaginal or anal probes connected to an external pulse generator.

The methods of pelvic floor electrical stimulation vary in location, stimulus frequency (Hz), stimulus intensity or amplitude (mA), pulse duration (duty cycle), treatments per day, number of treatment days per week, length of time for each treatment session, overall time period for device use and between clinic and home settings. In general, the stimulus frequency and other parameters are chosen based on the patient's clinical diagnosis.

Pelvic floor electrical stimulation with a non-implantable stimulator is covered for the treatment of stress and/or urge urinary incontinence in cognitively intact patients who have failed a documented trial of pelvic muscle exercise (PME) training.

A failed trial of PME training is defined as no clinically significant improvement in urinary continence after completing 4 weeks of an ordered plan of pelvic muscle exercises designed to increase periurethral muscle strength.

65-1 HYDROPHILIC CONTACT LENSES

Hydrophilic contact lenses are eyeglasses within the meaning of the exclusion in §l862(a)(7) of the law and are not covered when used in the treatment of nondiseased eyes with spherical ametrophia, refractive astigmatism, and/or corneal astigmatism. Payment may be made under the prosthetic device benefit, however, for hydrophilic contact lenses when prescribed for an aphakic patient.

Contractors are authorized to accept an FDA letter of approval or other FDA published material as evidence of FDA approval.

(See §45-7 for coverage of a hydrophilic lens as a corneal bandage.) Cross-reference: Intermediary Manual, §§3110.3, 3110.4, 3151, and 3157; Carriers Manual, §§2130, 2320; Hospital Manual, §§228.3, 228.4, 260.1 and 260.7.

65-3 SCLERAL SHELL

Scleral shell (or shield) is a catchall term for different types of hard scleral contact lenses.

A scleral shell fits over the entire exposed surface of the eye as opposed to a corneal contact lens which covers only the central non-white area encompassing the pupil and iris. Where an eye has been rendered sightless and shrunken by inflammatory disease, a scleral shell may, among other things, obviate the need for surgical enucleation and prosthetic implant and act to support the surrounding orbital tissue.

In such a case, the device serves essentially as an artificial eye. In this situation, payment may be made for a scleral shell under §1861(s)(8) of the law.

Scleral shells are occasionally used in combination with artificial tears in the treatment of "dry eye" of diverse etiology. Tears ordinarily dry at a rapid rate, and are continually replaced by the lacrimal gland. When the lacrimal gland fails, the half-life of artificial tears may be greatly prolonged by the use of the scleral contact lens as a protective barrier against the drying action of the atmosphere. Thus, the difficult and sometimes hazardous process of frequent installation of artificial tears may be avoided. The lens acts in this instance to substitute, in part, for the functioning of the diseased lacrimal gland and would be covered as a prosthetic device in the rare case when it is used in the treatment of "dry eye."

Cross-reference: HCFA-Pub. 13-3, §§3110.4, 3110.5; HCFA-Pub. 14-3, §§2130, 2133; HCFA- Pub. 10, §§210.4, 211

65-5 ELECTRONIC SPEECH AIDS

Electronic speech aids are covered under Part B as prosthetic devices when the patient has had a laryngectomy or his larynx is permanently inoperative. There are two types of speech aids. One operates by placing a vibrating head against the throat; the other amplifies sound waves through a tube which is inserted into the user's mouth. A patient who has had radical neck surgery and/or extensive radiation to the anterior part of the neck would generally be able to use only the "oral tube" model or one of the more sensitive and more expensive "throat contact" devices.

Cross-reference: HCFA-Pub. 13-3, §3110.4; HCFA-Pub. 14-3, §2130; HCFA-Pub. 10, §228.4

65-7 INTRAOCULAR LENSES (IOLs)

An intraocular lens, or pseudophakos, is an artificial lens which may be implanted to replace the natural lens after cataract surgery. Intraocular lens implantation services, as well as the lens itself,may be covered if reasonable and necessary for the individual. Implantation services may include hospital, surgical, and other medical services, including pre-implantation ultrasound (A-can) eye measurement of one or both eyes.

Cross-reference: HCFA Pub. 13-3, §§3110.4, 3151, and 3157; HCFA Pub.14-3, §2130; HCFA Pub. 10, §228.4

65-8 ELECTRICAL NERVE STIMULATORS

Two general classifications of electrical nerve stimulators are employed to treat chronic intractable pain: peripheral nerve stimulators and central nervous system stimulators.

A. Implanted Peripheral Nerve Stimulators.—Payment may be made under the prosthetic device benefit for implanted peripheral nerve stimulators. Use of this stimulator involves implantation of electrodes around a selected peripheral nerve. The stimulating electrode is connected by an insulated lead to a receiver unit which is implanted under the skin at a depth not greater than 1/2 inch. Stimulation is induced by a generator connected to an antenna unit which is attached to the skin surface over the receiver unit. Implantation of electrodes requires surgery and usually necessitates an operating room.

NOTE: Peripheral nerve stimulators may also be employed to assess a patient's suitability for continued treatment with an electric nerve stimulator. As explained in §35-46, such use of the stimulator is covered as part of the total diagnostic service furnished to the beneficiary rather than as a prosthesis.

B. Central Nervous System Stimulators (Dorsal Column and Depth Brain Stimulators).—The implantation of central nervous system stimulators may be covered as therapies for the relief of chronic intractable pain, subject to the following conditions:

1 Types of Implantations.—There are two types of implantations covered by this instruction:

a. Dorsal Column (Spinal Cord) Neurostimulation.—The surgical implantation of neurostimulator electrodes within the dura mater (endodural) or the percutaneous insertion of electrodes in the epidural space is covered.

b. Depth Brain Neurostimulation.—The stereotactic implantation of electrodes in the deep brain (e.g., thalamus and periaqueductal gray matter) is covered.

2. Conditions for Coverage.—No payment may be made for the implantation of dorsal column or depth brain stimulators or services and supplies related to such implantation, unless all of the conditions listed below have been met:

a. The implantation of the stimulator is used only as a late resort (if not a last resort) for patients with chronic intractable pain;

b. With respect to item a, other treatment modalities (pharmacological, surgical, physical, or psychological therapies) have been tried and did not prove satisfactory, or are judged to be unsuitable or contraindicated for the given patient;

c. Patients have undergone careful screening, evaluation and diagnosis by a multidisciplinary team prior to implantation. (Such screening must include psychological, as well as physical evaluation);

d. All the facilities, equipment, and professional and support personnel required for the proper diagnosis, treatment training, and followup of the patient (including that required to satisfy item c) must be available; and

e. Demonstration of pain relief with a temporarily implanted electrode precedes permanent implantation.

Contractors may find it helpful to work with PROs to obtain the information needed to apply these conditions to claims.

See Intermediary Manual, §3110.4 and §§35-20 and 35-27.

65-9 INCONTINENCE CONTROL DEVICE

A. Mechanical/Hydraulic Incontinence Control Devices. Mechanical/hydraulic incontinence control devices are accepted as safe and effective in the management of urinary incontinence in patients with permanent anatomic and neurologic dysfunctions of the bladder. This class of devices achieves control of urination by compression of the urethra. The materials used and the success rate may vary somewhat from device to device. Such a device is covered when its use is reasonable and necessary for the individual patient.

B. Collagen Implant.—A collagen implant, which is injected into the submucosal tissues of the urethra and/or the bladder neck and into tissues adjacent to the urethra, is a prosthetic device used in the treatment of stress urinary incontinence resulting from intrinsic sphincter deficiency (ISD). ISD is a cause of stress urinary incontinence in which the urethral sphincter is unable to contract and generate sufficient resistance in the bladder, especially during stress maneuvers.

Prior to collagen implant therapy, a skin test for collagen sensitivity must be administered and evaluated over a 4 week period.

In male patients, the evaluation must include a complete history and physical examination and a simple cystometrogram to determine that the bladder fills and stores properly. The patient then is asked to stand upright with a full bladder and to cough or otherwise exert abdominal pressure on his bladder. If the patient leaks, the diagnosis of ISD is established.

In female patients, the evaluation must include a complete history and physical examination (including a pelvic exam) and a simple cystometrogram to rule out abnormalities of bladder compliance and abnormalities of urethral support. Following that determination, an abdominal leak point pressure (ALLP) test is performed. Leak point pressure, stated in cm H2O, is defined as the intra-abdominal pressure at which leakage occurs from the bladder (around a catheter) when the bladder has been filled with a minimum of 150 cc fluid. If the patient has an ALLP of less than 100 cm H2O, the diagnosis of ISD is established.

To use a collagen implant, physicians must have urology training in the use of a cystoscope and must complete a collagen implant training program.

Coverage of a collagen implant, and the procedure to inject it, is limited to the following types of patients with stress urinary incontinence due to ISD:

* Male or female patients with congenital sphincter weakness secondary to conditions such as myelomeningocele or epispadias;

* Male or female patients with acquired sphincter weakness secondary to spinal cord lesions;
* Male patients following trauma, including prostatectomy and/or radiation; and
* Female patients without urethral hypermobility and with abdominal leak point pressures of 100 cm H2O or less.

Patients whose incontinence does not improve with 5 injection procedures (5 separate treatment sessions) are considered treatment failures, and no further treatment of urinary incontinence by collagen implant is covered. Patients who have a reoccurrence of incontinence following successful treatment with collagen implants in the past (e.g., 6-12 months previously) may benefit from additional treatment sessions. Coverage of additional sessions may be allowed but must be supported by medical justification.

See Intermediary Manual, §3110.4.

65-10 ENTERAL AND PARENTERAL NUTRITIONAL THERAPY COVERED AS PROSTHETIC DEVICE (Effective for items and services furnished on or after 07-11-84.)

There are patients who, because of chronic illness or trauma, cannot be sustained through oral feeding. These people must rely on either enteral or parenteral nutritional therapy, depending upon the particular nature of their medical condition.

Coverage of nutritional therapy as a Part B benefit is provided under the prosthetic device benefit provision, which requires that the patient must have a permanently inoperative internal body organ or function thereof. (See Intermediary Manual, §3110.4.) Therefore, enteral and parenteral nutritional therapy are not covered under Part B in situations involving temporary impairments. Coverage of such therapy, however, does not require a medical judgment that the impairment giving rise to the therapy will persist throughout the patient's remaining years. If the medical record, including the judgment of the attending physician, indicates that the impairment will be of long and indefinite duration, the test of permanence is considered met.

If the coverage requirements for enteral or parenteral nutritional therapy are met under the prosthetic device benefit provision, related supplies, equipment and nutrients are also covered under the conditions in the following paragraphs and the Intermediary Manual, §3110.4.

65-10.1 Parenteral Nutrition Therapy.—Daily parenteral nutrition is considered reasonable and necessary for a patient with severe pathology of the alimentary tract which does not allow absorption of sufficient nutrients to maintain weight and strength commensurate with the patient's general condition.

Since the alimentary tract of such a patient does not function adequately, an indwelling catheter is placed percutaneously in the subclavian vein and then advanced into the superior vena cava where intravenous infusion of nutrients is given for part of the day. The catheter is then plugged by the patient until the next infusion. Following a period of hospitalization, which is required to initiate parenteral nutrition and to train the patient in catheter care, solution preparation, and infusion technique, the parenteral nutrition can be provided safely and effectively in the patient's home by nonprofessional persons who have undergone special training. However, such persons cannot be paid for their services, nor is payment available for any services furnished by nonphysician professionals except as services furnished incident to a physician's service.

For parenteral nutrition therapy to be covered under Part B, the claim must contain a physician's written order or prescription and sufficient medical documentation to permit an independent conclusion that the requirements of the prosthetic device benefit are met and that parenteral nutrition therapy is medically necessary. An example of a condition that typically qualifies for coverage is a massive small bowel resection resulting in severe nutritional deficiency in spite of adequate oral intake. However, coverage of parenteral nutrition therapy for this and any other condition must be approved on an individual, case-by-case basis initially and at periodic intervals of no more than 3 months by the carrier's medical consultant or specially trained staff, relying on such medical and other documentation as the carrier may require. If the claim involves an infusion pump, sufficient evidence must be provided to support a determination of medical necessity for the pump. Program payment for the pump is based on the reasonable charge for the simplest model that meets the medical needs of the patient as established by medical documentation.

Nutrient solutions for parenteral therapy are routinely covered. However, Medicare pays for no more than one month's supply of nutrients at any one time. Payment for the nutrients is based on the reasonable charge for the solution components unless the medical record, including a signed statement from the attending physician, establishes that the beneficiary, due to his/her physical or mental state, is unable to safely or effectively mix the solution and there is no family member or other person who can do so. Payment will be on the basis of the reasonable charge for more expensive pre-mixed solutions only under the latter circumstances.

65-10.2 Enteral Nutrition Therapy.—Enteral nutrition is considered reasonable and necessary for a patient with a functioning gastrointestinal tract who, due to pathology to or nonfunction of the structures that normally permit food to reach the digestive tract, cannot maintain weight and strength commensurate with his or her general condition. Enteral therapy may be given by nasogastric, jejunostomy, or gastrostomy tubes and can be provided safely and effectively in the home by nonprofessional persons who have undergone special training. However, such persons cannot be paid for their services, nor is payment available for any services furnished by nonphysician professionals except as services furnished incident to a physician's service.

Typical examples of conditions that qualify for coverage are head and neck cancer with reconstructive surgery and central nervous system disease leading to interference with the neuromuscular mechanisms of ingestion of such severity that the beneficiary cannot be maintained with oral feeding. However, claims for Part B coverage of enteral nutrition therapy for these and any other conditions must be approved on an individual, case-by-case basis. Each claim must contain a physician's written order or prescription and sufficient medical documentation (e.g., hospital records, clinical findings from the attending physician) to permit an independent conclusion that the patient's condition meets the requirements of the prosthetic device benefit and that enteral nutrition therapy is medically necessary. Allowed claims are to be reviewed at periodic intervals of no more than 3 months by the contractor's medical consultant or specially trained staff, and additional medical documentation considered necessary is to be obtained as part of this review.

Medicare pays for no more than one month's supply of enteral nutrients at any one time.

If the claim involves a pump, it must be supported by sufficient medical documentation to establish that the pump is medically necessary, i.e., gravity feeding is not satisfactory due to aspiration, diarrhea, dumping syndrome. Program payment for the pump is based on the reasonable charge for the simplest model that meets the medical needs of the patient as established by medical documentation.

65-10.3 Nutritional Supplementation.—Some patients require supplementation of their daily protein and caloric intake. Nutritional supplements are often given as a medicine between meals to boost protein-caloric intake or the mainstay of a daily nutritional plan. Nutritional supplementation is not covered under Medicare Part B.

65-14 COCHLEAR IMPLANTATION

A cochlear implant device is an electronic instrument, part of which is implanted surgically to stimulate auditory nerve fibers, and part of which is worn or carried by the individual to capture, analyze and code sound. Cochlear implant devices are available in single channel and multi-channel models. The purpose of implanting the device is to provide an awareness and identification of sounds and to facilitate communication for persons who are profoundly hearing impaired.
Medicare coverage is provided only for those patients who meet all of the following selection guidelines.

A. General.—

* Diagnosis of bilateral severe-to-profound sensorineural hearing impairment with limited benefit from appropriate hearing (or vibrotactile) aids;
* Cognitive ability to use auditory clues and a willingness to undergo an extended program of rehabilitation;
* Freedom from middle ear infection, an accessible cochlear lumen that is structurally suited to implantation, and freedom from lesions in the auditory nerve and acoustic areas of the central nervous system;
* No contraindications to surgery; and
* The device must be used in accordance with the FDA-approved labeling.

B. Adults.—Cochlear implants may be covered for adults (over age 18) for prelinguistically, perilinguistically, and postlinguistically deafened adults. Postlinguistically deafened adults must demonstrate test scores of 30 percent or less on sentence recognition scores from tape recorded tests in the patient's best listening condition.

C. Children.—Cochlear implants may be covered for prelinguistically and postlinguistically deafened children aged 2 through 17. Bilateral profound sensorineural deafness must be demonstrated by the inability to improve on age appropriate closed-set word identification tasks with amplification.

65-16 TRACHEOSTOMY SPEAKING VALVE

A trachea tube has been determined to satisfy the definition of a prosthetic device, and the tracheostomy speaking valve is an add on to the trachea tube which may be considered a medically necessary accessory that enhances the function of the tube. In other words, it makes the system a better prosthesis. As such, a tracheostomy speaking valve is covered as an element of the trachea tube which makes the tube more effective.

70-1 CORSET USED AS HERNIA SUPPORT

A hernia support (whether in the form of a corset or truss) which meets the definition of a brace is covered under Part B under §1861(s)(9) of the Act.

See Intermediary Manual, §3110.5; Medicare Carriers Manual, §2133; and Hospital Manual, §228.5.

70-2 SYKES HERNIA CONTROL

Based on professional advice, it has been determined that the Sykes hernia control (a spring-type, U-shaped, strapless truss) is not functionally more beneficial than a conventional truss. Make program reimbursement for this device only when an ordinary truss would be covered. (Like all trusses, it is only of benefit when dealing with a reducible hernia). Thus, when a charge for this item is substantially in excess of that which would be reasonable for a conventional truss used for the same condition, base reimbursement on the reasonable charges for the conventional truss.

See Intermediary Manual, §3110.5; Medicare Carriers Manual, §2133; and Hospital Manual, §228.5.

MEDICARE CARRIERS MANUAL (MCM) REFERENCES

The following Medicare references refer to policy issues identified in the main body of the HCPCS code section. Medicare Carriers Manual references are identified with the term MCM: followed by the reference number(s). .

2000 COVERED MEDICAL AND OTHER HEALTH SERVICES

The supplementary medical insurance plan covers expenses incurred for the following medical and other health services:

1. Physician's services, including surgery, consultation, and office, and institutional calls, and services and supplies furnished incident to a physician's professional service;
2. Outpatient hospital services furnished incident to physicians services;
3. Outpatient diagnostic services furnished by a hospital;
4. Outpatient physical therapy; outpatient speech pathology services;
5. Diagnostic X-ray tests, laboratory tests, and other diagnostic tests;
6. X-ray, radium, and radioactive isotope therapy;
7. Surgical dressings, and splints, casts, and other devices used for reduction of fractures and dislocations;
8. Rental or purchase of durable medical equipment for use in the patient's home;
9. Ambulance service;
10. Prosthetic devices which replace all or part of an internal body organ;
11. Leg, arm, back and neck braces and artificial legs, arms, and eyes;
12. Certain medical supplies used in connection with home dialysis delivery systems;
13. Rural health clinic (RHC) services.
14. Ambulatory surgical center (ASC) services.

(See §2255 for provisions regarding supplementary medical insurance coverage of certain of these services when furnished to hospital and SNF inpatients.)

Supplementary medical insurance also provides coverage for home health visits for which the intermediary makes payment on the basis of the reasonable cost. Outpatient hospital services are also reimbursed by the intermediary.

Some medical services may be considered for coverage under more than one of the above enumerated categories. For example, EKGs can be covered as physician's services, services incident to a physician's service or as other diagnostic tests. It is sufficient to determine that the requirements for coverage under one category are met to permit payment.

Payment for physician services and medical and other health services rendered to beneficiaries is made on a reasonable charge basis. Make payment to the beneficiary, or the physician or supplier who renders the service, depending on whether the itemized bill or assignment method is used. Payment for medical services performed by a provider-based physician is made to the physician or beneficiary or, when the physician authorizes it, to the provider. When covered medical and other health services are furnished by a nonparticipating skilled nursing facility, make payment to the SNF or to the beneficiary on the basis of the reasonable charge.

An organization which furnishes medical and other health services on a prepayment basis may elect to be paid on the basis of reasonable costs in lieu of reasonable charges.

Payment may not be made under Part B for services furnished an individual if he is entitled to have payment made for those services under Part A. An individual is considered entitled to have payment made under Part A if the expenses incurred were used to satisfy a Part A deductible or coinsurance amount, or if payment would be made under Part A except for the lack of a request for payment or physician certification.
When covered Part B services are furnished by a participating hospital, skilled nursing facility, or home health agency, the intermediary makes payment on a reasonable cost basis to the provider only. Outpatient physical therapy or speech pathology providers are reimbursed on a reasonable cost basis by the designated intermediary or carrier.

Where covered Part B services are furnished by a nonparticipating hospital, the emergency intermediary makes payment on the basis of reasonable charges to the hospital or to the patient.

Membership dues, subscription fees, charges for service policies, insurance premium and other payments analogous to premiums which entitle enrollees to services or to repairs or replacement of devices or equipment or parts therefore without charge or at a reduced charge, are not considered expenses incurred for covered items or services furnished under such contracts or undertakings. Examples of such arrangements are memberships in ambulance companies, insurance for replacement of prosthetic lenses, and service contracts for durable medical equipment.

2005.1 Physicians' Expense for Surgery, Childbirth, and Treatment for Infertility

A. Surgery and Childbirth.—Skilled medical management is appropriate throughout the events of pregnancy, beginning with diagnosis, continuing through delivery and ending after the necessary postnatalcare. Similarly, in the event of termination of pregnancy,regardless of whether terminated spontaneously or for therapeutic reasons (i.e., where the life of the mother would be endangered if the fetus were brought to term), the need for skilled medical management and/or medical services is equally important as in those cases carried to full term.After the infant is delivered and is a separate individual, items and services furnished to the infant are not covered on the basis of the mother's eligibility.

   Most surgeons and obstetricians bill patients an all inclusive package charge intended to cover all services associated with the surgical procedure or delivery of the child. All expenses for surgical and obstetrical care, including preoperative/prenatal examinations and tests and postoperative/postnatal services are considered incurred on the date of surgery or delivery, as appropriate. This policy applies whether the physician bills on a package charge basis, or itemizes his/her bill separately for these items.

Occasionally, a physician's bill may include charges for additional services not directly related to the surgical procedure or the delivery. Such charges are considered incurred on the date the additional services are furnished.

The above policy applies only where the charges are imposed by one physician or by a clinic on behalf of a group of physicians. Where charges are imposed by more than one physician for surgical or obstetrical services, all preoperative/prenatal and postoperative/postnatal services performed by the physician who performed the surgery or delivery are considered incurred on the date of the surgery or delivery. Expenses for services rendered by other physicians are considered incurred on the date they were performed. for services rendered by other physicians are considered incurred on the date they were performed.

B. Treatment for Infertility.—Reasonable and necessary services associated with treatment forinfertility are covered under Medicare. Infertility is a condition sufficiently at variance with the usual state of health to make it appropriate for a person who normally is expected to be fertile to seek medical consultation and treatment. Coordinate with PROs to see that utilization guidelines are established for this treatment if inappropriate utilization or abuse is suspected.

2049 DRUGS AND BIOLOGICALS

The Medicare program provides limited benefits for outpatient drugs. The program covers drugs that are furnished "incident to" a physician's service provided that the drugs are not usually self-administered by the patients who take them.

Generally, drugs and biologicals are covered only if all of the following requirements are met:

* They meet the definition of drugs or biologicals (see §2049.1);
* They are of the type that are not usually self-administered by the patients who take them. (See §2049.2);
* They meet all the general requirements for coverage of items as incident to a physician's services (see § §2050.1 and 2050.3);
* They are reasonable and necessary for the diagnosis or treatment of the illness or injury for which they are administered according to accepted standards of medical practice (see §2049.4);
* They are not excluded as immunizations (see §2049.4.B); and
* They have not been determined by the FDA to be less than effective. (See §2049.4 D.)

Drugs that are usually self-administered by the patient, such as those in pill form, or are used for self-injection, are generally not covered by Part B. However, there are a limited number of self-administered drugs that are covered because the Medicare statute explicitly provides coverage. Examples of self-administered drugs that are covered include blood clotting factors, drugs used in immunosuppressive therapy, erythropoietin for dialysis patients, osteoporosis drugs for certain homebound patients, and certain oral cancer drugs.

(See §§2100.5 and 2130.D for coverage of drugs which are necessary to the effective use of DME or prosthetic devices.)

2049.1 Definition of Drug or Biological.--DRUGS AND BIOLOGICALS MUST BE DETERMINED TO MEET THE STATUTORY DEFINITION.

Section 1861(t)(1) provides that the terms "drugs" and "biologicals" "include only such drugs (including contrast agents) and biologicals, respectively, as are included (or approved for inclusion) in one of several pharmacopoeias (except for any drugs and biologicals unfavorably evaluated therein), or as are approved by the pharmacy and drug therapeutics committee (or equivalent committee) of the medical staff of the hospital furnishing such drugs and biologicals for use in such hospital." One such pharmacopeia is the United States Pharmacopeia, Drug Indications (USP DI). The inclusion of an item in the USP DI does not necessarily mean that the item is a drug or biological. The USP DI is a database of drug information developed by the U.S. Pharmacopeia but maintained by Micromedex, which contains medically accepted uses for generic and brand name drug products. Inclusion in such reference (or approval by a hospital committee) is a necessary condition for a product to be considered a drug or biological under the Medicare program, however, it is not enough. Rather, the product must also meet all other program requirements to be determined to be a drug or biological.

2049.2 Determining Self-Administration of Drug or Biological.—Whether a drug or biological is of a type which cannot be self-administered is based on the usual method of administration of the form of that drug or biological as furnished by the physician.

Whole blood is a biological which cannot be self-administered and is covered when furnished incident to a physician's services. Payment may also be made for blood fractions if all coverage requirements are satisfied. (See §2455 on Part B blood deductible.)

Medicare carriers have discretion in applying the criteria in this instruction in determining whether drugs are subject to this exclusion in their local areas. Carriers are to follow the instructions below when applying the exclusion for drugs that are usually self-administered by the patient. Each individual contractor must make its own individual determination on each drug. Contractors must continue to apply the policy that not only the drug is medically reasonable and necessary for any individual claim, but also that the route of administration is medically reasonable and necessary. That is, if a drug is available in both oral and injectable forms, the injectable form of the drug must be medically reasonable and necessary as compared to using the oral form. (See §2049.4.2)

For certain injectable drugs, it will be apparent due to the nature of the condition(s) for which they are administered or the usual course of treatment for those conditions, they are, or are not, usually self-administered. For example, an injectable drug used to treat migraine headaches is usually self-administered. On the other hand, an injectable drug, administered at the same time as chemotherapy, used to treat anemia secondary to chemotherapy is not usually self-administered.

Administered—The term "administered" refers only to the physical process by which the drug enters the patient's body. It does not refer to whether the process is supervised by a medical professional (for example, to observe proper technique or side-effects of the drug). Only injectable (including intravenous) drugs are eligible for inclusion under the "incident to" benefit. Other routes of administration including, but not limited to, oral drugs, suppositories, topical medications are all considered to be usually self-administered by the patient.

Usually—In arriving at a single determination as to whether a drug is usually self-administered, contractors should make a separate determination for each indication for a drug as to whether that drug is usually self-administered.

After determining whether a drug is usually self-administered for each indication, contractors should determine the relative contribution of each indication to total use of the drug (i.e., weighted average) in order to make an overall determination as to whether the drug is usually self-administered. For example, if a drug has three indications, is not self-administered for the first indication, but is self-administered for the second and third indications, and the first indication makes up 40% of total usage, the second indication makes up 30% of total usage, and the third indication makes up 30% of total usage, then the drug would be considered usually self-administered.

Reliable statistical information on the extent of self-administration by the patient may not always be available. Consequently, we offer the following guidance for each contractor's consideration in making this determination in the absence of such data:

1. Absent evidence to the contrary, drugs delivered intravenously should be presumed to be not usually self-administered by the patient.
2. Absent evidence to the contrary, drugs delivered by intramuscular injection should be presumed to be not usually self-administered by the patient. (For example, interferon beta-1a, tradename Avonex, when delivered by intramuscular injection is not usually self administered by the patient.) The contractor may consider the depth and nature of the particular intramuscular injection in applying this presumption.
3. Absent evidence to the contrary, drugs delivered by subcutaneous injection should be presumed to be self-administered by the patient.

In applying these presumptions, contractors should examine the use of the particular drug and consider the following factors:

A. Acute condition.—For the purposes of determining whether a drug is usually self-administered, an acute condition means a condition that begins over a short time period, is likely to be of short duration and/or the expected course of treatment is for a short, finite interval. A course of treatment consisting of scheduled injections lasting less than two weeks, regardless of frequency or route of administration, is considered acute. Evidence to support this may include Food and Drug administration (FDA) approval language, package inserts, drug compendia, and other information.

B. Frequency of administration.—How often is the injection given? For example, if the drug is administered once per month, it is less likely to be self-administered by the patient. However, if it is administered once or more per week, it is likely that the drug is self-administered by the patient.

By the patient—The term "by the patient" means Medicare beneficiaries as a collective whole. Include only the patients themselves and not other individuals (that is, do not include spouses, friends, or other care-givers). Base your determination on whether the drug is self-administered by the patient a majority of the time that the drug is used on an outpatient basis by Medicare beneficiaries for medically necessary indications. Ignore all instances when the drug is administered on an inpatient basis. Make this determination on a drug-by-drug basis, not on a beneficiary-by-beneficiary basis. In evaluating whether beneficiaries as a collective whole self-administer, do not consider individual beneficiaries who do not have the capacity to self-administer any drug due to a condition other than the condition for which they are taking the drug in question. For example, an individual afflicted with paraplegia or advanced dementia would not have the capacity to self-administer any injectable drug, so such individuals would not be included in the population upon which the determination for self-administration by the patient was based. Note that some individuals afflicted with a less severe stage of an otherwise debilitating condition would be included in the population upon which the determination for "self-administered by the patient" was based; for example, an early onset of dementia.

Evidentiary Criteria —In making a self-administration determination, contractors are only required to consider the following types of evidence: peer reviewed medical literature, standards of medical practice, evidence-based practice guidelines, FDA approved label, and package inserts. Contractors may also consider other evidence submitted by interested individuals or groups subject to their judgment.

Contractors should also use these evidentiary criteria when reviewing requests for making a determination as to whether a drug is usually self-administered, and requests for reconsideration of a pending or published determination.

Please note that prior to August 1, 2002, one of the principal factors used to determine whether a drug was subject to the self-administered exclusion was whether the FDA label contained instructions for self-administration. However, we note that under the standard in effect after August 1, 2002, the fact that the FDA label includes instructions for self-administration is not, by itself, a determining factor that a drug is subject to this exclusion.

Provider Notice of Non-Covered Drugs—Contractors must describe the process they will use to determine whether a drug is usually self-administered and thus does not meet the "incident to" benefit category. Contractors must place a description of the process on their Web site. Contractors must publish a list of the injectable drugs that are subject to the self-administered exclusion on their Web site, including the data and rationale that led to the determination. Contractors will report the workload associated with developing new coverage statements in CAFM 21208.

Contractors must provide notice 45 days prior to the date that these drugs will not be covered. During the 45-day time period, contractors will maintain existing medical review and payment procedures. After the 45-day notice, contractors may deny payment for the drugs subject to the notice.

Contractors must not develop local medical review policies (LMRPs) for this purpose because further elaboration to describe drugs that do not meet the 'incident to' and the 'not usually self-administered' provisions of the statute are unnecessary. Current LMRPs based solely on these provisions must be withdrawn. LMRPs that address the self-administered exclusion and other information may be reissued absent the self-administered drug exclusion material. Contractors will report this workload in CAFM 21206. However, contractors may continue to use and write LMRPs to describe reasonable and necessary uses of drugs that are not usually self-administered.

Conferences Between Contractors—Contractors' Medical Directors may meet and discuss whether a drug is usually self-administered without reaching a formal consensus. Each contractor uses its discretion as to whether or not it will participate in such discussions. Each contractor must make its own individual determinations, except that fiscal intermediaries may, at their discretion, follow the determinations of the local carrier with respect to the self-administered exclusion.

Beneficiary Appeals—If a beneficiary's claim for a particular drug is denied because the drug is subject to the "self-administered drug" exclusion, the beneficiary may appeal the denial. Because it is a "benefit category" denial and not a denial based on medical necessity, an Advance Beneficiary Notice (ABN) is not applicable. A "benefit category" denial (i.e., a denial based on the fact that there is no benefit category under which the drug may be covered) does not trigger the financial liability protection provisions of Limitation On Liability [under §1879 of the Act]. Therefore, physicians or providers may charge the beneficiary for an excluded drug. See Chapter XV of the Medicare Carrier Manual for more detail on the appeals process.

Provider and Physician Appeals—A physician accepting assignment may appeal a denial under the provisions found in §12000 of the Medicare Carriers Manual. See Chapter XV of the Medicare Carrier Manual for more detail on the appeals process.

Reporting Requirements—Each carrier must report to CMS, every September 1 and March 1, its complete list of injectable drugs that the contractor has determined are excluded when furnished incident to a physician's service on the basis that the drug is usually self-administered. We anticipate that contractors will review injectable drugs on a rolling basis and publish their list of excluded drugs as it is developed. For example, contractors should not wait to publish this list until every drug has been reviewed.

Contractors must send their exclusion list to the following e-mail address: drugdata@cms.hhs.gov. Below is an example of the Microsoft Excel template that should be submitted to CMS.

Carrier Name	State	Carrier ID #	HCPCS	Descriptor	Effective date of exclusion	End date of exclusion	Comments

2049.3 Incident-to Requirements.—In order for Medicare payment to be made for a drug, the "incident to" requirements are met. "Incident to" a physician's professional service means that the services are furnished as an integral, although incidental, part of the physician's personal professional services in the course of diagnosis or treatment of an illness or injury. See §2050.1 for more detail on incident-to requirements.

In order to meet all the general requirements for coverage under the incident-to provision, an FDA approved drug or biological must be furnished by a physician and administered by him/her or by auxiliary personnel employed by him/her under his/her personal supervision. The charge, if any, for the drug or biological must be included in the physician's bill, and the cost of the drug or biological must represent an expense to the physician. Drugs and biologicals furnished by other health professionals may also meet these requirements. (See §§2154, 2156, 2158 and 2160 for specific instructions.)

2049.4 Reasonableness and Necessity.—Use of the drug or biological must be safe and effective and otherwise reasonable and necessary. (See §2303.) Drugs or biologicals approved for marketing by the Food and Drug Administration (FDA) are considered safe and effective for purposes of this requirement when used for indications specified on the labeling. Therefore, you may pay for the use of an FDA approved drug or biological, if:

* It was injected on or after the date of the FDA's approval;
* It is reasonable and necessary for the individual patient; and
* All other applicable coverage requirements are met.

Deny coverage for drugs and biologicals which have not received final marketing approval by the FDA unless you receive instructions from CMS to the contrary. For specific guidelines on coverage of Group C cancer drugs, see the Coverage Issues Manual.

If there is reason to question whether the FDA has approved a drug or biological for marketing, obtain satisfactory evidence of FDA's approval. Acceptable evidence includes a copy of the FDA's letter to the drug's manufacturer approving the new drug application (NDA); or listing of the drug or biological in the FDA's Approved Drug Products or FDA Drug and Device Product Approvals; or a copy of the manufacturer's package insert, approved by the FDA as part of the labeling of the drug, containing its recommended uses and dosage, as well as possible adverse reactions and recommended precautions in using it. When necessary, the RO may be able to help in obtaining information.

An unlabeled use of a drug is a use that is not included as an indication on the drug's label as approved by the FDA. FDA approved drugs used for indications other than what is indicated on the official label may be covered under Medicare if the carrier determines the use to be medically accepted, taking into consideration the major drug compendia, authoritive medical literature and/or accepted standards of medical practice. In the case of drugs used in an anti-cancer chemotherapeutic regimen, unlabeled uses are covered for a medically accepted indication as defined in §2049.4.C.

Determinations as to whether medication is reasonable and necessary for an individual patient should be made on the same basis as all other such determinations (i.e., with the advice of medical consultants and with reference to accepted standards of medical practice and the medical circumstances of the individual case). The following guidelines identify three categories with specific examples of situations in which medications would not be reasonable and necessary according to accepted standards of medical practice.

1. Not for Particular Illness.—Medications given for a purpose other than the treatment of a particular condition, illness, or injury are not covered (except for certain immunizations).

   Exclude the charge for medications, e.g., vitamins, given simply for the general good and welfare of the patient and not as accepted therapy for a particular illness.

2. Medication given by injection (parenterally) is not covered if standard medical practice indicates that the administration of the medication by mouth(orally) is effective and is an accepted or preferred method of administration. For example, the accepted standards of medical practice for the treatment of certain diseases is to initiate therapy with parenteral penicillin and to complete therapy with oral penicillin. Exclude the entire charge for penicillin injections given after the initiation of therapy if oral penicillin is indicated unless there are special medical circumstances which justify additional injections.

3. Excessive Medications.—Medications administered for treatment of a disease which exceed the frequency or duration of injections indicated by accepted standards of medical practice are not covered. For example, the accepted standard of medical practice in the maintenance treatment of pernicious anemia is one vitamin B-12 injection per month. Exclude the entire charge for injections given in excess of this frequency unless there are special medical circumstances which justify additional injections.

Supplement the guidelines as necessary with guidelines concerning appropriate use of specific injections in other situations. Use the guidelines to screen out questionable cases for special review, further development or denial when the injection billed for would not be reasonable and necessary. Coordinate any type of drug treatment review with the PRO.

If a medication is determined not to be reasonable and necessary for diagnosis or treatment of an illness or injury according to these guidelines, exclude the entire charge (i.e., for both the drug and its administration). Also exclude from payment any charges for other services (such as office visits) which were primarily for the purpose of administering a noncovered injection (i.e., an injection that is not reasonable and necessary for the diagnosis or treatment of an illness or injury).

A. Antigens.—Payment may be made for a reasonable supply of antigens that have been prepared for a particular patient if: (1) the antigens are prepared by a physician who is a doctor of medicine or osteopathy, and (2) the physician who prepared the antigens has examined the patient and has determined a plan of treatment and a dosage regimen. Antigens must be administered in accordance with the plan of treatment and by a doctor of medicine or osteopathy or by a properly instructed person (who could be the patient) under the supervision of the doctor. he associations of allergists that HCFA consulted advised that a reasonable supply of antigens is onsidered to be not more than a 12-week supply of antigens that has been prepared for a particular patient at any one time. The purpose of the reasonable supply limitation is to assure that the antigens retain their potency and effectiveness over the period in which they are to be administered to the patient. (See §§2005.2 and 2050.2.)

B. Immunizations.—Vaccinations or inoculations are excluded as immunizations unless they are directly related to the treatment of an injury or direct exposure to a disease or condition, such as anti-rabies treatment, tetanus antitoxin or booster vaccine, botulin antitoxin, antivenin sera, or immune globulin. In the absence of injury or direct exposure, preventive immunization (vaccination or inoculation) against such diseases as smallpox, polio, diphtheria, etc., is not covered. However, pneumococcal, hepatitis B, and influenza virus vaccines are exceptions to this rule. (See items 1, 2, and 3.) In cases where a vaccination or inoculation is excluded from coverage, deny the entire charge.

1. Pneumococcal Pneumonia Vaccinations.—Furnished on or after May 1, 1981, the Medicare Part B program covers pneumococcal pneumonia vaccine and its administration when furnished in compliance with any applicable State law by any provider of services or any entity or individual with a supplier number. This includes revaccination of patients at highest risk of pneumococcal infection. Typically, these vaccines are administered once in a lifetime except for persons at highest risk. Effective July 1, 2000, Medicare does not require for coverage purposes that the vaccine must be ordered by a doctor of medicine or osteopathy. Therefore, the beneficiary may receive the vaccine upon request without a physician's order and without physician supervision.

An initial vaccine may be administered only to persons at high risk (see below) of pneumococcal disease. Revaccination may be administered only to persons at highest risk of serious Pneumococcal Pneumonia Vaccinations.—Effective for services pneumococcal infection and those likely to have a rapid decline in pneumococcal antibody levels, provided that at least 5 years have passed since receipt of a previous dose of pneumococcal vaccine.

Persons at high risk for whom an initial vaccine may be administered include all people age 65 and older; immunocompetent adults who are at increased risk of pneumococcal disease or its complications because of chronic illness (e.g., cardiovascular disease, pulmonary disease, diabetes mellitus, alcoholism, cirrhosis, or cerebrospinal fluid leaks); and individuals with compromised immune systems (e.g., splenic dysfunction or anatomic asplenia, Hodgkin's disease, lymphoma, multiple myeloma, chronic renal failure, HIV infection, nephrotic syndrome, sickle cell disease, or organ transplantation).

Persons at highest risk and those most likely to have rapid declines in antibody levels are those for whom revaccination may be appropriate. This group includes persons with functional or anatomic asplenia (e.g., sickle cell disease, splenectomy), HIV infection, leukemia, lymphoma, Hodgkin's disease, multiple myeloma, generalized malignancy, chronic renal failure, nephrotic syndrome, or other conditions associated with immunosuppression such as organ or bone marrow transplantation, and those receiving immuno-suppressive chemotherapy. Routine revaccination of people age 65 or older who are not at highest risk is not appropriate.

Those administering the vaccine should not require the patient to present an immunization record prior to administering the pneumococcal vaccine, nor should they feel compelled to review the patient's complete medical record if it is not available. Instead, provided that the patient is competent, it is acceptable for them to rely on the patient's verbal history to determine prior vaccination status. If the patient is uncertain about their vaccination history in the past 5 years, the vaccine should be given. However, if the patient is certain he/she was vaccinated in the last 5 years, the vaccine should not be given. If the patient is certain that the vaccine was given and that more than 5 years have passed since receipt of the previous dose, revaccination is not appropriate unless the patient is at highest risk.

2. Hepatitis B Vaccine.—With the enactment of P.L. 98-369, coverage under Part B was extended to hepatitis B vaccine and its administration, furnished to a Medicare beneficiary who is at high or intermediate risk of contracting hepatitis B. This coverage is effective for services furnished on or after September 1, 1984.

High-risk groups currently identified include (see exception below):

* End stage renal disease (ESRD) patients;

* Hemophiliacs who receive Factor VIII or IX concentrates; Clients of institutions for the mentally retarded;
* Persons who live in the same household as an Hepatitis B Virus (HBV) carrier; Homosexual men; and
* Illicit injectable drug abusers.
* Intermediate risk groups currently identified include:
* Staff in institutions for the mentally retarded; and
* Workers in health care professions who have frequent contact with blood or blood-derived body fluids during routine work.

EXCEPTION: Persons in the above-listed groups would not be considered at high or intermediate risk of contracting hepatitis B, however, if there is laboratory evidence positive for antibodies to hepatitis B. (ESRD patients are routinely tested for hepatitis B antibodies as part of their continuing monitoring and therapy.)

For Medicare program purposes, the vaccine may be administered upon the order of a doctor of medicine or osteopathy by home health agencies, skilled nursing facilities, ESRD facilities, hospital outpatient departments, persons recognized under the incident to physicians' services provision of law, and doctors of medicine and osteopathy.

A charge separate from the ESRD composite rate will be recognized and paid for administration of the vaccine to ESRD patients.

For ESRD laboratory tests, see Coverage Issues Manual, §50-17.

3. Influenza Virus Vaccine.—Effective for services furnished on or after May 1, 1993, the Medicare Part B program covers influenza virus vaccine and its administration when furnished in compliance with any applicable State law by any provider of services or any entity or individual with a supplier number. Typically, these vaccines are administered once a year in the fall or winter. Medicare does not require for coverage purposes that the vaccine must be ordered by a doctor of medicine or osteopathy. Therefore, the beneficiary may receive the vaccine upon request without a physician's order and without physician supervision.

C. Unlabeled Use For Anti-Cancer Drugs.—Effective January 1, 1994, unlabeled uses of FDA approved drugs and biologicals used in an anti-cancer chemotherapeutic regimen for a medically accepted indication are evaluated under the conditions described in this paragraph. A regimen is a combination of anti-cancer agents which has been clinically recognized for the treatment of a specific type of cancer. An example of a drug regimen is: Cyclophosphamide + vincristine + prednisone (CVP) for non-Hodgkin's lymphoma.

In addition to listing the combination of drugs for a type of cancer, there may be a different regimen or combinations which are used at different times in the history of the cancer (induction, prophylaxis of CNS involvement, post remission, and relapsed or refractory disease). A protocol may specify the combination of drugs, doses, and schedules for administration of the drugs. For purposes of this provision, a cancer treatment regimen includes drugs used to treat toxicities or side effects of the cancer treatment regimen when the drug is administered incident to a chemotherapy treatment. Contractors must not deny coverage based solely on the absence of FDA approved labeling for the use, if the use is supported by one of the following and the use is not listed as "not indicated" in any of the three compendia. (See note at the end of this subsection.)

1. American Hospital Formulary Service Drug Information.—Drug monographs are arranged in alphabetical order within therapeutic classifications. Within the text of the monograph, information concerning indications is provided, including both labeled and unlabeled uses. Unlabeled uses are identified with daggers. The text must be analyzed to make a determination whether a particular use is supported.

2. American Medical Association Drug Evaluations.—Drug evaluations are organized into sections and chapters that are based on therapeutic classifications. The evaluation of a drug provides information concerning indications, including both labeled and unlabeled uses. Unlabeled uses are not specifically identified as such. The text must be analyzed to make a determination whether a particular use is supported. In making these determinations, also refer to the AMA Drug Evaluations Subscription, Volume III, section 17 (Oncolytic Drugs), chapter 1 (Principles of Cancer Chemotherapy), tables 1 and 2.

   Table 1, Specific Agents Used In Cancer Chemotherapy, lists the anti-neoplastic agents which are currently available for use in various cancers. The indications presented in this table for a particular anti-cancer drug include labeled and unlabeled uses (although they are not identified as such). Any indication appearing in this table is considered to be a medically accepted use.

   Table 2, Clinical Responses To Chemotherapy, lists some of the currently preferred regimens for various cancers. The table headings include (1) type of cancer, (2) drugs or regimens currently preferred, (3) alternative or secondary drugs or regimens, and (4) other drugs or regimens with reported activity.

   A regimen appearing under the preferred or alternative/secondary headings is considered to be a medically accepted use.

   A regimen appearing under the heading "Other Drugs or Regimens With Reported Activity" is considered to be for a medically accepted use provided:

   * The preferred and alternative/secondary drugs or regimens are contraindicated; or
   * A preferred and/or alternative/secondary drug or regimen was used but was not tolerated or was ineffective; or

* here was tumor progression or recurrence after an initial response.

3. United States Pharmacopoeia Drug Information (USPDI).—Monographs are arranged in alphabetic order by generic or family name. Indications for use appear as accepted, unaccepted, or insufficient data. An indication is considered to be a medically accepted use only if the indication is listed as accepted. Unlabeled uses are identified with brackets. A separate indications index lists all indications included in USPDI along with the medically accepted drugs used in treatment or diagnosis.

4. A Use Supported by Clinical Research That Appears in Peer Reviewed Medical Literature.—This applies only when an unlabeled use does not appear in any of the compendia or is listed as insufficient data or investigational. If an unlabeled use of a drug meets these criteria, contact the compendia to see if a report regarding this use is forthcoming. If a report is forthcoming, use this information as a basis for your decision making. The compendium process for making decisions concerning unlabeled uses is very thorough and continuously updated. Peer reviewed medical literature includes scientific, medical, and pharmaceutical publications in which original manuscripts are published, only after having been critically reviewed for scientific accuracy, validity, and reliability by unbiased independent experts. This does not include in-house publications of pharmaceutical manufacturing companies or abstracts (including meeting abstracts)

   In determining whether there is supportive clinical evidence for a particular use of a drug, your medical staff (in consultation with local medical specialty groups) must evaluate the quality of the evidence in published peer reviewed medical literature. When evaluating this literature, consider (among other things) the following:

   * The prevalence and life history of the disease when evaluating the adequacy of the number of subjects and the response rate. While a 20 percent response rate may be adequate for highly prevalent disease states, a lower rate may be adequate for rare diseases or highly unresponsive conditions.
   * The effect on the patient's well-being and other responses to therapy that indicate effectiveness, e.g., a significant increase in survival rate or life expectancy or an objective and significant decrease in the size of the tumor or a reduction in symptoms related to the tumor. Stabilization is not considered a response to therapy.
   * The appropriateness of the study design. Consider:

     1. Whether the experimental design in light of the drugs and conditions under investigation is appropriate to address the investigative question. (For example, in some clinical studies, it may be unnecessary or not feasible to use randomization, double blind trials, placebos, or crossover.);

2. That nonrandomized clinical trials with a significant number of subjects may be a basis for supportive clinical evidence for determining accepted uses of drugs; and
3. That case reports are generally considered uncontrolled and anecdotal information and do not provide adequate supportive clinical evidence for determining accepted uses of drugs.

   Use peer reviewed medical literature appearing in the following publications:

* *American Journal of Medicine;*
* *Annals of Internal Medicine;*
* *The Journal of the American Medical Association;*
* *Journal of Clinical Oncology;*
* *Blood;*
* *Journal of the National Cancer Institute;*
* *The New England Journal of Medicine;*
* *British Journal of Cancer;*
* *British Journal of Hematology;*
* *British Medical Journal;*
* *Cancer*;
* *Drugs*;
* *European Journal of Cancer* (formerly *European Journal of Cancer and Clinical Oncology)*;
* *Lancet*; or
* *Leukemia.*

   You are not required to maintain copies of these publications. If a claim raises a question about the use of a drug for a purpose not included in the FDA approved labeling or the compendia, ask the physician to submit copies of relevant supporting literature

4. Unlabeled uses may also be considered medically accepted if determined by you to be medically accepted generally as safe and effective for the particular use.

   NOTE: If a use is identified as not indicated by HCFA or the FDA or if a use is specifically identified as not indicated in one or more of the three compendia mentioned or if you determine based on peer reviewed medical literature that a particular use of a drug is not safe and effective, the off- label usage is not supported and, therefore, the drug is not covered.

5. Less Than Effective Drug.—This is a drug that has been determined by the Food and Drug Administration (FDA) to lack substantial evidence of effectiveness for all labeled indications.

   Also, a drug that has been the subject of a Notice of an Opportunity for a Hearing (NOOH) published in the Federal Register before being withdrawn from the market, and for which the Secretary has not determined there is a compelling justification for its medical need, is considered less than effective. This includes any other drug product that is identical, similar, or related. Payment may not be made for a less than effective drug.

Because the FDA has not yet completed its identification of drug products that are still on the market,existing FDA efficacy decisions must be applied to all similar products once they are identified.

6. Denial of Medicare Payment for Compounded Drugs Produced in Violation of Federal Food, Drug, and Cosmetic Act.—The Food and Drug Administration (FDA) has found that, from time to time, firms established as retail pharmacies engage in mass production of compounded drugs, beyond the normal scope of pharmaceutical practice, in violation of the Federal Food, Drug, and Cosmetic Act (FFDCA). By compounding drugs on a large scale, a company may be operating as a drug manufacturer within the meaning of the FFDCA,without complying with requirements of that law. Such companies may be manufacturing drugs which are subject to the new drug application (NDA) requirements of the FFDCA, but for which FDA has not approved an NDA or which are misbranded or adulterated. If the manufacturing and processing procedures used by these facilities have not been approved by the FDA, the FDA has no assurance that the drugs these companies are producing are safe and effective. The safety and effectiveness issues pertain to such factors as chemical stability, purity, strength, bioequivalency, and biovailability.

   Section 1862(a)(1)(A) of the Act requires that drugs must be reasonable and necessary in order to by covered under Medicare. This means, in the case of drugs, they must have been approved for marketing by the FDA. Section 2049.4 instructs carriers to deny coverage for drugs that have not received final marketing approval by the FDA, unless instructed otherwise by HCFA. Section 2300.1 instructs carriers to deny coverage of services related to the use of noncovered drugs as well. Hence, if DME or a prosthetic device is used to administer a noncovered drug, coverage is denied for both the nonapproved drug and the DME or prosthetic device.

   In those cases in which the FDA has determined that a company is producing compounded drugs in violation of the FFDCA, Medicare does not pay for the drugs because they do not meet the FDA approval requirements of the Medicare program. In addition, Medicare does not pay for the DME or prosthetic device used to administer such a drug if FDA determines that a required NDA has not been approved or that the drug is misbranded or adulterated.

   HCFA will notify you when the FDA has determined that compounded drugs are being produced in violation of the FFDCA. Do not stop Medicare payment for such a drug unless you are notified that it is appropriate to do so through a subsequent instruction. In addition, if you or ROs become aware that other companies are possibly operating in violation of the FFDCA, notify:

Health Care Financing Administration
Bureau of Policy Development
Office of Physician and Ambulatory Care Policy
Baltimore, MD 21244-1850

2049.5 Self-Administered Drugs and Biologicals.—Drugs that are self-administered are not covered by Medicare Part B unless the statute provides for such coverage. This includes blood clotting factors,drugs used in immunosuppressive therapy, erythropoietin for dialysis patients, certain oral anti-cancer drugs, and oral anti-nausea drugs when used in certain situations.

A. Until January 1, 1995, immunosuppressive drugs are covered under Part B for a period of one year following discharge from a hospital for a Medicare covered organ transplant. HCFA interprets the 1-year period after the date of the transplant procedure to mean 365 days from the day on which an inpatient is discharged from the hospital. Beneficiaries are eligible to receive additional Part B coverage within 18 months after the discharge date for drugs furnished in 1995; within 24 months for drugs furnished in 1996; within 30 months for drugs furnished in 1997; and within 36 months for drugs furnished after 1997.

Covered drugs include those immunosuppressive drugs that have been specifically labeled as such and approved for marketing by the FDA, as well as those prescription drugs, such as prednisone, that are used in conjunction with immunosuppressive drugs as part of a therapeutic regimen reflected in FDA approved labeling for immunosuppressive drugs. Therefore, antibiotics, hypertensives, and other drugs that are not directly related to rejection are not covered. The FDA had identified and approved for marketing five specifically labeled immunosuppressive drugs. They are Sandimmune (cyclosporine),Sandoz Pharmaceutical; Imuran (azathioprine), Burroughs Wellcome; Atgam (antithymocyte globulin), Upjohn; and Orthoclone OKT3 (Muromonab-CD3), Ortho Pharmaceutical and, Prograf (tacrolimus), Fujisawa USA, Inc. You are expected to keep informed of FDA additions to the list of the immunosuppressive drugs.

B. Erythropoietin (EPO).—The statute provides that EPO is covered for the treatment of anemia for patients with chronic renal failure who are on dialysis. Coverage is available regardless of whether the drug is administered by the patient or the patient's caregiver. EPO is a biologically engineered protein which stimulates the bone marrow to make new red blood cells.

NOTE: Non-ESRD patients who are receiving EPO to treat anemia induced by other conditions such as chemotherapy or the drug zidovudine (commonly called AZT) must meet the coverage requirements in §2049.

EPO is covered for the treatment of anemia for patients with chronic renal failure who are on dialysis when:

* It is administered in the renal dialysis facility; or
* It is self-administered in the home by any dialysis patient (or patient caregiver) who is determined competent to use the drug and meets the other conditions detailed below.

NOTE: Payment may not be made for EPO under the incident to provision when EPO is administered in the renal dialysis facility. (See §5202.4.)

Medicare covers EPO and items related to its administration for dialysis patients who use EPO in the home when the following conditions are met.

1. Patient Care Plan.—A dialysis patient who uses EPO in the home must have a current care plan (a copy of which must be maintained by the designated back-up facility for Method II patients) for monitoring home use of EPO which includes the following:
   a. Review of diet and fluid intake for aberrations as indicated by hyperkalemia and elevated blood pressure secondary to volume overload;
   b. Review of medications to ensure adequate provision of supplemental iron;
   c. Ongoing evaluations of hematocrit and iron stores;
   d. Reevaluation of the dialysis prescription taking into account the patient's increased appetite and red blood cell volume;
   e. Method for physician and facility (including back-up facility for Method II patients) follow-up on blood tests and a mechanism (such as a patient log) for keeping the physician informed of the results;
   f. Training of the patient to identify the signs and symptoms of hypotension and hypertension; and
   g. The decrease or discontinuance of EPO if hypertension is uncontrollable.

2. Patient Selection.—The dialysis facility, or the physician responsible for all dialysis-related services furnished to the patient, must make a comprehensive assessment that includes the following:
   a. Pre-selection monitoring. The patient's hematocrit (or hemoglobin), serum iron, transferrin saturation, serum ferritin, and blood pressure must be measured.
   b. Conditions the patient must meet. The assessment must find that the patient meets the following conditions:
      (1) Is a dialysis patient;
      (2) Has a hematocrit (or comparable hemoglobin level) that is as follows:
         (a) For a patient who is initiating EPO treatment, no higher than 30 percent unless there is medical documentation showing the need for EPO despite a hematocrit (or comparable hemoglobin level) higher than 30 percent. Patients with severe angina, severe pulmonary distress, or severe hypotension may require EPO to prevent adverse symptoms even if they have higher hematocrit or hemoglobin levels.
         (b) For a patient who has been receiving EPO from the facility or the physician, between 30 and 36 percent; and

3. Is under the care of:
   a. A physician who is responsible for all dialysis-related services and who prescribes the EPO and follows the drug labeling instructions when monitoring the EPO home therapy; and
   b. A renal dialysis facility that establishes the plan of care and monitors the progress of the home EPO therapy.
   c. The assessment must find that the patient or a caregiver meets the following conditions:
      (1) Is trained by the facility to inject EPO and is capable of carrying out the procedure;
      (2) Is capable of reading and understanding the drug labeling; and
      (3) Is trained in, and capable of observing, aseptic techniques.
   d. Care and storage of drug. The assessment must find that EPO can be stored in the patient's residence under refrigeration and that the patient is aware of the potential hazard of a child's having access to the drug and syringes.

4. Responsibilities of Physician or Dialysis Facility.—The patient's physician or dialysis facility must:
   a. Develop a protocol that follows the drug label instructions;
   b. Make the protocol available to the patient to ensure safe and effective home use of EPO;
   c. Through the amounts prescribed, ensure that the drug on hand at any time does not exceed a 2-month supply; and
   d. Maintain adequate records to allow quality assurance for review by the network and State survey agencies. For Method II patients, current records must be provided to and maintained by the designated back-up facility.

See §5202.4 for information on EPO payment.

Submit claims for EPO in accordance with §§4273.1 and 4273.2.

C. Oral Anti-Cancer Drugs.—Effective January 1, 1994, Medicare Part B coverage is extended to include oral anti-cancer drugs that are prescribed as anti-cancer chemotherapeutic agents providing they have the same active ingredients and are used for the same indications as anti-cancer chemotherapeutic agents which would be covered if they were not self administered and they were furnished incident to a physician's service as drugs and biologicals.

   This provision applies only to the coverage of anti-neoplastic chemotherapeutic agents. It does not apply to oral drugs and/or biologicals used to treat toxicity or side effects such as nausea or bone marrow depression. Medicare will cover anti-neoplastic chemotherapeutic agents, the primary drugs which directly fight the cancer, and self-administered antiemetics which are necessary for the administration and absorption of the anti-neoplastic chemotherapeutic agents when a high likelihood of vomiting exists. The substitution of an oral form of an anti-neoplastic drug requires that the drug be retained for absorption. The antiemetics drug is covered as a necessary means for administration of the oral drug (similar to a syringe and needle necessary for injectable administration).

Oral drugs prescribed for use with the primary drug which enhance the anti-neoplastic effect of the primary drug or permit the patient to tolerate the primary anti-neoplastic drug in higher doses for longer periods are not covered. Self-administered antiemetics to reduce the side effects of nausea and vomiting brought on by the primary drug are not included beyond the administration necessary to achieve drug absorption.

In order to assure uniform coverage policy, regional carriers and FIs must be apprised of local carriers'anti-cancer drug medical review policies which may impact on future medical review policy development. Local carrier's current and proposed anti-cancer drug medical review polices should be provided by local carrier medical directors to regional carrier or FI medical directors, upon request.

For an oral anti-cancer drug to be covered under Part B, it must:

* Be prescribed by a physician or other practitioner licensed under State law to prescribe such drugs as anti-cancer chemotherapeutic agents;
* Be a drug or biological that has been approved by the Food and Drug Administration (FDA);
* Have the same active ingredients as a non-self-administrable anti-cancer chemotherapeutic drug or biological that is covered when furnished incident to a physician's service. The oral anti-cancer drug and the non-self-administrable drug must have the same chemical/generic name as indicated by the FDA's Approved Drug Products (Orange Book), Physician's Desk Reference (PDR), or an authoritative drug compendium; —or, effective January 1, 1999, be a prodrug—an oral drug ingested into the body that metabolizes into the same active ingredient that is found in the non-self-administrable form of the drug;
* Be used for the same indications, including unlabeled uses, as the non-self-administrable version of the drug; and
* Be reasonable and necessary for the individual patient.

D. Oral Anti-Nausea Drugs—Section 4557 of the Balanced Budget Act of 1997 amends §1861(s)(2) by extending the coverage of oral anti-emetic drugs under the following conditions:

* Coverage is provided only for oral drugs approved by FDA for use as anti-emetics; the oral anti-emetic(s) must either be administered by the treating physician or in accordance with a written order from the physician as part of a cancer chemotherapy regimen;
* Oral anti-emetic drug(s) administered with a particular chemotherapy treatment must be initiated within 2 hours of the administration of the chemotherapeutic agent and may be continued for a period not to exceed 48 hours from that time.

* The oral anti-emetic drug(s) provided must be used as a full therapeutic replacement for the intravenous anti-emetic drugs that would have otherwise been administered at the time of the chemotherapy treatment.

Only drugs pursuant to a physician's order at the time of the chemotherapy treatment qualify for this benefit. The dispensed number of dosage units may not exceed a loading dose administered within 2 hours of that treatment, plus a supply of additional dosage units not to exceed 48 hours of therapy. However, more than one oral anti-emetic drug may be prescribed and will be covered for concurrent usage within these parameters if more than one oral drug is needed to fully replace the intravenous drugs that would otherwise have been given.

Oral drugs that are not approved by the FDA for use as anti-emetics and which are used by treating physicians adjunctively in a manner incidental to cancer chemotherapy are not covered by this benefit and are not reimbursable within the scope of this benefit.

It is recognized that a limited number of patients will fail on oral anti-emetic drugs. Intravenous anti-emetics may be covered (subject to the rules of medical necessity) when furnished to patients who fail on oral anti-emetic therapy.

This coverage, effective for services on or after January 1, 1998, is subject to regular Medicare Part B coinsurance and deductible provisions.

NOTE: Existing coverage policies authorizing the administration of suppositories to prevent vomiting when oral cancer drugs are used are unchanged by this new coverage.

E. Hemophilia Clotting Factors.—Section 1861(s)(2)(I) of the Act provides Medicare coverage of blood clotting factors for hemophilia patients competent to use such factors to control bleeding without medical supervision, and items related to the administration of such factors. Hemophilia, a blood disorder characterized by prolonged coagulation time, Is caused by deficiency of a factor in plasma necessary for blood to clot. (The discovery in 1964 of a cryoprecipitate rich in antihemophilic factor activity facilitated management of acute bleeding episodes.) For purposes of Medicare Part B coverage, hemophilia encompasses the following conditions:

* Factor VIII deficiency (classic hemophilia);
* Factor IX deficiency (also termed plasma thromboplastin component (PTC) or Christmas factor deficiency); and
* Von Willebrand's disease.

Claims for blood clotting factors for hemophilia patients with these diagnoses may be covered if the patient is competent to use such factors without medical supervision.

The amount of clotting factors determined to be necessary to have on hand and thus covered under this provision is based on the historical utilization pattern or profile developed by the carrier for each patient. It is expected that the treating source; e.g., a family physician or comprehensive hemophilia diagnostic and treatment center, has such information. From this data, the contractor is able to make reasonable projections concerning the quantity of clotting factors anticipated to be needed by the patient over a specific period of time. Unanticipated occurrences involving extraordinary events, such as automobile accidents of inpatient hospital stays, will change this base line data and should be appropriately considered. In addition, changes in a patient's medical needs over a period of time require adjustments in the profile. (See §5245 for payment policies.)

2070.l Independent Laboratories.—Diagnostic laboratory services furnished by an independent laboratory are covered under medical insurance if the laboratory is an approved Independent Clinical Laboratory. (However, as is the case of all diagnostic services, in order to be covered these services must be related to a patient's illness or injury (or symptom or complaint) and ordered by a physician.

See §2020.l for the definition of a "physician".)

A. Definition of Independent.—An independent laboratory is one which is independent both of an attending or consulting physician's office and of a hospital which meets at least the requirements to qualify as an emergency hospital as defined in section l86l(e) of the Act. (A consulting physician is one whose services include history taking, examination of the patient, and, in each case, furnishing to the attending physician an opinion regarding diagnosis or treatment. A physician providing clinical laboratory services for patients of other physicians is not considered to be a consulting physician.)

A laboratory which is operated by or under the supervision of a hospital (or the organized medical staff of the hospital) which does not meet at least the definition of an emergency hospital is considered to be an independent laboratory. However, a laboratory serving hospital patients and operated on the premises of a hospital which meets the definition of an emergency hospital is presumed to be subject to the supervision of the hospital or its organized medical staff and is not an independent laboratory. A laboratory which a physician or group of physicians maintains for performing diagnostic tests in connection with his own or the group practice is also not considered to be an independent laboratory.

An out-of-hospital laboratory is ordinarily presumed to be independent unless there is written evidence establishing that it is operated by or under the supervision of a hospital which meets at least the definition of an emergency hospital or of the organized medical staff of such a hospital.

Where a laboratory operated on hospital premises is claimed to be independent or where an out-of-hospital facility is designated as a hospital laboratory, the RO makes the determination concerning the laboratory's status.

B. Clinical Defined.—A clinical laboratory is a laboratory where microbiological, serological, chemical, hematological, radiobioassay, cytological, immuno-hematological, or pathological examinations are performed on materials derived from the human body, to provide information for the diagnosis, prevention, or treatment of a disease or assessment of a medical condition.

C. Approval of Laboratories.—An approved independent clinical laboratory is one which is approved by the Secretary of Health, Education, and Welfare as meeting the specific conditions for coverage under the program. These require that: (l) where State or applicable local law provides for licensing of independent clinical laboratories, the laboratory is either licensed under such law or it is pproved as meeting the requirements for licensing laboratories; and (2) such laboratories also meet he health and safety requirements prescribed by the Secretary of Health, Education, and Welfare.

See "Conditions for Coverage of Services of Independent Laboratories. (HIRM l Subpart M)

Diagnostic laboratory tests performed by a laboratory of a nonparticipating hospital which meet the statutory definition of an emergency hospital are covered only if the laboratory meets the requirements set forth in the regulations for hospital laboratories.

Services rendered by an independent clinical laboratory are covered under medical insurance only if the laboratory has been approved under the program. Carriers are furnished lists of approved laboratories and their approved specialties by HCFA. If you have any reason to question the lists concerning additions or deletions of particular laboratories or specialties, clarifying information should be requested from the RO.

Laboratory Certification and Decertification

You must notify your physicians of the initial certification of the laboratories in your service areas and also furnished certification information about laboratories outside your service area upon request from individual physicians or clinics. This information is available from the RO (see § 2070.lD below). Where there are any changes in the certification of a laboratory, i.e., addition or deletion of tests for which the laboratory is certified, notify the physicians in your service areas of these changes.

When some or all of the services of an independent laboratory no longer meet the conditions for coverage, inform all physicians having an interest in the laboratory's certification status of the effective date of decertification, reasons for the decertification, and the applicability of the determination to the various categories of diagnostic tests performed by the independent laboratory. Notification to the physicians must be made prior to the termination date since you cannot honor any bill for services performed after the termination date.

If you issue a monthly bulletin or newsletter to physicians in your service area you may wish to use this vehicle to inform the physicians involved. If, in a particular instance, timely notification cannot be made by use of the regular monthly bulletin or newsletter, a special bulletin will be necessary. In cases where there are a limited number of physicians in a remote area, a notification to all physicians in your service area may not be necessary. In these situations, you may wish to limit the scope of the notification and use means other than the monthly newsletter. You must secure the prior approval of the regional office for limited notification.

For notices of decertification, you will receive a copy of the decertification letter to the laboratory from the RO. Language suitable for use in the carrier notices to physicians concerning the reasons for the decertification will also be supplied. The following information will be included in the notification:

1. Name and address of laboratory;

2. Effective date of decertification;

3. Which services are not covered (all or particular specialty(ies); and

4. Reason for decertification.

Your notification to the physicians should contain a statement that no payment can be made under title XVIII on behalf of Medicare patients receiving these services from the laboratory on or after the effective decertification dates.

A copy of all notifications to physicians concerning laboratory decertifications, whether by regular monthly newsletter or by a special bulletin, should be sent to the RO Contractor Operations Staff on the date of issuance.

NOTE: The notification to physicians also applies to services performed by suppliers of portable X-ray services (see §2070.4B).

D. The Specialty Provision.—One of the conditions for coverage of services of independent laboratories is that the laboratory agrees to perform tests for Medicare beneficiaries only in the specialties for which it is certified. Clinical laboratory services rendered in a specialty for which an independent laboratory is not certified are not covered and claims for payment of benefits for these services must be denied.

HCFA furnishes lists to the carriers showing specialties and subspecialties in which each laboratory has been certified. The lists are updated quarterly. Each carrier receives two lists showing the independent laboratories located in its service area: one list by provider number and the other list alphabetical. For information on laboratories not located within a carrier's service area, the RO's maintain national lists showing all approved laboratories. A key is furnished for interpreting the codes on the lists. See §§ 4110ff. for additional information.

Following is a list of covered clinical laboratory test procedures and calculations by specialty and subspecialty that may be performed by independent laboratories participating in the Medicare program (hospital laboratories are not currently approved by specialty/subspecialty). The list contains most of the common test procedures but is not considered all inclusive. Test procedures and calculations that may be performed in more than one specialty/subspecialty are asterisked and cross-referred.

This list is also used by State agencies of certification of the laboratories in the various specialty and subspecialty categories.

GLOSSARY OF LABORATORY TESTS AND CALCULATIONS LISTED BY CATEGORY

010 Historcompatibility Testing (Tissue Typing)

Antiglobulin Crossmatch for Transplantation
Antiglobulin microcytotoxicity Technique
Capillary Agglutination
Cell-mediated lympholysis Test
HLA Typing - Platelet Complement Fixation (FLCF)
HLA Typing - Lymphocyte Complement Fixation
HLA Typing - B27, specific B lymphocyte antigen
HLA Typing - Total
Leukocyte Aggregation Test (LAT)
Leukoagglutination or Phytohemagglutination
Lymphocyte Antibody Lymphocytolytic Interaction (LALI)
Lymphocyte - dependent antibody-mediated lysis (LDA)
Mixed Leukocyte Culture
Mixed Lymphocyte Reaction (Mixed Lymphocyte Culture)-MLR, MLC
Screening Sera for HLA antibodies
Detection of Leukocyte antibodies by the Complement Consumption Test
Separation of multiple HLA antibody specificities by platelet absorption and
acid elution
Other techniques: Target Cells
(terminology used) Killer Cells

100 MICROBIOLOGY

110 Bacteriology (with antimicrobial susceptibility

Acid-fast culture, primary isolation
Acid-fast culture, identification
Acid-fast smear
Antimicrobial susceptibility test (mycobacteriology)
Antimicrobial susceptibility test (general bacteriology)
Antogenous vaccine
Culture, primary isolation
Culture, identification
Culture, for Mycoplasma pneumoniae
Gram Smear
Leptospirosis (Blood, Urine and CSF)
*Mycoplasma pneumoniae CF test-220
PKU (Guthrie only)
Pyrogen test
Pyrogen test (Samples containing protein)

*Streptococcus MG agglutination-220
*Tularemia agglutination-220

120 Mycology

*Coccidiomycosis, Precipitin-220
Culture for Fungi Identification
Abscess
Blood
Bone Marrow
CSF (cerebrospinal fluid)
Eye
Skin, Hair, Nail
Sputum
Tissue Section
Vaginal
Culture, Primary isolation
*Histoplasma agglutionation-220
Mycelia Direct Examination—fungal smear

130 Parasitology

Blood Specimen for Filariasis
*Blood Specimen for Malaria-400
Purged Stool for Amebiasis
Routine Stool for Ova and Parasite
Scotch Tape Test for Enterobius Vermicularis
Stool, urine for Schistosomiasis toxoplasmosis
*Toxoplasmosis agglutionation-220
*Trichina agglutionation-l30
Vaginal Swab for Trichomonas vaginalis

140 Virology (including Rickettsiae and chlamydiae)
(isolation and identification)

150 Other

*Febrile Group-220
Fluorescent stains for bacterial identification
*Immunoflourescence Methods - 220
Phage typing for staphylococci/other bacterial organisms

200 SEROLOGY

210 Syphilis

Automated reagin test (ART)
Dark field Examination
Flourescent treponemal antibodies (FTA)
Kolmer, qual.
Kolmer, quant.
Rapid Plasma Reagin test (RPR Card Test)
Reagin Screen Test (RST)
Spinal Fluid, VDRL

VDRL (Venereal Disease Research Laboratory), qualitative slide

220 Serology-Other

Non-syphilis serology
(Diagnostic Immunology)
Alpha - 1 - antitrypsin
*Alpha - 1 - fetoprotein (AFP) - 330
Anti-deoxuribonuclease (ADNase)
Anti-mitrochonorial antibody
Anti-nuclear antibodies (ANA)
Anti-parietal cell antibody
Anti-skeltal muscle antibody
Anti-smooth muscle antibody
Anti-streptococcalhyaluronidase (ASH)
Anti-streptolysin O (ASO) Test
Anti-thyroglobulin antibodies
Anti-toxoplasmosis antibody
Beta-lc/Beta la globulin
Brucella Agglutination
*Carcinoembryonic Antigen Assay (CEA) - 330
*Coccidiomycosis, Precipitin-120
Cold Agglutinin
Complement, (Total Serum (C') & C'3 and components
C-reactive protein (CRP)
Free DNA Antibody
Free DNA Antigen
*Febrile group (Brucella, typhoid O & H, OX-19, OX-K and OX-2)-150
Gamma globulin, by salt pptn.
*Glucose-6 Phosphate Dehydrogenase (G-6-PD) - 130, 400
*Hepatitis B Antigen (HBsAg) - 330, 540
*Hepatitis B Antibody (Anti-HBs-330, 540
Heterophile antibodies (Presumptive)
Heterophile with absorptions (Differential)
*Histoplasma aggluatination - 120
l - Immunoglobulin Quantitation - See serum specific proteins
*Immunofluorescence Methods (Flourescent Antibody Techniques-
Identification of Group A streptococci;
Neisseria gonorrhoeae, etc) - 150
Infectious Mononucleosis
Leptospira agglutination
Lupus erythematosus - latex aggultination (LE)
*Mycoplasma pneumoniae CF test - 110
Ox cell hemolysin test
Q-Fever, Agglutination Titre
Q-Fever, Complement Fixation
Radioallergo Sorbent Test (RAST Test)
Rheumatoid Arthritis-latex fixation (RA)
Rose test
Rubella CF antibody
Bubella HI antibody
Serum Specific Proteins - Immunoglobulin quantitation
(IgG; IgA; IgM; IgD; IgE)
Sheep Cell Agglutination test for RA

*Streptococcus MG agglutination - 110
Thyroid auto-antibodies
*Trichina agglutination - 130
*Toxoplasmosis Agglutination - 130
*Tularemia agglutination - 110

300 CLINICAL CHEMISTRY - ROUTINE

310 Clinical Chemistry - Routine

Blood Urine, Stool, Cerebro-Spinal Fluid Chemistry
(includes electrophoresis and enzymes
Acetone-acetoacetic acid-serum
Acid mucopolysaccharides, qualitative
Acid phosphatase
Acidity, titration
Albumin
Albumin-globulin (A/G) ratio (calculation)
Aldolase
Alkaline phospahtase, serum
Alpha-hydroxybutyric dehydrogenase (HED)
Alpha-amino acid nitrogen
Delta-aminolevulinic acid (ALA)
Amino acids, fractionated quant.
p-aminohippuric acid (PAH)
Aminophylline
Ammonia, Blood Urine
Amylase, Serum, Urine
Arterial Blood pH
Ascorbic Acid (Vitamin C)
Atyherogenic Index (AI)
Bicarbonate
Bile Acids, fractionated
Bilirubin, total
Bilirubin, Total and Direct
Blood gas and pH (calculation) (Pco2; po2; % 02 saturation; base-total)
Boric Acid
Bromide
Bromsulfalcin, dye analysis only (BSP) – Sulfobromphthalein Excretion - Liver
BUN (Blood Urea Nitrogen)
Calcium, Serum, Urine, Feces
Carbon Dioxide Content
Carotene
Cephalin Flocculation
Ceruloplasmin
Chloride
Cholesterol, total
Cholesterol, total and esters
Cholinesterase, serum, plasma, RBC
Chondroitin sulfate, qual.
Citric acid, serum, urine
C02-combining power
Creatine phosphokinase (CPK) - also known as creatine kinase

Creatine, urine, serum
Creatinine, urine, serum
Creatinine Clearance
Cryoglobulins
Cystine
Diastase
Electrolytes (Na, K, Cl) - sodium, potassium, chloride
FATS, serum or stool
Fatty acids, unesterified
Folate, RBC, serum
Free Fatty acids
Galactose, by chromatography
Gamma glutamyl transpetidase (Gamma-GTP)
Globulins, total
Glucose
Glucose tolerance
*Glucose-6-Phosphate Dehydrogenase-220,400
Glutathione Reductase
Glycoprotein
Guanase
Haptoglobin
*Hemoglobin electrophoresis - 400
Hexosamine
Hippuric acid quant.
Histamine
Homogentisic acid quant.
Icterus index (calculation)
Indocyanine green excretion-liver dye test
Iron, total, serum, urine
Iron-binding capacity and total iron
Unsaturated iron binding capacity-UIBEL
Isocitric dehydrogenase (ICD)
Kynurenic and Xanthurenic acids
Lactic acid
Lactose tolerance test
LDH (lactic dehydrogenase), serum, CSF
LDH (fractionated)
LDH Isoenzymes by electrophoresis
Leucine aminopeptidase (LAP), serum, urine
Lipase
Lipid Profile-Phospholipids, cholesterol, triglycerides
Lipids, total and fractionated, serum
Lipids, total, feces
Lipids, total and split fat, feces
Lipids per dry weight, feces
B-Liporpotein screening
Lipoproteins by electrophoresis
Lipoproteins, phenotyping
Lipoproteins by ultracentrigufation
Lithium
Macroglobulin by ultracentrifugation
Magnesium, serum
Magnesium, urine
Manganese

Melanin, qualitative
Methylmalonic acid
Mucopolysaccharides, acid, qual.
Mucoprotein
Nitrogen, total, Urine, Feces
Non-esterified fatty acids (NEFA)
Non-protein nitrogen (NPN)
5'-Nucleotidase
Orinase Tolerance Test (Tolbutamide)
Ornithine carbamyl transferase (OCT)
Osmolatity by freezing point depression
Oxalate
Paraldehyde (as acetaldehyde)
PCO2
Pepsinogen
pH
Phenylpyruvic acid, qual.
Phosphoethanolamine by column chromatography
Phosphogalactose transferase
Phospholipids
Phospholipids, cholesterol, triglycerides
Phosphorus, Serum & Urine
PKU (exluding Guthrie method)
P02
Potassium, Serum, Urine, Feces
Protein, total
Protein, quant., urine, CSF
Protein fractionation by electrophoresis
Protoporphyrin, REC
Pyruvic acid
Reducing sugars by chromatography, qual., blood
Salicylates, serum, urine - 330
SGOT (Serum glutamic - oxalacetic transaminase) - also known as aspartate amino transferase
SGPT (Serum glutamic - pyruvic transaminase) - also know as alanine amino transferase
Silica, in lung tissue
Sodium, Serum, Urine, Feces
Spinal Fluid, Chlorides
Spinal Fluid, Sugar
Spinal Fluid, Total Protein
Split fat and total lipids, feces
Stercobilinogen
Sugars, qual., by paper chromatography
Sulfa level
Sulfate
Sweat Chlorides
Thiocyanate
Thymol Turbidity
Trichloracetic acid (TCA)
Trichlorethanol
Triglycerides
Triglycerides, phospholipids, cholesterol, total lipids
Tryspin

Tryptamine
Tryrosine
Urea clearance
Uric acid (phosphotungstate method)
Uropepsin
Vitamin A
Vitamin B2
*Vitamin Bl2-400
Xanthurenic and kynurenic acids
Xylose (for tolerance test)

320 URINALYSIS (Routine and Calculi)-Clinical Microscopy

Acetone-acetoacetic acid (urine)
Addis Count
Basic chemical profile
Qualitative glucose
Qualitative bile
Qualitative Ketone bodies
Qualitative blood
Qualitative nitrate
Qualitative protein (predominantly albumin)
pH
Specific gravity
Color and appearance
Bile, urine
Calculi, qualitative
Coproporphyrin
Diagnex Blue (Tubeless gastric)
Galactose (for tolerance test)
Hippuric acid
Homogentisic acid, qualitative
Microscopic examination of urine sediment
(cells, casts)
Myoglobin, semi-quantitive
Para-aminohippuric acid (PAH)
Pentose Sugar in urine (qual) screening
Phenosulfonphthalein excretion test-
renal function test (P.S.P.)
Porphobilinogen, quant.
Porphyrins, urine
Porphyrins, feces
Protein, Bence-Jones
Protoporphyrin
Reducing sugars by chromatography, qual., urine
*Serotonin, urine - 5HIAA - 330
Urinalysis (including Microscopic)
Urobilinogen, urine, feces
Uroporphyrin

320 CHEMISTRY - Other (including Toxiocology)

Alkaloids and other organic bases
*Alpha-l-fetoprotein - 220

Amphetamine
Anti-convulsant group
Antimony
Arsenic, quantitative
Barbiturates
Barbiturates, tissue, quant.
Beryllium
Bismuth
Blood Alcohol ethyl)
Bromides, serum
Bromides, urine
Cadmium
Carbon Monoxide (Carboxyhemoglobin)
*Carcinoembryonic Antigen Assay (CEA) - 220
Chloramphenicol (Chloromycetin)
Chromium
Codeine, urine
Copper, Serum, Urine
Cyanide
Darvon
Dicumarol
Digitalis
Digitoxin
Digoxin
Dilantin
Doriden (glutethimide)
Elavil
Ethyl Alcohol (ethanol)
Fluoride
Gentamicin (by RIA)
Gold
Heavy metals (arsenic, lead, mercury) - Reinsch Test
*Hepatitis B Antigen (HBsAg) - 220, 540
*Hepatitis B Antibody (Anti-HBs) - 220, 540
Hypnotic and Tranquilizer Screen
Lead
Librium
Meprobamate (Miltown, Equanil)
Mercury
Methaqualone
Minerals
Nickel
Nicotine
Phenacetin
Phenols
Phenothiazines
Quinidine
Reinsch Test
*Salicylates, serum, urine - 3l0
Selenium
Strychnine
Thallium
Theophylline
Trace Elements

Trofranil - Imipramine)
Valium
Volatiles by gas chromatography
(Acetaldehyde, acetone, ethanol, diethyl ether, isopropanol, methanol; other may be detected)
Zinc

330 CHEMISTRY - Other (Endrocrinology)

Adrenocorticotrophic hormone
Anti-diuretic hormone
Andrenaline-noradrenaline, total
Adrenaline-noradrenaline fractionation
A/E/DHA, by chromatography
Aldosterone
Calcitonin
Catecholamines, total
Chorionic gonadotropin, quant. BIOASSAY
Chorionic gonadodotropin, quant., IMMUNOASSAY
Cortiosol, plasma
11-Deoxy: 11-oxy ratio of 17-KGS
Dehydroepiandrosterone (DHA)
Estradiol receptor assay
Estriol, placental
Estrogens, total
Estrogens, fractionated (Brown method)
Estrogen receptor assay
Etiocholanolone, dehydroepiandrosterone, androsterone and total
17-Ketosteriods (A/E/DHA)
Ferminiminoglutamic acid (FIGLU)
Free thyroxine (Includes T4-by-column)
FSH (Follicle stimulating Hormone)
Gastrin
Growth hormone (GH OR HGH)
5-HIAA (5 OH-indoleacetic acid, serotonin metabolite)
Homovanillic Acid (HVA)
Human growth hormone (HGH)
Hydroxbutyric dehydrogenase (HBD)
17-Hydroxycorticosteroids, plasma (cortisol by fluorescence method)
17-Hydroxycorticosteroids, urine
11-R-Hydroxylase inhibition test
Hydroxyproline, free
Hydroxyproline, total
5-Hydroxytryptamine
Indole-3-Acetic Acid
Insulin
Insulin (for clearance test)
Inulin
Iodine, T4-by-column chromatography
Iodine, total, fluids, feces
Iodine, total inorganic and PBI
17-Ketosteroids, total, plasma, urine
17-Ketosteroids, beta: alpha ratio
17-Ketosteroids, separated by chromatography (7 compounds)

17-Ketogenic steroids (l7KGS)
Long-acting thyroid stimulator and Thyroid stimulating hormone (LATS and TSH)
Luteinizing hormone (LH)
Metanephrines (total)
11-Oxysteroids
Parathyroid hormone
PBI
PBI, total and inorganic iodine
Phenylalanine
Phenylketonuria (PKU) screening
Pituitary gonadotropins (FSH)
Placental estroil
Placidyl
Plasma cortisol
Pregnanediol
Pragnanetriol
Progesterone
Prolactin
Renin activity
Serotonin, Blood - 5HIAA, 5-hydroxyindoleacetic acid
*Serotonin metabolite, urine - 320
Testosterone
Tetrahydro compound S (THS)
Thyroid stimulating hormone
Thyroxine by column chromatography (T4)
Thyroxine, Free (T4)
Thyroxine by Murphy-Pattee method (T4)
Thyroxine-binding globulin (TBG)
Thyroxine-binding globulin (TBG) without T4 test)
Triiodothyronine (T3)
Vanillyl mandelic acid (VMA)

400 HEMATOLOGY

A2 hemoglobin
A2 and fetal hemoglobin
Basophillic stippling
*Blood specimen for malaria - 130
Cell count - spinal fluid
Complete Blood Count with Differential
Differential
Eosinophile Count
Erythrocyte Sedimentation Rate, Sed Rate
*Folate, R.B.C., Serum - 310
Fragility Test, erythrocytes
*G-6-PD (Glucose-6-Phosphate dehydrogenase) - 220, 310
Hemoglobin A2
Hemoglobin, Fetal
Hemoglobin, Fetal and A2
Hemoglobin-binding protein
*Hemoglobin electrophoresis - 310
Hematocrit
Hemoglobin (cyanmethemoglobin method)

Hemoglobin (iron assay)
Hemoglobin, plasma, urine
Indices, Wintrobe (calculation)
Methemalbumin (Schumm Test)
Platelet Count
Red Blood Count (Erythrocyte Count, RBC)
Reticulocyte Count
Screening test for DIC - Disseminated Intravascular Coagulation
Sickle Cell Preparation
Sulfhemoglobin, methemoglobin, and total Hgb
*Vitamin B-l2 - 310
White Blood Count (Leukocyte Count, WBC)

Coagulation Studies Hematology

Bleeding time (Duke) or Ivy and Clotting time (Lee and White)
Complete Coagulation Study
Factor Assays (Factor VIII, IX, VII, XI)
Fibrin-Fibrinogen l egradation Products
Fibrinogen
Partial Thromboplastin Time (APTT, PTT)
Prothrombin Time (Pro time, PT)
Prothrombin Consumption
Prothrombin Utilization
Tests for Circulating Anticoagulants

Cellular Study Hematology

Bone Marrow Aspirate
Eosinophile Smear
Leukocyte Alkaline Phosphatase
Lupus crythematosus Preparation (L.E. Pre)
*Blood Specimen for malaria - See 130 and for other parasites
Molecular abnormality studies
Hemoglobinopathy
Synovial Fluid - Cell Count or Differential

500 IMMUNOHEMATOLOGY

510 Immunohematology

A Subgrouping
Blood Grouping, A., B, O, and AB
Rh factor Including Du
Rh Cenotype (C, D, E, c, e)
*M+N Type - 540
*Husband's red cell genotype - 540

520 Antibody Indentification

*Antibody screening test - Indirect Coombs - 540
Antibody titration
Rh antibody titer and blocking antibodies

530 Compatibility Testing - Crossmatch

540 Blood Typing for paternity tests

Direct Coomb's Test
*Hepatitis B Antigen (HBsAg) - 220, 330
*Hepatitis B Antibody (Anti-HBs) - 220, 330
*Husband's Red Cell Genotype - 510
*Indirect Coombs - Antibody screening test - 520
*M + N typing - 510
Rho Gam Workup

600 PATHOLOGY

601 Histopathology

Tissue Decalcification
Bone Marrow Biopsy
Tissue Pathology
Surgical pathology
Frozen sections
Autopsy and sections

620 Oral Pathology

630 Exfoliative Cytology

Cytology - Female Genital Tract
Cytology - nongynecological fluid cytologies

700 PHYSIOLOGICAL TESTING

710 EKG Services

800 Radiobioassay and Nuclides Radiobioassay

Blood volume - RBC Mass (Cr 51)
I^{131} Therapy
Polonium
Schilling test (Cobalt 60 - labelled B-12)
Thyroid function studies (1131 Uptake) (IST-3)
Tritium

900 All Specialties And Subspecialties

*More than one specialty category

E. Certification Changes.—Each page of the lists of approved specialties also includes a column "Certification Changed" in which the following codes are used:

- "C" indicates a change in the laboratory's approved certification since the preceding listing.
- "A" discloses an accretion.

* "TERM" - Laboratory not approved for payment after the indicated date which follows the code.

The reason for termination also is given in the following codes:

1. Involuntary termination - no longer meets requirements
2. Voluntary withdrawal
3. Laboratory closed, merged with other interests, or organizational change
4. Ownership change with new ownership participating under different name
5. Ownership change with new owner not participating
6. Change in ownership - new provider number assigned
7. Involuntary termination - failure to abide by agreement
8. Former "emergency" hospital now fully participating

F. Carrier Contacts With Independent Clinical Laboratories.—An important role of the carrier is as a communicant of necessary information to independent clinical laboratories. Experience has shown that the failure to inform laboratories of Medicare regulations and claims processing procedures may have an adverse effect on prosecution of laboratories suspected of fraudulent activities with respect to tests performed by, or billed on behalf of, independent laboratories. United Stated Attorneys often have to prosecute under a handicap or may simply refuse to prosecute cases where there is no evidence that a laboratory has been specifically informed of Medicare regulations and claims processing procedures.

To assure that laboratories are aware of Medicare regulations and carrier's policy, carrier newsletters should be sent to independent laboratories when any changes are made in coverage policy or claims processing procedures. Additionally, to completely document efforts to fully inform independent laboratories of Medicare policy and their responsibilities, previously issued newsletters should be periodically re-issued to remind laboratories of existing requirements. Some items which should be discussed are the requirements to have the same fee schedule for Medicare and private patients, to specify whether the tests are manual or automated, to indicate the numeric designation 6 or 12 when billing for SMA tests, to document fully the medical necessity for pick-up of specimens from a skilled nursing facility or a beneficiary's home, and, in cases when a laboratory service is referred from one independent laboratory to another independent laboratory, to identify the laboratory actually performing the test.

Additionally, when carrier professional relations representatives make personal contacts with particular laboratories, they should prepare and retain reports of contact indicating dates, persons present, and issues discussed.

G. Independent Laboratory Service to a Patient in His Home or an Institution. —Where it is medically necessary for an independent laboratory to visit a patient to obtain a specimen or to perform EKGs, the service would be covered in the following circumstances:

1. Patient Confined to His Home.—If a patient is confined to his home or other place of residence used as his home, (see §2051.1 for the definition of a "homebound patient"), medical necessity would exist, for example, where a laboratory technician draws a blood specimen or takes an EKG tracing. However, where the specimen is a type which would require only the services of a messenger and would not require the skills of a laboratory technician, e.g., urine or sputum, a specimen pickup service would not be considered medically necessary.
2. Place of Residence is an Institution.—Medical necessity could also exist where the patient's place of residence is an institution including a skilled nursing facility, that does not perform venipunctures. This would apply even though the institution meets the basic definition of a skilled nursing facility and would not ordinarily be considered a beneficiary's home under the rules in § 2100.
3. (This policy is intended for independent laboratories only and does not expand the range of coverage of services to homebound patients under the incident to provision.) A trip by an independent laboratory technician to a facility (other than a hospital) for the purpose of performing a venipuncture or taking an EKG tracing is considered medically necessary only if (a) the patient was confined to the facility, and (b) the facility did not have on duty personnel qualified to perform this service. When facility personnel actually obtained and prepared the specimens for the independent laboratory to pick them up, the laboratory provides this pickup service as a service to the facility in the same manner as it does for physicians.

2070.4 Coverage of Portable X-ray Services Not Under the Direct Supervision of a Physician.-

A. Diagnostic X-ray Tests.—Diagnostic x-ray services furnished by a portable x-ray supplier are covered under Part B when furnished in a place or residence used as the patient's home and in nonparticipating institutions. These services must be performed under the general supervision of a physician and certain conditions relating to health and safety (as prescribed by the Secretary) must be met.

   Diagnostic portable x-ray services are also covered under Part B when provided in participating SNFs and hospitals, under circumstances in which they cannot be covered under hospital insurance, i.e., the services are not furnished by the participating institution either directly or under arrangements that provide for the institution to bill for the services. (See §2255 for reimbursement for Part B services furnished to inpatients of participating and nonparticipating institutions.)

B. Applicability of Health and Safety Standards.—The health and safety standards apply to all suppliers of portable x-ray services, except physicians who provide immediate personal supervision during the administration of diagnostic x-ray services. Payment is made only for services of approved suppliers who have been found to meet the standards. Notice of the coverage dates for services of approved suppliers are given to carriers by the RO.

When the services of a supplier of portable x-ray services no longer meet the conditions of coverage, physicians having an interest in the supplier's certification status must be notified. The notification action regarding suppliers of portable x-ray equipment is the same as required for decertification of independent laboratories, and the procedures explained in §2070.lC should be followed.

C. Scope of Portable X-Ray Benefit.—In order to avoid payment for services which are inadequate or hazardous to the patient, the scope of the covered portable x-ray benefit is defined as:

* Skeletal films involving arms and legs, pelvis, vertebral column, and skull;
* Chest films which do not involve the use of contrast media (except routine screening procedures and tests in connection with routine physical examinations); and
* Abdominal films which do not involve the use of contrast media.

D. Exclusions From Coverage as Portable X-Ray Services.— Procedures and examinations which are not covered under the portable x-ray provision include the following:

* Procedures involving fluoroscopy;
* Procedures involving the use of contrast media;
* Procedures requiring the administration of a substance to the patient or injection of a substance into the patient and/or special manipulation of the patient;
* Procedures which require special medical skill or knowledge possessed by a doctor of medicine or doctor of osteopathy or which require that medical judgment be exercised;
* Procedures requiring special technical competency and/or special equipment or materials;
* Routine screening procedures; and
* Procedures which are not of a diagnostic nature.

E. Reimbursement Procedure.

1. Name of Ordering Physician. — Assure that portable x-ray tests have been provided on the written order of a physician. Accordingly, if a bill does not include the name of the physician who ordered the service, that information must be obtained before payment may be made.

2. Reason Chest X-Ray Ordered. — Because all routine screening procedures and tests in connection with routine physical examinations are excluded from coverage under Medicare, all bills for portable x-ray services involving the chest contain, in addition to the name of the physician who ordered the service, the reason an x-ray test was required.

If this information is not shown, it is obtained from either the supplier or the physician. If the test was for an excluded routine service, no payment may be made.

See also §§4110 ff. for additional instructions on reviewing bills involving portable x-ray.

F. Electrocardiograms.—The taking of an electrocardiogram tracing by an approved supplier of portable x-ray services may be covered as an "other diagnostic test." The health and safety standards referred to in §2070.4B are thus also applicable to such diagnostic EKG services, e.g., the technician must meet the personnel qualification requirements in the Conditions for Coverage of Portable x-ray Services. (See §50-15 (Electrocardiographic Services) in the Coverage Issues Manual.)

2079 SURGICAL DRESSINGS, AND SPLINTS, CASTS, AND OTHER DEVICES USED FOR REDUCTIONS OF FRACTURES AND DISLOCATIONS

Surgical dressings are limited to primary and secondary dressings required for the treatment of a wound caused by, or treated by, a surgical procedure that has been performed by a physician or other health care professional to the extent permissible under State law. In addition, surgical dressings required after debridement of a wound are also covered, irrespective of the type of debridement, as long as the debridement was reasonable and necessary and was performed by a health care professional who was acting within the scope of his or her legal authority when performing this function. Surgical dressings are covered for as long as they are medically necessary.
Primary dressings are therapeutic or protective coverings applied directly to wounds or lesions either on the skin or caused by an opening to the skin. Secondary dressing materials that serve a therapeutic or protective function and that are needed to secure a primary dressing are also covered. Items such as adhesive tape, roll gauze, bandages, and disposable compression material are examples of secondary dressings. Elastic stockings, support hose, foot coverings, leotards, knee supports, surgical leggings, gauntlets, and pressure garments for the arms and hands are examples of items that are not ordinarily covered as surgical dressings. Some items, such as transparent film, may be used as a primary or secondary dressing.

If a physician, certified nurse midwife, physician assistant, nurse practitioner, or clinical nurse specialist applies surgical dressings as part of a professional service that is billed to Medicare, the surgical dressings are considered incident to the professional services of the health care practitioner. (See sections 2050.1, 2154, 2156, 2158, and 2160.) When surgical dressings are not covered incident to the services of a health care practitioner and are obtained by the patient from a supplier (e.g., a drugstore, physician, or other health care practitioner that qualifies as a supplier) on an order from a physician or other health care professional authorized under State law or regulation to make such an order, the surgical dressings are covered separately under Part B.

2100 DURABLE MEDICAL EQUIPMENT - GENERAL

Expenses incurred by a beneficiary for the rental or purchase of durable medical equipment (DME) are reimbursable if the following three requirements are met. The decision whether to rent or purchase an item of equipment resides with the beneficiary.

A. The equipment meets the definition of DME (§2100.1); and

B. The equipment is necessary and reasonable for the treatment of the patient's illness or injury or to improve the functioning of his malformed body member (§2100.2); and

C. The equipment is used in the patient's home (§2100.3).

Payment may also be made under this provision for repairs, maintenance, and delivery of equipment as well as for expendable and nonreusable items essential to the effective use of the equipment subject to the conditions in §2100.4.

See §2105 and its appendix for coverage guidelines and screening list of DME. See §4105.3 for models of payment: decisions as to rental or purchase, lump sum and periodic payments, etc. Where covered DME is furnished to a beneficiary by a supplier of services other than a provider of services, reimbursement is made by the carrier on the basis of the reasonable charge. If the equipment is furnished by a provider of services, reimbursement is made to the provider by the intermediary on a reasonable cost basis; see Coverage Issues Appendix 25-1 for hemodialysis equipment and supplies.

2100.1 Definition of Durable Medical Equipment.—Durable medical equipment is equipment which a) can withstand repeated use, and b) is primarily and customarily used to serve a medical purpose, and c) generally is not useful to a person in the absence of an illness or injury; and d) is appropriate for use in the home.
All requirements of the definition must be met before an item can be considered to be durable medical equipment.

A. Durability.—An item is considered durable if it can withstand repeated use, i.e., the type of item which could normally be rented. Medical supplies of an expendable nature such as, incontinent pads, lambs wool pads, catheters, ace bandages, elastic stockings, surgical face masks, irrigating kits, sheets and bags are not considered "durable" within the meaning of the definition. There are other items which, although durable in nature, may fall into other coverage categories such as braces, prosthetic devices, artificial arms, legs, and eyes.

B. Medical Equipment.—Medical equipment is equipment which is primarily and customarily used for medical purposes and is not generally useful in the absence of illness or injury. In most instances, no development will be needed to determine whether a specific item of equipment is medical in nature. However, some cases will require development to determine whether the item constitutes medical equipment. This development would include the advice of local medical organizations (hospitals, medical schools, medical societies) and specialists in the field of physical medicine and rehabilitation. If the equipment is new on the market, it may be necessary, prior to seeking professional advice, to obtain information from the supplier or manufacturer explaining the design, purpose, effectiveness and method of using the equipment in the home as well as the results of any tests or clinical studies that have been conducted.

1. Equipment Presumptively Medical.—Items such as hospital beds, wheelchairs, hemodialysis equipment, iron lungs, respirators, intermittent positive pressure breathing machines, medical regulators, oxygen tents, crutches, canes, trapeze bars, walkers, inhalators, nebulizers, commodes, suction machines and traction equipment presumptively constitute medical equipment. (Although hemodialysis equipment is a prosthetic device (§ 2130), it also meets the definition of DME, and reimbursement for the rental or purchase of such equipment for use in the beneficiary's home will be made only under the provisions for payment applicable to DME. See 25-1 and 25-2 of the Coverage Issues Appendix for coverage of home use of hemodialysis.)

NOTE: There is a wide variety in type of respirators and suction machines. The carrier's medical staff should determine whether the apparatus specified in the claim is appropriate for home use.

2. Equipment Presumptively Nonmedical.—Equipment which is primarily and customarily used for a nonmedical purpose may not be considered "medical" equipment for which payment can be made under the medical insurance program. This is true even though the item has some remote medically related use. For example, in the case of a cardiac patient, an air conditioner might possibly be used to lower room temperature to reduce fluid loss in the patient and to restore an environment conducive to maintenance of the proper fluid balance. Nevertheless, because the primary and customary use of an air conditioner is a nonmedical one, the air conditioner cannot be deemed to be medical equipment for which payment can be made.

   Other devices and equipment used for environmental control or to enhance the environmental setting in which the beneficiary is placed are not considered covered DME. These include, for example, room heaters, humidifiers, dehumidifiers, and electric air cleaners. Equipment which basically serves comfort or convenience functions or is primarily for the convenience of a person caring for the patient, such as elevators, stairway elevators, and posture chairs do not constitute medical equipment. Similarly,physical fitness equipment, e.g., an exercycle; first-aid or precautionary-type equipment, e.g., present portable oxygen units; self-help devices, e.g., safety grab bars; and training equipment, e.g., speech teaching machines and braille training texts, are considered nonmedical in nature.

3. Special Exception Items.—Specified items of equipment may be covered under certain conditions even though they do not meet the definition of DME because they are not primarily and customarily used to serve a medical purpose and/or are generally useful in the absence of illness or injury. These items would be covered when it is clearly established that they serve a therapeutic purpose in an individual case and would include:

a. Gel pads and pressure and water mattresses (which generally serve a preventive purpose) when prescribed for a patient who had bed sores or there is medical evidence indicating that he is highly susceptible to such ulceration; and
b. Heat lamps for a medical rather than a soothing or cosmetic purpose, e.g., where the need for heat therapy has been established.

In establishing medical necessity (§2100.2) for the above items, the evidence must show that the item is included in the physician's course of treatment and a physician is supervising its use. (See also Appendix to § 2105.)

NOTE: The above items represent special exceptions and no extension of coverage to other items should be inferred.

2100.4 Repairs, Maintenance, Replacement, and Delivery.—Under the circumstances specified below, payment may be made for repair, maintenance, and replacement of medically required DME, including equipment which had been in use before the user enrolled in Part B of the program. However, do not pay for repair, maintenance, or replacement of equipment in the frequent and substantial servicing or oxygen equipment payment categories. In addition, payments for repair and maintenance may not include payment for parts and labor covered under a manufacturer's or supplier's warranty.

A. Repairs.— To repair means to fix or mend and to put the equipment back in good condition after damage or wear. Repairs to equipment which a beneficiary owns are covered when necessary to make the equipment serviceable. However, do not pay for repair of previously denied equipment or equipment in the frequent and substantial servicing or oxygen equipment payment categories. If the expense for repairs exceeds the estimated expense of purchasing or renting another item of equipment for the remaining period of medical need, no payment can be made for the amount of the excess. (See subsection C where claims for repairs suggest malicious damage or culpable neglect.)

Since renters of equipment recover from the rental charge the expenses they incur in maintaining in working order the equipment they rent out, separately itemized charges for repair of rented equipment are not covered. This includes items in the frequent and substantial servicing, oxygen equipment, capped rental, and inexpensive or routinely purchased payment categories which are being rented.

A new Certificate of Medical Necessity (CMN) and/or physician's order is not needed for repairs. For replacement items, see Subsection C below.

B. Maintenance.—Routine periodic maintenance, such as testing, cleaning, regulating and checking of the beneficiary's equipment is not covered. Such routine maintenance is generally expected to be done by the owner rather than by a retailer or some other person who charges the beneficiary. Normally, purchasers of DME are given operating manuals which describe the type of servicing an owner may perform to properly maintain the equipment. It is reasonable to expect that beneficiaries will perform this maintenance. Thus, hiring a third party to do such work is for the convenience of the beneficiary and is not covered.

However, more extensive maintenance which, based on the manufacturers' recommendations, is to be performed by authorized technicians, is covered as repairs for medically necessary equipment which a beneficiary owns. This might include, for example, breaking down sealed components and performing tests which require specialized testing equipment not available to the beneficiary. Do not pay for maintenance of purchased items that require frequent and substantial servicing or oxygen equipment. See §5102.2.G.

Since renters of equipment recover from the rental charge the expenses they incur in maintaining in working order the equipment they rent out, separately itemized charges for maintenance of rented equipment are generally not covered. Payment may not be made for maintenance of rented equipment other than the maintenance and servicing fee established for capped rental items in §5102.1.E.4.

A new CMN and/or physician's order is not needed for covered maintenance.

C. Replacement.—Replacement refers to the provision of an identical or nearly identical item. Situations involving the provision of a different item because of a change in medical condition are not addressed in this section.

Equipment which the beneficiary owns or is a capped rental item may be replaced in cases of loss or irreparable damage. Irreparable damage refers to a specific accident or to a natural disaster (e.g., fire, flood, etc.). A physician's order and/or new Certificate of Medical Necessity (CMN), when required, is needed to reaffirm the medical necessity of the item.

Irreparable wear refers to deterioration sustained from day-to-day usage over time and a specific event cannot be identified. Replacement of equipment due to irreparable wear takes into consideration the reasonable useful lifetime of the equipment. If the item of equipment has been in continuous use by the patient on either a rental or purchase basis for the equipment's useful lifetime, the beneficiary may elect to obtain a new piece of equipment. Replacement may be reimbursed when a new physician order and/or new CMN, when required, is needed to reaffirm the medical necessity of the item.

The reasonable useful lifetime of durable medical equipment is determined through program instructions. In the absence of program instructions, carriers may determine the reasonable useful lifetime of equipment, but in no case can it be less than 5 years. Computation of the useful lifetime is based on when the equipment is delivered to the beneficiary, not the age of the equipment. Replacement due to wear is not covered during the reasonable useful lifetime of the equipment. During the reasonable useful lifetime, Medicare does cover repair up to the cost of replacement (but not actual replacement) for medically necessary equipment owned by the beneficiary. (See subsection A.)

Charges for the replacement of oxygen equipment, items that require frequent and substantial servicing or inexpensive or routinely purchased items which are being rented are not covered.

Cases suggesting malicious damage, culpable neglect or wrongful disposition of equipment as discussed in §2100.6 should be investigated and denied where the DMERC/Carrier determines that it is unreasonable to make program payment under the circumstances.

D. Delivery.—Payment for delivery of DME whether rented or purchased is generally included in the fee schedule allowance for the item. See §5105 for the rules that apply to making reimbursement for exceptional cases.

E. Leased Renal Dialysis Equipment.—Generally, where renal dialysis equipment is leased directly from the manufacturer, the rental charge is closely related to the manufacturer's cost of the equipment which means it does not include a margin for recovering the cost of repairs beyond the initial warranty period.

In view of physical distance and other factors which may make it impractical for the manufacturer to perform repairs, it is not feasible to make the manufacturer responsible for all repairs and include a margin for the additional costs. Therefore, reimbursement may be made for the repair and maintenance of home dialysis equipment leased directly from the manufacturer (or other party acting essentially as an intermediary between the patient and the manufacturer for the purpose of assuming the financial risk) if the rental charge does not include a margin to recover these costs, and then only when the patient is free to secure repairs locally in the most economical manner.

Where, on the other hand, a third party is in the business of medical equipment retail supply and rental, the presumption that there is a margin in the rental charge for dialysis equipment to cover the costs of repair services will be retained. The exclusion from coverage of separately itemized repair charges will, therefore, continue to be applied in these situations, and the patient must look to the supplier to perform (or cover the cost of) necessary repairs, maintenance, and replacement of the home dialysis equipment.

In all cases, whether the dialysis equipment is being purchased, is owned outright, or is being leased, Medicare payment is to be made only after the initial warranty period has expired. Generally, reimbursement for repairs, maintenance, and replacement parts for medically necessary home dialysis equipment may be made in a lump sum payment. However, where extensive repairs are required and the charge for repairing the item represents a substantial proportion of the purchase price of a replacement system, exercise judgment with respect to a possible need to make periodic payments, instead of a lump-sum payment, for repair of such equipment.

As in the case of the maintenance of purchased DME, routine periodic servicing of leased dialysis equipment, including most testing and cleaning, is not covered. While reimbursement will be made for more extensive maintenance and necessary repairs of leased dialysis equipment, the patient or family member is expected to perform those services for which the training for home or self-dialysis would have qualified them, e.g., replacement of a light bulb.

Reasonable charges for travel expenses related to the repair of leased dialysis equipment are covered if the repairman customarily charges for travel and this is a common practice among other repairman in the area. When a repair charge includes an element for travel, however, the location of other suitably qualified repairmen will be considered in determining the allowance for travel.

NOTE: The above coverage instructions pertain to a special case and no extension of such coverage with respect to other items should be inferred.

2100.5 Coverage of Supplies and Accessories.— Reimbursement may be made for supplies, e.g., oxygen (see §60-4 in the Coverage Issues Manual for the coverage of oxygen in the home), that are necessary for the effective use of durable medical equipment. Such supplies include those drugs and biologicals which must be put directly into the equipment in order to achieve the therapeutic benefit of the durable medical equipment or to assure the proper functioning of the equipment, e.g., tumor chemotherapy agents used with an infusion pump or heparin used with a home dialysis system. However, the coverage of such drugs or biologicals does not preclude the need for a determination that the drug or biological itself is reasonable and necessary for treatment of the illness or injury or to improve the functioning of a malformed body member.

In the case of prescription drugs, other than oxygen, used in conjunction with durable medical equipment, prosthetic, orthotics, and supplies (DMEPOS) or prosthetic devices, the entity that dispenses the drug must furnish it directly to the patient for whom a prescription is written. The entity that dispenses the drugs must have a Medicare supplier number, must possess a current license to dispense prescription drugs in the State in which the drug is dispensed, and must bill and receive payment in its own name.

A supplier that is not the entity that dispenses the drugs cannot purchase the drugs used in conjunction with DME for resale to the beneficiary. Payments made for drugs provided on or after December 1, 1996 to suppliers not having a valid pharmacy license to dispense prescription drugs must be recouped.

2120.1 Vehicle and Crew Requirement

A. The Vehicle.—The vehicle must be a specially designed and equipped automobile or other vehicle (in some areas of the United States this might be a boat or plane) for transporting the sick or injured. It must have customary patient care equipment including a stretcher, clean linens, first aid supplies, oxygen equipment, and it must also have such other safety and lifesaving equipment as is required by State or local authorities.

B. The Crew.—The ambulance crew must consist of at least two members. Those crew members charged with the care or handling of the patient must include one individual with adequate first aid training, i.e., training at least equivalent to that provided by the standard and advanced Red Cross first aid courses. Training "equivalent" to the standard and advanced Red Cross first aid training courses included ambulance service training and experience acquired in military service, successful completion by the individual of a comparable first aid course furnished by or under the sponsorship of State or local authorities, an educational institution, a fire department, a hospital, a professional organization, or other such qualified organization. On-the-job training involving the administration of first aid under the supervision of or in conjunction with trained first aid personnel for a period of time sufficient to assure the trainee's proficiency in handling the wide range of patient care services that may have to be performed by a qualified attendant can also be considered as "equivalent training."

C. Verification of Compliance.—In determining whether the vehicles and personnel of each supplier meet all of the above requirements, carriers may accept the supplier's statement (absent information to the contrary) that its vehicles and personnel meet all of the requirements if (l) the statement describes the first aid, safety, and other patient care items with which the vehicles are equipped, (2) the statement shows the extent of first aid training acquired by the personnel assigned to those vehicles, (3) the statement contains the supplier's agreement to notify the carrier of any change in operation which could affect the coverage of his ambulance services, and (4) the information provided indicates that the requirements are met. The statement must be accompanied by documentary evidence that the ambulance has the equipment required by State and local authorities. Documentary evidence could include a letter from such authorities, a copy of a license, permit certificate, etc., issued by the authorities. The statement and supporting documentation would be kept on file by the carrier.

When a supplier does not submit such a statement or whenever there is a question about a supplier's compliance with any of the above requirements for vehicle and crew (including suppliers who have completed the statement), carriers should take appropriate action including, where necessary, on-site inspection of the vehicles and verification of the qualifications of personnel to determine whether the ambulance service qualifies for reimbursement under Medicare. Since the requirements described above for coverage of ambulance services are applicable to the overall operation of the ambulance supplier's service, it is not required that information regarding personnel and vehicles be obtained on an individual trip basis.

D. Ambulance of Providers of Services.—The Part A intermediary is responsible for the processing of claims for ambulance service furnished by participating hospitals, skilled nursing facilities and home health agencies and has the responsibility to determine the compliance of provider's ambulance and crew. Since provider ambulance services furnished "under arrangements" with suppliers can be covered only if the supplier meets the above requirements, the Part A intermediary may ask the carrier to identify those suppliers who meet the requirements.

E. Equipment and Supplies.—As mentioned above, the ambulance must have customary patient care equipment and first aid supplies. Reusable devices and equipment such as backboards, neckboards and inflatable leg and arm splints are considered part of the general ambulance service and would be included in the charge for the trip. On the other hand, separate reasonable charge based on actual quantities used may be recognized for nonreusable items and disposable supplies such as oxygen, gauze and dressings required in the care of the patient during his trip.

2125 COVERAGE GUIDELINES FOR AMBULANCE SERVICE CLAIMS

Reimbursement may be made for expenses incurred by a patient for ambulance service provided the following conditions have been met:

A. Patient was transported by an approved supplier of ambulance services.
B. The patient was suffering from an illness or injury which contraindicated transportation by other means. (section 2120.2A)
C. The patient was transported from and to points listed below.(section 2120.3)

   1. From patient's residence (or other place where need arose) to hospital or skilled nursing home.
   2. Skilled nursing home to a hospital or hospital to a skilled nursing home.
   3. Hospital to hospital or skilled nursing home to skilled nursing home.
   4. From a hospital or skilled nursing home to patient's residence.
   5. Round trip for hospital or participating skilled nursing facility inpatients to the nearest hospital or nonhospital treatment facility

   A patient's residence is the place where he makes his home and dwells permanently, or for an extended period of time. A skilled nursing home is one which is listed in the Directory of Medical Facilities as a participating SNF or as an institution which meets section 1861(j)(1) of the law. Ambulance service to a physician's office or a physician-directed clinic is not covered. (See section 2120.3G where a stop is made at a physician's office enroute to a hospital and 2120.3C for additional exceptions.)

2130 PROSTHETIC DEVICES

A. General.—Prosthetic devices (other than dental) which replace all or part of an internal body organ (including contiguous tissue), or replace all or part of the function of a permanently inoperative or malfunctioning internal body organ are covered when furnished on a physician's order. This does not require a determination that there is no possibility that the patient's condition may improve sometime in the future. If the medical record, including the judgment of the attending physician, indicates the condition is of long and indefinite duration, the test of permanence is considered met. (Such a device may also be covered under §2050.l as a supply when furnished incident to a physician's service.)

   Examples of prosthetic devices include cardiac pacemakers, prosthetic lenses (see subsection B), breast prostheses (including a surgical brassiere) for postmastectomy patients, maxillofacial devices and devices which replace all or part of the ear or nose. A urinary collection and retention system with or without a tube is a prosthetic device replacing bladder function in case of permanent urinary incontinence. The Foley catheter is also considered a prosthetic device when ordered for a patient with permanent urinary incontinence. However, chucks, diapers, rubber sheets, etc., are supplies that are not covered under this provision. (Although hemodialysis equipment is a prosthetic device, payment for the rental or purchase of such equipment for use in the home is made only under the provisions for payment applicable to durable medical equipment (see §4105ff) or the special rules that apply to the ESRD program.)

NOTE: Medicare does not cover a prosthetic device dispensed to a patient prior to the time at which the patient undergoes the procedure that makes necessary the use of the device. For example, do not make a separate Part B payment for an intraocular lens (IOL) or pacemaker that a physician, during an office visit prior to the actual surgery, dispenses to the patient for his/her use. Dispensing a prosthetic device in this manner raises health and safety issues. Moreover, the need for the device cannot be clearly established until the procedure that makes its use possible is successfully performed. Therefore, dispensing a prosthetic device in this manner is not considered reasonable and necessary for the treatment of the patient's condition.

Colostomy (and other ostomy) bags and necessary accouterments required for attachment are covered as prosthetic devices. This coverage also includes irrigation and flushing equipment and other items and supplies directly related to ostomy care, whether the attachment of a bag is required.

Accessories and/or supplies which are used directly with an enteral or parenteral device to achieve the therapeutic benefit of the prosthesis or to assure the proper functioning of the device are covered under the prosthetic device benefit subject to the additional guidelines in the Coverage Issues Manual §§65-10 - 65-10.3.

Covered items include catheters, filters, extension tubing, infusion bottles, pumps (either food or infusion), intravenous (I.V) pole, needles, syringes, dressings, tape, Heparin Sodium (parenteral only), volumetric monitors (parenteral only), and parenteral and enteral nutrient solutions. Baby food and other regular grocery products that can be blenderized and used with the enteral system are not covered. Note that some of these items, e.g., a food pump and an I.V. pole, qualify as DME. Although coverage of the enteral and parenteral nutritional therapy systems is provided on the basis of the prosthetic device benefit, the payment rules relating to rental or purchase of DME apply of such items. (See §4105.3.) Code claims in accordance with the HCFA Common rocedure Coding System (HCPCS).

The coverage of prosthetic devices includes replacement of and repairs to such devices as explained in subsection D.

B. Prosthetic Lenses.—The term "internal body organ" includes the lens of an eye. Prostheses replacing the lens of an eye include post-surgical lenses customarily used during convalescence from eye surgery in which the lens of the eye was removed. In addition, permanent lenses are also covered when required by an individual lacking the organic lens of the eye because of surgical removal or congenital absence. Prosthetic lenses obtained on or after the beneficiary's date of entitlement to supplementary medical insurance benefits may be covered even though the surgical removal of the crystalline lens occurred before entitlement.

1. Prosthetic Cataract Lenses.—Make payment for one of the following prosthetic lenses or combinations of prosthetic lenses when determined to be medically necessary by a physician (see §2020.25 for coverage of prosthetic lenses prescribed by a doctor of optometry) to restore essentially the vision provided by the crystalline lens of the eye:

   * prosthetic bifocal lenses in frames;
   * prosthetic lenses in frames for far vision, and prosthetic lenses in frames for near vision; or
   * when a prosthetic contact lens(es) for far vision is prescribed (including cases of binocular and monocular aphakia), make payment for the contact lens(es) and prosthetic lenses in frames for near vision to be worn at the same time as the contact lens(es), and prosthetic lenses in frames to be worn when the contacts have been removed.

   Make payment for lenses which have ultraviolet absorbing or reflecting properties, in lieu of payment for regular (untinted) lenses, if it has been determined that such lenses are medically reasonable and necessary for the individual patient.

   Do not make payment for cataract sunglasses obtained in addition to the regular (untinted) prosthetic lenses since the sunglasses duplicate the restoration of vision function performed by the regular prosthetic lenses.

2. Payment for IOLs Furnished in Ambulatory Surgical Centers (ASCs). Effective for services furnished on or after March 12, 1990, payment for IOLs inserted during or subsequent to cataract surgery in a Medicare certified ASC is included with the payment for facility services that are furnished in connection with the covered surgery. Section 5243.3 explains payment procedures for ASC facility services and the IOL allowance.
3. Limitation on Coverage of Conventional Lenses.—Make payment for no more than one pair of conventional eyeglasses or conventional contact lenses furnished after each cataract surgery with insertion of an IOL.

C. Dentures.—Dentures are excluded from coverage. However, when a denture or a portion thereof is an integral part (built-in) of a covered prosthesis (e.g., an obturator to fill an opening in the palate), it is covered as part of that prosthesis.

D. Supplies, Repairs, Adjustments, and Replacement.—Make payment for supplies that are necessary for the effective use of a prosthetic device (e.g., the batteries needed to operate an artificial larynx). Adjustment of prosthetic devices required by wear or by a change in the patient's condition is covered when ordered by a physician. To the extent applicable, follow the provisions relating to the repair and replacement of durable medical equipment in §2100.4 for the repair and replacement of prosthetic devices. (See §2306.D in regard to payment for devices replaced under a warranty.) Regardless of the date that the original eyewear was furnished (i.e., whether before, on, or after January 1, 1991), do not pay for replacement of conventional eyeglasses or contact lenses covered under subsection B.3.

Necessary supplies, adjustments, repairs, and replacements are covered even when the device had been in use before the user enrolled in Part B of the program, so long as the device continues to be medically required.

2133 LEG, ARM, BACK, AND NECK BRACES, TRUSSES, AND ARTIFICIAL LEGS, ARMS, AND EYES

These appliances are covered when furnished incident to physicians' services or on a physician's order. A brace includes rigid and semi-rigid devices which are used for the purpose of supporting a weak or deformed body member or restricting or eliminating motion in a diseased or injured part of the body. Elastic stockings, garter belts, and similar devices do not come within the scope of the definition of a brace. Back braces include, but are not limited to, special corsets, e.g., sacroiliac, sacrolumbar, dorsolumbar corsets and belts. A terminal device (e.g., hand or hook) is covered under this provision whether an artificial limb is required by the patient. (See §2323.) Stump stockings and harnesses (including replacements) are also covered when these appliances are essential to the effective use of the artificial limb.

Adjustments to an artificial limb or other appliance required by wear or by a change in the patient's condition are covered when ordered by a physician. To the extent applicable, follow the provisions in §2100.4 relating to the repair and replacement of durable medical equipment for the repair and replacement of artificial limbs, braces, etc. Adjustments, repairs and replacements are covered even when the item had been in use before the user enrolled in Part B of the program so long as the device continues to be medically required.

2134 THERAPEUTIC SHOES FOR INDIVIDUALS WITH DIABETES

Coverage of therapeutic shoes (depth or custom-molded) along with inserts for individuals with diabetes is available as of May 1, 1993.These diabetic shoes are covered if the requirements as specified in this section concerning certification and prescription are fulfilled. In addition, this benefit provides for a pair of diabetic shoes even if only one foot suffers from diabetic foot disease. Each shoe is equally equipped so that the affected limb, as well as the remaining limb, is protected.

Claims for therapeutic shoes for diabetics are processed by the Durable Medical Equipment Regional Carriers (DMERCs.)

A. Definitions.—The following items may be covered under the diabetic shoe benefit:

   1. Custom-Molded Shoes.—Custom-molded shoes are shoes that are:

      * Constructed over a positive model of the patient's foot; Made from leather or other suitable material of equal quality;
      * Have removable inserts that can be altered or replaced as the patient's condition warrants; and
      * Have some form of shoe closure.

   2. Depth Shoes.—Depth shoes are shoes that:

* Have a full length, heel-to-toe filler that, when removed, provides a minimum of 3/16 inch of additional depth used to accommodate custom-molded or customized inserts;
* Are made from leather or other suitable material of equal quality;
* Have some form of shoe closure; and
* Are available in full and half sizes with a minimum of 3 widths so that the sole is graded to the size and width of the upper portions of the shoes according to the American standard last sizing schedule or its equivalent. (The American standard last sizing schedule is the numerical shoe sizing system used for shoes sold in the United States.)

3. Inserts.—Inserts are total contact, multiple density, removable inlays that are directly molded to the patient's foot or a model of the patient's foot and that are made of a suitable material with regard to the patient's condition.

B. Coverage.—

1. Limitations.—For each individual, coverage of the footwear and inserts is limited to one of the following within one calendar year:

   * No more than one pair of custom-molded shoes (including inserts provided with such shoes) and two additional pairs of inserts; or
   * No more than one pair of depth shoes and three pairs of inserts (not including the non-customized removable inserts provided with such shoes).

2. Coverage of Diabetic Shoes and Brace.—Orthopedic shoes, as stated in §2323.D, generally are not covered. This exclusion does not apply to orthopedic shoes that are an integral part of a leg brace. In situations in which an individual qualifies for both diabetic shoes and a leg brace, these items are covered separately. Thus, the diabetic shoes may be covered if the requirements for this section are met, while the brace may be covered if the requirements of section 2133 are met.

3. Substitution of Modifications for Inserts.—An individual may substitute modification(s) of custom-molded or depth shoes instead of obtaining a pair(s) of inserts in any combination. Payment for the modification(s) may not exceed the limit set for the inserts for which the individual is entitled. The following is a list of the most common shoe modifications available, but it is not meant as an exhaustive list of the modifications available for diabetic shoes:

   * Rigid Rocker Bottoms. These are exterior elevations with apex positions for 51 percent to 75 percent distance measured from the back end of the heel. The apex is a narrowed or pointed end of an anatomical structure. The apex must be positioned behind the metatarsal heads and tapering off sharply to the front tip of the sole. Apex height helps to eliminate pressure at the metatarsal heads.

Rigidity is ensured by the steel in the shoe. The heel of the shoe tapers off in the back in order to cause the heel to strike in the middle of the heel.

* Roller Bottoms (Sole or Bar). These are the same as rocker bottoms, but the heel is tapered from the apex to the front tip of the sole.
* Metatarsal Bars.—An exterior bar is placed behind the metatarsal heads in order to remove pressure from the metatarsal heads. The bars are of various shapes, heights, and construction depending on the exact purpose.
* Wedges (Posting). Wedges are either of hind foot, fore foot, or both and may be in the middle or to the side. The function is to shift or transfer weight bearing upon standing or during ambulation to the opposite side for added support, stabilization, equalized weight distribution, or balance.
* Offset Heels. This is a heel flanged at its base either in the middle, to the side, or a combination, that is then extended upward to the shoe in order to stabilize extreme positions of the hind foot.
* Other modifications to diabetic shoes include, but are not limited to:
* Flared heels;
* Velcro closures; and Inserts for missing toes.

4. Separate Inserts. Inserts may be covered and dispensed independently of diabetic shoes if the supplier of the shoes verifies in writing that the patient has appropriate footwear into which the insert can be placed. This footwear must meet the definitions found above for depth shoes and custom-molded shoes.

C. Certification. The need for diabetic shoes must be certified by a physician who is a doctor of medicine or a doctor of osteopathy and who is responsible for diagnosing and treating the patient's diabetic systemic condition through a comprehensive plan of care. This managing physician must:

* Document in the patient's medical record that the patient has diabetes;
* Certify that the patient is being treated under a comprehensive plan of care for his or her diabetes, and that he or she needs diabetic shoes; and
* Document in the patient's record that the patient has one or more of the following conditions:

  - Peripheral neuropathy with evidence of callus formation;
  - History of pre-ulcerative calluses;
  - History of previous ulceration;
  - Foot deformity;
  - Previous amputation of the foot or part of the foot; or
  - Poor circulation.

D. Prescription. Following certification by the physician managing the patient's systemic diabetic condition, a podiatrist or other qualified physician who is knowledgeable in the fitting of diabetic shoes and inserts may prescribe the particular type of footwear necessary.

E. Furnishing Footwear. The footwear must be fitted and furnished by a podiatrist or other qualified individual such as a pedorthist, an orthotist, or a prosthetist. The certifying physician may not furnish the diabetic shoes unless he or she is the only qualified individual in the area. It is left to the discretion of each carrier to determine the meaning of "in the area."

F. Payment. For 1994, payment for diabetic shoes and inserts is limited to 80 percent of the reasonable charge, up to a limit of $348 for one pair of custom-molded shoes including any initial inserts, $59 for each additional pair of custom-molded shoe inserts, $116 for one pair of depth shoes, and $59 for each pair of depth shoe inserts. These limits are based on 1988 amounts that were set forth in §1833(o) of the Act and then adjusted by the same percentage increases allowed for DME for fee screen limits by applying the same update factor that is applied to DME fees, except that if the updated limit is not a multiple of $1, it is rounded to the nearest multiple of $1.

Although percentage increase in payment for diabetic shoes are the same percentage increases that are used for payment of DME through the DME fee schedule, the shoes are not subject to DME coverage rules or the DME fee schedule. In addition, diabetic shoes are neither considered DME nor orthotics, but a separate category of coverage under Medicare Part B. (See §1861(s)(12) and §1833(o) of the Act.)

Payment for the certification of diabetic shoes and for the prescription of the shoes is considered to be included in the payment for the visit or consultation during which these services are provided. If the sole purpose of an encounter with the beneficiary is to dispense or fit the shoes, then no payment may be made for a visit or consultation provided on the same day by the same physician. Thus, a separate payment is not made for certification of the need for diabetic shoes, the prescribing of diabetic shoes, or the fitting of diabetic shoes unless the physician documents that these services were not the sole purpose of the visit or consultation.

2210 PAYABLE PHYSICAL THERAPY (PT)

A. General.-To be covered PT services, the services must relate directly and specifically to an active written treatment regimen established by the physician after any needed consultation with the qualified physical therapist and must be reasonable and necessary to the treatment of the individual's illness or injury.Effective July 18, 1984, a plan of treatment for OPT services may be established by either the physician or the qualified physical therapist providing such services.Services related to activities for the general good and welfare of patients, e.g., general exercises to promote overall fitness and flexibility and activities to provide diversion or general motivation, do not constitute PT services for Medicare purposes.

Services furnished beneficiaries must constitute PT where entitlement to benefits is at issue.Since the OPT benefit under Part B provides coverage only of PT services, payment can be made only for those services which constitute PT.

B. Reasonable and Necessary.-To be considered reasonable and necessary the following conditions must be met:

* The services must be considered under accepted standards of medical practice to be a specific and effective treatment for the patient's condition.
* The services must be of such a level of complexity and sophistication or the condition of the patient must be such that the services required can be safely and effectively performed only by a qualified physical therapist or under his supervision. Services which do not require the performance or supervision of a physical therapist are not considered reasonable or necessary PT services, even if they are performed or supervised by a physical therapist.(When you determine the services furnished were of a type that could have been safely and effectively performed only by a qualified physical therapist or under his supervision, presume that such services were properly supervised.However, this assumption is rebuttable, and, if in the course of processing claims you find that PT services are not being furnished under proper supervision, deny the claim and bring this matter to the attention of the Division of Survey and Certification of the RO.)
* The development, implementation, management, and evaluation of a patient care plan constitute skilled physical therapy services when, because of the beneficiary's condition, those activities require the skills of a physical therapist to meet the beneficiary's needs, promote recovery, and ensure medical safety.Where the skills of a physical therapist are needed to manage and periodically reevaluate the appropriateness of a maintenance program because of an identified danger to the patient, those reasonable and necessary management and evaluation services could be covered, even if the skills of a therapist are not needed to carry out the activities performed as part of the maintenance program.
* While a beneficiary's particular medical condition is a valid factor in deciding if skilled physical therapy services are needed, a beneficiary's diagnosis or prognosis should never be the sole factor in deciding that a service is or is not skilled.The key issue is whether the skills of a physical therapist are needed to treat the illness or injury, or whether the services can be carried out by nonskilled personnel.
* A service that ordinarily would be performed by nonskilled personnel could be considered a skilled physical therapy service in cases in which there is clear documentation that, because of special medical complications, a skilled physical therapist is required to perform or supervisethe service.However, the importance of a particular service to a beneficiary or the frequency with which it must be performed does not, by itself, make a nonskilled service into a skilled service.
* There must be an expectation that the patient's condition will improve significantly in a reasonable (and generally predictable) period of time, or the services must be necessary for the establishment of a safe and effective maintenance program required in connection with a specific disease state.
* The amount, frequency, and duration of the services must be reasonable.

NOTE:Claims for PT services denied because they are not considered reasonable and necessary are excluded by §1862(a)(1) of the Act and are thus subject to consideration under the waiver of liability provision in §1879 of the Act.(See §7300.10.)

2210.1 Restorative Therapy

To constitute physical therapy a service must, among other things, be reasonable and necessary to the treatment of the individual's illness.If an individual's expected restoration potential would be insignificant in relation to the extent and duration of physical therapy services required to achieve such potential, the physical therapy would not be considered reasonable and necessary.In addition, there must be an expectation that the patient's condition will improve significantly in a reasonable (and generally predictable) period of time.However, if at any point in the treatment of an illness it is determined that the expectations will not materialize the services will no longer be considered reasonable and necessary; and they, therefore, should be excluded from coverage under §l862(a)(l) of the Act.

Skilled physical therapy may be needed, and improvement in a patient's condition may occur, even where a patient's full or partial recovery is not possible.For example, a terminally ill patient may begin to exhibit self care, mobility, and/or safety dependence requiring skilled physical therapy services.The fact that full or partial recovery is not possible does not necessarily mean that skilled physical therapy is not needed to improve the patient's condition. The deciding factors are always whether the services are considered reasonable, effective treatments for the patient's condition and require the skills of a physical therapist, or whether they can be safely and effectively carried out by nonskilled personnel without physical therapy supervision.

2210.2 Maintenance Programs.

The repetitive services required to maintain function generally do not involve complex and sophisticated physical therapy procedures, and, consequently, the judgment and skill of a qualified physical therapist are not required for safety and effectiveness.
However, in certain instances, the specialized knowledge and judgment of a qualified physical therapist may be required to establish a maintenance program intended to prevent or minimize deterioration caused by a medical condition, if the program is to be safely carried out and the treatment aims of the physician achieved.Establishing such a program is a skilled service.For example, a Parkinson patient who has not been under a restorative physical therapy program may require the services of a physical therapist to determine what type of exercises will contribute the most to maintain the patient's present functional level.In such situations, the initial evaluation of the patient's needs, the designing by the qualified physical therapist of a maintenance program which is appropriate to the capacity and tolerance of the patient and the treatment objectives of the physician, the instruction of the patient or family members in carrying out the program, and such infrequent reevaluations as may be required would constitute physical therapy.

While a patient is under a restorative physical therapy program, the physical therapist should reevaluate his/her condition when necessary and adjust any exercise program the patient is expected to carry out himself/herself or with the aid of supportive personnel to maintain the function being restored.Consequently, by the time it is determined that no further restoration is possible, i.e., by the end of the last restorative session, the physical therapist will have already designed the maintenance program required and instructed the patient or supportive personnel in the carrying out of the program.Therefore, where a maintenance program is not established until after the restorative physical therapy program has been completed, it would not be considered reasonable and necessary for the treatment of the patient's condition and would be excluded from coverage under §1862(a)(1) of the Act.

The repetitive services required to maintain function sometimes involve the use of complex and sophisticated therapy procedures, and, consequently, the judgment and skill of a physical therapist might be required for the safe and effective rendition of such services.

EXAMPLE:Where there is an unhealed, unstable fracture which requires regular exercise to maintain function until the fracture heals, the skills of a physical therapist would be needed to ensure that the fractured extremity is maintained in proper position and alignment during maintenance range of motion exercises.

2210.3 Application of Guidelines

The following discussion illustrates the application of the above guidelines to some of the more common physical therapy modalities and procedures utilized in the treatment of patients:

1. Hot Pack, Hydrocollator, Infra-Red Treatments, Paraffin Baths and Whirlpool Baths.-Heat treatments of this type and whirlpool baths do not ordinarily require the skills of a qualified physical therapist.However, in a particular case the skills, knowledge, and judgment of a qualified physical therapist might be required in such treatments or baths, e.g., where the patient's condition is complicated by circulatory deficiency, areas of desensitization, open wounds, or other complications. Also, if such treatments are given prior to but as an integral part of a skilled physical therapy procedure, they would be considered part of the physical therapy service.
2. Gait Training.-Gait evaluation and training furnished a patient whose ability to walk has been impaired by neurological, muscular, or skeletal abnormality require the skills of a qualified physical therapist.However, if gait evaluation and training cannot reasonably be expected to improve significantly the patient's ability to walk, such services would not be considered reasonable and necessary. Repetitive exercises to improve gait or maintain strength and endurance, and assistive walking, such as provided in support for feeble or unstable patients, are appropriately provided by supportive personnel, e.g., aides or nursing personnel and do not require the skills of a qualified physical therapist.
3. Ultrasound, Shortwave, and Microwave Diathermy Treatments.-These modalities must always be performed by or under the supervision of a qualified physical therapist, and therefore, such treatments constitute physical therapy.
4. Range of Motion Tests.-Only the qualified physical therapist may perform range of motion tests and, therefore, such tests would constitute physical therapy.

5. Therapeutic Exercises.-Therapeutic exercises which must be performed by or under the supervision of a qualified physical therapist due either to the type of exercise employed or to the condition of the patientwould constitute physical therapy.Range of motion exercises require the skills of a qualified physical therapist only when they are part of the active treatment of a specific disease which has resulted in a loss or restriction of mobility (as evidenced by physical therapy notes showing the degree of motion lost and the degree to be restored) and such exercises, either because of their nature or the condition of the patient, may only be performed safely and effectively by or under the supervision of a qualified physical therapist.Generally, range of motion exercises which are not related to the restoration of a specific loss of function but rather are related to the maintenance of function (see §2210.2) do not require the skills of a qualified physical therapist.

2303 SERVICES NOT REASONABLE AND NECESSARY

Items and services which are not reasonable and necessary for the diagnosis or treatment of illness or injury, or to improve the functioning of a malformed body member; e.g., payment cannot be made for the rental of a special hospital bed to be used by the patient in his home unless it was a reasonable and necessary part of the patient's treatment. See also §2318.

2320 ROUTINE SERVICES AND APPLIANCES

Routine physical checkups; eyeglasses, contact lenses, and eye examinations for the purpose of prescribing, fitting or changing eyeglasses; eye refractions; hearing aids and examinations for hearing aids; and immunizations are not covered.

The routine physical checkup exclusion applies to (a) examinations performed without relationship to treatment or diagnosis for a specific illness, symptom, complaint, or injury, and (b) examinations required by third parties such as insurance companies, business establishments, or Government agencies.

(If the claim is for a diagnostic test or examination performed solely for the purpose of establishing a claim under title IV of Public Law 91-173 (Black Lung Benefits), advise the claimant to contact his/her Social Security office regarding the filing of a claim for reimbursement under that program.)

The exclusions apply to eyeglasses or contact lenses and eye examinations for the purpose of prescribing, fitting, or changing eyeglasses or contact lenses for refractive errors. The exclusions do not apply to physician services (and services incident to a physician's service) performed in conjunction with an eye disease (e.g., glaucoma or cataracts) or to postsurgical prosthetic lenses which are customarily used during convalescence from eye surgery in which the lens of the eye was removed or to permanent prosthetic lenses required by an individual lacking the organic lens of the eye, whether by surgical removal or congenital disease. Such prosthetic lens is a replacement for an internal body organ (the lens of the eye). (See §2130.)

The coverage of services rendered by an ophthalmologist is dependent on the purpose of the examination rather than on the ultimate diagnosis of the patient's condition. When a beneficiary goes to an ophthalmologist with a complaint or symptoms of an eye disease or injury, the ophthalmologist's services (except for eye refractions) are covered regardless of the fact that only eyeglasses were prescribed. However, when a beneficiary goes to his/her ophthalmologist for an eye examination with no specific complaint, the expenses for the examination are not covered even though as a result of such examination the doctor discovered a pathologic condition.

In the absence of evidence to the contrary, you may carrier may assume that an eye examination performed by an ophthalmologist on the basis of a complaint by the beneficiary or symptoms of an eye disease was not for the purpose of prescribing, fitting, or changing eyeglasses.

Expenses for all refractive procedures, whether performed by an ophthalmologist (or any other physician) or an optometrist and without regard to the reason for performance of the refraction, are excluded from coverage. (See §§4125 and 5217 for claims review and reimbursement instructions concerning refractive services.)

With the exception of vaccinations for pneumococcal pneumonia, hepatitis B, and influenza, which are specifically covered under the law, vaccinations or inoculations are generally excluded as immunizations unless they are directly related to the treatment of an injury or direct exposure such as antirabies treatment, tetanus antitoxin or booster vaccine, botulin antitoxin, antivenin, or immune globulin.

2323 FOOT CARE AND SUPPORTIVE DEVICES FOR FEET

NOTE: See §4281 for the relationship between foot care and the coverage and billing of the diagnosis and treatment of peripheral neuropathy with loss of protective sensation (LOPS) in people with diabetes.

A. Exclusion of Coverage.—The following foot care services are generally excluded from coverage under both Part A and Part B. Exceptions to this general exclusion for limited treatment of routine foot care services are described in subsections A.2 and B. (See §4120 for procedural instructions in applying foot care exclusions.)

1. Treatment of Flat Foot.—The term “flat foot” is defined as a condition in which one or more arches of the foot have flattened out. Services or devices directed toward the care or correction of such conditions, including the prescription of supportive devices, are not covered.

2. Treatment of Subluxation of Foot.—Subluxations of the foot are defined as partial dislocations or displacements of joint surfaces, tendons ligaments, or muscles of the foot. Surgical or nonsurgical treatments undertaken for the sole purpose of correcting a subluxated structure in the foot as an isolated entity are not covered.

This exclusion does not apply to medical or surgical treatment of subluxation of the ankle joint (talo-crural joint). In addition, reasonable and necessary medical or surgical services, diagnosis, or treatment for medical conditions that have resulted from or are associated with partial displacement of structures is covered. For example, if a patient has osteoarthritis that has resulted in a partial displacement of joints in the foot, and the primary treatment is for the osteoarthritis, coverage is provided.

3. Routine Foot Care.—Except as provided in subsection B, routine foot care is excluded from coverage. Services that normally are considered routine and not covered by Medicare include the following:
   * The cutting or removal of corns and calluses;
   * The trimming, cutting, clipping, or debriding of nails; and
   * Other hygienic and preventive maintenance care, such as cleaning and soaking the feet, the use of skin creams to maintain skin tone of either ambulatory or bedfast patients, and any other service performed in the absence of localized illness, injury, or symptoms involving the foot.

B. Exceptions to Routine Foot Care Exclusion.—

1. Necessary and Integral Part of Otherwise Covered Services.—In certain circumstances, services ordinarily considered to be routine may be covered if they are performed as a necessary and integral part of otherwise covered services, such as diagnosis and treatment of ulcers, wounds, or infections.
2. Treatment of Warts on Foot.—The treatment of warts (including plantar warts) on the foot is covered to the same extent as services provided for the treatment of warts located elsewhere on the body.
3. Presence of Systemic Condition.—The presence of a systemic condition such asmetabolic, neurologic, or peripheral vascular disease may require scrupulous foot care by a professional that in the absence of such condition(s) would be considered routine (and, therefore, excluded from coverage). Accordingly, foot care that would otherwise be considered routine may be covered when systemic condition(s) result in severe circulatory embarrassment or areas of diminished sensation in the individual's legs or feet. (See subsection C.)

   In these instances, certain foot care procedures that otherwise are considered routine (e.g., cutting or removing corns and calluses, or trimming, cutting, clipping, or debriding nails) may pose a hazard when performed by a nonprofessional person on patients with such systemic conditions. (See §4120 for procedural instructions.)
4. Mycotic Nails.—In the absence of a systemic condition, treatment of mycotic nails may be covered.

   The treatment of mycotic nails for an ambulatory patient is covered only when the physician attending the patient's mycotic condition documents that (1) there is clinical evidence of mycosis of the toenail, and (2) the patient has marked limitation of ambulation, pain, or secondary infection resulting from the thickening and dystrophy of the infected toenail plate.

   The treatment of mycotic nails for a nonambulatory patient is covered only when the physician attending the patient's mycotic condition documents that (1) there is clinical evidence of mycosis of the toenail, and (2) the patient suffers from pain or secondary infection resulting from the thickening and dystrophy of the infected toenail plate.

   For the purpose of these requirements, documentation means any written information that is required by the carrier in order for services to be covered. Thus, the information submitted with claims must be substantiated by information found in the patient's medical record. Any information, including that contained in a form letter, used for documentation purposes is subject to carrier verification in order to ensure that the information adequately justifies coverage of the treatment of mycotic nails. (See §4120 for claims processing criteria.)

C. Systemic Conditions.—Although not intended as a comprehensive list, the following metabolic, neurologic, and peripheral vascular diseases (with synonyms in parentheses) most commonly represent the underlying conditions that might justify coverage for routine foot care.

- * Diabetes mellitus
- * Arteriosclerosis obliterans (A.S.O., arteriosclerosis of the extremities, occlusive peripheral arteriosclerosis)
- * Buerger's disease (thromboangiitis obliterans)
- * Chronic thrombophlebitis
- * Peripheral neuropathies involving the feet
- * Associated with malnutrition and vitamin deficiency
- * Malnutrition (general, pellagra)
- * Alcoholism
- * Malabsorption (celiac disease, tropical sprue)
- * Pernicious anemia
- * Associated with carcinoma
- * Associated with diabetes mellitus
- * Associated with drugs and toxins
- * Associated with multiple sclerosis
- * Associated with uremia (chronic renal disease)
- * Associated with traumatic injury
- * Associated with leprosy or neurosyphilis
- * Associated with hereditary disorders
- * Hereditary sensory radicular neuropathy
- * Angiokeratoma corporis diffusum (Fabry's)
- * Amyloid neuropathy

When the patient's condition is one of those designated by an asterisk (*), routine procedures are covered only if the patient is under the active care of a doctor of medicine or osteopathy who documents the condition.

D. Supportive Devices for Feet.—Orthopedic shoes and other supportive devices for the feet generally are not covered. However, this exclusion does not apply to such a shoe if it is an integral part of a leg brace (see §2133), and its expense is included as part of the cost of the brace. Also, this exclusion does not apply to therapeutic shoes furnished to diabetics. (See §2134.)

E. Coding.—You are responsible for informing all medical specialties that codes and policies for routine foot care and supportive devices for the feet are not exclusively for the use of podiatrists. These codes must be used to report foot care services regardless of the specialty of the physician who furnishes the services. Instruct physicians to use the most appropriate code available when billing for routine foot care.

2455 MEDICAL INSURANCE BLOOD DEDUCTIBLE

A. General.—Program payment under Part B may not be made for the first three units of whole blood, or packed red cells, received by a beneficiary in a calendar year. For purpose of the blood deductible, a unit of whole blood means a pint of whole blood. The term whole blood means human blood from which none of the liquid or cellular components has been removed. Where packed red cells are furnished, a unit of packed red cells is considered equivalent to a pint of whole blood. After the three unit deductible has been satisfied, payment may be made for all blood charges, subject to the normal coverage and reasonable charge criteria.

NOTE: Blood is a biological and can be covered under Part B only when furnished incident to a physician's services. (See §§2050.1ff. for a more complete explanation of services rendered "incident to a physician's services.")

B. Application of the Blood Deductible.—The blood deductible applies only to whole blood or packed red cells. Other components of blood such as platelets, fibrinogen, plasma, gamma globulin, and serum albumin are not subject to the blood deductible. These components of blood are covered biologicals.

The blood deductible involves only the charges for the blood (or packed red cells). Charges for the administration of blood or packed cells are not subject to the blood deductible. Accordingly, although payment may not be made for the first three pints of blood and/or units of packed red cells furnished to a beneficiary in a calendar year, payment may be made (subject to the cash deductible) for the administration charges for all covered pints or units including the first three furnished in a calendar year.

The blood deductible applies only to the first three pints and/or units furnished in a calendar year, even though more than one physician or clinic furnished blood. Furthermore, to count toward the deductible, the blood must be covered with respect to all applicable criteria (i.e., it must be medically necessary, it must be furnished incident to a physician's services, etc.). (See §2050.5.)

C. Physician or Supplier Right to Charge for Deductible Blood.—A physician or other supplier who accepts assignment may bill a beneficiary the reasonable charge for unreplaced deductible blood (i.e., any of the first three units in a calendar year) but may not charge for blood which has been replaced.

Once a physician or supplier accepts a replacement unit of whole blood or packed red cells from a beneficiary or another individual acting on his behalf, the beneficiary may not be charged for the blood.

When a supplier accepts blood donated in advance, in anticipation of need by a specific beneficiary, whether the beneficiary's own blood, that is, an autologous donation, or blood furnished by another individual or blood assurance group, such donations are considered replacement for units subsequently furnished the beneficiary.

D. Distinction Between Blood Charges and Blood Administration Charges.—Since the blood deductible applies only to charges for blood and does not apply to charges for blood administration, these two charges must be considered separately. Where a bill for unreplaced blood shows only a single blood charge, break down the charge between blood and blood administration in accordance with the supplier's customary charges for these items. If the supplier does not customarily bill separately for blood and for blood administration, the portion of the single charge that is considered to be a charge for blood is determined by reference to the established reasonable charge in the locality as it applies to blood. The remainder of the charge is considered a blood administration charge.

E. Relationship to Other Deductibles.—Part B payment for all blood administration charges and for blood charges after the beneficiary has received three pints and/or units in a calendar year is subject to the annual cash deductible and coinsurance provisions. Expenses incurred in meeting the Part B blood deductible do not count as incurred expenses under Part B for purposes of meeting the cash deductible or for purposes of payment.

There is also a Part A blood deductible applicable to the first three pints of whole blood or equivalent units of packed red cells received by a beneficiary in a benefit period. The Part A and Part B blood deductibles are applied separately.

F. Example of Application of the Part B Blood Deductible.—In 1991, a beneficiary received three pints of blood from a physician for which the total charge is $100 per pint. (The physician does not specify how much of the charge is for blood, and how much is for blood administration.) The physician accepted assignment and submitted a claim for Part B payment.

Determine that the beneficiary has not met any part of the Part B blood deductible and has met only $40 of the cash deductible. You determine that the physician's customary charge for blood administration is $50 per unit and that it is reasonable. Consequently, charges for blood administration are $50 per unit or a total of $150 for the three units furnished and charges for blood are $50 per unit or a total of $150 for the three units furnished. The beneficiary replaces one pint of blood. Since the beneficiary had not met any of the Part B blood deductible, none of the $150 in blood charges are payable nor may any of such charges be applied to satisfy the annual cash deductible ($100). Of the $150 in blood administration charges, $60 is applied to satisfy the beneficiary's unmet cash deductible and a payment of $72 is made on the remaining $90 in charges ($90 x 80%). Since the physician accepted assignment and since the beneficiary replaced one pint of blood, the physician may charge the beneficiary the reasonable charge only for the two remaining deductible pints.

3045.4 Effect of Assignment Upon Purchase of Cataract Glasses from Participating Physician or Supplier.--A pair of cataract glasses is comprised of two distinct products: a professional product (the prescribed lenses) and a retail commercial product (the frames). The frames serve not only as a holder of lenses but also as an article of personal apparel. As such, they are usually selected on the basis of personal taste and style. Although Medicare will pay only for standard frames, most patients want deluxe frames. Participating physicians and suppliers cannot profitably furnish such deluxe frames unless they can make an extra (non-covered) charge for the frames even though they accept assignment.

Therefore, a participating physician or supplier (whether an ophthalmologist, optometrist, or optician) who accepts assignment on cataract glasses with deluxe frames may charge the Medicare patient the difference between his usual charge to private pay patients for glasses with standard frames and his usual charge to such patients for glasses with deluxe frames, in addition to the applicable deductible and coinsurance on glasses with standard frames, if all of the following requirements are met:

A. The participating physician or supplier has standard frames available, offers them for sale to the patient, and explains to the patient the price and other differences between standard and deluxe frames.

B. The participating physician or supplier obtains from the patient (or his representative) and keeps on file the following signed and dated statement:

Name of Patient Medicare Claim Number

Having been informed that an extra charge is being made by the physician or supplier for deluxe frames, that this extra charge is not covered by Medicare, and that standard frames are available for purchase from the physician or supplier at no extra charge, I have chosen to purchase deluxe frames.

____________________________ ____________

Signature Date

C. The participating physician or supplier itemizes on his claim his actual charge for the lenses, his actual charge for the standard frames, and his actual extra charge for the deluxe frames (charge differential).

Once the assigned claim for deluxe frames has been processed, the carrier will explain the extra charge for the deluxe frames on the EOMB, as indicated in the following example.

		BILLED	**APPROVED**
CATARACT LENSES	JULY 20, 1985	$200.00	$175.00

APPROVED AMOUNT LIMITED BY ITEM 5C ON BACK

STANDARD FRAMES	JULY 20, 1985	$ 20.00	$ 15.00

APPROVED AMOUNT LIMITED BY ITEM 5C ON BACK DR. JONES AGREED TO CHARGE NO MORE FOR THE ABOVE SERVICES THAN THE AMOUNT APPROVED BY MEDICARE.

EXTRA CHARGE DELUXE	JULY 20, 1985	$ 35.00	$ 00.00

MEDICARE DOES NOT PAY THE EXTRA CHARGE FOR DELUXE FRAMES.

TOTAL APPROVED AMOUNT $190.00
MEDICARE PAYMENT (80% OF THE APPROVED AMOUNT) $152.00

WE ARE PAYING A TOTAL OF $152.00 TO DR. JONES FOR THE ABOVE SERVICES. YOU ARE RESPONSIBLE FOR THE DIFFERENCE OF $38.00 BETWEEN THE APPROVED AMOUNT AND THE MEDICARE PAYMENT, PLUS THE EXTRA CHARGE OF $35.00 FOR DELUXE FRAMES.

4107 DURABLE MEDICAL EQUIPMENT - BILLING AND PAYMENT CONSIDERATIONS UNDER THE FEE SCHEDULE

The Omnibus Budget Reconciliation Act of 1987 requires that payment for DME, prosthetics and orthotics be made under fee schedules effective January 1, 1989. The allowable charge is limited to the lower of the actual charge for the equipment, or the fee schedule amount. The equipment is categorized into one of six classes:

* Inexpensive or other routinely purchased DME;
* Items requiring frequent and substantial servicing;
* Customized items;
* Prosthetic and orthotic devices;
* Capped rental items; or
* Oxygen and oxygen equipment.

The fee schedule allowances for each class are determined in accord with §§5102ff

4107.6 Written Order Prior to Delivery.--Ensure that your system will pay for the equipment listed below only when the supplier has a written order in hand prior to delivery. Otherwise, do not pay for that item even if a written order is subsequently furnished. However, you can pay for a similar item if it is subsequently provided by an unrelated supplier which has a written order in hand prior to delivery. The HCPCS codes for the equipment requiring a written order are:

B0180
B0181
B0182
B0183
B0184
B0185
B0188
B0189
B0190
B0192
B0195
B0620
B0720
B0730
B1230

4107.8 EOMB Messages.--The following EOMB messages are suggested: (See §§7012ff. for other applicable messages.)

A. General.—

* "This is the maximum approved amount for this item." (Use when payment is reduced for a line item.)

B. Inexpensive/Frequently Purchased Equipment.—

* "The total approved amount for this item is ______________ whether this item is purchased or rented." (Use in first month.)
* "This is your next to last rental payment."
* "This is your last rental payment."
* "This item has been rented up to the Medicare payment limit."
* "The approved amount has been reduced by the previously approved rental amounts."

C. Items Requiring Frequent and Substantial Servicing.—Use the general rental messages in §4107.8A, if applicable. If the beneficiary has purchased the item prior to June 1, 1989, follow §7014.6. If the beneficiary purchase an item in this category on or after June 1, 1989, use the following message:

* "This equipment can only be paid for on a rental basis."

D. Customized Items and Other Prosthetic and Orthotic Devices.—

* "The total approved amount for this item is ____________."

E. Capped Rental Items.—

* "Under a provision of Medicare law, monthly rental payments for this item can continue for up to 15 months from the first rental month or until the equipment is no longer needed, whichever comes first."
* "If you no longer are using this equipment or have recently moved and will rent this item from a different supplier, please contact our office." (Use on beneficiary's EOMB.)
* "This is your next to last rental payment."
* "This is your last rental payment."
* "This item has been rented up to the 15 month Medicare payment limit."
* "Your equipment supplier must supply and service this item for as long as you continue to need it."
* "Medicare cannot pay for maintenance and/or servicing of this item until 6 months have elapsed since the end of the 15th paid rental month."
* If the beneficiary purchased a capped rental item prior to June 1, 1989, follow §7014.6.

If the beneficiary purchased a capped rental item on or after June 1, 1989, use the following denial message:

* "This equipment can only be paid for on a rental basis." F. Oxygen and Oxygen Equipment.—
* "The monthly allowance includes payment for all covered oxygen contents and supplies." "Payment for the amount of oxygen supplied has been reduced or denied based on the patient's medical condition." (To supplier after medical review.)
* "The approved amount has been reduced to the amount allowable for medically necessary oxygen therapy." (To beneficiary.)
* "Payment denied because the allowance for this item is included in the monthly payment amount."
* "Payment denied because Medicare oxygen coverage requirements are not met." If the beneficiary purchased an oxygen system prior to June 1, 1989, follow §7014.6. If the beneficiary purchased an oxygen system on or after June 1, 1989, use the following denial message:
* "This item can only be paid for on a rental basis."

G. Items Requiring a Written Order Prior to Delivery.—

* "Payment is denied because the supplier did not obtain a written order from your doctor prior to the delivery of this item."

4107.9 Oxygen HCPCS Codes Effective 1/1/89.--

NEW	OLD	DEFINITION
Q0036 notes (1) and (8)	E1377-E1385, E1397	Oxygen concentrator, See High humidity
Q0038 See note (2)	E0400, E0405	Oxygen contents, gaseous, per unit (for use with owned gaseous stationary systems or when both a stationary and portable gaseous system are owned; 1 unit = 50 cubic ft.)
Q0039 See note (2)	E0410, E0415O	Oxygen contents, liquid, per unit, (for use with owned stationary liquid systems or when both a stationary and portable liquid system are owned; 1 unit = 10 lbs.)
Q0040 See note (2)	E0416	Portable oxygen contents, per unit (for use only with portable gaseous systems when no stationary gas system is used; 1 unit = 5 cubic ft.)
Q0041 See note (2)	None	Portable oxygen contents, liquid, per unit (for use only with portable liquid systems when no stationary liquid system is used; 1 unit = 1 lb.)
Q0042	E0425	Stationary compressed See note (3)gas system rental, includes contents (per unit), regulator with flow gauge, humidifier, nebulizer, cannula or mask & tubing; 1 unit = 50 cubic ft.
E0425 See notes (4) and (8)	Same	No change
E0430 See notes (8) and (9)	Same	No change
E0435 See notes (7) and 8	Same	No change in terminology, but and (8)see note (7).

Q0043	E0440	Stationary liquid (see note (3) oxygen system rental), includes contents (per unit), use of reservoir, contents indicator, flowmeter, humidifier, nebulizer, cannula or mask and tubing; 1 unit of contents = 10 lbs.
B0440 See note (4)	Same	No change
E0455	Same	No change See note (6)
E0555 See note (6)	Same	No change
E0580	Same	No change See note (6)
E1351	Same	No change See note (6)
E1352 See note (6)	Same	No change
E1353	Same See notes (6) and (8)	No change
E1354 See note (6)	Same	No change
E1371	Same See note (6)	No change
E1374 See note (6)	Same	No change
E1400 See note (1) and (8)	E1388-E1396	Same as Q0014
E1401 See notes (1) and (8)	E1388-E1396	Same as Q0015
E1402	Same	No change
E1403	Same	No change
E1404	Same	No change
E1405	Q0037	Combine the fee See note (10)schedule amounts for the stationary oxygen system and the nebulizer with a compressor and heater (code E0585) to determine the fee schedule amount to apply to oxygen enrichers with a heater (code E1405)
E1406	Q0037	Combine the fee schedule amounts for the stationary oxygen system and the nebulizer with only a compressor (i.e., without a heater, code E0570) to determine the fee schedule amount to apply to oxygen enrichers without a heater (code E1406)

4120 FOOT CARE

NOTE: See §4281 for the relationship between foot care and the coverage and billing of the diagnosis and treatment of peripheral neuropathy with loss of protective sensation (LOPS) in people with diabetes.

4120.1 Application of Foot Care Exclusions to Physicians' Services.--The exclusion of foot care is determined by the nature of the service (§2323). Thus, reimbursement for an excluded service should be denied whether performed by a podiatrist, osteopath, or a doctor of medicine, and without regard to the difficulty or complexity of the procedure.

When an itemized bill shows both covered services and noncovered services not integrally related to the covered service, the portion of charges attributable to the noncovered services should be denied. (For example, if an itemized bill shows surgery for an ingrown toenail and also removal of calluses not necessary for the performance of toe surgery, any additional charge attributable to removal of the calluses should be denied.)

In reviewing claims involving foot care, the carrier should be alert to the following exceptional situations:

1. Payment may be made for incidental noncovered services performed as a necessary and integral part of, and secondary to, a covered procedure. For example, if trimming of toenails is required for application of a cast to a fractured foot, the carrier need not allocate and deny a portion of the charge for the trimming of the nails. However, a separately itemized charge for such excluded service should be disallowed. When the primary procedure is covered the administration of anesthesia necessary for the performance of such procedure is also covered.

2. Payment may be made for initial diagnostic services performed in connection with a specific symptom or complaint if it seems likely that its treatment would be covered even though the resulting diagnosis may be one requiring only noncovered care.

4173 POSITRON EMISSION TOMOGRAPHY (PET) SCANS

BACKGROUND:

For dates of service on or after March 14, 1995, Medicare covers one use of PET scans, imaging of the perfusion of the heart using Rubidium 82 (Rb 82).

For dates of service on or after January 1, 1998, Medicare expanded coverage of PET scans for the characterization of solitary pulmonary nodules and for the initial staging of lung cancer, conditioned upon its ability to effect the management and treatment of patients with either suspected or demonstrated lung cancer. All other uses of PET scans remain not covered by Medicare.

Beginning for dates of service on or after July 1, 1999, Medicare will cover PET scans for evaluation of recurrent colorectal cancer in patients with levels of carinoembryonic antigen (CEA), staging lymphoma (both Hodgkins and non-Hodgkins) in place of a Gallium study or lymphangiogram, and for the staging of recurrent melanoma prior to surgery.

See Coverage Issues Manual §50-36 for specific coverage criteria for PET scans. Regardless of any other terms or conditions, all uses of PET scans, in order to be covered by Medicare program, must meet the following conditions:

* Scans must be performed using PET scanners that have either been approved or cleared for marketing by the FDA as PET scanners;
* Submission of claims for payment must include any information Medicare requires to assure that the PET scans performed were: (a) reasonable and necessary; (b) did not unnecessarily duplicate other covered diagnostic tests, and (c) did not involve investigational drugs or procedures using investigational drugs, as determined by the Food and Drug Administration (FDA); and
* The PET scan entity submitting claims for payment must keep such patient records as Medicare requires on file for each patient for whom a PET scan claim is made.

4173.1 Conditions for Medicare Coverage of PET Scans for Noninvasive Imaging of the Perfusion of the Heart.--Pet scans done at rest or with pharmacological stress used for noninvasive imaging of the perfusion of the heart for the diagnosis management of patients with known or suspected coronary artery disease using the FDA-approved radiopharmaceutical Rubidium 82 (Rb 82) are covered for services performed on or after March 15, 1995, provided such scans meet either of the two following conditions:

* The PET scan, whether rest alone or rest with stress, is used in place of, but not in addition to, a single photon emission computed tomography (SPECT); or
* The PET scan, whether rest alone or rest with stress, is used following a SPECT that was found inconclusive. In these cases, the PET scan must have been considered necessary in order to determine what medical or surgical intervention is required to treat the patient. (For purposes of this requirement, an inconclusive test is a test whose results are equivocal, technically uninterpretable, or discordant with a patient's other clinical data.)

NOTE: PET scans using Rubidium 82, whether rest or stress are not covered by Medicare for routine screening of asymptomatic patients, regardless of the level of risk factors applicable to such patients.

4173.2 Conditions of Coverage of PET Scans for Characterization of Solitary Pulmonary Nodules (SPNs) and PET Scans Using FDG to Initially Stage Lung Cancer

PET scans using the glucose analog 2-[fluorine-18]-fluoro-2-deoxy-D-glucose(FDG) are covered for services on or after January 1, 1998, subject to the condition and limitations described in CIM 50-36.

NOTE: A Tissue Sampling Procedure (TSP) should not be routinely covered in the case of a negative PET scan for characterization of SPNs, since the patient is presumed not to have a malignant lesion, based upon the PET scan results. Claims for a TSP after a negative PET must be submitted with documentation in order to determine if the TSP is reasonable and necessary in spite of a negative PET. Claims submitted for a TSP after a negative PET without documentation should be denied. Physicians should discuss with their patients the implications of this decision, both with respect to the patient's responsibility for payment for such a biopsy if desired, as well as the confidence the physician has in the results of such PET scans, prior to ordering such scans for this purpose. This physician-patient decision should occur with a clear discussion and understanding of the sensitivity and specificity trade-offs between a computerized tomography (CT) and PET scans. In cases where a TSP is performed, it is the responsibility of the physician ordering the TSP to provide sufficient documentation of the reasonableness and necessity for such procedure or procedures. Such documentation should include, but is not necessarily limited to, a description of the features of the PET scan that call into question whether it is an accurate representation of the patient's condition, the existence of other factors in the patient's condition that call into question the accuracy of the PET scan, and such other information as the contractor deems necessary to determine whether the claim for the TSP should be covered and paid.

In cases of serial evaluation of SPNs using both CT and regional PET chest scanning, such PET scans will not be covered if repeated within 90 days following a negative PET scan.

4173.3 Conditions of Coverage of PET Scans for Recurrence of Colorectal Cancer, Staging and Characterization of Lymphoma, and Recurrence of Melanoma

Medicare adds coverage for these three new indications for PET, one for evaluation of recurrent colorectal cancer in patients with rising levels of carcinoembryonic antigen (CEA), one for staging of lymphoma (both Hodgkins and non-Hodgkins) when the PET scan substitutes for a Gallium scan, and one for the detection of recurrent melanoma, provided certain conditions are met. All three indications are covered only when using the radiopharmaceutical FDA (2-[fluorine-18]-fluoro-2deoxy-D-glucose), and are further predicated on the legal availability of FDG for use in such scans.

4173.4 Billing Requirements for PET Scans.--

A. Effective for Services on or After January 1, 1998, Claims for Characterizing SPNs Should Include.-

NOTE: PET scans are not covered by Medicare for routine screening of asymptomatic patients, regardless of the level of risk factors applicable to such patients.

B. Effective for services on or after January 1, 1998, claims for staging metastatic non-small-cell lung carcinoma (NSCLC) must include:

- Since this service is covered only in those cases in which a primary cancerous lung tumor has been confirmed, claims for PET must show evidence of the detection of such primary lung tumor. For example, a diagnosis code indicating the existence of a primary tumor or any other evidence you deem appropriate. A surgical pathology report which documents the presence of an NSCLC must be kept on file with the provider. If you deem it necessary, contact the provider for a copy of this documentation.

* Whole body PET scan results and results of concurrent CT and follow-up lymph node biopsy. In order to ensure that the PET scan is properly coordinated with other diagnostic modalities, claims must include both (1) the results of concurrent thoracic CT, which is necessary for anatomic information, and (2) the results of any lymph node biopsy performed to finalize whether the patient will be a surgical candidate.

NOTE: A lymph node biopsy is not covered in the case of a negative CT and negative PET where the patient is considered a surgical candidate, given the presumed absence of metastatic NSCLC.

C. Effective for dates of service on or after July 1, 1999 PET claims for the following conditions must include:

* Recurring colorectal cancer with rising CEA:
  — A statement or other evidence of previous colorectal tumor;
  — The results of the concurrent CT, which is necessary for anatomic information; and
  — The necessary procedure codes and/or modifiers.
* Staging or restaging of lymphoma in place of a Gallium study or lymphangiogram:
  — A statement or other evidence of previously-made diagnosis of lymphoma;
  — The results of the concurrent CT, which is necessary for anatomic information; and
  — The date of the last Gallium scan or lymphangiogram when done in the same facility as the PET scan.

* Recurrent Melanoma prior to surgery:
  — A statement or other evidence of previous melanoma;
  — The results of the concurrent CT, which is necessary for anatomic information; and
  — The date of the last Gallium scan when done in the same facility as the PET scan.

As with any claim but particularly in view of the limitations on this coverage, you may decide to conduct post-payment reviews to determine that the use of PET scans is consistent with this instruction. PET scan facilities must keep patient record information on file for each Medicare patient for whom a PET scan claim is made. These medical records will be used in any post payment reviews and must include the information necessary to substantial the need for the PET scan.

4173.5 HCPCS and Modifiers for PET Scans.--Providers should use HCPCS codes G0030 through G0047 to indicate the conditions under which a PET scan was done for imaging of the perfusion of the heart. These codes represent the global service, so providers performing just the technical or professional component of the test should use modifier TC or 26, respectively. The following codes should be reported for PET scans used for the imaging of the lungs:

- G0125—PET lung imaging of solitary pulmonary nodules using 2-fluorine-18]-fluoro-2deoxy-D-glucose (FDG), following CT (71250/71260 or 71270); or
- G0126—PET lung imaging of solitary pulmonary nodules using 2-[fluorine-18]-fluoro-2 deoxy-D-glucose (FDG), following CT (71250/71260 or 71270); for initial staging of pathologically diagnosed NSCLC, or
- G0163—Positron Emission Tomography (PET), whole body, for recurrence of colorectal or colorectal metastatic cancer; or
- G0164—Positron Emission Tomography (PET), whole body, for staging and characterization of lymphoma; or
- G0165—Positron Emission Tomography (PET), whole body, for recurrence of melanoma or melanoma metastic cancer

NOTE: The payment for the radio tracer, or radio pharmaceutical is included in the relative value units of the technical components of the above procedure codes. Do not make any separate payments for these agents for PET scans.
In addition, providers must indicate the results of the PET scan and the previous test using a two digit modifier. (The modifier is not required for technical component-only billings or billings to the intermediary.) The first character should indicate the result of the PET scan; the second character should indicate the results of the prior test. Depending on the procedure codes with which the modifiers are used, the meaning of the modifier will be apparent. The test result modifiers and their descriptions are as follows:

Modifier	Description
N	Negative;
E	Equivocal;
P	Positive, but not suggestive of, extensive ischemia or not suggestive of malignant single pulmonary nodule; and
S	Positive and suggestive of; extensive ischemia (greater than 20 percent of the left ventricle) or malignant single pulmonary nodule.

These modifiers may be used in any combination.

4173.6 Claims Processing Instructions for PET Scan Claims.--

A. FDA Approval.—PET scans are covered only when performed at a PET imaging center with a PET scanner that has been approved or cleared by the FDA. When submitting the claim, the provider is certifying this and must be able to produce a copy of this approval upon request. An official approval letter need not be submitted with the claim.

You may consider conducting a review on a post-payment basis to verify, based on a sample of PET scan claims, that the PET scan was performed at a center with a PET scanner which was approved or cleared for marketing.

B. EOMB and Remittance Messages.—Providers must indicate the results of the PET scan and the previous test using a two-digit modifier as specified in §4173.4. Deny assigned claims received prior to April 1, 1996 without such modifier, using the following EOMB message:

C. "Your service was denied because information required to make payment was missing. We have asked your provider to resubmit a claim with the missing information so that it may be reprocessed." (Message 9.33)

Deny unassigned claims received prior to April 1, 1996, without the two-digit modifier using the following EOMB message:

"Medicare cannot pay for this service because the claim is missing information/documentation. Please ask your provider to submit a new, complete claim to us." (Messages 9.8 and 9.15)

Claims received on or after April 1, 1996, without the two-digit modifier must be returned as unprocessable. (See §3005.)

Use the following remittance message for assigned claims:

"The procedure code is inconsistent with the modifier used, or a required modifier is missing." (Reason Code 4)

Assigned claims for dates of service on or after January 1, 1998, without the proper documentation must be denied using the following EOMB message:

D. Type of Service.—The type of service for the PET scan codes in the "G" range is 4, Diagnostic Radiology.

4175.5 Medicare Summary Notices (MSNs) and Explanation of Medicare Benefits (EOMB) and Remittance Advise Messages.--Use the following MSN or EOMB messages where appropriate.

If a claim is denied because it was submitted by a physician, other than the hospice patient's designated attending physician, who treated the beneficiary for the terminal condition use:

* MSN #27.13, "According to Medicare hospice requirements this service is not covered because the service was provided by a non-attending physician."
* EOMB #20.4, "According to Medicare hospice requirements this service is not covered because the service was provided by a non-attending physician."
* The Spanish version of the above message is:
* Según requisitos de hospicio de Medicare este servicio no se cubre debido a que el servicio fue proporcionado por un médico no primario.
* When the claim is being denied per the above reason, use the following code in the remittance advice message.
* Remark Code N90, "Covered only when performed by the attending physician."

4182 PROSTATE CANCER SCREENING TESTS AND PROCEDURES

The following sections summarize coverage requirements and detail claims processing procedures for prostate cancer screening tests and procedures.

4182.1 Coverage Summary.--Sections 1861(s)(2)(P) and 1861(oo) of the Social Security Act (as added by §4103 of the Balanced Budget Act of 1997), provide for coverage of certain prostate cancer screening tests and procedures subject to certain coverage, frequency, and payment limitations.

Effective for services furnished on or after January 1, 2000, Medicare will cover prostate cancer screening tests and procedures for the early detection of prostate cancer. Coverage currently consists of the following tests and procedures furnished to an individual for the early detection of prostate cancer:

A. Screening Digital Rectal Examination.—This test is a clinical examination of an individual's prostate for nodules or other abnormalities of the prostate; and

B. Screening Prostate Specific Antigen (PSA) Blood Test.—This test detects the marker for adenocarcinoma of the prostate.

For more information regarding coverage of prostate cancer screening tests and procedures, refer to §50-55 of the Coverage Issues Manual.

4182.2 Requirements for Submitting Claims

Submit claims for prostate cancer screening tests on Health Insurance Claim Form HCFA-1500 or electronic equivalent. Follow the general instructions in §2010, Purpose of Health Insurance Claim Form HCFA1500, Medicare Carriers Manual, Part 4, Chapter 2.

4182.3 HCPCS Codes and Payment Requirements

The following table lists coverable codes and services for prostate cancer screening tests and procedures. Pay for these services according to the appropriate fee schedule when all of the requirements noted are met.

HCPCS (TOS)	Description	Requirements	Methodology/ Fee Schedule
G0102; TOS=1	Prostate cancer screening; digital rectal exam	1. Performed on a male Medicare beneficiary over 50 years of age (i.e., for services starting at least one day after the beneficiary attained age 50).	Refer to the Physician's fee schedule. 1. Apply deductible and coinsurance.
		2. Performed by one of the following, who is authorized under State law to perform the examination, is fully knowledgeable about the beneficiary, and is responsible for explaining the results of the examination to the beneficiary: a. Doctor of medicine or osteopathy b. Qualified physician assistant c. Qualified nurse practitioner d. Qualified clinical nurse specialist e. Qualified certified nurse midwife 3. Performed at a frequency no greater than once every 12 months (See §4182.4).	2. Claims from physicians for these examinations where assignment was not taken are subject to the Medicare limiting charge. (See §7555.) 3. Correct Coding Initiative requirements apply. See §4182.6.

G0103; TOS=5	Prostate cancer screening; PSA test	1. Performed on a male Medicare beneficiary over 50 years of age (i.e., for services starting at least one day after the beneficiary attained age 50)	1. Refer to the clinical laboratory fee schedule; payment for this test is the same as for code "84153, PSA; total."
		2. Ordered by one of the following, who is authorized under State law to perform the examination, is fully knowledgeable about the beneficiary, and is responsible for explaining the results of the examination to the beneficiary: a. Physician (doctor of medicine or osteopathy) b. Qualified physician assistant c. Qualified nurse practitioner d. Qualified clinical nurse specialist e. Qualified certified nurse midwife 3. Performed at a frequency no greater than once every 12 months. (See §4182.4.)	2. Do not apply deductible and coinsurance.

4182.4 Calculating the Frequency.--Once a beneficiary has received any (or all) of the covered prostate cancer screening test/procedures, he may receive another (or all) of such test/procedures after 11 full months have passed. To determine the 11-month period, start your count beginning with the month after the month in which any (or all) of the previous covered screening test/procedures was performed.

EXAMPLE: The beneficiary received a screening PSA test on February 25, 2000. Start your count beginning March 2000. The beneficiary is eligible to receive another screening PSA test on February 1, 2001 (the month after 11 months have passed.)

4182.5 CWF Edits.--CWF will edit prostate cancer screening tests and procedures for age, frequency, sex, and valid HCPCS code.

4182.6 Correct Coding Requirements.--Billing and payment for a Digital Rectal Exam (DRE) (G0102) is to be bundled into the payment for a covered E/M service (CPT codes 99201-99456 and 99499) when the two services are furnished to a patient on the same day. If the DRE is the only service or is provided as part of an otherwise noncovered service, HCPCS code G0102 would be payable separately if all other coverage requirements are met.

4182.7 Diagnosis Coding Requirements.--There are no specific diagnosis requirements for prostate screening tests and procedures. However, prostate cancer screening digital rectal examinations and screening Prostate Specific Antigen (PSA) blood tests must be billed using screening ("V") code V76.44 (Special Screening for Malignant Neoplasms, Prostate)

4182.8 Denial Messages.--

A. Remittance Advice Notices.—If the claim for a screening prostate antigen test or screening digital rectal examination is being denied because the patient is not over 50 years of age, use existing American National Standard Institute (ANSI) X12-835 claim adjustment reason code 6 "the procedure code is inconsistent with the patient's age", at the line level along with line level Remark Code M140 "Service not covered until after the patient's 50th birthday, i.e., no coverage prior to the day after the patient's 50th birthday"

   If the claim for a screening prostate antigen test or screening digital rectal examination is being denied because the time period between the test/procedure has not passed, use existing ANSI X12-835 claim adjustment reason code 119 "Benefit maximum for this time period has been reached" at the line level.

   If the claim for a screening prostate antigen test or screening digital rectal examination is being denied due to the absence of diagnosis code V76.44 on the claim, use existing ANSI X-12-835 claim adjustment reason code 47, "This (these) diagnosis (es) is (are) not covered, missing, or invalid."

B. Medicare Summary Notice (MSN) and Explanation of Your Medicare Benefits (EOMB) Messages.—If the claim for a screening prostate specific antigen test or screening digital rectal examination is being denied because the patient is not over 50 years of age, the following new line (May 2000) MSN or EOMB message:

C. "This service is not covered until after the beneficiary's 50th birthday." (MSN Message 18.19, EOMB Message 18.27)

The Spanish version of this MSN or EOMB message should read: "Este servicio no está cubierto hasta después de que el beneficiario cumpla 50 años."

If a claim for screening prostate specific antigen test or screening digital rectal examination is being denied because the minimum time period between the same test or procedure has not elapsed, use the following MSN or EOMB message:

"Service is being denied because it has not been [12/24/48] months since your last [test/procedure] of this kind." (MSN Message 18.14, EOMB Message 18.23)

The Spanish version of this MSN or EOMB message should read: "Este servicio está siendo denegado ya que no han transcurrido [12, 24, 48] meses desde el último [examen/procedimiento] de esta clase."

4270 ESRD BILL PROCESSING PROCEDURES

Physicians, independent laboratories, and beneficiaries must submit claims (Form CMS-1500, Form CMS-1490Sor electronic equivalent) to their local carrier for services furnished to end stage renal disease (ESRD) beneficiaries. Suppliers of Method II dialysis equipment and supplies will submit their claims (Form CMS-1500 or electronic equivalent) to the appropriate Durable Medical Equipment Regional Carriers (DMERCs). All ESRD facilities must submit their claims to their appropriate fiscal intermediary (FI).

4270.2 Bill Review of Laboratory Services.--See §5114.1 for a detailed description of payment for outpatient clinical diagnostic laboratory tests using fee schedules and for specimen collection fees.

All laboratory tests not included under the ESRD composite rate payment and performed by an independent laboratory for dialysis patients of independent dialysis facilities must be billed by the independent laboratory to carriers. The fee schedule applies to all clinical diagnostic tests except for tests already included under the ESRD composite rate payment. These tests are reimbursed only through the composite rate paid by the intermediary.

Laboratory tests not included under the ESRD composite rate payment, including all laboratory tests furnished to home dialysis patients who have selected payment Method II (see §4271), are billed to and paid by you at the fee schedule, if the tests are performed by an independent laboratory for an independent dialysis facility patient.

For purposes of the fee schedule, clinical diagnostic laboratory services include all laboratory tests listed in codes 80002-89399 of the Current Procedural Terminology Fourth Edition (CPT-4) with the following exceptions:

85095-85109:	Codes dealing with bone marrow smears and biopsies
85120	Bone marrow transplant
88000-88130:	Certain cytopathology services
88160-88199	Certain cytopathology services
88260-88299:	Cytogenetic studies
88300-88399	Surgical pathology services

Where tests not included in the composite rate are performed, the lab includes all tests (both those included in the composite rate and those that meet the frequency guidelines) on the bill. The tests listed below are included in the composite rate if their frequency does not exceed that which is indicated. Do not pay for tests up to the frequency described as they are paid under the composite rate. Tests in excess of the frequency may be paid unless you determine they are not medically necessary. Medical documentation is required to substantiate the frequency. A diagnosis of renal disease is not sufficient. The nature of the illness or injury (diagnosis, complaint, or symptom) requiring the performance of the test(s) must be present on the claim. A diagnosis from the ICD-9-CM coding system may be shown in lieu of a narrative description.

1. Laboratory Tests For Hemodialysis, Peritoneal Dialysis, and CCPD Included in the Composite Rate

2. Per Treatment

All hematocrit or hemoglobin and clotting time tests furnished incident to dialysis treatments.

3. Weekly

- Prothrombin time for patients on anti-coagulant therapy
- Serum Creatinine
- Weekly or Thirteen Per Quarter
- BUN

4. Monthly

Serum Calcium	Serum Bicarbonate	Alkaline Phosphatase
Serum Chloride	Serum Phosphorous	AST, SGOT
Total Protein	Serum Potassium	LDH
CBC	Serum Albumin	

Monthly Laboratory Tests For CAPD Included in the Composite Rate

BUN	Magnesium	Alkaline Phosphatase
Creatinine	Phosphate	LDH
Sodium	Potassium	AST, SGOT
CO2	TotalProtein	HCT
Calcium	Albumin	Hgb Dialysate Protein

A. Automated Profile Tests.—Clinical laboratory tests can be performed individually or in groups on automated profile equipment. If a clinical laboratory test is performed individually, it is paid in accordance with §§5114ff. If clinical laboratory tests are performed as part of an automated profile, then the following procedure applies:

1. Determine which of the laboratory tests in the automated profile are included under the composite rate and which are separately billable ESRD laboratory tests.

2. Determine the payment allowance of the automated profile by comparing it to the total payment allowances of the covered laboratory tests in the automated profile when the medically necessary tests in the profile are performed individually. The payment allowance of the automated profile is the lower of these two amounts. (See §5114.1.L.) If the payment allowance for the automated profile containing only the medically necessary tests is lower, you must determine the percentage of covered tests included under the composite rate payment. If 50 percent or more of the covered tests are included under the composite rate payment, then the entire profile is included within the composite payment. In this case, no separate payment in addition to the composite rate is made for any of the separately billable tests. If more than 50 percent of the covered tests are separately billable, the entire automated profile is considered separately billable. In this case, the entire automated profile is paid for in addition to the ESRD composite rate.

   If the lower payment allowance is the payment allowance of the laboratory tests taken individually, the tests may be billed individually. In this case, the tests included under the composite rate are not billed or paid separately, and the tests that are not included under the composite rate are billed and paid separately.

B. Separately Billable Tests Furnished by Hospital-Based Facilities.—Hospital-based facilities are paid for the separately billable ESRD laboratory tests furnished to their outpatients following the same rules that apply to all other Medicare covered outpatient laboratory services furnished by a hospital.

C. Separately Billable Tests Furnished to Patients of Independent Dialysis Facilities.—All separately billable ESRD clinical laboratory services furnished to patients of independent dialysis facilities must be billed by and reimbursed to the person or entity that performs the laboratory test in accordance with usual Medicare program rules. Independent dialysis facilities with the appropriate clinical laboratory certification may perform and bill their intermediary for separately billable laboratory services. Independent dialysis facilities are paid for separately billable clinical laboratory tests according to the Medicare laboratory fee schedule for independent laboratories.

   Following are tests not included in the composite rate which may be paid at the frequency shown without medical documentation. Tests in excess of that frequency require medical documentation. A diagnosis of ESRD alone is not sufficient medical documentation. The nature of the illness or injury (diagnosis, complaint, or symptom) requiring the performance of the test(s) must be present on the claim. A diagnosis from the ICD-9-CM coding system may be shown in lieu of a narrative description.

Guidelines for Separately Billable Tests for Hemodialysis, IPD, and CCPD

- Serum Aluminum: one every 3 months
- Serum Ferritin: one every 3 months

Guidelines for CAPD (every 3 months)

- WBC
- RBC
- Platelet count

4273 CLAIMS FOR PAYMENT FOR EPOETIN ALFA (EPO)

Effective June 1, 1989, the drug EPO is covered under Part B if administered incident to a physician's services. EPO is used to treat anemia associated with chronic renal failure, including patients on dialysis and those who are not on dialysis.

4273.1 Completion of Initial Claim for EPO.—The following information is required. Due to space limitations, some items must be documented on a separate form. Therefore, initial claims are generally submitted on paper unless your electronic billers are able to submit supplemental documentation with EMC claims. Return incomplete assigned claims in accordance with §3311.

Develop incomplete unassigned claims.

A. Diagnoses.—The diagnoses must be submitted according to ICD-9-CM and correlated to the procedure. This information is in Items 23A and 24D, of the Form HCFA-1500.

B. Hematocrit (HCT)/Hemoglobin (Hgb).—There are special HCPCS codes for reporting the injection of EPO. These allow the simultaneous reporting of the patient's latest HCT or Hgb reading before administration of EPO.

   Instruct the physician and/or staff to enter a separate line item for injections of EPO at different HCT/Hgb levels. The Q code for each line items is entered in Item 24C.

   1. Code Q9920 - Injection of EPO, per 1,000 units, at patient HCT of 20 or less/Hgb of 6.8 or less.

   2. Codes Q9921 through Q9939 - Injection of EPO, per 1,000 units, at patient HCT of 21 to 39/Hgb of 6.9 to 13.1.

      For HCT levels of 21 or more, up to a HCT of 39/Hgb of 6.9 to 13.1, a Q code that includes the actual HCT levels is used. To convert actual Hgb to corresponding HCT values for Q code reporting, multiply the Hgb value by 3 and round to the nearest whole number. Use the whole number to determine the appropriate Q code.

      EXAMPLES: If the patient's HCT is 25/Hgb is 8.2-8.4, Q9925 must be entered on the claim. If the patient's HCT is 39/Hgb is 12.9-13.1, Q9939 is entered.

   3. Code Q9940 - Injection of EPO, per 1,000 units at patient HCT of 40 or above. A single line item may include multiple doses of EPO administered while th patient's HCT level remained the same.

C. Units Administered.—The standard unit of EPO is 1,000. The number of 1,000 units administered per line item is included on the claim. The physician's office enters 1 in the units field for each multiple of 1,000 units. For example, if 12,000 units are administered, 12 is entered. This information is shown in Item 24F (Days/Units) on Form HCFA-1500.

In some cases, the dosage for a single line item does not total an even multiple of 1,000. If this occurs, the physician's office rounds down supplemental dosages of 0 to 499 units to the prior 1,000 units. Supplemental dosages of 500 to 999 are rounded up to the next 1,000 units.

EXAMPLES: A patient's HCT reading on August 6 was 22/Hgb was 7.3.The patient received 5,000 units of EPO on August 7, August 9 and August 11, for a total of 15,000 units. The first line of Item 24 of Form HCFA-1500 shows:

Dates of Service	Procedure Code	Days or Units
8/7-8/11	Q9922	15

On September 13, the patient's HCT reading increased to 27/Hgb increased to 9. The patient received 5,100 units of EPO on September 13, September 15, and September 17, for a total of 15,300 units. Since less than 15,500 units were given, the figure is rounded down to 15,000. This line on the claim form shows:

Dates of Service	Procedure Code	Days or Units
9/13-9/17	Q9927	15

On October 16, the HCT level increased to 33/Hgb increased to 11.The patient received doses of 4,850 units on October 16, October 18, and October 20 for a total of 14,550 units. Since more than 14,500 units were administered, the figure is rounded up to 15,000. Form HCFA-1500 shows:

Dates of Service	Procedure Code	Days or Units
10/16-10/20	Q9933	15

D. Date of the patient's most recent HCT or Hgb.

E. Most recent HCT or Hgb level prior to initiation of EPO therapy.

F. Date of most recent HCT or Hgb level prior to initiation of EPO therapy.

G Patient's most recent serum creatinine, within the last month, prior to initiation of EPO therapy. H. Date of most recent serum creatinine prior to initiation of EPO therapy.

I. Patient's weight in kilograms.

J. Patient's starting dose per kilogram. (The usual starting dose is 50-100 units per kilogram.) When a claim is submitted on Form HCFA-1500, these items are submitted on a separate document. It is not necessary to enter them into your claims processing system. This information is used in utilization review.

4273.2 Completion of Subsequent Claims for EPO.--Subsequent claims include the following:

A. Diagnoses.

B. Hematocrit or Hemoglobin.—This is indicated by the appropriate Q code. Claims include a EJ modifier to the Q code. This allows you to identify subsequent claims which do not require as much information as initial claims and prevent unnecessary development.

C. Number of units administered.—See §4273.1 for a description of these items. Subsequent claims may be submitted electronically. See §3023.7 for including the number of units in standard format EMC claims.

4450. PARENTERAL AND ENTERAL NUTRITION (PEN)

PEN coverage is determined by information provided by the attending physician and the PEN supplier. A certification of medical necessity (CMN) contains pertinent information needed to ensure consistent coverage and payment determinations nationally. A completed CMN must accompany and support the claims for PEN to establish whether coverage criteria are met and to ensure that the PEN provided is consistent with the attending physician's prescription.

The medical and prescription information on a PEN CMN can be completed most appropriately by the attending physician, or from information in the patient's records by an employee of the physician for the physician's review and signature. Although PEN suppliers may assist in providing PEN items they cannot complete the CMN since they do not have the same access to patient information needed to properly enter medical or prescription information.

A. Scheduling and Documenting Certifications and Recertifications of Medical Necessity for PEN.--A PEN CMN must accompany the initial claim submitted. The initial certification is valid for three months. Establish the schedule on a case-by-case basis for recertifying the need for PEN therapy. A change in prescription for a beneficiary past the initial certification period does not restart the certification process. A period of medical necessity ends when PEN is not medically required for two consecutive months. The entire certification process, if required, begins after the period of two consecutive months have elapsed.

B. Initial Certifications.--In reviewing the claim and the supporting data on the CMN, compare certain items, especially pertinent dates of treatment. For example, the start date of PEN coverage cannot precede the date of physician certification. The estimated duration of therapy must be contained on the

CMN. Use this information to verify that the test of permanence is met. Once coverage is established, the estimated length of need at the start of PEN services will determine the recertification schedule. (See §4450 A.)

Verify that the information shown on the certification supports the need for PEN supplies as billed. A diagnosis must show a functional impairment that precludes the enteral patient from swallowing and the parenteral patient from absorbing nutrients.

The attending physician and/or his/her designated employee are in a position to accurately complete the patient's medical information including:

- The patient's general condition, estimated duration of therapy, and other treatments or therapies (see §3329 B.2.);
- The patient's clinical assessment relating to the need for PEN therapy (see §3329 B.3.); and
- The nutritional support therapy (i.e., the enteral or parenteral formulation). (See §3329 B.4.)

Initial assigned claims with the following conditions can be denied without development:

- Inappropriate or missing diagnosis or functional impairment;
- Estimated duration of therapy is less than 90 consecutive days;
- Duration of therapy is not listed;
- Supplies have not been provided;
- Supplies were provided prior to onset date of therapy; and
- Stamped physician's signature.

Develop unassigned claims for missing or incomplete information. (See §3329 C.)

Review all claims with initial certifications and recertifications before payment is authorized.

C. Revised Certifications/Change in Prescription.--Remind suppliers to submit revised certifications if the attending physician changes the PEN prescription. A revised certification is appropriate when:

- There is a change in the attending physician's orders in the category of nutrients and/or calories prescribed;
- There is a change by more than one liter in the daily volume of parenteral solutions;
- There is a change from home-mix to pre-mix or pre-mix to home-mix parenteral solutions;
- There is a change from enteral to parenteral or parenteral to enteral therapy; or
- There is a change in the method of infusion (e.g., from gravity-fed to pump-fed).

Do not adjust payments on PEN claims unless a revised or renewed certification documents the necessity for the change. Adjust payments timely, if necessary, for supplies since the PEN prescription was changed.

Do not exceed payment levels for the most current certification or recertification if a prescription change is not documented by a new recertification.

Adjust your diary for scheduled recertifications. When the revised certification has been considered, reschedule the next recertification according to the recertification schedule. (See § 4450 A.)

D. Items Requiring Special Attention.--

1. Nutrients.--Category IB of enteral nutrients contains products that are natural intact protein/protein isolates commonly known as blenderized nutrients. Additional documentation is required to justify the necessity of Category IB nutrients. The attending physician must provide sufficient information to indicate that the patient:

   - Has an intolerance to nutritionally equivalent (semi-synthetic) products;
   - Had a severe allergic reaction to a nutritionally equivalent (semi-synthetic) product; or
   - Was changed to a blenderized nutrient to alleviate adverse symptoms expected to be of permanent duration with continued use of semi-synthetic products.

   Also, enteral nutrient categories III through VI require additional medical justification for coverage.

   Parenteral nutrition may be either "self-mixed" (i.e., the patient is taught to prepare the nutrient solution aseptically) or "pre-mixed" (i.e., the nutrient solution is prepared by trained professionals employed or contracted by the PEN supplier). The attending physician must provide information to justify the reason for "pre-mixed" parenteral nutrient solutions.

2. Prospective Billing.--Pay for no more than a one-month supply of parenteral or enteral nutrients for any one prospective billing period. Claims submitted retroactively may include multiple months.

3. Pumps.--Enteral nutrition may be administered by syringe, gravity, or pump. The attending physician must specify the reason that necessitates the use of an enteral feeding pump. Ensure that the equipment for which payment is claimed is consistent with that prescribed (e.g., expect a claim for an I.V. pole, if a pump is used).

Effective April 1, 1990, claims for parenteral and enteral pumps are limited to rental payments for a total of 15 months during a period of medical need. A period of medical need ends when enteral or parenteral nutrients are not medically necessary for two consecutive months.

Do not allow additional rental payments once the 15-month limit is reached, unless the attending physician changes the prescription between parenteral and enteral nutrients.

Do not continue rental payments after a pump is purchased unless the attending physician changes the prescription between parenteral and enteral nutrients.

Do not begin a new 15-month rental period when a patient changes suppliers. The new supplier is entitled to the balance remaining on the 15-month rental period.

Effective October 1, 1990, necessary maintenance and servicing of pumps after the 15-month rental limit is reached, includes repairs and extensive maintenance that involves the breaking down of sealed components or performing tests that require specialized testing equipment not available to the beneficiary or nursing home.

4. Supplies.--Enteral care kits contain all the necessary supplies for the enteral patient using the syringe, gravity, or pump method of nutrient administration. Parenteral nutrition care kits and their components are considered all inclusive items necessary to administer therapy during a monthly period.

   Compare the enteral feeding care kits on the claim with the method of administration indicated on the CMN.

   - Reduce the allowance to the amount paid for a gravity-fed care kit when billed for a pump feeding kit in the absence of documentation or unacceptable documentation for a pump.
   - Limit payment to a one-month supply.
   - Deny payment for additional components included as part of the PEN supply kit.

5. Attending Physician Identification.--A CMN must contain the attending physician's Unique Physician Identification Number (UPIN) and be signed and dated by the attending physician. A stamped signature is unacceptable.

   Deny certifications and recertifications altered by "whiting out" or "pasting over" and entering new data. Consider suppliers that show a pattern of altering CMNs for educational contact and/or audit.

Be alert to certifications from suppliers who have questionable utilization or billing practices or who are under sanction. Consider an audit of any such situations.

4471 PAYMENT FOR IMMUNOSUPPRESSIVE DRUGS

Beginning January 1, 1987, Medicare pays for FDA approved immunosuppressive drugs and for drugs used in immunosuppressive therapy.(See §2050.5.)Generally, pay for self-administered immunosuppressive drugs that are specifically labeled and approved for marketing as such by the FDA, or identified in FDA-approved labeling for use in conjunction with immunosuppressive drug therapy.This benefit is subject to the Part B deductible and coinsurance provision and is limited to the 1-year period after the date of the transplant.Pay for immunosuppressive drugs which are provided outside the 1-year period if they are covered under another provision of the law (e.g., as inpatient hospital services or are furnished incident to a physician's service).

"One-year period after the date of the transplant" means 365 days from the day on which an inpatient is discharged from the hospital.From surgery until hospital discharge, payment for these drugs is included in Medicare's Part A payment to the hospital.If the same patient receives a subsequent transplant operation within 365 days, the period begins anew.

Prescriptions generally should be nonrefillable and limited to a 30 day supply.The 30 day guideline is necessary because dosage frequently diminishes over a period of time, and further, it is not uncommon for the physician to change the prescription from one drug to another.Also, these drugs are expensive and the coinsurance liability on unused drugs could be a financial burden to the beneficiary.Unless there are special circumstances, do not consider a supply of drugs in excess of 30 days to be reasonable and necessary.

4471.1 Routing Claims

Route claims for immunosuppressive drugs and any supporting documentation to one of two specialty carriers.Process your part of the claim and notify the beneficiary, and if needed, the physician and supplier of the transfer.The specialty carrier to which to route the claim is based upon the drug supplier's home office.

If the supplier's home office is west of the Mississippi river or in Minnesota:

TransAmerica Occidental Life Insurance Company
Medicare Immuno Drug Claims
P.O. Box 60549
Los Angeles, CA90060-0549

If the supplier's home office is east of the Mississippi river, excluding Minnesota:

Blue Cross and Blue Shield of South Carolina
Medicare Immunosuppressive Drug Unit PEN Claims
P.O. Box 102401
Columbia, SC29224

Notify all suppliers regularly of the billing address for the specialty carriers for submission of immunosuppressive drug claims.

4471.2 Determination of Eligibility

Benefit eligibility is limited to the l-year period following the date of the beneficiary's discharge from a hospital or transplant center after a Medicare covered kidney, heart or liver transplant.(See §5249.)The specialty carrier consults one of three alternative sources of information to determine the date of kidney transplant:

HCFA compiles and furnishes in hardcopy or tape format to specialty carriers a monthly listing of beneficiaries who have received kidney transplants.HCFA's system is not yet equipped to handle heart and liver transplant data.The initial listing includedall beneficiaries who had received a kidney transplant since January 1, 1986.It is updated monthly.The listing includes:

* HICN under which benefits are paid.
* Last name, first name, and middle initial of person receiving benefits.
* Month, day, and year of beneficiary's most recent kidney transplant (MMDDYY).
* Month, day, and year that beneficiary died (MMDDYY)
* Month, day, and year of kidney transplant failure (MMDDYY).
* Intermediaries send copies of the Part A Medicare Benefit Notice which contains the date of transplant to the specialty carriers.The specialty carriers maintain the data and release it to area carriers upon request.

If you are unable to locate the beneficiary's transplant information above, refer to the discharge date listed on the prescription form.The prescription form, or facsimile thereof, should accompany the initial claim and indicate the date of discharge.You may contact the prescribing physician for substantiation of the discharge date.If you do not have any eligibility information other than the prescription regarding the discharge date, you may pay for 1 month's supply of immunosuppressive drugs based upon the discharge date listed.If the information obtained indicates transplant failure, do not approve payment for drugs in subsequent periods.

4471.3 Reasonable Charge Determinations

For purposes of establishing customary and prevailing charges, the United States is considered a single locality structure.

Since immunosuppressive drugs have not been previously covered, there is no existing charge data base for determining customary or prevailing charges.Therefore, the normal gap filling techniques in §5022 are not appropriate.

To establish reimbursement for the initial 3 month coverage period; i.e., January 1, 1987 through March 31, 1987, use available drug pricing data.Sources for pricing ingredient costs may include the Drug Topics Red Book, the American Druggist Blue Book, or manufacturers price lists.Also consider the appropriateness of an additional charge for administration.

During the initial 3 month interim coverage period, gather charge data and use it to establish customary and prevailing charges.Establish and maintain reasonable charge screens until a general revision is made to the reasonable charge screens at the beginning of the new fee screen year, i.e., January 1, 1988.Then use the charge data for the period January 1 through June 30, 1987 as the base year to calculate reasonable charges.

Adjust prevailing charges if they are grossly deficient or excessive in comparison to data from other sources.(See §5246 for determining appropriateness of charges.)For example, prevailing charges may be adjusted where they appear grossly excessive in relation to charge data from mail order pharmacies reflecting substantial discounts over published prices.

4471.4 HCPCS Codes

The following HCPCS codes are assigned:

Code	Definition
Q0004	Azathioprine (e.g., Imuran) - oral, tab, 50 mg., 100s ea.
Q0005	Azathioprine (e.g.,Imuran) - parenteral, vial, 100 mg., 20 ml. ea.
Q0006	Cyclosporine (e.g.,Sandimmune) - oral, sol; 100 mg/ml., 50 ml., ea.
Q0007	Cyclosporine (e.g., Sandimmune) - parenteral amp, I.V, 250 mg., 5 ml., 10s ea UD
Q0008	Lymphocyte Immune Globulin, Antithymocyte Globulin (e.g., Atgam) - parenteral, amp, 50 mg./ml., 5 ml.ea.
Q0009	Monoclonal Antibodies (eg Muromonab C D3; Orthoclone) -parenteral, amp, 5 mg./5 ml., 5 ml. ea.

5102.3 Transition to Fee Schedule-Relationship to Prior Rules.—

A. Comparability and Inherent Reasonableness Limitations.—Effective January 1, 1989, until further notice, you may no longer apply the comparable circumstances provision contained in §5026. Between January 1, 1989 and December 31, 1990, you may not apply the special limitations provision contained in §5246.

B. Purchase of Items Requiring Frequent and Substantial Servicing or Capped Rental Items.-

1. Purchase Prior to January 1, 1989.—If the beneficiary purchased an item of equipment in either of these two categories (see §5102.1.B or E) prior to January 1, 1989, pay the reasonable and necessary charges for

maintenance and servicing of this equipment. In the event the item of equipment needs to be replaced on or after June 1, 1989, pay on a rental basis according to the instructions in §5102.1.B. or E.

If the beneficiary purchased the equipment even though you determined that rental was more economical under the rent/purchase guidelines, or if the beneficiary made an approved purchase on an installment plan, make payment on an installment basis until the purchase price has been reached or medical necessity terminated. If the purchase price has not been reached by January 1, 1989, continue paying on an installment basis but at the monthly fee schedule amount until the purchase price is reached, the purchase price fee schedule calculated under prior instructions is reached, or the medical necessity ends, whichever occurs first. The limitation on total payments to 15 months rental (as described in §5102.1.E) does not apply.

2. Purchase On Or After June 1, 1989.—If a beneficiary purchased an item of equipment that requires frequent and substantial servicing on or after June 1, 1989, do not make payment. Also, do not make payment for maintenance and servicing or for replacement of items in either category that are purchased on or after June 1, 1989.

   If a beneficiary purchased an item of equipment in the capped rental category between June 1, 1989 and April 30, 1991, do not make payment. Also, do not make payment for maintenance and servicing. However, see §5102.1.E.5 or 6 for payment of purchase options after April 30, 1991 and for payment of replacement of items purchased between June 1, 1989 and April 30, 1991.

3. Purchase Between January 1, 1989 and June 1, 1989.—If a beneficiary purchased an item of equipment in either category after December 31, 1988, but before June 1, 1989, pay monthly installments equivalent to the rental fee schedule amounts until the medical necessity ends, the purchase price fee schedule calculated under prior instructions is reached, or the actual purchase charge has been reached, whichever occurs first. Pay the reasonable and necessary charges for maintenance and servicing of this equipment. In the event the item of equipment needs to be replaced on or after June 1, 1989, pay on a rental basis according to the instructions in §5102.1.B. or E. Payment may be made for purchase even if the purchase was preceded by a period of rental.

   However, total payments for rental plus purchase of capped rental items may not exceed the amount that would have been paid had the equipment been continuously rented for 15 months. (Therefore, if a purchase occurs during a period of continuous use after 15 months of rentals have been paid, no payment may be made other than the reasonable and necessary charges for servicing as described in §5102.1.E.4.)

C. Purchase of Oxygen Equipment.—

1. Purchase Prior to June 1, 1989.—If the beneficiary purchased stationary or portable oxygen equipment (see §5102.1.F) prior to June 1, 1989, pay the reasonable and necessary charges for maintenance and servicing of this equipment. In the event the item of equipment needs to be replaced on or after June 1, 1989, pay on a rental basis according to the instructions in §5102.1.F. If the beneficiary purchased the equipment even though you determined that rental was more economical under the rent/purchase guidelines, or if the beneficiary made an approved purchase on an installment plan, make payment on an installment basis until the purchase price had been reached or medical necessity terminated. If the purchase price has not been reached by June 1, 1989, continue paying on an installment basis (see §5102.1.F.9) but at the monthly fee schedule amount until the purchase price is reached or the medical necessity ends,whichever occurs first.

2. Purchase On Or After June 1, 1989.—If a beneficiary purchased stationary or portable oxygen equipment on or after June 1, 1989, do not make payment for the equipment. However, make payment for the contents in accordance with §5102.1.F.4 or 5. Also, do not make payment for maintenance and servicing or for replacement of oxygen equipment that is purchased on or after June 1, 1989.

D. 15-Month Ceiling.—For purposes of computing the 10-month purchase option or the 15-month period for capped rental items, begin counting the first month that the beneficiary continuously rented the equipment. For example, if the beneficiary began renting the equipment in July 1988, the rental month which begins in January 1989 is counted as the beneficiary's 7th month of rental. Therefore, if the equipment has been continuously rented prior to October 2, 1987, no further rental payments are made since the 15-month period is terminated before January 1, 1989. The maintenance and service provision in §5102.1.E.4 begins July 1, 1989.

If the beneficiary has reached (on a date of service prior to January 1989) the purchase price limitation on a rental claim, do not make any further purchase or rental payments until the useful life has elapsed according to the instructions in §5102.1.E.7. However, for capped rental items previously rented that have reached the purchase cap under the rent/purchase rules, pay claims for maintenance and servicing fees in accordance with §5102.1.E.4 effective July 1, 1989.

E. Oxygen.—Claims for oxygen contents provided after May 31, 1989, but prior to the start of the June equipment rental month, may be paid in either of the following two ways. Either continue paying the reasonable charge payment amount for contents through the end of the May monthly rental period; or pay the reasonable charge payment amount for contents through the end of May and pay the actual charge for contents up to the fee schedule allowance for oxygen contents only, as prorated for the period June 1 through the end of the May rental period. Begin paying the appropriate full fee schedule amount at the beginning of the new rental period. For example, a beneficiary's rental period began May 15, 1989. Pay on a reasonable charge basis from May 15 through June 14; or pay on a reasonable charge basis from May 15 through May 31, 1989 and pay the actual charge up to 14/31 of the oxygen contents fee (established in §5102.1.F.4) from June 1 through June 14, 1989. Pay the lesser of the full fee schedule amount or actual charge beginning June 15, 1989.

F. Purchase Options For Capped Rental Items.—

1. Electric Wheelchairs.—If the beneficiary purchases an electric wheelchair prior to May 1, 1991, pay for the wheelchair as a routinely purchased item in accordance with §5102.1.A. If the beneficiary elects to rent an electric wheelchair prior to May 1, 1991, pay the rental fee schedule amount not to exceed the purchase price in accordance with §5102.1.A. If, on May 1,1991, the purchase price has not been reached, convert the monthly fee schedule amount from routinely purchased to capped rental. As such, each month's rental before and after conversion must be counted toward the 10 month purchase option in §5102.1.E.6 and the 15 month rental cap in §5102.1.E.2.

2. All Other Capped Rental Items.—If the beneficiary purchased a capped rental item prior to May 1, 1991, do not make payment. If the beneficiary rented a capped rental item prior to May 1, 1991, pay the rental fee schedule amount not to exceed the 15 month rental cap in accordance with §5102.1.E.2.Each month's rental must be counted toward the 10 month purchase option in §5102.1.E.6 and the 15 month rental cap in §5102.1.E.2.

5114 PAYMENT FOR DIAGNOSTIC LABORATORY SERVICES

This section sets out payment rules for diagnostic laboratory services, i.e., (1) outpatient clinical diagnostic laboratory tests subject to the fee schedule, and (2) other diagnostic laboratory tests.

Regardless of whether a diagnostic laboratory test is performed in a physician's office, by an independent laboratory, or by a hospital laboratory for its outpatients or nonpatients, it is considered a laboratory service.When a hospital laboratory performs diagnostic laboratory tests for nonhospital patients, the laboratory is functioning as an independent laboratory.Also, when physicians and laboratories perform the same test, whether manually or with automated equipment, the services are deemed similar.

The laboratory services for which this instruction applies are those listed in §2070.1.D. The tests are not subject to the economic index under the guidelines in §5020.3.A.Any test not listed in §2070.1.D is considered a physicians' service, is subject to the economic index as described in §5020.3.A, and is not considered in implementing this instruction. The only exceptions are as specified in §5020.3.A. For example, the taking of an EKG is a laboratory service when billed separately; but an EKG interpretation alone, as well as the taking of an EKG billed with interpretation, is a physician service subject to the economic index.Similarly, clinical laboratory services not subject to the fee schedule (see '5114.1) included in office visits for which a single prevailing charge screen is maintained are subject to the economic index.

Clinical diagnostic laboratory tests subject to the fee schedule are specifically delineated in §5114.1.B.

Other diagnostic laboratory tests are laboratory tests other than clinical diagnostic laboratory tests subject to fee schedule reimbursement.Such tests include EKGs and physiological testing.
Payment for clinical diagnostic laboratory tests subject to the fee schedule is made in accordance with the instructions in §5114.1.

Generally, payment for other diagnostic laboratory tests is made in accordance with the reasonable charge methodology.Special payment rules for physicians who do not personally perform or supervise other diagnostic laboratory tests but who bill for such tests are referenced in §5258.In accordance with '5262, payment for diagnostic radiology tests is made on a fee schedule basis.

5114.1 Payment for Outpatient Clinical Diagnostic Laboratory Tests Using Fee Schedules and for Specimen Collection

Under Part B, for services rendered on or after July 1, 1984, clinical diagnostic laboratory tests performed in a physician's office, by an independent laboratory, or by a hospital laboratory for its outpatients are reimbursed on the basis of fee schedules.

The fee schedules are established on a carrierwide basis (not to exceed a statewide basis). National fee schedules may be established beginning January 1, 1990.

The lowest charge level provisions no longer apply to clinical diagnostic laboratory tests. In addition, §5100.2.C no longer applies.This section provides that laboratory tests furnished to CAPD End Stage Renal Disease (ESRD) patients dialyzing at home are billed in the same way as any other test furnished home patients.The reasonable charge criteria were used for tests performed by an independent laboratory for the home patient.Since clinical diagnostic laboratory tests are no longer paid in accordance with the reasonable charge criteria, the fee schedule now applies to laboratory tests performed for the home ESRD dialysis patient described in §4270.2 when the tests are not covered under the ESRD composite rate.

A. Application of Fee Schedule.-The fee schedule applies to all clinical diagnostic laboratory tests except:

   * Laboratory tests furnished to a hospital inpatient whose stay is covered under Part A.
   * Laboratory tests provided by a hospital for an inpatient of such hospital that are payable under Part B (due to lack of Part A coverage) continue to be reimbursed on a reasonable cost basis.
   * Laboratory tests performed by a Skilled Nursing Facility (SNF) for its own SNF inpatients and reimbursed under Part A or Part B and any laboratory tests furnished under arrangements to an SNF inpatient with Part A coverage.(The only covered source for laboratory services furnished under Part A is the SNF itself or a hospital with which the facility has a transfer agreement in effect.)Continue to reimburse such

tests on a reasonable cost basis.All Part B tests, furnished by a laboratory other than the SNF's own are reimbursable only to the laboratory under the fee schedule; and

* Laboratory tests furnished by hospital-based or independent ESRD dialysis facilities that are included under the ESRD composite rate payment.(See §4270.2 for discussion of laboratory tests included in composite rate payment.)These tests are reimbursed only through this payment. Never pay anyone else for these tests.Laboratory tests that are not included under the ESRD composite rate payment and are performed by an independent laboratory for dialysis patients of independent dialysis facilities are billed to you and paid at the fee schedule.This procedure applies to all laboratory tests furnished to home dialysis patients who have selected payment Method II.(See §4271.)
* Laboratory tests furnished by hospitals in States or areas which have been granted demonstration waivers of Medicare reimbursement principles for outpatient services.The State of Maryland has been granted such demonstration waivers.This also may apply to hospitals in States granted approval for alternative payment methods for paying for hospital outpatient services under §1886© of the Act.
* Laboratory tests furnished to inpatients of a hospital with a waiver under §602(k) of the 1983 Amendments to the Act.(See '2255.)This section of the Act provides that an outside supplier may bill under Part B for laboratory and other nonphysician services furnished to inpatients that are otherwise paid only though the hospital.Part B payment to the outside supplier for laboratory tests furnished to inpatients under the 602(k) waiver is made at 80 percent of the reasonable charge if the claim is unassigned or at 100 percent of the reasonable charge if the claim is assigned. The fee schedule does apply to any tests furnished by the outside supplier to hospital outpatients and to nonhospital patients.
* Laboratory tests furnished to patients of rural health clinics under an all inclusive rate.
* Laboratory tests provided by a participating health maintenance organization (HMO) or health care prepayment plan (HCPP) to an enrolled member of the plan.
* Laboratory test furnished by a hospice.

B. Clinical Diagnostic Laboratory Services Subject to Fee Schedule.-For purposes of the fee schedule, clinical diagnostic laboratory services include laboratory tests listed in codes 80002-89399 of the Current Procedural Terminology, Fourth Edition (CPT-4), 1991 printing.Certain tests, however, are required to be performed by a physician and are therefore exempt from the fee schedule.These tests include:

80500-80502 Clinical pathology consultation

85095-85109 Codes dealing with bone marrow smears and biopsies

86077-86079 Blood bank services

88000-88125 Certain cytopathology services

88160-88199 Certain cytopathology services

88300-88399 Surgical pathology services

Some CPT-4 codes in the 80000 series are not clinical diagnostic laboratory tests.Such codes include codes for procedures, services, blood products and autotransfusions.Other codes for tests primarily associated with the provision of blood products are also not considered clinical diagnostic tests.

These codes include the various blood crossmatching techniques. The following codes are never subject to fee schedule limitations:

85060

86012

86013

86016-86019

86024

86034

86068

86070

86100

86120

86128

861300

86265-86267

86455-86585

86595

89100-89105

89130-89141

89350

89360

The following codes are not subject to fee schedule limitations when they are submitted for payment on the same bill with charges for blood products:

86011

86014

86031-86033

86080

86082-86095

86105

If no blood product is provided and billed on the same claim, these codes are subject to the fee schedule.

The following codes that delineate allergy, organ or disease oriented panels/profilesare not currently subject to the national limitation amounts because laboratories do not always utilize the same array or number of tests in a particular panel.However, the national limitation amount applies to each test included in the panel/profile.(See §§5114.1.F and 5114.l.G.)

80050-80099

86421-86422

Know which individual tests have been performed when claims are received using panel/profile codes.This does not need to be reported on each bill as long as you are confident that every laboratory reporting a panel or profile uses a consistent set of tests.If there is variation in content of the panel or profile, establish a uniform definition and require laboratories that do not comply with this definition to identify the individual tests when billing the panel or profile.

The following codes for unlisted or not otherwise classified clinical diagnostic laboratory tests are not subject to the national limitation amounts.

81099

84999

85999

86999

87999

88299

89399

Please note that for purposes of the fee schedule, clinical diagnostic laboratory tests include some services described as anatomic pathology services in CPT-4 (i.e., certain cervical, vaginal, or peripheral blood smears).Use the CPT-4 code 85060 only when a physician interprets an abnormal peripheral blood smear for a hospital inpatient or a hospital outpatient, and the hospital is responsible for the technical component.When a physician interpretation of an abnormal peripheral blood smear is billed by an independent laboratory, it is considered a complete or global service, and the service is not billed under the CPT-4 code 85060.A physician interpretation of an abnormal peripheral blood smear performed by an independent laboratory is considered a routine part of the ordered hematology service (i.e., those tests that include a different white blood count).

HCPCS code 88150 (cervical or vaginal smears) included both screening and interpretation in CPT-4 1986 terminology while the CPT-4 1987 terminology includes only screening.A new code, 88151, was added for those smears which require physician interpretation. Code 88151 is treated and priced in the same manner as you previously treated code 88150.Code 88151 with a "26" modifier is paid when a physician performs an interpretation of an abnormal smear for a hospital inpatient or outpatient, and the hospital is responsible for the technical component.No longer recognize the "26" modifier for code 88150.Price code 88151(26) as you would have priced code 88150(26) if the coding terminology had not been revised.Independent laboratories bill under code 88150 for normal smears and under code 88151 for abnormal smears.However, the fee schedule amount is equivalent.

Certain blood gas levels are determined either by invasive means through use of a blood specimen for a clinical diagnostic laboratory test or by noninvasive means through ear or pulse oximetry which is not considered a clinical diagnostic laboratory test.Use CPT-4 code 82792 for invasive oximetry. Use

HCPCS code M0592 for ear and pulse oximetry. Code M0592 is not subject to fee schedules. (See Coverage Issues Manual, §60-4C, for coverage requirements and Medicare Carriers Manual §5246.6 for pricing consideration.)

Services excluded from the fee schedule when billed by an independent laboratory are reimbursable under existing reasonable charge rules and assignment may be taken on a case-by-case basis unless the laboratory enrolls as a participating supplier in which event assignment is mandatory.Where a service is performed by a physician for a hospital inpatient or outpatient and meets the definition of a physician service under §8318-B, the service is subject to the Medicare Economic Index and the limitation on physician fees under §9331 of the Omnibus Budget Reconciliation Act of 1986.Such service, however, when billed by an independent laboratory as a laboratory service for a nonhospital patient (e.g., surgical pathology) is not considered a physician service for purposes of the Medicare Economic Index or the limitation on physician fees.

C. Calculation of Fee Schedule Amounts.-Set the fee schedule amounts at 60 percent of the prevailing charges for laboratory tests performed in physicians' offices by independent laboratories and for laboratory tests performed by hospital laboratories for nonhospital patients for the fee screen year beginning July 1, 1984.For hospital outpatient laboratory tests, the fee schedule amount is established at 62 percent of the prevailing charges.Beginning January 1, 1987, the fee schedule amount of 62 percent is paid for outpatient laboratory services only if provided by a qualified hospital laboratory, as described below.Beginning April 1, 1988, the fee schedule amount of 62 percent is payable only in a qualified hospital laboratory located in a sole community hospital. For this purpose, a qualified hospital laboratory is one which provides some clinical diagnostic laboratory tests 24 hours a day, 7 days a week, in order to serve a hospital's emergency room which is available to provide services 24 hours a day, 7 days week.To meet this requirement, a hospital must have physicians physically present or available within 30 minutes through a medical staff call roster to handle emergencies 24 hours a day, 7 days a week.Hospital laboratory personnel must be on duty or on call at all times to provide testing for the emergency room.

The prevailing charge is calculated as the 75th percentile of the customary charges, weighted by frequency, that were determined for the fee screen year beginning on July 1, 1984, for both physicians and independent laboratories (including hospital laboratories acting as independent laboratories) in (1) your existing service area or (2) no more than one State where your service area includes more than one entire State.In several instances, e.g., Kansas City and Washington, D.C. metropolitan areas, the area of a carrier includes portions of more than one State and that area is used in determining the prevailing charge.

Effective April 1, 1988, the fee schedules for certain automated tests, and for tests (with the exception of cytopathology) that were subject to the lowest charge level (LCL) provision prior to July 1, 1984, are adjusted in accordance with §5114.1.F.

Any rounding of initial fee schedule amounts is handled in the same manner as rounding for the application of the Medicare Economic Index.(See §5021.)

Where a hospital laboratory acts as an independent laboratory, i.e., performs tests for persons who are nonhospital patients or, where, commencing January 1, 1987, the hospital laboratory is not a qualified hospital laboratory, the services are reimbursed using the 60 percent of prevailing charge fee schedule or the adjusted fee schedule (see §5114.1.F), as appropriate.A hospital outpatient is a person who has not been admitted by the hospital as an inpatient but is registered on the hospital records as an outpatient and receives services (rather than supplies alone) from the hospital.Where a tissue sample, blood sample, or specimen is taken by personnel who are not employed by the hospital and is sent to the hospital for performance of tests, the tests are not outpatient hospital services since the patient does not directly receive services from the hospital.Where the hospital uses the category "day patient," i.e., an individual who receives hospital services during the day and is not expected to be lodged in the hospital at midnight, the individual is classified as an outpatient.

The fee schedule amounts are adjusted annually to reflect changes in the Consumer Price Index (CPI) for all Urban Consumers (U.S. city average).For laboratory tests performed on or after July 1, 1985 through December 31, 1986, the fee schedules are increased 4.1 percent.Beginning January 1, 1987, CPI adjustments are made January 1 of each year instead of July 1.The annualized index changes are as follows:

FSY	Annual Adjustment by Percent
1986	4.1
1987	5.4
1988	.0
1989	4.0
1990	4.7
1991	2.0
1992	2.0
1993	2.0

Information regarding the index changes for subsequent periods is furnished to you in time to make the necessary adjustments.In applying the annual adjustment, round calculations to the nearest penny.

The provisions in §5020.3.A provide for using the economic index to limit the prevailing charges for office visits combined with clinical laboratory tests for which you maintained a single prevailing charge screen.Since clinical diagnostic laboratory tests are no longer paid on the basis of the customary and prevailing charge criteria, do not allow the combination of laboratory tests with the physician's office visit in one prevailing charge.The fee schedule is used in determining the payment amount allowed for the laboratory tests, and the regular reasonable charge criteria and economic index are used for the office visit.

The codes and terminology in HCPCS are used in the fee schedule to identify and describe the laboratory tests.If you have not yet converted your coding systems to HCPCS, identify the equivalent tests in your own systems and use HCPCS codes for those services in establishing the fee schedules.

D. Specimen Collection Fee.-Separate charges made by physicians (except for services furnished to dialysis patients as indicated below), independent laboratories (except for services furnished to dialysis patients as indicated below), or hospital laboratories for drawing or collecting specimens are allowed up to $3 whether the specimens are referred to physicians or other laboratories for testing.This fee is not paid to anyone who has not actually extracted the specimen from the patient.Only one collection fee is allowed for eachpatient encounter, regardless of the number of specimens drawn.When a series of specimens is required to complete a single test (e.g., glucose tolerance test), the series is treated as a single encounter.A specimen collection fee is allowed in circumstances such as drawing a blood sample through venipuncture (i.e., inserting into a vein a needle with syringe or vacutainer to draw the specimen) or collecting a urine sample by catheterization.

A specimen collection fee for physicians is allowed only when (1) it is the accepted and prevailing practice among physicians in the locality to make separate charges for drawing or collecting a specimen, and (2) it is the customary practice of the physician performing such services to bill separate charges for them.

A specimen collection fee is not allowed when the cost of collecting the specimen is minimal, such as a throat culture or a routine capillary puncture for clotting or bleeding time.Stool specimen collection for an occult blood test is usually done by the patients at home, and a fee for such collection is not allowed.When a stool specimen is collected during a rectal examination, the collection is an incidental byproduct of that examination. Costs such as gloves are related to the rectal examination and compensated for in the payment for the visit.Payment for performing the test is separate from the specimen collection fee.Costs such as media (e.g., the slides) and labor are included in the payment for the test.

You no longer have authority to make payment for routine handling charges where a specimen is referred by one laboratory to another.Preparatory services, e.g., where a referring laboratory prepares a specimen before transfer to a reference laboratory, are considered an integral part of the testing process, and the costs of such services are included in the charge for the total testing service.

A specimen collection fee is allowed when it is medically necessary for a laboratory technician to draw a specimen from either a nursing home patient or homebound patient. The technician must personally draw the specimen, e.g., venipuncture or urine sample by catheterization.A specimen collection fee is not allowed in situations where a patient is not in a nursing facility or confined to his or her home. When a laboratory performs the specimen collection, it may receive payment both for the draw and for the associated travel to obtain the specimen(s) for testing.Payment may be made to the laboratory even if the nursing facility has on-duty personnel qualified to perform the specimen collection.When the nursing home performs the specimen collection, it may only receive payment for the draw.Specimen collection performed by nursing home personnel for patients covered under Part A is paid for as part of the facility's payment for its reasonable costs, not on the basis of the specimen collection fee.

Special rules apply when services are furnished to dialysis patients.ESRD facilities are only paid by intermediaries.Therefore, never pay a specimen collection fee to an ESRD facility.The specimen collection fee is not allowed when a physician or one of the physician's employees draws the specimen from the dialysis patient because it is included in the Monthly Capitation Payment (MCP).(See §5037.)Independent laboratories are not paid the specimen collection fee for specimens collected that are used in performing a laboratory test reimbursed under the composite rate.If a home dialysis patient selects reimbursement Method II (see §4271) and all other criteria for payment are met, pay an independent laboratory the specimen collection fee for specimens collected from the patient.

The coinsurance and deductible provisions do not apply to the specimen collection fee where 100 percent of the fee schedule amount is payable on the basis of an assignment to the persons or entities drawing the specimen.For services (including specimen collection) rendered on or after January 1, 1987, payment to laboratories or physicians is only made on the basis of an assignment.For services rendered prior to January 1, 1987, acceptance of an assignment is optional for physicians.However, the coinsurance and deductible is applied to the specimen collection fee where a physician collects the specimen and does not accept assignment.

Complex vascular injection procedures, such as arterial punctures and venesections, are not subject either to this specimen collection policy or to the assignment provisions.

E. Who Can Bill and Receive Payment for Clinical Laboratory Tests.-

1. General

It is your responsibility to determine whether the laboratory services were performed in the office of the physician or by another laboratory.If they were performed by another laboratory, payment may be made only if the laboratory performed tests in the specialties for which it is certified under the program.(See §2070.1.D.)

When Part B payment for clinical laboratory tests is subject to the fee schedule, payment is only made to the person or entity which performed or supervised the performance of the tests, except as follows:

* Payment may be made to an independent laboratory (if it meets the special conditions below) or hospital laboratory for tests performed by another laboratory on specimens referred to it by the first laboratory. Section 3102.F describes the guidelines regarding jurisdiction for payment of independent laboratory services.

* Payment may be made to one physician for tests performed or supervised by another physician with whom he shares his practice, i.e., where the two physicians are members of a medical group whose physicians bill in their own names rather than in the name of the group.Where the medical group bills in the name of the group for the services of the physician who performed or supervised the performance of these tests, payment is made to the group if the claim is assigned or, for services rendered on or before December 31, 1986, to the beneficiary if the claim is not assigned. See §2070.1 regarding the determination of when a laboratory is considered independent.
* Payment may only be made to the beneficiary, including home dialysis patients under Method II (see §4271), when:
  - For services rendered on or before December 31, 1986, on the basis of an itemized bill of a physician or medical group for tests performed or supervised by that physician or group, where the physician or group is not required to meet the conditions of coverage of an independent laboratory because during any calendar year the physician or medical group performs the tests on less than 100 specimens in any particular category on referral from other physicians not in the same practice; and neither the physician or group has entered into an agreement to be a participating physician or supplier; or
  - On the basis of an itemized bill of a rural health clinic for tests performed for a nonpatient of the clinic where the rural health clinic is not required to meet the conditions of coverage of an independent laboratory because, during any calendar year, the clinic performs tests on less than 100 specimens in a particular category on referral from outside physicians.

Except as noted above, unless a laboratory, physician or medical group accepts assignment, no Part B payment may be made for laboratory tests.Laboratories, physicians or medical groups that have entered into a participation agreement must accept assignment.Effective January 1, 1988, sanctions of double the violative charges, civil money penalties (up to $2,000 per violation) and/or disbarment from the program for a period of up to 5 years may be imposed on physicians and laboratories with the exception of rural health clinic laboratories that knowingly, willfully, and repeatedly bill patients on an unassigned basis.However, sole community physicians and physicians who are the sole source of an essential specialty in a community are not excluded from the program.Whenever you are notified of a sanction action, follow the procedures contained in §4165 regarding processing of claims after the imposition of a sanction.(See §§3040.3 and 3040.4 for processing instructions for claims which have been inadvertently submitted as unassigned.)

For purposes of this section, the term assignment includes assignment in the strict sense of the term as well as the procedure under which payment is made, after the death of the beneficiary, to the person or entity which furnished the service, on the basis of that person's or entity's agreement to accept the approved charge or fee you determine as the full charge or fee for the service.

When payment is made under the above rules to the beneficiary but the beneficiary is deceased, follow §7201 and §A7201.If the beneficiary has a legal guardian or representative payee, follow §7050.If an approved health benefits plan pays for the test on behalf of the beneficiary, follow §7065.

Ordinarily a physician or laboratory does not bill the Medicare program for noncovered tests.However, if the beneficiary (or his representative) contends that a clinical diagnostic laboratory test which a physician or laboratory believes is noncovered may be covered, the physician or laboratory must file a claim that includes the test, to effectuate the beneficiary's right to a determination.The physician or laboratorynotes on the claim that he or it believes that the test is noncovered and is including it at the beneficiary's insistence.

Before furnishing a beneficiary a test which the physician or laboratory believes is excluded from coverage as not reasonable and necessary (rather than excluded from coverage as part of a routine physical checkup), the physician or laboratory obtains a statement from the beneficiary (or his representative) that the physician or laboratory has informed him of the noncoverage of the test and that there is a charge for the test.This is needed to protect the physician or laboratory against possible liability for the test under the limitation of liability provision.

2. Special Conditions for Referring Laboratories In accordance with §6111(b) of OBRA of 1989 as amended by §4154 of OBRA of 1990, a referring laboratory may bill for tests for Medicare beneficiaries performed on or after May 1, 1990, by a reference laboratory only if it meets any one of the following three exceptions:

   * The rural hospital exception.The referring laboratory is located in, or is part of, a rural hospital;
   * The ownership related exception (formerly, the subsidiary related exception). The referring laboratory and reference laboratory are ownership related. That is:
     - The referring laboratory is wholly-owned by the reference laboratory; or
     - The referring laboratory wholly owns the reference laboratory; or
     - Both the referring laboratory and the reference laboratory are wholly-owned subsidiaries of the same entity; or
     - The 30 percent exception

   * For services rendered from May 1, 1990 through April 30, 1991, no more than 30 percent of the clinical diagnostic laboratory tests billed annually by the referring laboratory may be performed by another laboratory other than an ownership related laboratory.

* For services rendered on or after January 1, 1991, no more than 30 percent of the clinical diagnostic laboratory tests for which the referring laboratory receives requests annually may be performed by another laboratory, other than an ownership related laboratory described above.

EXAMPLE: A laboratory receives requests for 200 tests, performs 70 tests, and refers 130 tests to a non-related laboratory.The laboratory bills Medicare for the 70 tests it performed and 30 of the tests it referred.Before January 1, 1991, the laboratory would have met the 30 percent exception.Since only the referred tests that the laboratory billed itself would have been counted, no more than 30 percent of the tests (30/100) are counted, and the laboratory may receive Medicare payment for the tests for which it bills.However, under the amended rule, all referred tests are counted. Thus, 65 percent (130/200) of the tests are considered referred tests and, since this exceeds the 30 percent standard, the laboratory may not bill for any referred tests for Medicare beneficiaries.

Effective with services rendered on or after January 1, 1991, deny bills from a referring laboratory for tests performed by a reference laboratory unless you are informed in writing by the referring laboratory that it meets one of the exceptions.

If it is later found that a referring laboratory does not, in fact, meet an exception criterion recoup payment for the referred tests improperly billed. For services rendered between January 1, 1991 and April 30, 1991, there is a date overlap in the criteria for a referring laboratory to meet the 30 percent exception.Therefore, payments made to referring laboratories for referred tests performed between January 1, 1991 and April 30, 1991 are subject to recoupment if the referring laboratory fails to meet either of the 30 percent criteria.

NOTE:This provision of §6111(b) of OBRA of 1989 has no effect on hospitals that are paid under §1833(h)(5)(A)(iii).

F. Adjusted Fee Schedule.-Beginning April 1, 1988, the 1987 fee schedules for automated tests, and for tests (with the exception of cytopathology) that were subject to the LCL provision prior to July 1, 1984, are reduced by 8.3 percent.To determine the adjusted fee schedules, multiply the 1987 fee schedules by .9170 (100 percent of the 1987 fee schedule minus 8.3 percent).

The automated tests subject to the adjusted fee schedules tests are listed in codes 80002-80019 of the 1990 printing of the CPT-4.

The adjusted fee schedules also apply to the following tests that were subject to the LCL provision prior to the establishment of the fee schedule methodology.The current CPT-4 codes are provided.

Test	1989 CPT-4 Code
Cholesterol, Serum	82465

Complete Blood Count	85022 85031
Hemoglobin	85018
Hematocrit	85014
Prothrombin Time	85610
Sedimentation Rate (ESR)	85650 85651
Glucose	82947 82948
Urinalysis	81000*
Blood Uric Acid	84550
Blood Urea Nitrogen	84520
White Blood Cell Count	85048

*If 81002 and 81015 are both billed, pay as though the combined service (81000) had been billed.

Where these adjusted fee schedule tests are part of allergy, disease or organ panels/profiles, you must assure that your fee for the panel/profiledoes not exceed the sum of the fees for the individual components after accounting for the reductions due to the adjustment.

G. National Limitation Amount.-The Consolidated Omnibus Budget Reconciliation Act (COBRA) requires national limitation amounts to be applied to the payments for outpatient clinical diagnostic laboratory services.For services rendered on or after July 1, 1986 and before April 1, 1988, the national limitation amount is 115 percent of the median of all the fee schedules established for a test for each laboratory code (separately calculated for 60 and 62 percent fee schedules).HCFA furnished you a tape file of these initial national limitation amounts for each HCPCS code for both the 60 and 62 percent fee schedules.For laboratory tests performed on or after January 1, 1987 through March 31, 1988, the initial national limitation amounts are increased by 5.4 percent and the result is the 1987 national limitation amount.

For laboratory tests performed on or after April 1, 1988 and before January 1, 1990, the national limitation amount is 100 percent of the median of all the fee schedules established for a test for each laboratory code (separately calculated for 60 and 62 percent fee schedules).The 100 percent national limitation amount for automated tests and tests formerly subject to the LCL limit, is determined by reducing the current national limitation amount by 8.3 percent (i.e., by multiplying the national limitation by .9170) and multiplying this result by .8696 (100 percent divided by 115 percent).In a single step computation, the 1987 national limitation amount is multiplied by .7974 (.9170 x .8696).For all other tests, the 100 percent national limitation amount is determined by multiplying the 1987 national limitation amount by .8696 (100 percent divided by 115 percent).Each HCFA regional office has a listing of the computed 1988 national limitation amounts which is available to you.

For laboratory tests performed on or after January 1, 1990 and before January 1, 1991, the national limitation amount is 93 percent of the median of all the fee schedules established for a test for each laboratory code (separately calculated for 60 and 62 percent fee schedules).

For laboratory tests performed on or after January 1, 1991, the national limitation amount is 88 percent of the median of all the fee schedules established for a test for each laboratory code (separately calculated for 60 and 62 percent fee schedules).

Currently, no specific national limitation amounts apply to allergy, organ, or disease oriented panels/profiles.However, the individual tests that comprise such panels are subject to the national limitation and where applicable, to the adjusted fee schedule. Ensure that the payment allowance for the panel/profile, therefore, does not exceed the lower of (l) the sum of the applicable fee schedule amounts (or national limitation amounts, if lower) for the individual tests included in the panel/profile, or (2) the sum of the fee schedule amount you have established for the panel/profile.

You are responsible for applying the national limitations in calculating your payment allowances. The national limitation amounts are computed to the nearest cent.Do not round in applying these limits.Do not use the national limitation amounts to fill gaps in your prevailing charge screens for clinical laboratory tests.Establish a fee schedule for each HCPCS code that requires gap filling and then apply the national limitation amount.

H. Summary of Payment Rules for Clinical Diagnostic Laboratory Tests.-The following rules apply in determining the amount of Part B payment for clinical laboratory tests:

- For tests performed by an independent laboratory, by a hospital or SNF laboratory (for a nonpatient of the hospital or SNF), or by a physician or medical group, the payment is the lesser of the actual charge, the fee schedule amount or the national limitation amount and the Part B deductible and coinsurance do not apply.
- If payment is made to a hospital for tests furnished for an outpatient of that hospital, the payment is the lesser of the actual charge, the fee schedule amount, or the national limitation amount and Part B deductible and coinsurance do not apply.
- For tests performed by a reference laboratory, the payment is the lesser of the actual charge by the billing laboratory, the fee schedule amount or the national limitation amount.Existing carrier jurisdiction rules apply.Part B deductible and coinsurance do not apply.
- If payment is made to a beneficiary for services prior to January 1, 1987 (see §5114.1.E.3) on the basis of an unassigned itemized bill from a physician, medical group or rural health clinic, the payment is 80 percent of the lesser of the fee schedule, the actual charge or the national limitation amount and Part B deductible and coinsurance applies.
- If payment is made to a participating hospital for tests performed for an inpatient of that hospital without Part A coverage, payment is made on a cost basis and is subject to Part B deductible and coinsurance.
- If payment is made to a participating SNF for tests performed by that SNF for an inpatient of the SNF, payment is made on a cost basis and is subject to Part B deductible and coinsurance.

- If payment is made to a hospital-based or independent dialysis facility for laboratory tests included under the composite rate payment and performed for a patient of that facility, the facility's composite rate payment includes payment for these tests and is subject to the Part B deductible and coinsurance.
- If payment is made to a rural health clinic for laboratory tests performed for a patient of that clinic, payment is made as part of the all-inclusive rate and is subject to Part B deductible and coinsurance.
- If payment is made to a hospital which has been granted a waiver of Medicare reimbursement principles for outpatient services, Part B deductible and coinsurance apply unless otherwise waived as part of an approved waiver.
- If payment is made to a participating HMO or HCPP for laboratory tests performed for a patient who is not a member, payment is the lesser of the actual charge, the national limitation amount or the fee schedule amount and the Part B deductible and coinsurance do not apply.

I. Coordination Between Intermediaries, Carriers, and the Railroad Retirement Board (RRB).-Furnish copies of fee schedules and updates (including national limitation amounts where applicable) to Medicare fiscal intermediaries and to the appropriate Travelers RRB office.(See §4540.)Provide updates at least 30 days prior to the scheduled implementation.The fiscal intermediaries and the RRB use the fee schedules in paying for hospital laboratory tests performed for outpatients of the hospital and for persons who are not patients of the hospital.The Travelers RRB offices use the fee schedules in paying for outpatient clinical diagnostic laboratory tests.Fiscal intermediaries and the Travelers RRB consult with carriers on filling gaps in fee schedules for certain tests.If intermediaries or the Travelers RRB offices have bills for payment on laboratory tests that are not in the fee schedule, they consult with the carriers that gave them the fee schedules. If those carriers are unable to help the intermediaries, the carriers consult with other nearby carriers. HCPCS contains the American Medical Association's CPT-4 (Physician's Current Procedural Terminology).For those entities which are not familiar with HCPCS but have used the CPT-4, the coding and terminology for laboratory tests are the same in both HCPCS and the CPT-4.The CPT-4 may be used before receipt of the HCPCS.

J. Application of Fee Schedules to Medicaid.-Furnish copies of the fee schedules and the annual update (including national limitation amounts where applicable) to State agencies.Provide updates at least 30 days prior to the scheduled implementation.To obtain Federal matching funds for clinical diagnostic laboratory services, State Medicaid agencies may not pay more for the services and specimen collections than are paid for them under Medicare.This applies to payments for calendar quarters beginning on or after October 1, 1984.

Since the fee schedule provisions have been implemented on a carrierwide basis, a State may have more than one carrier servicing Medicare beneficiaries residing there.A Medicaid agency for such a State may, if it deems necessary, use the fee schedules of either one or both of the carriers to meet the Federal fund matching requirement.State Medicaid agencies may consult with ROs concerning the fee schedule, the national limitation amounts and specimen collection provisions.

K. Travel Allowance.-In addition to a specimen collection fee allowed under §5114.1.D, a travel allowance can also be made to cover the costs of travel to collect a specimen from a nursing home or homebound patient.The additional allowance can be made only where a specimen collection fee is also payable, i.e., no travel allowance is made where the technician merely performs a messenger service to pick up a specimen drawn by a physician or nursing home personnel.The travel allowance may not be paid to a physician unless the trip to the home or nursing home was solely for the purpose of drawing a specimen.Otherwise travel costs are considered to be associated with the other purposes of the trip.Since a travel allowance can now be paid routinely, the differential specimen collection amount formerly allowed when a specimen is collected from a single patient rather than multiple patients (i.e., $5 rather than $3) is discontinued.

The allowance is intended to cover the estimated travel costs of collecting a specimen and is an allowance reflecting the technician's salary and travel costs.The following HCPCS codes are used for travel allowances:

P9603--Travel allowance - one way, in connection with medically necessary laboratory specimen collection drawn from homebound or nursing home bound patient; prorated miles actually traveled (carrier allowance on per mile basis); or

P9604--Travel allowance - one way, in connection with medically necessary laboratory specimen collection drawn from homebound or nursing home bound patient; prorated trip charge (carrier allowance on flat fee basis).

Identify round trip travel by use of modifier LR.

If you determine that it results in equitable payment, you may extend your former payment allowances for additional travel (such as to a distant rural nursing home) to all circumstances where travel is required.This might be appropriate, for example, if your former payment allowance was on a per mile basis.Otherwise you must establish an appropriate allowance.If you decide to establish a new allowance, one method is to consider developing a travel allowance consisting of:

- The current Federal mileage allowance for operating personal automobiles, plus
- A personnel allowance per mile to cover personnel costs based on an estimate of average hourly wages and average driving speed.

For your convenience, a chronology of mileage rates from July 1, 1984 to date is listed below:

Mileage Rate	From	To
20.5 cents	July 1, 1984	July 31, 1987
21 cents	August 1, 1987	August 13, 1988
22.5 cents	August 14, 1988	September 16, 1989

24 cents	September 17, 1989	June 29, 1991
25 cents	June 30, 1991	

Travel allowance amounts claimed by suppliers are prorated by the total number of patients (including Medicare and non Medicare patients) from whom specimens are drawn or picked up on a given trip.

EXAMPLE 1:On October 1, 1989, a carrier determines that the average technician is paid $9 per hour and estimates 45 miles per hour as the average speed driven or $.20 per mile. This amount plus the Federal mileage allowance of $0.24 per mile results in a total allowance of $0.44 per mile.A laboratory technician makes a trip to two nursing homes involving a total mileage of 20 miles and draws specimens from three patients, Medicare as well as non- Medicare patients.In addition, specimens that were not drawn by the technician are picked up from two patients.A travel allowance per Medicare claim of $1.76 can be made (20 miles round trip x $0.44 per mile divided by 5). The supplier bills 4 miles (20 miles) 5) under code P9603LR.

EXAMPLE 2:The carrier, through a review of the laboratory records, estimates that on average four specimens are drawn or picked up each trip, and that the average trip is 30 miles including both round trips and one way trips.Assuming the same facts as Example 1 (i.e., $9 per hour and 45 miles per hour), the carrier establishes a flat travel allowance of $3.30.Suppliers bill code P9604 and are paid $3.30 regardless of actual distance or number of patients served.

In keeping with the principles of §5024 and §5200, a payment in addition to the routine travel allowance determined under this section may be allowed to cover the additional costs of travel to collect a specimen from a nursing home or homebound patient when clinical diagnostic laboratory tests are needed on an emergency basis outside the general business hours of the laboratory making the collection.

L. Laboratory Tests Utilizing Automated Equipment.-Because of the numerous technological advances and innovations in the clinical laboratory field and the increased availability of automated testing equipment to all entities that perform clinical diagnostic laboratory tests, no distinction is generally made in determining payment allowances (i.e., the lower of the respective fee schedules or the national limitations) for such tests between (1) the sites where the service is performed, i.e., physician's office or other laboratory, or (2) the method of the testing process used, whether manual or automated.

When physicians and laboratories perform the same test, whether manually or with automated equipment, the services are considered similar.

1. Determining Payment for Automated Tests.-The common automated tests comprise specific groupings of blood chemistries which enable physicians to more accurately diagnose their patients' medical problems.

   The following list contains some of the tests which can be and are frequently done as groups and combinations on automated profile equipment.

Albumin
Alanine
Aminotransferase (ALT,SGPT)
Alkaline phosphatase
Aspartate aminotransferase
Bilirubin, direct (AST, SGOT)
Bilirubin, total
Carbon dioxide content
Calcium
Chloride
Cholesterol
Creatinine
Glucose(sugar)
Creatine kinase (CK, CPK)
GammaGlutamylTransferase (GGT)
Lactate dehydrogenase (LDH, LD)
Phosphorus
Potassium
Protein, total
Sodium
Triglyceride
Urea nitrogen (BUN)
Uric Acid

While the component tests in automated profiles may vary somewhat from one laboratory to another, or from one physician's office or clinic to another, group together those profile tests which can be performed at the same time on the same equipment for purposes of developing appropriate payment allowances.For Medicare payment purposes, the tests on this list must be grouped together when billed separately and considered automated profile tests.While laboratory entities may bill additional tests using automated profile codes and be paid according to §5114.1, the above listed 22 tests are the only tests that you may group into automated profiles if they are billed separately. Future revisions to this list will be made through manual revisions.

Payment is made only for those tests in an automated profile that meet Medicare coverage rules.Where only some of the tests in a profile of tests are covered, payment cannot exceed the amount that would have been paid if only the covered tests had been ordered.For example, the use of the 12-channel serum chemistry test to determine the blood sugar level in a proven case of diabetes is unreasonable because the results of a blood sugar test performed separately provides the essential information.Normally, the payment allowance for a blood sugar test is lower than the payment allowance for the automated profile of tests.In no event, however, may payment for the covered tests exceed the payment allowance for the profile.

Periodically, at least annually, remind physicians and suppliers that you will review claims for patterns of high utilization of automated profiles with large number of tests and if your review shows that the documentation does not support Medicare coverage that you will pursue recoupment.Encourage physicians to target their test ordering to only those tests that are related to specific symptoms or disease conditions.Remind physicians of Medicare coverage rules that require that payment may be made only for medically necessary tests and that payment is not made for routine screening tests.As a general rule, you may assume that where a physician orders automated profile tests on a test-by-test basis (i.e., not as part of a profile or custom panel), each of the tests is covered. (See §7517.1.)If, after analysis, you find that a pattern of overutilization exists, even if tests were individually ordered, follow the procedures of §7517.2 to aid you in ameliorating the problems.

2. Separately Billed Tests That Are Commonly Part of Automated Test Profiles.-If you receive claims for laboratory services in which the physician or laboratory has separately billed for tests that are available as part of anautomated profile test, make the following determinations:

- If the sum of the payment allowance for the separately billed tests exceeds the payment allowance for the profile that includes these tests, make payment at the lesser amount for the profile.Conversely, the payment allowance for a profile cannot exceed the payment allowances for the individual tests.
- The limitation that payment for individual tests not exceed the payment allowance for an automated profile is applied whether or not a particular laboratory has the automated equipment.A higher amount may be paid in unusual circumstances where justified or where individual tests are unavailable on automated equipment.(See §5024.)Suppliers are to provide a detailed explanation to you of the justification for a higher level of payment.Review to determine if unusual circumstances exist and warrant a higher payment amount.
- When one or more automated profile tests are performed for a patient on the same day, determine whether to base payment on an automated profile that includes such tests rather than to base payment on the individual or separately billed tests. For example,compare the allowance for code 80002 of the Current Procedural Terminology - Fourth Edition (CPT-4) for the above determination when one or two tests from the commonly performed automated tests are included on a claim.

M. Organ or Disease Oriented Panels.-The American Medical Association (AMA) is responsible for the nomenclature of codes in the Current Procedural Terminology (CPT). The AMA has developed codes for panels of tests commonly ordered together and related through their use to diagnose a disease state or to evaluate an organ system.The tests listed in the CPT with each panel code are the defined components of that code for Medicare purposes.

Payment for panels is the same as found in subsection L. Payment for the total panel cannot exceed the allowance for individual tests.All Medicare coverage rules apply.

5114.2 Review of Laboratory Test Results by Physician

Reviewing results of laboratory tests, phoning results to patients, filing such results, etc., are services which are covered by the program, and payment for these services is included in the payment for the evaluation and management (E and M) services to the patient. Visit services entail a wide range of components and activities that may vary somewhat from patient to patient. The CPT-4 lists different levels of E and M services for both new and established patients and describes services which are included as part of E and M services.Such activities include obtaining, reviewing, and analyzing appropriate diagnostic tests.

Payment may not be made for the services to the extent that they exceed the frequency of such testing that is indicated by accepted standards of medical practice as appropriate care for the patient's condition.Therefore, establish appropriate processing procedures to ensure that payment is made for a reasonable and necessary frequency of such services.

15022 PAYMENT CONDITIONS FOR RADIOLOGY SERVICES

A. Professional Component (PC).—Pay for the PC of radiology services furnished by a physician to an individual patient in all settings under the fee schedule for physician services regardless of the specialty of the physician who performs the service. For services furnished to hospital patients, pay only if the services meet the conditions for fee schedule payment in §15014.C.1 and are identifiable, direct, and discrete diagnostic or therapeutic services to an individual patient, such as an interpretation of diagnostic procedures and the PC of therapeutic procedures. The interpretation of a diagnostic procedure includes a written report.

B. Technical Component TC).—

1. Hospital Patients.—Do not pay for the TC of radiology services furnished to Hospital patients. Payments for physicians' radiological services to the hospital, e.g., Aministrative orsupervisory services, and for provider services needed to produce the radiology service is made by the intermediary as provider services through various payment mechanisms.

2. Services Not Furnished in Hospitals.—Pay under the fee schedule for the TC of radiology services furnished to beneficiaries who are not patients of any hospital in a physician's office, a freestanding imaging or radiation oncology center, or other setting that is not part of a hospital.

3. Services Furnished in Leased Departments.—In the case of procedures furnished in a leased hospital radiology department to a beneficiary who is neither an inpatient nor an outpatient of any hospital, e.g., the patient

is referred by an outside physician and is not registered as a hospital outpatient, both the PC and the TC of the services are payable under the fee schedule.

4. Purchased TC Services.—Apply the purchased services limitation as set forth in §15048 to the TC of radiologic services other than screening mammography procedures.

5. Computerized Axial Tomography (CT) Procedures.—Do not reduce or deny payment for medically necessary multiple CT scans of different areas of the body that are performed on the same day.

   The TC RVUs for CT procedures that specify "with contrast" include payment for high osmolar contrast media. When separate payment is made for low osmolar contrast media under the conditions set forth in subsection F.1, reduce payment for the contrast media as set forth in subsection F.2.

6. Magnetic Resonance Imaging (MRI) Procedures.—Do not make additional payments for 3 or more MRI sequences. The RVUs reflect payment levels for 2 sequences.

   The TC RVUs for MRI procedures that specify "with contrast" include payment for paramagnetic contrast media. Do not make separate payment under code A4647.

   A diagnostic technique has been developed under which an MRI of the brain or spine is first performed without contrast material, then another MRI is performed with a standard (0.1mmol/kg) dose of contrast material and, based on the need to achieve a better image, a third MRI is performed with an additional double dosage (0.2mmol/kg) of contrast material. When the high-dose contrast technique is utilized:

   * Do not pay separately for the contrast material used in the second MRI procedure;
   * Pay for the contrast material given for the third MRI procedure through supply code A4643 when billed with CPT codes 70553, 72156, 72157, and 72158;
   * Do not pay for the third MRI procedure. For example, in the case of an MRI of the brain, if CPT code 70553 (without contrast material, followed by with contrast material(s) and further sequences) is billed, make no payment for CPT code 70551 (without contrast material(s)), the additional procedure given for the purpose of administering the double dosage, furnished during the same session. Medicare does not pay for the third procedure (as distinguished from the contrast material) because the CPT definition of code 70553 includes all further sequences; and
   * Do not apply the payment criteria for low osmolar contrast media in subsection F to billings for code A4643.

7. Stressing Agent.—Make separate payment under code J1245 for pharmacologic stressing agents used in connection with nuclear medicine and cardiovascular stress testing procedures furnished to beneficiaries in settings in which TCs are payable. Such an agent is classified as a supply and covered as an integral part of the diagnostic test. However, pay for code J1245 under the policy for determining payments for "incident to" drugs.

C. Nuclear Medicine (CPT 78000 Through 79999).—

1. Payments for Radionuclides.—The TC RVUs for nuclear medicine procedures (CPT codes 78XXX for diagnostic nuclear medicine, and codes 79XXX for therapeutic nuclear medicine) do not include the radionuclide used in connection with the procedure. These substances are separately billed under codes A4641 and A4642 for diagnostic procedures and code 79900 for therapeutic procedures and are paid on a "By Report" basis depending on the substance used. In addition, CPT code 79000 is separately payable in connection with certain clinical brachytherapy procedures. (See subsection D.3.)

2. Application of Multiple Procedure Policy (CPT Modifier 51).—Apply the multiple procedure reduction as set forth in §15038 to the following nuclear medicine diagnostic procedures: codes 78306, 78320, 78803, 78806, and 78807.

3. Generation and Interperetation of Automated Data.—Payment for CPT codes 78890 and 78891 is bundled into payments for the primary procedure.

4. Positron Emission Tomography (PET) Scans (HCPCS Codes G0030-G0047).—For procedures furnished on or after March 14, 1995, pay for PET procedure of the heart under the limited coverage policy set forth in §50-36 of the Coverage Issues Manual (HCFA Pub. 6) using the billing instructions in §4173 of the Medicare Carriers Manual.

D. Radiation Oncology (Therapeutic Radiology) (CPT 77261-77799).—

1. Weekly Radiation Therapy Management (CPT 77419-77430).—Pay for a physician's weekly treatment management services under codes 77419, 77420, 77425, and 77430. Instruct billing entities to indicate on each claim the number of fractions for which payment is sought.

   A weekly unit of treatment management is equal to five fractions or treatment sessions. A week for the purpose of making payments under these codes is comprised of five fractions regardless of the actual time period in which the services are furnished. It is not necessary that the radiation therapist personally examine the patient during each fraction for the weekly treatment management code to be payable. Multiple fractions representing two or more treatment sessions furnished on the same day may be counted as long as there has been a distinct break in therapy sessions, and the fractions are of the character usually furnished on different days. If, at the final billing of the treatment course, there are three or four fractions beyond a multiple of five, those three or four fractions are paid for as a week. If there are one or two fractions beyond a multiple of five, consider payment for these services as having been made through prior payments.

EXAMPLE:

18 fractions	=	4 weekly services
62 fractions	=	12 weekly services
8 fractions	=	2 weekly services
6 fractions	=	1 weekly service

If billings have occurred which indicate that the treatment course has ended (and, therefore, the number of residual fractions has been determined), but treatments resume, adjust your payments for the additional services consistent with the above policy.

EXAMPLE:

8 fractions = payment for 2 weeks

2 additional fractions are furnished by the same physician. No additional Medicare payment is made for the 2 additional fractions.

There are situations in which beneficiaries receive a mixture of simple (code 77420), intermediate (code 77425), and complex (code 77430) treatment management services during a course of treatment. In such cases, pay under the weekly treatment management code that represents the more frequent of the fractions furnished during the five-fraction week. For example, an intermediate weekly treatment management service is payable when, in a grouping of five fractions, a beneficiary receives three intermediate and two simple fractions.

2. Services Bundled Into Treatment Management Codes.—Make no separate payment for any of the following services rendered by the radiation oncologists or in conjunction with radiation therapy:

11920:	Tattooing, intradermal introduction of insoluble opaque pigments to correct color defects of skin; 6.0 sq. cm or less
11921:	6.1 to 20.0 sq. cm
11922:	each additional 20.0 sq. cm
16000:	Initial treatment, first degree burn, when no more than local treatment is required 16010: Dressings and/or debridement, initial or subsequent; under anesthesia, small 16015: under anesthesia, medium or large, or with major debridement
16020:	without anesthesia, office or hospital, small
16025:	without anesthesia, medium (e.g., whole face or whole extremity)
16030:	without anesthesia, large (e.g., more than one extremity)
36425:	Venipuncture, cut down age 1 or over

53670: Catheterization, urethra; simple

53675: complicated (may include difficult removal of balloon catheter)

99211: Office or other outpatient visit, established patient; Level I

99212: Level II

99213: Level III

99214: Level IV

99215: Level V

99238: Hospital discharge day management

99281: Emergency department visit, new or established patient; Level I

99282: Level II

99283: Level III

99284: Level IV

99285: Level V

90780: IV infusion therapy, administered by physician or under direct supervision of physician; up to one hour

90781: each additional hour, up to eight (8) hours

90841: Individual medical psychotherapy by a physician, with continuing medical diagnostic evaluation, and drug management when indicated, including psychoanalysis, insight oriented, behavior modifying or supportive psychotherapy; time unspecified

90843: approximately 20 to 30 minutes

90844: approximately 45 to 50 minutes

90847: Family medical psychotherapy (conjoint psychotherapy) by a physician, with continuing medical diagnostic evaluation, and drug management when indicated

99050: Services requested after office hours in addition to basic service

99052: Services requested between 10:00 PM and 8:00 AM in addition to basic service

99054: Services requested on Sundays and holidays in addition to basic service

99058: Office services provided on an emergency basis

99071: Educational supplies, such as books, tapes, and pamphlets, provided by the physician for the patient's education at cost to physician

99090: Analysis of information data stored in computers (e.g., ECG, blood pressures, hematologic data)

99150: Prolonged physician attendance requiring physician detention beyond usual service (e.g., operative standby, monitoring ECG, EEG, intrathoracic pressures, intravascular pressures, blood gases during surgery, standby for newborn care following caesarean section); 30 minutes to one hour

99151: more than one hour

99180: Hyperbaric oxygen therapy initial

99182: Subsequent

99185: Hypothermia; regional

99371: Telephone call by a physician to patient or for consultation or medical management or for coordinating medical management with other health care professionals; simple or brief (e.g., to report on tests and/or laboratory results, to clarify or alter previous instructions, to integrate new information from other health professionals into the medical treatment plan, or to adjust therapy)

99372: intermediate (e.g., to provide advice to an established patient on a new problem, to initiate therapy that can be handled by telephone, to discuss test results in detail, to coordinate medical management of a new problem in an established patient, to discuss and evaluate new information and details, or to initiate a new plan of care)

99373: complex or lengthy (e.g., lengthy counseling session with anxious or distraught patient, detailed or prolonged discussion with family members regarding seriously ill patient, lengthy communication necessary to coordinate complex services or several different health professionals working on different aspects of the total patient care plan)

* Anesthesia (whatever code billed)
* Care of infected skin (whatever code billed)
* Checking of treatment charts
* Verification of dosage, as needed (whatever code billed)
* Continued patient evaluation, examination,written progress notes, as needed (whatever code billed)
* Final physical examination (whatever code billed)
* Medical prescription writing (whatever code billed
* Nutritional
* Pain management (whatever code billed)
* Review & revision of treatment plan (whatever code billed)
* Routine medical management of unrelated problem (whatever code billed)
* Special care of ostomy (whatever code billed)
* Written reports, progress note (whatever code billed)
* Follow-up examination and care for 90 days after last treatment (whatever code billed)

3. Radiation Treatment Delivery (CPT 77401-77417).—Pay for these TC services on a daily basis under CPT codes 77401-77416 for radiation treatment delivery. Do not use local codes and RVUs in paying for the TC of radiation oncology services. Multiple treatment sessions on the same day are payable as long as there has been a distinct break in therapy

services, and the individual sessions are of the character usually furnished on different days. Pay for CPT code 77417 (Therapeutic radiology port film(s)) on a weekly (5 fractions) basis.

4. Clinical Brachytherapy (CPT Codes 77750-77799).—Apply the bundled services policy in §15022.D.2. to procedures in this family of codes other than CPT code 77776. For procedures furnished in settings in which you make TC payments, pay separately for the expendable source associated with these procedures under CPT code 79900 except in the case of remote afterloading high intensity brachytherapy procedures (CPT codes 77781-77784). In the 4 codes cited, the expendable source is included in the RVUs for the TC of the procedures.

5. Radiation Physics Services (CPT Codes 77300-77399).—Until further notice, pay for the PC and TC of CPT codes 77300-77334 and 77739 on the same basis as you pay for radiologic services generally. For PC billings in all settings, presume that the radiologist participated in the provision of the service, e.g., reviewed/validated the physicist's calculation. CPT codes 77336 and 77370 are technical services only codes that are payable by carriers only in settings in which TCs are payable.

F. Supervision and Interpretation (S&I) Codes and Interventional Radiology.—

1. Physician Presence.—Radiologic S&I codes are used to describe the personal supervision of the performance of the radiologic portion of a procedure by one or more physicians and the interpretation of the findings. In order to bill for the supervision aspect of the procedure, the physician must be present during its performance. This kind of personal supervision of the performance of the procedure is a service to an individual beneficiary and differs from the type of general supervision of the radiologic procedures performed in a hospital for which intermediaries pay the costs as physician services to the hospital. The interpretation of the procedure may be performed later by another physician. In situations in which a cardiologist, for example, bills for the supervision (the "S") of the S&I code, and a radiologist bills for the interpretation (the "I") of the code, both physicians should use a -52 modifier indicating a reduced service, e.g., the interpretation only. Pay no more for the fragmented S&I code than you would if a single physician furnished both aspects of the procedure.

2. Multiple Procedure Reduction.—Make no multiple procedure reductions in the S&I or primary nonradiologic codes in these types of procedures, or in any procedure codes for which the descriptor and RVUs reflect a multiple service reduction. For additional procedure codes that do not reflect such a reduction, apply the multiple procedure reductions set forth in §15038.

G. Low Osmolar Contrast Media (LOCM) (HCPCS Codes A4644-A4646).—

1. Payment Criteria.—Make separate payments for LOCM (HCPCS codes A4644, A4645, and A4646) in the case of all medically necessary intrathecal radiologic procedures furnished to nonhospital patients. In the case of intraarterial and intravenous radiologic procedures, pay separately for LOCM only when it is used for nonhospital patients with one or more of the following characteristics:

   * A history of previous adverse reaction to contrast material, with the exception of a sensation of heat, flushing, or a single episode of nausea or vomiting;
   * A history of asthma or allergy;
   * Significant cardiac dysfunction including recent or imminent cardiac decompensation, severe arrhythmia, unstable angina pectoris, recent myocardial infarction, and pulmonary hypertension;
   * Generalized severe debilitation; or
   * Sickle cell disease.

   If the beneficiary does not meet any of these criteria, the payment for contrast media is considered to be bundled into the TC of the procedure, and the beneficiary may not be billed for LOCM.

2. Payment Level.—A LOCM pharmaceutical is considered to be a supply which is an integral part of the diagnostic test. However, determine payment in the same manner as for a drug furnished incident to a physician's service with the following additional requirement. Reduce the lower of the estimated actual acquisition cost or the national average wholesale price by 8 percent to take into account the fact that the TC RVUs of the procedure codes reflect less expensive contrast media.

H. Services of Portable X-Ray Suppliers.—Services furnished by portable X-ray suppliers (see §2070.4) may have as many as four components.

1. Professional Component.—Pay the PC of radiologic services furnished by portable X-ray suppliers on the same basis as other physician fee schedule services.

2. Technical Component.—Pay the TC of radiology services furnished by portable X-ray suppliers under the fee schedule on the same basis as TC services generally.

3. Transportation Component (HCPCS Codes R0070-R0076).—This component represents the transportation of the equipment to the patient. Establish local RVUs for the transportation R codes based on your knowledge of the nature of the service furnished. Allow only a single transportation payment for each trip the portable X-ray supplier makes to a particular location. When more than one Medicare patient is X-rayed at the same location, e.g., a nursing home, prorate the single fee schedule transportation payment among all

patients receiving the services. For example, if two patients at the same location receive X-rays, make one-half of the transportation payment for each.

Use any information regarding the number of patients X-rayed in each location that the supplier visits during each trip that the supplier of the X-ray may volunteer on the bill or claim for payment. If such information is not indicated, assume that at least four patients were X-rayed at the same location, and pay only one-fourth of the fee schedule payment amount for any one patient. Advise the suppliers in your area regarding the way in which you use this information.

NOTE: No transportation charge is payable unless the portable X-ray equipment used was actually transported to the location where the X-ray was taken. For example, do not allow a transportation charge when the X-ray equipment is stored in a nursing home for use as needed. However, a set-up payment (see subsection G.4) is payable in such situations. Further, for services furnished on or after January 1, 1997, make no separate payment under HCPCS code R0076 for the transportation of EKG equipment by portable X-ray suppliers or any other entity.

4. Set-Up Component (HCPCS Code Q0092).—Pay a set-up component for each radiologic procedure (other than retakes of the same procedure) during both single patient and multiple patient trips under Level II HCPCS code Q0092.Do not make the set-up payment for EKG services furnished by the portable X-ray supplier.

15030 SUPPLIES

Make a separate payment for supplies furnished in connection with a procedure only when one of the two following conditions exists:

A. HCPCS codes A4550, A4200, and A4263 are billed in conjunction with the appropriate procedure in the Medicare Physician Fee Schedule Data Base (place of service is physician's office); or

B. The supply is a pharmaceutical or radiopharmaceutical diagnostic imaging agent (including codes A4641 through A4647); pharmacologic stressing agent (code J1245); or therapeutic radionuclide (CPT code 79900). The procedures performed are:

* Diagnostic radiologic procedures (including diagnostic nuclear medicine) requiring pharmaceutical or radiopharmaceutical contrast media and/or pharmocological stressing agent,
* Other diagnostic tests requiring a pharmacological stressing agent,
* Clinical brachytherapy procedures (other than remote afterloading high intensity brachytherapy procedures (CPT codes 77781 through 77784) for which the expendable source is included in the TC RVUs), or
* Therapeutic nuclear medicine procedures.

15360 ECHOCARDIOGRAPHY SERVICES (CODES 93303 - 93350)

Separate Payment for Contrast Media.—Effective October 1, 2000, physicians may separately bill for contrast agents used in echocardiography. Physicians should use HCPCS Code A9700 (Supply of injectable contrast material for use in echocardiography, per study). The type of service code is 9. This code will be carrier-priced.

APPENDIX E: PQRS REFERENCES

The measure specifications contained in this section are intended for claims-based and registry reporting of individual measures for the Physician Quality Reporting System (PQRS—formerly known as Physician Quality Reporting Initiative or PQRI). Each measure is assigned a unique number. This section contains only those PQRS measures that specifically include HCPCS codes.

DENOMINATOR CODES (ELIGIBLE CASES) AND NUMERATOR QUALITY-DATA CODES

Quality measures consist of a numerator and a denominator that permit the calculation of the percentage of a defined patient population that receive a particular process of care or achieve a particular outcome. The denominator population is defined by demographic information, certain International Classification of Diseases, Ninth Revision, Clinical Modification (ICD-9-CM) diagnosis, Current Procedural Terminology (CPT) and Healthcare Common Procedure Coding System (HCPCS) codes specified in the measure that are submitted by individual eligible professionals as part of a claim for covered services under the PFS. If the specified denominator codes for a measure are not included on the patient's claim (for the same date of service) as submitted by the individual eligible professional, then the patient does not fall into the enominator population, and the Physician Quality Reporting measure does not apply to the patient. Some measure specifications are adapted as needed for implementation in Physician Quality Reporting in agreement with the measure developer. For example, CPT codes for non-covered services such as preventive visits are not included in the denominator. Also, the denominators for measures groups have been modified to provide common denominator codes for all measures within the group.

Physician Quality Reporting measure specifications include specific instructions regarding CPT Category I modifiers, place of service codes, and other detailed information. Each eligible professional should carefully review the measure's denominator coding to determine whether codes submitted on a given claim meet denominator inclusion criteria.

If the patient does fall into the denominator population, the applicable Quality Data Codes or QDCs (CPT Category II codes or G-codes) that define the numerator should be submitted to satisfactorily report quality data for a measure. When a patient falls into the denominator, but the measure specifications define circumstances in which a patient may be appropriately excluded, CPT Category II code modifiers such as 1P, 2P and 3P or G-codes are available to describe medical, patient, system, or other reasons for performance exclusion. When the performance exclusion does not apply, a measure-specific CPT Category II reporting modifier 8P or HCPCS G-code may be used to indicate that the process of care was not provided for a reason not otherwise specified.

Each measure specification provides detailed reporting information.

MEASURE SPECIFICATION FORMAT

- Measure title
- Reporting option available for each measure (claims-based or registry)
- Measure description
- Instructions on reporting including frequency, timeframes, and applicability
- Denominator statement and coding
- Numerator statement and coding options
- Definition(s) of terms where applicable

DIABETES MELLITUS MEASURES GROUP OVERVIEW

2013 PQRS OPTIONS FOR MEASURES GROUPS: CLAIMS, REGISTRY

2013 PQRS MEASURES IN DIABETES MELLITUS MEASURES GROUP:

#1. Diabetes Mellitus: Hemoglobin A1c Poor Control

#2. Diabetes Mellitus: Low Density Lipoprotein (LDL-C) Control

#3. Diabetes Mellitus: High Blood Pressure Control

#117. Diabetes Mellitus: Dilated Eye Exam

#119. Diabetes Mellitus: Medical Attention for nephropathy #163. Diabetes Mellitus: Foot Exam

INSTRUCTIONS FOR REPORTING: (These instructions apply to both Claims and Registry reporting, unless otherwise specified.)

• Indicate your intention to report the Diabetes Mellitus Measures Group by submitting the measures group-specific intent G-code at least once during the reporting period when billing a patient claim for the 20 Patient Sample Method. It is not necessary to submit the measures group-specific intent G-code on more than one claim. It is not necessary to submit the measures group-specific intent G-code for registry-based submissions.

G8485: I intend to report the Diabetes Mellitus Measures Group

• Select patient sample method:

20 Patient Sample Method via claims: 20 unique Medicare Part B FFS (fee for service) patients meeting patient sample criteria for the measures group.

OR

20 Patient Sample Method via registries: 20 unique patients (a majority of which must be Medicare Part B FFS patients) meeting patient sample criteria for the measures group during the reporting period (January 1 through December 31, 2013 **OR** July 1 through December 31, 2013).

• Patient sample criteria for the Diabetes Mellitus Measures Group are patients aged 18 through 75 years with a specific diagnosis of diabetes accompanied by a specific patient encounter:

The following diagnosis codes indicating diabetes mellitus:

ICD-9-CM: 250.00, 250.01, 250.02, 250.03, 250.10, 250.11, 250.12, 250.13, 250.20, 250.21, 250.22, 250.23, 250.30, 250.31, 250.32, 250.33, 250.40, 250.41, 250.42, 250.43, 250.50, 250.51, 250.52, 250.53, 250.60, 250.61, 250.62, 250.63, 250.70, 250.71, 250.72, 250.73, 250.80, 250.81, 250.82, 250.83, 250.90, 250.91, 250.92, 250.93, 357.2, 362.01, 362.02, 362.03, 362.04, 362.05, 362.06, 362.07, 366.41, 648.00, 648.01, 648.02, 648.03, 648.04

ICD-10-CM [Reference ONLY/Not Reportable]: E10.10, E10.11, E10.21, E10.22, E10.29, E10.311, E10.319, E10.321, E10.329, E10.331, E10.339, E10.341, E10.349, E10.351, E10.359, E10.36, E10.39, E10.40, E10.41, E10.42, E10.43, E10.44, E10.49, E10.51, E10.52, E10.59, E10.610, E10.618, E10.620, E10.621, E10.622, E10.628, E10.630, E10.638, E10.641, E10.649, E10.65, E10.69, E10.8, E10.9, E11.00, E11.01, E11.21, E11.22, E11.29, E11.311, E11.319, E11.321, E11.329, E11.331, E11.339, E11.341, E11.349, E11.351, E11.359, E11.36, E11.39, E11.40, E11.41, E11.42, E11.43, E11.44, E11.49, E11.51, E11.52, E11.59, E11.610, E11.618, E11.620, E11.621, E11.622, E11.628, E11.630, E11.638, E11.641, E11.649, E11.65, E11.69, E11.8, E11.9, O24.011, O24.012, O24.013, O24.019, O24.02, O24.03, O24.111, O24.112, O24.113, O24.119, O24.12, O24.13

Accompanied by

One of the following patient encounter codes: 97802, 97803, 97804, 99201, 99202, 99203, 99204, 99205, 99212, 99213, 99214, 99215, 99304, 99305, 99306, 99307, 99308, 99309, 99310, 99324, 99325, 99326, 99327, 99328, 99334, 99335, 99336, 99337, 99341, 99342, 99343, 99344, 99345, 99347, 99348, 99349, 99350, G0270, G0271, G0402

• Report quality-data codes (QDCs) on **all** measures within the Diabetes Mellitus Measures Group for each patient within the sample.

• Instructions for quality-data code reporting for each of the measures within the Diabetes Mellitus Measures Group are displayed on the next several pages. If all quality actions for the patient have been performed for all the measures within the group, the following composite G-code may be reported in lieu of the individual quality-data codes for each of the measures within the group. Please note that Measure #1 (Diabetes Mellitus: Hemoglobin A1c Poor Control) is a poor control or inverse measure, therefore, the **composite G-code should only**

be reported when the patient's **most recent hemoglobin A1c Level ≤ 9.0%** and all of the other quality actions for this measures group have been performed. It is not necessary to submit the following composite G-code for registry-based submissions.

Composite G-code G8494: All quality actions for the applicable measures in the Diabetes Mellitus Measures Group have been performed for this patient

• To report satisfactorily the Diabetes Mellitus Measures Group requires **all** measures for each patient within the eligible professional's patient sample to be reported a minimum of once during the reporting period.

• Measures groups containing a measure with a 0% performance rate will not be counted as satisfactorily reporting the measures group. The recommended clinical quality action must be performed on at least one patient for each measure within the measures group reported by the eligible professional. When a lower rate indicates better performance, such as Measure #1, a 0% performance rate will be counted as satisfactorily reporting (100% performance rate would not be considered satisfactorily reporting). Performance exclusion quality-data codes are not counted in the performance denominator. If the eligible professional submits all performance exclusion quality-data codes, the performance rate would be 0/0 and would be considered satisfactorily reporting.

• When using the 20 Patient Sample Method via claims, report all measures for the 20 unique Medicare Part B FFS patients seen. When using the 20 Patient Sample Method via registries, report all measures for the 20 unique patients seen, a majority of which must be Medicare Part B FFS patients.

• For claims-based submissions, the Carrier/MAC remittance advice notice sent to the practice will show a denial remark code (N365) for the line item on the claim containing **G8485** (and **G8494** if reported) as well as all other line items containing QDCs. N365 indicates the code is not payable and is used for reporting/informational purposes only. Other services/codes on the claim will not be affected by the addition of a measures group-specific intent G-code or other QDCs. The N365 remark code does NOT indicate whether the QDC is accurate for that claim or for the measure the eligible professional is attempting to report, but does indicate that the QDC was processed and transmitted to the NCH.

MEASURE #3 (NQF 0061): DIABETES MELLITUS: HIGH BLOOD PRESSURE CONTROL

DESCRIPTION:

Percentage of patients aged 18 through 75 years with diabetes mellitus who had most recent blood pressure in control (less than 140/90 mmHg)

NUMERATOR:

Patients whose most recent blood pressure < 140/90 mmHg

Numerator Instructions: To describe both systolic and diastolic blood pressure values, **two CPT II codes must be reported** – 1) One to describe the systolic value; AND 2) One to describe the diastolic value. If there are multiple blood pressures on the same date of service, use the lowest systolic and lowest diastolic blood pressure on that date as the representative blood pressure.

NUMERATOR NOTE: The performance period for this measure is 12 months.

Numerator Quality-Data Coding Options for Reporting Satisfactorily: Most Recent Blood Pressure Measurement Performed

Systolic codes **(Select one (1) code from this section): G8919:** Most recent systolic blood pressure < 140 mmHg

OR

G8920: Most recent systolic blood pressure ≥ 140 mmHg **AND**

Diastolic pressure **(Select one (1) code from this section):**

G8921: Most recent diastolic blood pressure < 90 mmHg

OR

G8922: Most recent diastolic blood pressure ≥ 90 mmHg

OR

Blood Pressure Measurement not Performed, Reason not Otherwise Specified

Append a reporting modifier (**8P**) to CPT Category II code **2000F** to report circumstances when the action described in the numerator is not performed and the reason is not otherwise specified. **2000F *with* 8P: No** documentation of blood pressure measurement

MEASURE #119 (NQF 0062): DIABETES MELLITUS: MEDICAL ATTENTION FOR NEPHROPATHY

DESCRIPTION:

Percentage of patients aged 18 through 75 years with diabetes mellitus who received urine protein screening or medical attention for nephropathy during at least one office visit within 12 months

NUMERATOR:

Patients who have a nephropathy screening during at least one office visit within 12 months

Numerator Instructions: This measure is looking for a nephropathy screening test or evidence of nephropathy.

Numerator Quality-Data Coding Options for Reporting Satisfactorily: Nephropathy Screening Performed

CPT II 3060F: Positive microalbuminuria test result documented and reviewed

OR

CPT II 3061F: Negative microalbuminuria test result documented and reviewed

OR

CPT II 3062F: Positive macroalbuminuria test result documented and reviewed

OR

CPT II 3066F: Documentation of treatment for nephropathy (eg, patient receiving dialysis, patient being treated for ESRD, CRF, ARF, or renal insufficiency, any visit to a nephrologist)

OR

G8506: Patient receiving angiotensin converting enzyme (ACE) inhibitor or angiotensin receptor blocker (ARB) therapy

OR

Nephropathy Screening not Performed, Reason not Otherwise Specified

Append a reporting modifier (**8P**) to CPT Category II code **3060F or 3061F or 3062F** to report circumstances when the action described in the numerator is not performed and the reason is not otherwise specified.

3060F or 3061F or 3062F *with* 8P: Nephropathy screening was **not** performed, reason not otherwise specified

CHRONIC KIDNEY DISEASE (CKD) MEASURES GROUP OVERVIEW

2013 PQRS OPTIONS FOR MEASURES GROUPS: CLAIMS, REGISTRY

2013 PQRS MEASURES IN THE CHRONIC KIDNEY DISEASE (CKD) MEASURES GROUP:

#110. Preventive Care and Screening: Influenza Immunization
#121. Adult Kidney Disease: Laboratory Testing (Lipid Profile)

#122. Adult Kidney Disease: Blood Pressure Management

#123. Adult Kidney Disease: Patients On Erythropoiesis-Stimulating Agents (ESA) - Hemoglobin Level > 12.0 g/Dl

INSTRUCTIONS FOR REPORTING: (These instructions apply to both Claims and Registry reporting, unless otherwise specified.)

Indicate your intention to report the CKD Measures Group by submitting the measures group-specific intent G-code at least once during the reporting period when billing a patient claim for the 20 Patient Sample Method. It is not necessary to submit the measures group-specific intent G-code on more than one claim. It is not necessary to submit the measures group-specific intent G-code for registry-based submissions.

G8487: I intend to report the Chronic Kidney Disease (CKD) Measures Group

• Select patient sample method:

20 Patient Sample Method via claims: 20 unique Medicare Part B FFS (fee for service) patients meeting patient sample criteria for the measures group.

OR

20 Patient Sample Method via registries: 20 unique patients (a majority of which must be Medicare Part B FFS patients) meeting patient sample criteria for the measures group during the reporting period (January 1 through December 31, 2013 **OR** July 1 through December 31, 2013).

• Patient sample criteria for the CKD Measures Group are patients aged 18 years and older with a specific diagnosis of CKD accompanied by a specific patient encounter:

One of the following diagnosis codes indicating stage 4 or 5 chronic kidney disease:

ICD-9-CM: 585.4, 585.5

ICD-10-CM [Reference ONLY/Not Reportable]: N18.4, N18.5

Accompanied by

One of the following patient encounter codes: 99201, 99202, 99203, 99204, 99205, 99212, 99213, 99214, 99215, 99304, 99305, 99306, 99307, 99308, 99309, 99310, 99324, 99325, 99326, 99327, 99328, 99334, 99335, 99336, 99337, 99341, 99342, 99343, 99344, 99345, 99347, 99348, 99349, 99350

• Report quality-data codes (QDCs) on **all applicable** measures within the CKD Measures Group for each patient within the eligible professional's patient sample. Report measures #122 and #123 once during the month the patient is included in the patient sample population. For these measures, subsequent months do not need to be reported.

• Measure #122 only needs to be reported when the patient also has the following diagnosis code indicating Proteinuria:

ICD-9-CM: 791.0

ICD-10-CM [Reference ONLY/Not Reportable]: R80.1 R80.8, R80.9

Instructions for quality-data code reporting for each of the measures within the CKD Measures Group are displayed on the next several pages. If all quality actions for the patient have been performed for all the measures within the group, the following composite G-code may be reported in lieu of the individual quality-data codes for each of the measures within the group. It is not necessary to submit the following composite G-code for registry-based submissions.

Composite G-code G8495: All quality actions for the applicable measures in the CKD Measures Group have been performed for this patient

• To report satisfactorily the CKD Measures Group requires **all applicable** measures for each patient within the eligible professional's patient sample to be reported a minimum of once during the reporting period.

• Measure #110 only needs to be reported a minimum of once during the reporting period when the patient's visit included in the patient sample population is between January and March for the 2012-2013 influenza season **OR** between October and December for the 2013-2014 influenza season. When the patient's office visit is between April and September, Measure #110 is not applicable and will not affect the eligible provider's reporting or performance rate. Measure #110 need only be reported on patients 18 years and older.

• Measures groups containing a measure with a 0% performance rate will not be counted as satisfactorily reporting the measures group. The recommended clinical quality action must be performed on at least one patient for each measure within the measures group reported by the eligible professional. If a measure within a measures group is not applicable to a patient, the patient would not be counted in the performance denominator for that measure (e.g., Preventive Care Measures Group - Measure #39: Screening or Therapy for Osteoporosis for Women Aged 65 Years and Older would not be applicable to male patients according to the patient sample criteria). If the measure is not applicable for all patients within the sample, the performance rate would be 0/0 and would be considered satisfactorily reporting. Performance exclusion quality-data codes are not counted in the performance denominator. If the eligible professional submits all performance exclusion quality-data codes, the performance rate would be 0/0 and would be considered satisfactorily reporting. When a lower rate indicates better performance, such as Measure #123, a 0% performance rate will be counted as satisfactorily reporting (100% performance rate would not be considered satisfactorily reporting).

• When using the 20 Patient Sample Method via claims, report all applicable measures for the 20 unique Medicare Part B FFS patients seen. When using the 20 Patient Sample Method via registries, report all applicable measures for the 20 unique patients seen, a majority of which must be Medicare Part B FFS patients.

• For claims-based submissions, the Carrier/MAC remittance advice notice sent to the practice will show a denial remark code (N365) for the line item on the claim containing **G8487** (and **G8495** if reported) as well as all other line items containing QDCs. N365 indicates that the code is not payable and is used for reporting/informational purposes only. Other services/codes on the claim will not be affected by the addition of a measures group-specific intent G-code or other QDCs. The N365 remark code does NOT indicate whether the QDC is accurate for that claim or for the measure the eligible professional is attempting to report, but does indicate that the QDC was processed and transmitted to the NCH.

MEASURE #110 (NQF 0041): PREVENTIVE CARE AND SCREENING: INFLUENZA IMMUNIZATION

DESCRIPTION:

Percentage of patients aged 6 months and older seen for a visit between October 1 and March 31 who received an influenza immunization OR who reported previous receipt of an influenza immunization

NUMERATOR:

Patients who received an influenza immunization OR who reported previous receipt of influenza immunization

Numerator Instructions:

• If reporting this measure between January 1, 2013 and March 31, 2013, G-code **G8482** should be reported when the influenza immunization is ordered or administered to the patient during the months of August, September, October, November, and December of 2012 or January, February, and March of 2013 for the flu season ending March 31, 2013.

• If reporting this measure between October 1, 2013 and December 31, 2013, G-code **G8482** should be reported when the influenza immunization is ordered or administered to the patient during the months of August, September, October, November, and December of 2013 for the flu season ending March 31, 2014.

• Influenza immunizations administered during the month of August or September of a given flu season (either 2012-2013 flu season OR 2013-2014 flu season) can be reported when a visit occurs during the flu season (October 1 - March 31). In these cases, **G8482** should be reported.

Definition:

Previous Receipt - Receipt of the current season's influenza immunization from another provider OR from same provider prior to the visit to which the measure is applied (typically, prior vaccination would include influenza vaccine given since August 1st).

Numerator Quality-Data Coding Options for Reporting Satisfactorily: Influenza Immunization Administered

G8482: Influenza immunization administered or previously received

OR

Influenza Immunization not Administered for Documented Reasons

G8483: Influenza immunization was not ordered or administered for reasons documented by clinician (e.g., patient allergy or other medical reason, patient declined or other patient reasons, or other system reasons)

OR

Influenza Immunization Ordered or Recommended, but not Administered

G0919: Influenza immunization ordered or recommended (to be given at alternate location or alternate provider); vaccine not available at time of visit

OR

Influenza Immunization not Administered, Reason not Given

G8484: Influenza immunization was **not** ordered or administered, reason not given

MEASURE #121: ADULT KIDNEY DISEASE: LABORATORY TESTING (LIPID PROFILE)

DESCRIPTION:

Percentage of patients aged 18 years and older with a diagnosis of CKD (stage 3, 4 or 5, not receiving Renal Replacement Therapy [RRT]) who had a fasting lipid profile performed at least once within a 12-month period

NUMERATOR:

Patients who had a fasting lipid profile performed at least once within a 12-month period

Definition:

RRT (Renal Replacement Therapy): For the purposes of this measure, RRT includes hemodialysis, peritoneal dialysis, and kidney transplantation

Numerator Quality-Data Coding Options for Reporting Satisfactorily: Fasting Lipid Profile Performed

G8725: Fasting lipid profile performed (Triglycerides, LDL-C, HDL-C, and Total Cholesterol)

OR

Fasting Lipid Profile not Performed, for Documented Reason

G8726: Clinician has documented reason for not performing fasting lipid profile (e.g., patient declined, other patient reasons)

OR

Fasting Lipid Profile not Performed, Reason not Given G8728: Fasting lipid profile **not** performed, reason not given

MEASURE #122: ADULT KIDNEY DISEASE: BLOOD PRESSURE MANAGEMENT

DESCRIPTION:

Percentage of patient visits for those patients aged 18 years and older with a diagnosis of CKD (stage 3, 4 or 5, not receiving Renal Replacement Therapy [RRT]) and documented proteinuria with a blood pressure < 130/80 mmHg OR ≥ 130/80 mmHg with a documented plan of care

NUMERATOR:

Patient visits with blood pressure < 130/80 mmHg OR ≥ 130/80 mmHg and with a documented plan of care

Numerator Instructions: If multiple blood pressure measurements are taken at a single visit, use the most recent measurement taken at that visit.

Definitions:

Proteinuria - > 300 mg of albumin in the urine per 24 hours OR albumin creatinine ratio (ACR) > 300 mcg/mg creatinine OR protein to creatinine ratio > 0.3 mg/mg creatinine

Plan of Care - A documented plan of care should include one or more of the following: recheck blood pressure within 90 days; initiate or alter pharmacologic therapy for blood pressure control; initiate or alter non-pharmacologic therapy (lifestyle changes) for blood pressure control; documented review of patient's home blood pressure log which indicates that patient's blood pressure is or is not well controlled

RRT (Renal Replacement Therapy) - For the purposes of this measure, RRT includes hemodialysis, peritoneal dialysis, and kidney transplantation

NUMERATOR NOTE: The correct combination of numerator code(s) must be reported on the claim form in order to properly report this measure. The "correct combination" of codes may require the submission of multiple numerator codes.

Numerator Quality-Data Coding Options for Reporting Satisfactorily: Patient Visits with Blood Pressure < 130/80 mmHg

*(One G-code [***G8476***] is required on the claim form to submit this numerator option)* **G8476:** Most recent blood pressure has a systolic measurement of < 130 mmHg and a diastolic measurement of < 80 mmHg

OR

Blood Pressure Plan of Care Documented for Patient Visits with Systolic Blood Pressure

≥ 130 mmHg and/or Diastolic Blood Pressure ≥ 80 mmHg (If either systolic blood pressure is ≥ 130 mmHg OR diastolic blood pressure is ≥ 80 mmHg, patient requires a plan of care)**:**

*(One G-code & one CPT II code [***G8477 & 0513F***] are required on the claim form to submit this numerator option)*

G8477: Most recent blood pressure has a systolic measurement of ≥ 130 mmHg and/or a diastolic measurement of ≥ 80 mmHg

AND

CPT II 0513F: Elevated blood pressure plan of care documented

OR

Blood Pressure Measurement not Performed, Reason not Given

*(One G-code [***G8478***] is required on the claim form to submit this numerator option)* **G8478:** Blood pressure measurement **not** performed or documented, reason not given

OR

Elevated Blood Pressure Plan of Care not Documented for Patient Visits with Systolic Blood Pressure ≥ 130 mmHg and/or Diastolic Blood Pressure ≥ 80 mmHg, Reason not Otherwise Specified

*(One CPT II code & one G-code [***0513F-8P & G8477***] are required on the claim form to submit this numerator option)*

Append a reporting modifier (**8P**) to CPT Category II code **0513F** to report circumstances when the action described in the numerator is not performed and the reason is not otherwise specified. **0513F** ***with*** **8P: No** documentation of elevated blood pressure plan of care, reason not otherwise specified

AND

G8477: Most recent blood pressure has a systolic measurement of ≥ 130 mmHg and/or a diastolic measurement of ≥ 80 mmHg

MEASURE #123: ADULT KIDNEY DISEASE: PATIENTS ON ERYTHROPOIESIS- STIMULATING AGENT (ESA) -HEMOGLOBIN LEVEL > 12.0 G/DL

DESCRIPTION:

Percentage of calendar months within a 12-month period during which a hemoglobin level is measured for patients aged 18 years and older with a diagnosis of advanced CKD (stage 4 or 5, not receiving RRT [Renal Replacement Therapy]) or End Stage Renal Disease (ESRD) (who are on hemodialysis or peritoneal dialysis) who are also receiving ESA therapy AND have a hemoglobin level > 12.0 g/dL

NUMERATOR:

Calendar months during which patients have a hemoglobin level > 12.0 g/dL

Numerator Instructions: The hemoglobin values used for this measure should be the most recent (last) hemoglobin value recorded for each calendar month

For performance, a lower rate indicates better performance/control.

Definition:

RRT (Renal Replacement Therapy): For the purposes of this measure, RRT includes hemodialysis, peritoneal dialysis, and kidney transplantation

NUMERATOR NOTE: *The correct combination of numerator code(s) must be reported on the claim form in order to properly report this measure. The "correct combination" of codes may require the submission of multiple numerator codes.*

Numerator Quality-Data Coding Options for Reporting Satisfactorily: Most Recent Hemoglobin level > 12.0 g/dL

*(One G-code and one CPT II code [***G0908 and 4171F***] are required on the claim form to submit this numerator option)*

G0908: Most Recent Hemoglobin (Hgb) level > 12.0 g/dL **AND**

CPT II 4171F: Patient receiving erythropoiesis-stimulating agents (ESA) therapy

OR

Hemoglobin Level Measurement not Performed, Reason not Given

*(One G-code and one CPT II code [***G0909 and 4171F***] are required on the claim form to submit this numerator option)*

G0909: Hemoglobin level measurement **not** documented, reason not given

AND

CPT II 4171F: Patient receiving erythropoiesis-stimulating agents (ESA) therapy

OR

Documented Clinical Reason Patient is not Receiving Erythropoiesis-Stimulating Agent (ESA) Therapy, Patient is not Eligible

*(One CPT II code [***4172F***] is required on the claim form to submit this numerator option)* **CPT II 4172F:** Patient not receiving erythropoiesis-stimulating agents (ESA) therapy

OR

Most Recent Hemoglobin Level ≤12.0 g/dL

*(One G-code and one CPT II code [***G0910 and 4171F***] are required on the claim form to submit this numerator option)*

G0910: Most Recent Hemoglobin Level ≤ 12.0 g/dL

AND

CPT II 4171F: Patient receiving erythropoiesis-stimulating agents (ESA) therapy

PREVENTIVE CARE MEASURES GROUP OVERVIEW

2013 PQRS OPTIONS FOR MEASURES GROUPS: CLAIMS, REGISTRY

2013 PQRS MEASURES IN THE PREVENTIVE CARE MEASURES GROUP:

#39. Screening or Therapy for Osteoporosis for Women Aged 65 Years and Older
#48. Urinary Incontinence: Assessment of Presence or Absence of Urinary Incontinence in Women Aged 65 Years and Older
#110. Preventive Care and Screening: Influenza Immunization
#111. Preventive Care and Screening: Pneumonia Vaccination for Patients 65 Years and Older
#112. Preventive Care and Screening: Breast Cancer Screening

#113. Preventive Care and Screening: Colorectal Cancer Screening
#128. Preventive Care and Screening: Body Mass Index (BMI) Screening and Follow-Up
#173. Preventive Care and Screening: Unhealthy Alcohol Use – Screening
#226. Preventive Care and Screening: Tobacco Use: Screening and Cessation Intervention

INSTRUCTIONS FOR REPORTING: (These instructions apply to both Claims and Registry reporting, unless otherwise specified.)

• Indicate your intention to report the Preventive Care Measures Group by submitting the measures group-specific intent G-code at least once during the reporting period when billing a patient claim for the 20 Patient Sample Method. It is not necessary to submit the measures group-specific intent G-code on more than one claim. It is not necessary to submit the measures group-specific intent G-code for registry-based submissions.

G8486: I intend to report the Preventive Care Measures Group

• Select patient sample method:

20 Patient Sample Method via claims: 20 unique Medicare Part B FFS (fee for service) patients meeting patient sample criteria for the measures group.

OR

20 Patient Sample Method via registries: 20 unique patients (a majority of which must be Medicare Part B FFS patients) meeting patient sample criteria for the measures group during the reporting period (January 1 through December 31, 2013 **OR** July 1 through December 31, 2013).

• Patient sample criteria for the Preventive Care Measures Group are for patients aged 50 years and older with a specific patient encounter:

One of the following patient encounter codes: 99201, 99202, 99203, 99204, 99205, 99212, 99213, 99214, 99215

• Report quality-data codes (QDCs) on **all applicable** measures within the Preventive Care Measures Group for each patient within the eligible professional's patient sample.

Applicable measures contain patient demographic criteria specific to the measure. For example, Screening or Therapy for Osteoporosis is applicable to *women aged 65 years and older* within the sample population, while the Influenza Vaccination measure within this group is applicable to *all patients* aged 50 years and older. Eligible professionals may find it more efficient to report all measures in the group for each patient within their sample. Reporting measure(s) from the group that are inapplicable to an individual patient will not affect the eligible provider's reporting or performance rate.

• Inst ructions for quality-data code reporting for each of the measures within the Preventive Care Measures Group are displayed on the next several pages. If all quality actions for the patient have been performed for all the measures within the group, the following composite G-code may be reported in lieu of the individual quality- data codes for each of the measures within the group. It is not necessary to submit the following composite G-code for registry-based submissions.

Composite G-code G8496: All quality actions for the applicable measures in the Preventive Care Measures Group have been performed for this patient

• To report satisfactorily the Preventive Care Measures Group, it requires **all applicable** measures for each patient within the eligible professional's patient sample to be reported a minimum of once during the reporting period.

• Measure #110 need only be reported a minimum of once during the reporting period when the patient's visit included in the patient sample population is between January and March for the 2012-2013 influenza season **OR** between October and December for the 2013-2014 influenza season. When the patient's office visit is between April and September, Measure #110 is not applicable and will not affect the eligible provider's reporting or performance rate.

• Measures groups containing a measure with a 0% performance rate will not be counted as satisfactorily reporting the measures group. The recommended clinical quality action must be performed on at least one patient for each measure within the measures group reported by the eligible professional. Performance exclusion quality-data codes are not counted in the performance denominator. If the eligible professional submits all performance exclusion quality-data codes, the performance rate would be 0/0 and would be considered satisfactorily reporting. If a measure within a measures group is not applicable to a patient, the patient would not be counted in the performance denominator for that measure (e.g., Preventive Care Measures Group - Measure #39: Screening or Therapy for Osteoporosis for Women Aged 65 Years and Older would not be applicable to male patients according to the patient sample criteria). If the measure is not applicable for all patients within the sample, the performance rate would be 0/0 and would be considered satisfactorily reporting.

• When using the 20 Patient Sample Method via claims, report all measures for the 20 unique Medicare Part B FFS patients seen. When using the 20 Patient Sample Method via registries, report all measures for the 20 unique patients seen, a majority of which must be Medicare Part B FFS patients.

• For claims-based submissions, the Carrier/MAC remittance advice notice sent to the practice will show a denial remark code (N365) for the line item on the claim containing **G8486** (and **G8496** if reported) as well as all other line items containing N365 indicates that the code is not payable and is used for reporting/informational purposes only. Other services/codes on the claim will not be affected by the addition of a measures group-specific intent G-code or other QDCs. The N365 remark code does NOT indicate whether the QDC is accurate for that claim or for the measure the eligible professional is attempting to report, but does indicate that the QDC was processed and transmitted to the NCH.

MEASURE #39 (NQF 0046): SCREENING OR THERAPY FOR OSTEOPOROSIS FOR WOMEN AGED 65 YEARS AND OLDER

DESCRIPTION:

Percentage of female patients aged 65 years and older who have a central dual-energy X-ray absorptiometry (DXA) measurement ordered or performed at least once since age 60 or pharmacologic therapy prescribed within 12 months

NUMERATOR:

Patients who had a central DXA measurement ordered or performed at least once since age 60 or pharmacologic therapy prescribed within 12 months

Definitions:

Pharmacologic Therapy – U.S. Food and Drug Administration approved pharmacologic options for osteoporosis prevention and/or treatment of postmenopausal osteoporosis include, in alphabetical order: bisphosphonates (alendronate, ibandronate, and risedronate), calcitonin, estrogens (estrogens and/or hormone therapy), parathyroid hormone [PTH (1-34), teriparatide], and selective estrogen receptor modules or SERMs (raloxifene).

Prescribed – Includes patients who are currently receiving medication(s) that follow the treatment plan recommended at an encounter during the reporting period, even if the prescription for that medication was ordered prior to the encounter.

Numerator Quality-Data Coding Options for Reporting Satisfactorily:

Central DXA Measurement Ordered or Performed or Pharmacologic Therapy Prescribed G8399: Patient with central Dual-energy X-Ray Absorptiometry (DXA) results documented or ordered or pharmacologic therapy (other than minerals/vitamins) for osteoporosis prescribed

OR

Central DXA Measurement not Ordered or Performed or Pharmacologic Therapy not Prescribed for Documented Reasons

G8401: Clinician documented that patient was not an eligible candidate for screening or therapy

OR

Central DXA Measurement not Ordered or Performed or Pharmacologic Therapy not Prescribed, Reason not Given

G8400: Patient with central Dual-energy X-Ray Absorptiometry (DXA) results **not** documented or **not** ordered or pharmacologic therapy (other than minerals/vitamins) for osteoporosis not prescribed, reason not given

MEASURE #110 (NQF 0041): PREVENTIVE CARE AND SCREENING: INFLUENZA IMMUNIZATION

DESCRIPTION:

Percentage of patients aged 6 months and older seen for a visit between October 1 and March 31 who received an influenza immunization OR who reported previous receipt of an influenza immunization

NUMERATOR:

Patients who received an influenza immunization OR who reported previous receipt of influenza immunization

Numerator Instructions:

• If reporting this measure between January 1, 2013 and March 31, 2013, G-code **G8482** should be reported when the influenza immunization is ordered or administered to the patient during the months of August, September, October, November, and December of 2012 or January, February, and March of 2013 for the flu season ending March 31, 2013.

• If reporting this measure between October 1, 2013 and December 31, 2013, G-code **G8482** should be reported when the influenza immunization is ordered or administered to the patient during the months of August, September, October, November, and December of 2013 for the flu season ending March 31, 2014.

• Influenza immunizations administered during the month of August or September of a given flu season (either 2012-2013 flu season OR 2013-2014 flu season) can be reported when a visit occurs during the flu season (October 1 - March 31). In these cases, **G8482** should be reported.

Definition:

Previous Receipt - Receipt of the current season's influenza immunization from another provider OR from same provider prior to the visit to which the measure is applied (typically, prior vaccination would include influenza vaccine given since August 1st).

Numerator Quality-Data Coding Options for Reporting Satisfactorily: Influenza Immunization Administered

G8482: Influenza immunization administered or previously received

OR

Influenza Immunization not Administered for Documented Reasons

G8483: Influenza immunization was not ordered or administered for reasons documented by clinician (e.g., patient allergy or other medical reason, patient declined or other patient reasons, or other system reasons)

OR

Influenza Immunization Ordered or Recommended, but not Administered

G0919: Influenza immunization ordered or recommended (to be given at alternate location or alternate provider); vaccine not available at time of visit

OR

Influenza Immunization not Administered, Reason not Given

G8484: Influenza immunization was **not** ordered or administered, reason not given

MEASURE #128 (NQF 0421): PREVENTIVE CARE AND SCREENING: BODY MASS INDEX (BMI) SCREENING AND FOLLOW-UP

DESCRIPTION:

Percentage of patients aged 18 years and older with a calculated BMI in the past six months or during the current visit documented in the medical record AND if the most recent BMI is **outside of normal parameters**, a follow-up plan is documented within the past six months or during the current visit

Normal Parameters: Age 65 years and older BMI $\geq$ 23 and < 30
Age 18 – 64 years BMI $\geq$ 18.5 and < 25

NUMERATOR:

Patients with BMI calculated within the past six months or during the current visit and a follow-up plan documented within the past six months or during the current visit if the BMI is outside of normal parameters

Definitions:

BMI – Body mass index (BMI) is expressed as weight/height (BMI; kg/m^2) and is commonly used to classify weight categories.

Calculated BMI – Requires an eligible professional or their staff to measure both the height and weight. Self-reported values cannot be used. BMI is calculated either as weight in pounds divided by height in inches squared,

·Ampicillin/sulba ctam	·Cefuroxime	·Gentamicin
·Aztreonam	·Ciprofloxacin	·Levofloxacin
·Cefazolin	·Clindamycin	·Metronidazole
·Cefmetazole	·Ertapenem	·Moxifloxacin
·Cefotetan	·Erythromycin base	·Neomycin
·Cefoxitin	·Gatifloxacin	·Vancomycin

multiplied by 703, or as weight in kilograms divided by height in meters squared.

Follow-Up Plan – Proposed outline of treatment to be conducted as a result of a BMI out of normal parameters. Such follow-up may include but is not limited to: documentation of a future appointment, education, referral (such as, a registered dietician, nutritionist, occupational therapist, physical therapist, primary care provider, exercise physiologist, mental health professional, or surgeon), pharmacological interventions, dietary supplements, exercise counseling, or nutrition counseling.

Not Eligible/Not Appropriate for BMI Measurement or Follow-Up Plan – A patient is **not** eligible if one or more of the following reasons exists:

- Patient is receiving palliative care

- Patient is pregnant

- Patient refuses BMI measurement

- If there is any other reason documented in the medical record by the provider explaining why BMI measurement or follow-up plan was not appropriate

- Patient is in an urgent or emergent medical situation where time is of the essence and to delay treatment would jeopardize the patient's health status

Numerator Note: *The most recent quality code submitted will be used for performance calculation.*

Calculated BMI or follow-up plan for BMI outside of normal parameters that is documented in the medical record may be reported if done in the provider's office/facility or if obtained by the provider from outside medical records within the past six months.

The documented follow-up interventions must be related to the BMI outside of normal parameters, example: "Patient referred to nutrition counseling for BMI above normal parameters".

Numerator Quality-Data Coding Options for Reporting Satisfactorily: BMI Calculated as Normal, No Follow-Up Plan Required

*(One G- code [**G84xx**] is required on the claim form to submit this numerator option)* **G8420:** Calculated BMI within normal parameters and documented

OR

BMI Calculated Above Normal Parameters, Follow-Up Documented

G8417: Calculated BMI above normal parameters and a follow-up plan was documented

OR

BMI Calculated Below Normal Parameters, Follow-Up Documented

G8418: Calculated BMI below normal parameters and a follow-up plan was documented

OR

BMI not Calculated, Patient not Eligible/not Appropriate

*(One G- code [***G8422 or G8938***] is required on the claim form to submit this numerator option)*

G8422: Patient not eligible for BMI calculation

OR

BMI Calculated, Patient not Eligible/not Appropriate for Follow-up Plan

G8938: BMI is calculated, but patient not eligible for follow-up plan

OR

BMI not Calculated, Reason not Given

*(One G- code [***G84xx***] is required on the claim form to submit this numerator option)*

G8421: BMI not calculated

OR

BMI Calculated Outside Normal Parameters, Follow-Up Plan not Documented, Reason not Given

G8419: Calculated BMI outside normal parameters, no follow-up plan documented

CORONARY ARTERY BYPASS GRAFT (CABG) MEASURES GROUP OVERVIEW

2013 PQRS OPTIONS FOR MEASURES GROUPS:

REGISTRY ONLY

2013 PQRS MEASURES IN CORONARY ARTERY BYPASS GRAFT (CABG) MEASURES GROUP:

#43. Coronary Artery Bypass Graft (CABG): Use of Internal Mammary Artery (IMA) in Patients with Isolated CABG Surgery

#44. Coronary Artery Bypass Graft (CABG): Preoperative Beta-Blocker in Patients with Isolated CABG Surgery
#164. Coronary Artery Bypass Graft (CABG): Prolonged Intubation
#165. Coronary Artery Bypass Graft (CABG): Deep Sternal Wound Infection Rate
#166. Coronary Artery Bypass Graft (CABG): Stroke
#167. Coronary Artery Bypass Graft (CABG): Postoperative Renal Failure
#168. Coronary Artery Bypass Graft (CABG): Surgical Re-Exploration
#169. Coronary Artery Bypass Graft (CABG): Anti-Platelet Medications at Discharge
#170. Coronary Artery Bypass Graft (CABG): Beta-Blockers Administered at Discharge
#171. Coronary Artery Bypass Graft (CABG): Anti-Lipid Treatment at Discharge

INSTRUCTIONS FOR REPORTING: (These instructions apply to registry reporting. Do not report this measures group via claims.)

• It is not necessary to submit the measures group-specific intent G-code for registry-based submissions. However, the measures group-specific intent G-code has been created for registry only measures groups for use by registries that utilize claims data.

G8544: I intend to report the Coronary Artery Bypass Graft (CABG) Measures Group

• Report the patient sample method:

20 Patient Sample Method: 20 unique procedures (patients – a majority of which must be Medicare Part B FFS [fee for service] patients) meeting patient sample criteria for the measures group during the reporting period (January 1 through December 31, 2013 **OR** July 1 through December 31, 2013).

• Patient sample criteria for the CABG Measures Group are patients aged 18 years and older that have a specific procedure for isolated CABG performed:

One of the following procedure codes indicating coronary artery bypass graft: 33510, 33511, 33512, 33513, 33514, 33516, 33517, 33518, 33519, 33521, 33522, 33523, 33533, 33534, 33535, 33536

• Measure #167 need only be reported when the patient does not have a history renal failure or a baseline serum creatinine ≥ 4.0 mg/dL. Measure #169, #170, and #171 need only be reported when the patient is not deceased prior to discharge. Therefore, these measures are only applicable to a patient when these additional criteria are indicated.

• Report a numerator option on **all applicable** measures within the CABG Measures Group for each procedure (patient) within the eligible professional's patient sample.

Instructions for qualifying numerator option reporting for each of the measures within the CABG Measures Group are displayed on the next several pages. The following composite G-code has been created for registry only measures groups for use by registries that utilize claims data. This composite G-code may be reported in lieu of the individual quality-data codes for each of the measures within the group, if all quality actions for the patient have been performed for all the measures within the group. However, it is not necessary to submit the following composite G-code for registry-based submissions.

Composite G-code G8497: All quality actions for the applicable measures in the Coronary Artery Bypass Graft (CABG) Measures Group have been performed for this patient

• To report satisfactorily the CABG Measures Group it requires **all applicable** measures for each patient within the eligible professional's patient sample to be reported each time an isolated CABG procedure is performed during the reporting period.

• Measures groups containing a measure with a 0% performance rate will not be counted as satisfactorily reporting the measures group. The recommended clinical quality action must be performed on at least one patient for each measure within the measures group reported by the eligible professional. Performance exclusion quality-data codes are not counted in the performance denominator. If the eligible professional submits all performance exclusion quality-data codes, the performance rate would be 0/0 and would be considered satisfactorily reporting. If a measure within a measures group is not applicable to a patient, the patient would not be counted in the performance denominator for that measure (e.g., Preventive Care Measures Group - Measure #39: Screening or Therapy for Osteoporosis for Women would not be applicable to male patients according to the patient sample criteria). If the measure is not applicable for all patients within the sample, the performance rate would be 0/0 and would be considered satisfactorily reporting. When a lower rate indicates better performance, such as Measure #164, a 0% performance rate will be counted as satisfactorily reporting (100% performance rate would not be considered satisfactorily reporting).

• When using the 20 Patient Sample Method, report all applicable measures for the 20 unique procedures performed (patients seen) a majority of which must be Medicare Part B FFS procedures (patients) for the 12-month or 6-month reporting period.

MEASURE #164 (NQF 0129): CORONARY ARTERY BYPASS GRAFT (CABG): PROLONGED INTUBATION

DESCRIPTION:

Percentage of patients aged 18 years and older undergoing isolated CABG surgery who require intubation > 24 hours

NUMERATOR:

Patients undergoing isolated CABG who require intubation > 24 hours

Numerator Instructions: For performance, a lower rate indicates better performance.

Numerator Options:

Prolonged intubation (> 24 hrs) required **(G8569)**

OR

Prolonged intubation (> 24 hrs) not required **(G8570)**

MEASURE #165 (NQF 0130): CORONARY ARTERY BYPASS GRAFT (CABG): DEEP STERNAL WOUND INFECTION RATE

DESCRIPTION:

Percentage of patients aged 18 years and older undergoing isolated CABG surgery who, within 30 days postoperatively, develop deep sternal wound infection involving muscle, bone, and/or mediastinum requiring operative intervention

NUMERATOR:

Patients who, within 30 days postoperatively, develop deep sternal wound infection involving muscle, bone, and/or mediastinum requiring operative intervention. Patient must have **ALL** of the following conditions: 1. wound opened with excision of tissue (incision and drainage) or re-exploration of mediastinum, 2. positive culture unless patient is on antibiotics at time of culture or no culture obtained, and 3. treatment with antibiotics beyond perioperative prophylaxis

Numerator Instructions: For performance, a lower rate indicates better performance.

Numerator Options:

Development of deep sternal wound infection within 30 days postoperatively **(G8571)**

OR

No deep sternal wound infection **(G8572)**

MEASURE #166 (NQF 0131): CORONARY ARTERY BYPASS GRAFT (CABG): STROKE

DESCRIPTION:

Percentage of patients aged 18 years and older undergoing isolated CABG surgery who have a **postoperative** stroke (i.e., any confirmed neurological deficit of abrupt onset caused by a disturbance in blood supply to the brain) that did not resolve within 24 hours

NUMERATOR:

Patients who have a postoperative stroke (i.e., any confirmed neurological deficit of abrupt onset caused by a disturbance in blood supply to the brain) that did not resolve within 24 hours

Numerator Instructions: For performance, a lower rate indicates better performance.

Numerator Options:

Stroke following isolated CABG surgery **(G8573)**

OR

No stroke following isolated CABG surgery **(G8574)**

MEASURE #167 (NQF 0114): CORONARY ARTERY BYPASS GRAFT (CABG): POSTOPERATIVE RENAL FAILURE

DESCRIPTION:

Percentage of patients aged 18 years and older undergoing isolated CABG surgery (without pre-existing renal failure) who develop postoperative renal failure or require dialysis

NUMERATOR:

Patients who develop postoperative renal failure or require dialysis; (Definition of renal failure/dialysis requirement - patient had acute renal failure or worsening renal function resulting in one of the following: 1) increase of serum creatinine to ≥ 4.0 mg/dL or 3x most recent preoperative creatinine level, or 2) a new requirement for dialysis postoperatively)

Numerator Instructions: For performance, a lower rate indicates better performance.

Numerator Options:

Developed postoperative renal failure or required dialysis **(G8575)**

OR

No postoperative renal failure/dialysis not required **(G8576)**

MEASURE #168 (NQF 0115): CORONARY ARTERY BYPASS GRAFT (CABG): SURGICAL RE-EXPLORATION

DESCRIPTION:

Percentage of patients aged 18 years and older undergoing isolated CABG surgery who require a return to the operating room (OR) during the current hospitalization for mediastinal bleeding with or without tamponade, graft occlusion, valve dysfunction, or other cardiac reason

NUMERATOR:

Patients who require a return to the OR during the current hospitalization for mediastinal bleeding with or without tamponade, graft occlusion, valve dysfunction, or other cardiac reason

Numerator Instructions: For performance, a lower rate indicates better performance.

Numerator Options:

Re-exploration required due to mediastinal bleeding with or without tamponade, graft occlusion, valve dysfunction, or other cardiac reason **(G8577)**

OR

Re-exploration **not** required due to mediastinal bleeding with or without tamponade, graft occlusion, valve dysfunction, or other cardiac reason **(G8578)**

MEASURE #169 (NQF 0116): CORONARY ARTERY BYPASS GRAFT (CABG): ANTIPLATELET MEDICATIONS AT DISCHARGE

DESCRIPTION:

Percentage of patients aged 18 years and older undergoing isolated CABG surgery who were discharged on antiplatelet medication

NUMERATOR:

Patients who were discharged on antiplatelet medication

Numerator Options:

Antiplatelet medication at discharge **(G8579)**

OR

Antiplatelet medication contraindicated **(G8580)**

OR

No antiplatelet medication at discharge **(G8581)**

MEASURE #170 (NQF 0117): CORONARY ARTERY BYPASS GRAFT (CABG): BETA-BLOCKERS ADMINISTERED AT DISCHARGE

DESCRIPTION:

Percentage of patients aged 18 years and older undergoing isolated CABG surgery who were discharged on beta-blockers

NUMERATOR:

Patients who were discharged on beta-blockers

Numerator Options:

Beta-blocker at discharge **(G8582)**

OR

Beta-blocker contraindicated **(G8583)**

OR

No beta-blocker at discharge **(G8584)**

MEASURE #171 (NQF 0118): CORONARY ARTERY BYPASS GRAFT (CABG): ANTI-LIPID TREATMENT AT DISCHARGE

DESCRIPTION:

Percentage of patients aged 18 years and older undergoing isolated CABG surgery who were discharged on a statin or other lipid-lowering regimen

NUMERATOR:

Patients who were discharged on a statin or other lipid-lowering regimen

Numerator Options:

Anti-lipid treatment at discharge **(G8585)**

OR

Anti-lipid treatment contraindicated **(G8586)**

OR

No anti-lipid treatment at discharge **(G8587)**

RHEUMATOID ARTHRITIS (RA) MEASURES GROUP OVERVIEW

2013 PQRS OPTIONS FOR MEASURES GROUPS: CLAIMS, REGISTRY

2013 PQRS MEASURES IN RHEUMATOID ARTHRITIS (RA) MEASURES GROUP:

#108. Rheumatoid Arthritis (RA): Disease Modifying Anti-Rheumatic Drug (DMARD) Therapy
#176. Rheumatoid Arthritis (RA): Tuberculosis Screening
#177. Rheumatoid Arthritis (RA): Periodic Assessment of Disease Activity
#178. Rheumatoid Arthritis (RA): Functional Status Assessment
#179. Rheumatoid Arthritis (RA): Assessment and Classification of Disease Prognosis
#180. Rheumatoid Arthritis (RA): Glucocorticoid Management

INSTRUCTIONS FOR REPORTING: (These instructions apply to both Claims and Registry reporting, unless otherwise specified.)

• Indicate your intention to report the RA Measures Group by submitting the measures group-specific intent G-code at least once during the reporting period when billing a patient claim for the 20 Patient Sample Method. It is not necessary to submit the measures group-specific intent G-code on more than one claim. It is not necessary to submit the measures group-specific intent G-code for registry-based submissions.

G8490: I intend to report the Rheumatoid Arthritis Measures Group

• Select patient sample method:

20 Patient Sample Method via claims: 20 unique Medicare Part B FFS (fee for service) patients meeting patient sample criteria for the measures group.

OR

20 Patient Sample Method via registries: 20 unique patients (a majority of which must be Medicare Part B FFS patients) meeting patient sample criteria for the measures group during the reporting period (January 1 through December 31, 2013 **OR** July 1 through December 31, 2013).

• Patient sample criteria for the RA Measures Group are patients aged 18 years and older with a specific diagnosis of RA accompanied by a specific patient encounter:

One of the following diagnosis codes indicating rheumatoid arthritis:

ICD-9-CM: 714.0, 714.1, 714.2, 714.81

ICD-10-CM [Reference ONLY/Not Reportable]: M05.00, M05.011, M05.012, M05.019, M05.021, M05.022, M05.029, M05.031, M05.032,

M05.039, M05.041, M05.042, M05.049, M05.051, M05.052, M05.059, M05.061, M05.062, M05.069, M05.071, M05.072, M05.079, M05.09, M05.111, M05.112, M05.119, M05.121, M05.122, M05.129, M05.131, M05.132, M05.139, M05.141, M05.142, M05.149, M05.151, M05.152, M05.159, M05.161, M05.162, M05.169, M05.171, M05.172, M05.179, M05.19, M05.20, M05.211, M05.212, M05.219, M05.221, M05.222, M05.229, M05.231, M05.232, M05.239, M05.241, M05.242, M05.249, M05.251, M05.252, M05.259, M05.261, M05.262, M05.269, M05.271, M05.272, M05.279, M05.29, M05.30, M05.311, M05.312, M05.319, M05.321, M05.322, M05.329, M05.331, M05.332, M05.339, M05.341, M05.342, M05.349, M05.351, M05.352, M05.359, M05.361, M05.362, M05.369, M05.371, M05.372, M05.379, M05.39, M05.40, M05.411, M05.412, M05.419, M05.421, M05.422, M05.429, M05.431, M05.432, M05.439, M05.441, M05.442, M05.449, M05.451, M05.452, M05.459, M05.461, M05.462, M05.469, M05.471, M05.472, M05.479, M05.49, M05.50, M05.511, M05.512, M05.519, M05.521, M05.522, M05.529, M05.531, M05.532, M05.539, M05.541, M05.542, M05.549, M05.551, M05.552, M05.559, M05.561, M05.562, M05.569, M05.571, M05.572, M05.579, M05.59, M05.60, M05.611, M05.612, M05.619, M05.621, M05.622, M05.629, M05.631, M05.632, M05.639, M05.641, M05.642, M05.649, M05.651, M05.652, M05.659, M05.661, M05.662, M05.669, M05.671, M05.672, M05.679, M05.69, M05.70, M05.711, M05.712, M05.719, M05.721, M05.722, M05.729, M05.731, M05.732, M05.739, M05.741, M05.742, M05.749, M05.751, M05.752, M05.759, M05.761, M05.762, M05.769, M05.771, M05.772, M05.779, M05.79, M05.80, M05.811, M05.812, M05.819, M05.821, M05.822, M05.829, M05.831, M05.832, M05.839, M05.841, M05.842, M05.849, M05.851, M05.852, M05.859, M05.861, M05.862, M05.869, M05.871, M05.872, M05.879, M05.89, M05.9, M06.00, M06.011, M06.012, M06.019, M06.021, M06.022, M06.029, M06.031, M06.032, M06.039, M06.041, M06.042, M06.049, M06.051, M06.052, M06.059, M06.061, M06.062, M06.069, M06.071, M06.072, M06.079, M06.08, M06.09, M06.1, M06.30, M06.311, M06.312, M06.319, M06.321, M06.322, M06.329, M06.331, M06.332, M06.339, M06.341, M06.342, M06.349, M06.351, M06.352, M06.359, M06.361, M06.362, M06.369, M06.371, M06.372, M06.379, M06.38, M06.39

Accompanied by

One of the following patient encounter codes: 99201, 99202, 99203, 99204, 99205, 99212, 99213, 99214, 99215, 99341, 99342, 99343, 99344, 99345, 99347, 99348, 99349, 99350, G0402

• Report quality-data codes (QDCs) on **all** measures within the RA Measures Group for each patient within the eligible professional's patient sample.

• Instructions for quality-data code reporting for each of the measures within the RA Measures Group are displayed on the next several pages. If all quality actions for the patient have been performed for all the measures within the group, the following composite G-code may be reported in lieu of the individual quality-data codes for each of the measures within the group. It is not necessary to submit the following composite G-code for registry-based submissions.

Composite G-code G8499: All quality actions for the applicable measures in the Rheumatoid Arthritis Measures Group have been performed for this patient

• To report satisfactorily the RA Measures Group it requires **all** measures for each patient within the eligible professional's patient sample to be reported a minimum of once during the reporting period.

• Measures groups containing a measure with a 0% performance rate will not be counted as satisfactorily reporting the measures group. The recommended clinical quality action must be performed on at least one patient for each measure within the measures group reported by the eligible professional. Performance exclusion quality-data codes are not counted in the performance denominator. If the eligible professional submits all performance exclusion quality-data codes, the performance rate would be 0/0 and would be considered satisfactorily reporting.

• When using the 20 Patient Sample Method via claims, report all measures for the 20 unique Medicare Part B FFS patients seen. When using the 20 Patient Sample Method via registries, report all measures for the 20 unique patients seen, a majority of which must be Medicare Part B FFS patients.

• For claims-based submissions, the Carrier/MAC remittance advice notice sent to the practice will show a denial remark code (N365) for the line item on the claim containing **G8490** (and **G8499** if reported) as well as all other line items containing QDCs. N365 indicates that the code is not payable and is used for reporting/informational purposes only. Other services/codes on the claim will not be affected by the addition of a measures group-specific intent G-code or other QDCs. The N365 remark code does NOT indicate whether the QDC is accurate for that claim or for the measure the eligible professional is attempting to report, but does indicate that the QDC was processed and transmitted to the NCH.

MEASURE #108 (NQF 0054): RHEUMATOID ARTHRITIS (RA): DISEASE MODIFYING ANTI-RHEUMATIC DRUG (DMARD) THERAPY

DESCRIPTION:

Percentage of patients aged 18 years and older who were diagnosed with RA and were prescribed, dispensed, or administered at least one ambulatory prescription for a DMARD

NUMERATOR:

Patients who were prescribed, dispensed, or administered at least one disease modifying anti-rheumatic drug (DMARD)

Definitions:

Prescribed – May include prescription given to the patient for DMARD therapy at one or more visits in the 12-month period OR patient already taking DMARD therapy as documented in current medication list.

The DMARDs listed below are considered DMARDs for the purposes of this measure.

Note: J codes should only be used to identify if the appropriate DMARD therapy was prescribed to the patient. CPT II codes are used when reporting this measure

Numerator Quality-Data Coding Options for Reporting Satisfactorily: DMARD Prescribed, Dispensed, or Administered

CPT II 4187F: Disease modifying anti-rheumatic drug therapy prescribed, dispensed, or administered

OR

DMARD not Prescribed, Dispensed, or Administered for Medical Reasons

Append a modifier (**1P**) to CPT Category II code **4187F** to report documented circumstances that appropriately exclude patients from the denominator.

4187F *with* 1P: Documentation of medical reason(s) for not prescribing, dispensing, or administering disease modifying anti-rheumatic drug therapy

OR

DMARD not Prescribed, Dispensed, or Administered, Reason not Otherwise Specified Append a reporting modifier (**8P**) to CPT Category II code **4187F** to report circumstances when the action described in the numerator is not performed and the reason is not otherwise specified. **4187F *with* 8P:** Disease modifying anti-rheumatic drug therapy was **not** prescribed, dispensed, or administered, reason not otherwise specified

PERIOPERATIVE CARE MEASURES GROUP OVERVIEW

2013 PQRS OPTIONS FOR MEASURES GROUPS: CLAIMS, REGISTRY

2013 PQRS MEASURES IN PERIOPERATIVE CARE MEASURES GROUP:

#20. Perioperative Care: Timing of Prophylactic Parenteral Antibiotic – Ordering Physician
#21. Perioperative Care: Selection of Prophylactic Antibiotic – First OR Second Generation Cephalosporin
#22. Perioperative Care: Discontinuation of Prophylactic Parenteral Antibiotics (Non-Cardiac Procedures)
#23. Perioperative Care: Venous Thromboembolism (VTE) Prophylaxis (When Indicated in ALL Patients)

INSTRUCTIONS FOR REPORTING: (These instructions apply to both Claims and Registry reporting, unless otherwise specified.)

• Indicate your intention to report the Perioperative Care Measures Group by submitting the measures group-specific intent G-code at least once during the reporting period when billing a patient claim for the 20 Patient Sample Method. It is not necessary to submit the measures group-specific intent G-code on more than one claim. It is not necessary to submit the measures group-specific intent G-code for registry-based submissions.

G8492: I intend to report the Perioperative Care Measures Group

• Select patient sample method:

20 Patient Sample Method via claims: 20 unique Medicare Part B FFS (fee for service) procedures (patients) meeting patient sample criteria for the measures group.

OR

20 Patient Sample Method via registries: 20 unique procedures (patients - a majority of which must be Medicare Part B FFS patients) meeting patient sample criteria for the measures group during the reporting period (January 1 through December 31, 2013 **OR** July 1 through December 31, 2013).

• Patient sample criteria for the Perioperative Care Measures Group are patients aged 18 years and older that have a specific surgical procedure performed:

One of the following surgical procedure codes: 0236T, 15734, 15830, 15832, 15833, 15834, 15835, 15836, 15837, 19260, 19271, 19272, 19300, 19305, 19306, 19307, 19316, 19318, 19324, 19361, 19364, 19366, 19367, 19368, 19369, 19380, 21627, 21632, 21740, 21750, 21805, 21825, 22558, 22600, 22612, 22630, 27080, 27125, 27130, 27132, 27134, 27137, 27138, 27158, 27202, 27235, 27236, 27244, 27245, 27269, 27280, 27282, 27440, 27441, 27442, 27443, 27445, 27446, 27447, 27880, 27881, 27882, 27884, 27886, 27888, 31760, 31766, 31770, 31775, 31786, 31805, 32096, 32097, 32098, 32100, 32110, 32120, 32124, 32140, 32141, 32150, 32215, 32220, 32225, 32310, 32320, 32440, 32442, 32445, 32480, 32482, 32484, 32486, 32488, 32491, 32505, 32506, 32507, 32800, 32810, 32815, 32900, 32905, 32906, 32940, 33020, 33025, 33030, 33031, 33050, 33300, 33310, 33320, 33877, 33880, 33881, 33883, 33886, 33889, 33891, 34051, 34800, 34802, 34803, 34804, 34805, 34812, 34820, 34825, 34830, 34831, 34832, 34833, 34834, 34900, 35011, 35013, 35021, 35081, 35082, 35091, 35092, 35102, 35103, 35131, 35141, 35142, 35151, 35152, 35206, 35216, 35246, 35266, 35271, 35276, 35301, 35311, 35363, 35371, 35372, 35460, 35512, 35521, 35522, 35523, 35525, 35526, 35533, 35537, 35538, 35539, 35540, 35556, 35558, 35565, 35566, 35570, 35571, 35572, 35583, 35585, 35587, 35601, 35606, 35612, 35616, 35621, 35623, 35626, 35631, 35632, 35633, 35634, 35636, 35637, 35638, 35642, 35645, 35646, 35647, 35650, 35654, 35656, 35661, 35663, 35665, 35666, 35671, 36830, 37224, 37225, 37226, 37227, 37228, 37229, 37230, 37231, 37235, 37616, 37617, 38100, 38101, 38115, 38120, 38381, 38571, 38572, 38700, 38720, 38724, 38740, 38745, 38746, 38747, 38760, 38765, 38770, 38780, 39000, 39010, 39200, 39220, 39545, 39561, 43020, 43030, 43045, 43100, 43101, 43107, 43108, 43112, 43113, 43116, 43117, 43118, 43121, 43122, 43123, 43124, 43130, 43135, 43279, 43280, 43281, 43282, 43300, 43305, 43310, 43312, 43313, 43314, 43320, 43325, 43327, 43328, 43330, 43331, 43332, 43333, 43334, 43335, 43336, 43337,

43340, 43341, 43350, 43351, 43352, 43360, 43361, 43400, 43401, 43405, 43410, 43415, 43420, 43425, 43496, 43500, 43501, 43502, 43510, 43520, 43605, 43610, 43611, 43620, 43621, 43622, 43631, 43632, 43633, 43634, 43635, 43640, 43641, 43644, 43645, 43651, 43652, 43653, 43800, 43810, 43820, 43825, 43830, 43832, 43840, 43843, 43845, 43846, 43847, 43848, 43850, 43855, 43860, 43865, 43870, 43880, 44005, 44010, 44020, 44021, 44050, 44055, 44120, 44125, 44126, 44127, 44130, 44140, 44141, 44143, 44144, 44145, 44146, 44147, 44150, 44151, 44155, 44156, 44157, 44158, 44160, 44180, 44186, 44187, 44188, 44202, 44204, 44205, 44206, 44207, 44208, 44210, 44211, 44212, 44227, 44300, 44310, 44312, 44314, 44316, 44320, 44322, 44340, 44345, 44346, 44602, 44603, 44604, 44605, 44615, 44620, 44625, 44626, 44640, 44650, 44660, 44661, 44680, 44700, 45000, 45020, 45110, 45111, 45112, 45113, 45114, 45116, 45119, 45120, 45121, 45123, 45126, 45130, 45135, 45136, 45150, 45160, 45171, 45172, 45395, 45397, 45400, 45402, 45540, 45541, 45550, 45560, 45562, 45563, 45800, 45805, 45820, 45825, 47100, 47120, 47122, 47125, 47130, 47140, 47141, 47142, 47350, 47400, 47420, 47425, 47460, 47480, 47560, 47561, 47562, 47563, 47564, 47570, 47600, 47605, 47610, 47612, 47620, 47630, 47700, 47701, 47711, 47712, 47715, 47720, 47721, 47740, 47741, 47760, 47765, 47780, 47785, 47800, 47801, 47802, 47900, 48000, 48001, 48020, 48100, 48102, 48105, 48120, 48140, 48145, 48146, 48148, 48150, 48152, 48153, 48154, 48155, 48500, 48510, 48520, 48540, 48545, 48547, 48548, 48554, 48556, 49000, 49002, 49010, 49020, 49021, 49040, 49041, 49060, 49203, 49204, 49205, 49215, 49220, 49250, 49320, 49321, 49322, 49323, 49505, 49507, 49568, 50320, 50340, 50360, 50365, 50370, 50380, 57267, 58150, 58152, 58180, 58200, 58210, 58240, 58260, 58262, 58263, 58267, 58270, 58275, 58280, 58285, 58290, 58291, 58292, 58293, 58294, 58951, 58953, 58954, 58956, 60521, 60522, 61312, 61313, 61315, 61510, 61512, 61518, 61548, 61697, 61700, 62230, 63015, 63020, 63047, 63056, 63081, 63267, 63276, 64746

NOTE: CPT Category I procedure codes billed by surgeons performing surgery on the same patient, submitted with modifier 62 (indicating two surgeons, i.e., dual procedures) will be included in the denominator population. Both surgeons participating in PQRS will be fully accountable for the clinical action described in the measure.

• Report quality-data codes (QDCs) on **all** measures within the Perioperative Care Measures Group for each procedure (patient) within the eligible professional's patient sample.

• Instructions for quality-data code reporting for each of the measures within the Perioperative Care Measures Group are displayed on the next several pages. If all quality actions for the patient have been performed for all the measures within the group, the following composite G-code may be reported in lieu of the individual quality-data codes for each of the measures within the group. It is not necessary to submit the following composite G-code for registry-based submissions.

Composite G-code G8501: All quality actions for the applicable measures in the Perioperative Care Measures Group have been performed for this patient

• To report satisfactorily the Perioperative Care Measures Group it requires **all** measures for each patient within the eligible professional's patient sample to be reported each time a surgical procedure is performed during the reporting period.

• Measures groups containing a measure with a 0% performance rate will not be counted as satisfactorily reporting the measures group. The recommended clinical quality action must be performed on at least one patient for each measure within the measures group reported by the eligible professional. Performance exclusion quality-data codes are not counted in the performance denominator. If the eligible professional submits all performance exclusion quality-data codes, the performance rate would be 0/0 and would be considered satisfactorily reporting.

• When using the 20 Patient Sample Method via claims, report all measures for the 20 unique Medicare Part B FFS procedures performed (patients seen). When using the 20 Patient Sample Method via registries, report all measures for the 20 unique procedures performed (patients seen), a majority of which must be Medicare Part B FFS patients.

• For claims-based submissions, the Carrier/MAC remittance advice notice sent to the practice will show a denial remark code (N365) for the line item on the claim containing **G8492** (and **G8501** if reported) as well as all other line items containing QDCs. N365 indicates that the code is not payable and is used for reporting/informational purposes only. Other services/codes on the claim will not be affected by the addition of a measures group-specific intent G-code or other QDCs. The N365 remark code does NOT indicate whether the QDC is accurate for that claim or for the measure the eligible professional is attempting to report, but does indicate that the QDC was processed and transmitted to the NCH.

MEASURE #20 (NQF 0270): PERIOPERATIVE CARE: TIMING OF PROPHYLACTIC PARENTERAL ANTIBIOTIC ORDERING PHYSICIAN

DESCRIPTION:

Percentage of surgical patients aged 18 years and older undergoing procedures with the indications for prophylactic parenteral antibiotics, who have an order for prophylactic parenteral antibiotic to be given within one hour (if fluoroquinolone or vancomycin, two hours), prior to the surgical incision (or start of procedure when no incision is required)

NUMERATOR:

Surgical patients who have an order for prophylactic parenteral antibiotic to be given within one hour (if fluoroquinolone or vancomycin, two hours) prior to the surgical incision (or start of procedure when no incision is required)

Numerator Instructions: There must be documentation of order (written order, verbal order, or standing order/protocol) specifying that prophylactic parenteral antibiotic is to be given within one hour (if fluoroquinolone or vancomycin, two hours) prior to the surgical incision (or start of procedure when no incision is required) OR documentation that prophylactic parenteral antibiotic *has* been given within one hour (if fluoroquinolone or vancomycin, two hours) prior to the surgical incision (or start of procedure when no incision is required).

Numerator Note: *In the event surgery is delayed, as long as the patient is redosed (if clinically appropriate) the numerator coding should be applied.*

Numerator Quality-Data Coding Options for Reporting Satisfactorily:

Table 1A: The antimicrobial drugs listed below are considered prophylactic parenteral antibiotics for the purposes of this measure. ***G8632*** *should be reported when antibiotics from this table were not ordered.*

• Ampicillin/ sulbactam • Aztreonam • Cefazolin • Cefmetazole • Cefotetan • Cefoxitin	• Cefuroxime • Ciprofloxacin • Clindamycin • Ertapenem • Erythromycin base • Gatifloxacin	• Gentamicin • Levofloxacin • Metronidazole • Moxifloxacin • Neomycin • Vancomycin

Documentation of Order for Prophylactic Parenteral Antibiotic (written order, verbal order, or standing order/protocol)

G8629: Documentation of order for prophylactic parenteral antibiotics to be given within one hour (if fluoroquinolone or vancomycin, two hours) prior to surgical incision (or start of procedure when no incision is required)

OR

Documentation that Prophylactic Parenteral Antibiotic has been Given within One Hour Prior to the Surgical Incision (or start of procedure when no incision is required)

G8630: Documentation that administration of prophylactic parenteral antibiotic was initiated within one hour (if fluoroquinolone or vancomycin, two hours) prior to surgical incision (or start of procedure when no incision is required), as ordered

OR

Order for Prophylactic Parenteral Antibiotic not Given for Documented Reasons

G8631: Clinician documented that patient was not an eligible candidate for ordering prophylactic parenteral antibiotics to be given within one hour (if fluoroquinolone or vancomycin, two hours) prior to the surgical incision (or start of procedure when no incision is required)

OR

Order for Administration of Prophylactic Parenteral Antibiotic not Given, Reason not Given G8632: Prophylactic parenteral antibiotics were **not** ordered to be given or given within one hour (if fluoroquinolone or vancomycin, two hours) prior to the surgical incision (or start of procedure when no incision is required), reason not given

BACK PAIN MEASURES GROUP OVERVIEW

2013 PQRS OPTIONS FOR MEASURES GROUPS: CLAIMS, REGISTRY

2013 PQRS MEASURES IN BACK PAIN MEASURES GROUP:

#148.Back Pain: Initial Visit
#149.Back Pain: Physical Exam
#150.Back Pain: Advice for Normal Activities
#151,Back Pain: Advice Against Bed Rest

INSTRUCTIONS FOR REPORTING: (These instructions apply to both Claims and Registry reporting, unless otherwise specified.)

• Indicate your intention to report the Back Pain Measures Group by submitting the measures group-specific intent G-code at least once during the reporting period when billing a patient claim for the 20 Patient Sample Method. It is not necessary to submit the measures group-specific intent G-code on more than one claim. It is not necessary to submit the measures group-specific intent G-code for registry-based submissions.

G8493: I intend to report the Back Pain Measures Group

• Select patient sample method:

20 Patient Sample Method via claims: 20 unique Medicare Part B FFS (fee for service) patients meeting patient sample criteria for the measures group.

OR

20 Patient Sample Method via registries: 20 unique patients (a majority of which must be Medicare Part B FFS patients) meeting patient sample criteria for the measures group during the reporting period (January 1 through December 31, 2013 **OR** July 1 through December 31, 2013).

• Patient sample criteria for the Back Pain Measures Group are patients aged 18 through 79 years with a specific diagnosis for back pain accompanied by a specific patient encounter **OR** patients aged 18-79 years that have a specific back surgical procedure performed:

One of the following diagnosis codes indicating back pain:

ICD-9-CM: 721.3, 721.41, 721.42, 721.90, 722.0, 722.10, 722.11, 722.2, 722.30, 722.31, 722.32, 722.39, 722.4, 722.51, 722.52, 722.6, 722.70, 722.71, 722.72, 722.73, 722.80, 722.81, 722.82, 722.83, 722.90, 722.91, 722.92,

722.93, 723.0, 724.00, 724.01, 724.02, 724.09, 724.2, 724.3, 724.4, 724.5, 724.6, 724.70, 724.71, 724.79, 738.4, 738.5, 739.3, 739.4, 756.12, 846.0, 846.1, 846.2, 846.3, 846.8, 846.9, 847.2

ICD-10-CM [Reference ONLY/Not reportable]: M43.00, M43.10, M43.27, M43.28, M46.40, M46.41, M46.42, M46.43, M46.44, M46.45, M46.46, M46.47, M46.48, M46.49, M47.14, M47.15, M47.16, M47.17, M47.18, M47.20, M47.26, M47.27, M47.28, M47.816, M47.817, M47.818, M47.819, M47.896, M47.897, M47.898, M47.899, M47.9, M48.00, M48.01, M48.02, M48.03, M48.04, M48.05, M48.06, M48.07, M48.08, M50.00, M50.01, M50.02, M50.03, M50.20, M50.21, M50.22, M50.23, M50.30, M50.31, M50.32, M50.33, M50.80, M50.81, M50.82, M50.83, M50.90, M50.91, M50.92, M50.93, M51.04, M51.05, M51.06, M51.07, M51.14, M51.15, M51.16, M51.17, M51.24, M51.26, M51.27, M51.34, M51.35, M51.36, M51.37, M51.44, M51.45, M51.47, M51.87, M51.9, M53.2X7, M53.2X8, M53.86, M53.87, M53.88, M54.14, M54.15, M54.16, M54.17, M54.30, M54.31, M54.32, M54.40, M54.41, M54.42, M54.5, M54.89, M54.9, M96.1, M99.03, M99.04, M99.20, M99.21, M99.22, M99.23, M99.24, M99.25, M99.26, M99.27, M99.28, M99.29, M99.30, M99.31, M99.32, M99.33, M99.34, M99.35, M99.36, M99.37, M99.38, M99.39, M99.40, M99.41, M99.42, M99.43, M99.44, M99.45, M99.46, M99.47, M99.48, M99.49, M99.50, M99.51, M99.52, M99.53, M99.54, M99.55, M99.56, M99.57, M99.58, M99.59, M99.60, M99.61, M99.62, M99.63, M99.64, M99.65, M99.66, M99.67, M99.68, M99.69, M99.70, M99.71, M99.72, M99.73, M99.74, M99.75, M99.76, M99.77, M99.78, M99.79, M99.83, M99.84, Q76.2, S33.5XXA, S33.6XXA, S33.8XXA, S33.9XXA

AND

One of the following patient encounter codes: 97001, 97002, 99201, 99202, 99203, 99204, 99205, 99212, 99213, 99214, 99215

OR

One of the following back surgical procedure codes: 22210, 22214, 22220, 22222, 22224, 22226, 22532, 22533, 22534, 22548, 22554, 22556, 22558, 22585, 22590, 22595, 22600, 22612, 22614, 22630, 22632, 22818, 22819, 22830, 22840, 22841, 22842, 22843, 22844, 22845, 22846, 22847, 22848, 22849, 63001, 63003, 63005, 63011, 63012, 63015, 63016, 63017, 63020, 63030, 63035, 63040, 63042, 63043, 63044, 63045, 63046, 63047, 63048, 63055, 63056, 63057, 63064, 63066, 63075, 63076, 63077, 63078, 63081, 63082, 63085, 63086, 63087, 63088, 63090, 63091, 63101, 63102, 63103, 63170, 63172, 63173, 63180, 63182, 63185, 63190, 63191, 63194, 63195, 63196, 63197, 63198, 63199, 63200

• Report quality-data codes (QDCs) on **all** measures within the Back Pain Measures Group for each patient within the eligible professional's patient sample.

• Instructions for quality-data code reporting for each of the measures within the Back Pain Measures Group are displayed on the next several pages. If all quality actions for the patient have been performed for all the measures within the group, the following composite G-code may be reported in lieu of the individual quality-data codes for each of the measures within the group. It is not necessary to submit the following composite G-code for registry-based submissions.

Composite G-code G8502: All quality actions for the applicable measures in the Back Pain Measures Group have been performed for this patient

• To report satisfactorily the Back Pain Measures Group for the 20 Patient Sample Method it requires **all** measures for each patient within the sample to be reported where **the initial visit** to the clinician for **each episode** of back pain or each surgery for back pain that occurred during the corresponding reporting period. If the patient's initial visit for this episode of back pain occurred prior to the beginning of the reporting period, report that the visit in the sample is a subsequent visit for the episode and this will **not** count toward the 20 patient sample. This measures group may be reported by more than one clinician if multiple clinicians evaluate or treat the patient for the back pain episode.

• Measures groups containing a measure with a 0% performance rate will not be counted as satisfactorily reporting the measures group. The recommended clinical quality action must be performed on at least one patient for each measure within the measures group reported by the eligible professional.

• When using the 20 Patient Sample Method via claims, report all measures for 20 unique Medicare Part B FFS patients seen. When using the 20 Patient Sample Method via registries, report all measures for 20 unique patients seen, a majority of which must be Medicare Part B FFS patients.

• For claims-based submissions, the Carrier/MAC remittance advice notice sent to the practice will show a denial remark code (N365) for the line item on the claim containing **G8493** (and **G8502** if reported) as well as all other line items containing QDCs. N365 indicates that the code is not payable and is used for reporting/informational purposes only. Other services/codes on the claim will not be affected by the addition of a measures group-specific intent G-code or other QDCs. The N365 remark code does NOT indicate whether the QDC is accurate for that claim or for the measure the eligible professional is attempting to report, but does indicate that the QDC was processed and transmitted to the NCH.

HEPATITIS C MEASURES GROUP OVERVIEW

2013 PQRS OPTIONS FOR MEASURES GROUPS: CLAIMS, REGISTRY

2013 PQRS MEASURES IN HEPATITIS C MEASURES GROUP:

#84. Hepatitis C: Ribonucleic Acid (RNA) Testing Before Initiating Treatment
#85. Hepatitis C: HCV Genotype Testing Prior to Treatment
#86. Hepatitis C: Antiviral Treatment Prescribed
#87. Hepatitis C: HCV Ribonucleic Acid (RNA) Testing at Week 12 of Treatment
#89. Hepatitis C: Counseling Regarding Risk of Alcohol Consumption
#90. Hepatitis C: Counseling Regarding Use of Contraception Prior to Antiviral Therapy

#183. Hepatitis C: Hepatitis A Vaccination in Patients with HCV
#184. Hepatitis C: Hepatitis B Vaccination in Patients with HCV

INSTRUCTIONS FOR REPORTING: (These instructions apply to both Claims and Registry reporting, unless otherwise specified.)

• Indicate your intention to report the Hepatitis C Measures Group by submitting the measures group-specific intent G-code at least once during the reporting period when billing a patient claim for the 20 Patient Sample Method. It is not necessary to submit the measures group-specific intent G-code on more than one claim. It is not necessary to submit the measures group-specific intent G-code for registry-based submissions.

G8545: I intend to report the Hepatitis C Measures Group

• Select patient sample method:

20 Patient Sample Method via claims: 20 unique Medicare Part B FFS (fee for service) patients meeting patient sample criteria for the measures group.

OR

20 Patient Sample Method via registries: 20 unique patients (a majority of which must be Medicare Part B FFS patients) meeting patient sample criteria for the measures group during the reporting period (January 1 through December 31, 2013 **OR** July 1 through December 31, 2013).

• Patient sample criteria for the Hepatitis C Measures Group are patients aged 18 years and older with a specific diagnosis of chronic hepatitis C accompanied by a specific patient encounter:

One of the following diagnosis codes indicating chronic hepatitis C: ICD-9-CM: 070.54

ICD-10-CM [Reference ONLY/Not Reportable]: B18.2

Accompanied by

One of the following patient encounter codes: 99201, 99202, 99203, 99204, 99205, 99212, 99213, 99214, 99215

• Report quality-data codes (QDCs) on **all applicable** measures within the Hepatitis C Measures Group for each patient within the eligible professional's patient sample.

Applicable measures contain patient demographic criteria specific to the measure. For example, Counseling Regarding Use of Contraception Prior to Antiviral Therapy is applicable to female patients *aged 18 through 44 years and all men aged 18 years and older* within the sample population, while the Antiviral Treatment Prescribed measure within this group is applicable to *all patients* aged 18 years and older. Eligible professionals may find it more efficient to report all measures in the group for each patient within their sample. Reporting measure(s) from the group that are inapplicable to an individual patient will not affect the eligible provider's reporting or performance rate.

• Instructions for quality-data code reporting for each of the measures within the Hepatitis C Measures Group are displayed on the next several pages. If all quality actions for the patient have been performed for all measures within the group, the following composite G-code may be reported in lieu of the individual quality-data codes for each of the measures within the group. It is not necessary to submit the following composite G-code for registry-based submissions.

Composite G-code G8549: All quality actions for the applicable measures in the Hepatitis C Measures Group have been performed for this patient

• To report satisfactorily the Hepatitis C Measures Group it requires **all applicable** measures for each patient within the eligible professional's patient sample to be reported a minimum of once during the reporting period.

• Measures groups containing a measure with a 0% performance rate will not be counted as satisfactorily reporting the measures group. The recommended clinical quality action must be performed on at least one patient for each measure within the measures group reported by the eligible professional. Performance exclusion quality-data codes are not counted in the performance denominator. If the eligible professional submits all performance exclusion quality-data codes, the performance rate would be 0/0 and would be considered satisfactorily reporting. If a measure within a measures group is not applicable to a patient, the patient would not be counted in the performance denominator for that measure (e.g., Preventive Care Measures Group - Measure #39: Screening or Therapy for Osteoporosis for Women would not be applicable to male patients according to the patient sample criteria). If the measure is not applicable for all patients within the sample, the performance rate would be 0/0 and would be considered satisfactorily reporting.

• When using the 20 Patient Sample Method via claims, report all measures for the 20 unique Medicare Part B FFS patients seen. When using the 20 Patient Sample Method via registries, report all measures for the 20 unique patients seen, a majority of which must be Medicare Part B FFS patients.

• For claims-based submissions, the Carrier/MAC remittance advice notice sent to the practice will show a denial remark code (N365) for the line item on the claim containing **G8545** (and **G8549** if reported) as well as all other line items containing QDCs. N365 indicates that the code is not payable and is used for reporting/informational purposes only. Other services/codes on the claim will not be affected by the addition of a measures group-specific intent G-code or other QDCs. The N365 remark code does NOT indicate whether the QDC is accurate for that claim or for the measure the eligible professional is attempting to report, but does indicate that the QDC was processed and transmitted to the NCH.

MEASURE #85 (NQF 0396): HEPATITIS C: HCV GENOTYPE TESTING PRIOR TO TREATMENT

DESCRIPTION:

Percentage of patients aged 18 years and older with a diagnosis of chronic hepatitis C who are receiving antiviral treatment for whom HCV genotype testing was performed prior to initiation of antiviral treatment

NUMERATOR:

Patients for whom HCV genotype testing was performed prior to initiation of antiviral treatment

NUMERATOR NOTE: *The correct combination of numerator code(s) must be reported on the claim form in order to properly report this measure. The "correct combination" of codes may require the submission of multiple numerator codes.*

Numerator Quality-Data Coding Options for Reporting Satisfactorily: Hepatitis C Genotype Testing Performed

*(One CPT II code & one G-code [***3266F & G8459***] are required on the claim form to submit this numerator option)*

CPT II 3266F: Hepatitis C genotype testing documented as performed prior to initiation of antiviral treatment for Hepatitis C

AND

G8459: Clinician documented that patient is receiving antiviral treatment for Hepatitis C

OR

If patient is not eligible for this measure because patient is not receiving antiviral treatment, report:

*(One G-code [***G8458***] is required on the claim form to submit this numerator option)*

G8458: Clinician documented that patient is not an eligible candidate for genotype testing; patient not receiving antiviral treatment for Hepatitis C

OR

Genotype Testing not Performed, Reason not Otherwise Specified

*(One CPT II code & one G-code [***3266F-8P & G8459***] are required on the claim form to submit this numerator option)*

Append a reporting modifier (**8P**) to CPT Category II code **3266F** to report circumstances when the action described in the numerator is not performed and the reason is not otherwise specified. **3266F** ***with*** **8P:** Hepatitis C genotype testing was **not** documented as performed prior to initiation of antiviral treatment for Hepatitis C, reason not otherwise specified

AND

G8459: Clinician documented that patient is receiving antiviral treatment for Hepatitis C

MEASURE #87 (NQF 0398): HEPATITIS C: HCV RIBONUCLEIC ACID (RNA) TESTING AT WEEK 12 OF TREATMENT

DESCRIPTION:

Percentage of patients aged 18 years and older with a diagnosis of chronic hepatitis C who are receiving antiviral treatment for whom quantitative HCV RNA testing was performed at no greater than 12 weeks from the initiation of antiviral treatment

NUMERATOR:

Patients for whom quantitative HCV RNA testing was performed at no greater than 12 weeks from the initiation of antiviral treatment

Definition:

12 Weeks from Initiation – Patients for whom testing was performed between 4-12 weeks from the initiation of antiviral treatment will meet the numerator for this measure (depending upon the specific antiviral therapy used).

NUMERATOR NOTE: The correct combination of numerator code(s) must be reported on the claim form in order to properly report this measure. The "correct combination" of codes may require the submission of multiple numerator codes.

Numerator Quality-Data Coding Options for Reporting Satisfactorily: Hepatitis C Quantitative RNA Testing at 12 weeks

*(One CPT II code & one G-code [***3220F & G8461***] are required on the claim form to submit this numerator option)*

CPT II 3220F: Hepatitis C quantitative RNA testing documented as performed at 12 weeks from initiation of antiviral treatment

AND

G8461: Patient receiving antiviral treatment for Hepatitis C

OR

Hepatitis C Quantitative RNA Testing not Performed at 12 Weeks for Medical or Patient Reasons

*(One CPT II code & one G-code [***3220F-xP & G8461***] are required on the claim form to submit this numerator option)*

Append a modifier (**1P or 2P**) to CPT Category II code **3220F** to report documented circumstances that appropriately exclude patients from the denominator.

3220F *with* 1P: Documentation of medical reason(s) for not performing quantitative HCV RNA at 12 weeks from initiation of antiviral treatment

3220F *with* 2P: Documentation of patient reason(s) for not performing quantitative HCV RNA at 12 weeks from initiation of antiviral treatment

AND

G8461: Patient receiving antiviral treatment for Hepatitis C

OR

If patient is not eligible for this measure because patient is not receiving antiviral treatment, report:

*(One G-code [***G8460***] is required on the claim form to submit this numerator option)*

G8460: Clinician documented that patient is not an eligible candidate for quantitative RNA testing at week 12; patient not receiving antiviral treatment for Hepatitis C

OR

Hepatitis C Quantitative RNA Testing not Performed at 12 Weeks, Reason not Otherwise Specified

*(One CPT II code & one G-code [***3220F-8P & G8461***] are required on the claim form to submit this numerator option)*

Append a reporting modifier (**8P**) to CPT Category II code **3220F** to report circumstances when the action described in the numerator is not performed and the reason is not otherwise specified. **3220F *with* 8P:** Hepatitis C quantitative RNA testing was **not** documented as performed at 12 weeks from initiation of antiviral treatment, reason not otherwise specified

AND

G8461: Patient receiving antiviral treatment for Hepatitis C

MEASURE #90 (NQF 0394): HEPATITIS C: COUNSELING REGARDING USE OF CONTRACEPTION PRIOR TO ANTIVIRAL THERAPY

DESCRIPTION:

Percentage of female patients aged 18 through 44 years and all men aged 18 years and older with a diagnosis of chronic hepatitis C who are receiving antiviral treatment who were counseled regarding contraception prior to the initiation of treatment

NUMERATOR:

Patients who were counseled regarding contraception prior to the initiation of treatment

NUMERATOR NOTE: *The correct combination of numerator code(s) must be reported on the claim form in order to properly report this measure. The "correct combination" of codes may require the submission of multiple numerator codes.*

Numerator Quality-Data Coding Options for Reporting Satisfactorily: Counseling Regarding Contraception Received

*(One CPT II code & one G-code [***4159F & G8463***] are required on the claim form to submit this numerator option)*

CPT II 4159F: Counseling regarding contraception received prior to initiation of antiviral treatment

AND

G8463: Patient receiving antiviral treatment for Hepatitis C documented

OR

Counseling Regarding Contraception not Received for Medical Reason

*(One CPT II code & one G-code [***4159F-1P & G8463***] are required on the claim form to submit this numerator option)*

Append a modifier (**1P**) to CPT Category II code **4159F** to report documented circumstances that appropriately exclude patients from the denominator.

4159F *with* 1P: Documentation of medical reason(s) for not counseling patient regarding contraception

AND

G8463: Patient receiving antiviral treatment for Hepatitis C documented

OR

If patient is not eligible for this measure because patient is not receiving antiviral treatment, report:

*(One G-code [***G8462***] is required on the claim form to submit this numerator option)*

G8462: Clinician documented that patient is not an eligible candidate for counseling regarding contraception prior to antiviral treatment; patient not receiving antiviral treatment for Hepatitis C

OR

Counseling Regarding Contraception not Received, Reason not Otherwise Specified

*(One CPT II code & one G-code [***4159F-8P & G8463***] are required on the claim form to submit this numerator option)*

Append a reporting modifier (**8P**) to CPT Category II code **4159F** to report circumstances when the action described in the numerator is not performed and the reason is not otherwise specified. **4159F *with* 8P:** Counseling regarding contraception **not** received prior to initiation of antiviral treatment, reason not otherwise specified

AND

G8463: Patient receiving antiviral treatment for Hepatitis C documented

HEART FAILURE (HF) MEASURES GROUP OVERVIEW

2013 PQRS OPTIONS FOR MEASURES GROUPS: REGISTRY ONLY

2013 PQRS MEASURES IN HEART FAILURE (HF) MEASURES GROUP:

#5. Heart Failure: Angiotensin-Converting Enzyme (ACE) Inhibitor or Angiotensin Receptor Blocker (ARB) Therapy for Left Ventricular Systolic Dysfunction (LVSD)
#8. Heart Failure: Beta-Blocker Therapy for Left Ventricular Systolic Dysfunction (LVSD)
#198. Heart Failure: Left Ventricular Ejection Fraction (LVEF) Assessment
#226. Preventive Care and Screening: Tobacco Use: Screening and Cessation Intervention

INSTRUCTIONS FOR REPORTING: (These instructions apply to registry reporting. Do not report this measures group via claims.)

• It is not necessary to submit the measures group-specific intent G-code for registry-based submissions. However, the measures group-specific intent G-code has been created for registry only measures groups for use by registries that utilize claims data.

G8548: I intend to report the Heart Failure (HF) Measures Group

• Report the patient sample method:

20 Patient Sample Method: 20 unique patients (a majority of which must be Medicare Part B FFS [fee for service] patients) meeting patient sample criteria for the measures group during the reporting period (January 1 through December 31, 2013 **OR** July 1 through December 31, 2013).

• Patient sample criteria for the HF Measures Group are patients aged 18 years and older with a specific diagnosis of HF accompanied by a specific patient encounter:

One of the following diagnosis codes indicating heart failure:

ICD-9-CM: 402.01, 402.11, 402.91, 404.01, 404.03, 404.11, 404.13, 404.91, 404.93, 428.0, 428.1, 428.20, 428.21, 428.22, 428.23, 428.30, 428.31, 428.32, 428.33, 428.40, 428.41, 428.42, 428.43, 428.9

ICD-10-CM [Reference ONLY/Not Reportable]: I11.0, I13.0, I13.2, I50.1, I50.20, I50.21, I50.22, I50.23, I50.30, I50.31, I50.32, I50.33, I50.40, I50.41, I50.42, I50.43, I50.9

Accompanied by

One of the following patient encounter codes: 99201, 99202, 99203, 99204, 99205, 99212, 99213, 99214, 99215, 99304, 99305, 99306, 99307, 99308, 99309, 99310, 99324, 99325, 99326, 99327, 99328, 99334, 99335, 99336, 99337, 99341, 99342, 99343, 99344, 99345, 99347, 99348, 99349, 99350

• Report a numerator option on **all applicable** measures within the HF Measures Group for each patient within the eligible professional's patient sample.

• Instructions for qualifying numerator option reporting for each of the measures within the HF Measures Group are displayed on the next several pages. The following composite G-code has been created for registry only measures groups for use by registries that utilize claims data. This composite G-code may be reported in lieu of the individual quality-data codes for each of the measures within the group, if all quality actions for the patient have been performed for all the measures within the group. However, it is not necessary to submit the following composite G-code for registry-based submissions.

Composite G-code G8551: All quality actions for the applicable measures in the Heart Failure (HF) Measures Group have been performed for this patient

• To report satisfactorily the HF Measures Group it requires **all applicable** measures for each patient within the eligible professional's patient sample to be reported a minimum of once during the reporting period.

• Measures #5 and #8 are represented differently from the corresponding individual measures. Therefore the individual measures are specified and analyzed in a slightly different manner than the same measures contained within the measures group. Use the measure specifications as defined within the measures group for reporting purposes in order to satisfactorily report the measures group.

• Measures groups containing a measure with a 0% performance rate will not be counted as satisfactorily reporting the measures group. The recommended clinical quality action must be performed on at least one patient for each measure within the measures group reported by the eligible professional. Performance exclusion quality-data codes are not counted in the performance denominator. If the eligible professional submits all performance exclusion quality-data codes, the performance rate would be 0/0 and would be considered satisfactorily reporting.

• When using the 20 Patient Sample Method, report all applicable measures for the 20 unique patients seen a majority of which must be Medicare Part B FFS patients for the 12-month or 6-month reporting period.

MEASURE #8 (NQF 0083): HEART FAILURE: BETA-BLOCKER THERAPY FOR LEFT VENTRICULAR SYSTOLIC DYSFUNCTION (LVSD)

DESCRIPTION:

Percentage of patients aged 18 years and older with a diagnosis of heart failure (HF) with a current or prior left ventricular ejection fraction (LVEF) < 40% who were prescribed beta-blocker therapy either within a 12 month period when seen in the outpatient setting OR at **each** hospital discharge

NUMERATOR:

Patients who were prescribed beta-blocker therapy either within a 12 month period when seen in the outpatient setting or at each hospital discharge

NUMERATOR NOTE: *The reporting numerator options contained within this specification are represented differently than the corresponding individual measure. Reference this specification only in order to satisfactorily report the measures group.*

For purposes of the Heart Failure Measures Group, hospital discharge codes are not included as part of the common denominator. This measure should only be reported on those patients seen in the outpatient setting.

Numerator Instructions: The left ventricular systolic dysfunction may be determined by quantitative or qualitative assessment, which may be current or historical. Examples of a quantitative or qualitative assessment may include an echocardiogram: 1) that provides a numerical value of left ventricular systolic dysfunction or 2) that uses descriptive terms such as moderately or severely depressed left ventricular systolic function. Any current or prior ejection fraction study documenting LVSD can be used to identify patients. LVEF < 40% corresponds to qualitative documentation of moderate dysfunction or severe left ventricular systolic dysfunction.

Definitions:

Prescribed – Outpatient Setting: May include prescription given to the patient for beta-blocker therapy at one or more visits in the measurement period OR patient already taking beta-blocker therapy as documented in current medication list.

Prescribed – Inpatient Setting: May include prescription given to the patient for beta-blocker therapy at discharge OR beta-blocker therapy to be continued after discharge as documented in the discharge medication list.

Beta-blocker Therapy for Patients with Prior LVEF < 40% – Should include bisoprolol, carvedilol, or sustained release metoprolol succinate.

Numerator Options:

Beta-blocker therapy prescribed **(G8450)**

AND

Left ventricular ejection fraction (LVEF) < 40% or documentation of moderately or severely depressed left ventricular systolic function **(G8923)**

OR

Clinician documented patient with left ventricular ejection fraction (LVEF) < 40% or documentation as moderately or severely depressed left ventricular systolic function was not eligible candidate for beta-blocker therapy (e.g., low blood pressure, fluid overload, asthma, patients recently treated with an intravenous positive inotropic agent, allergy, intolerance, other medical reasons, patient declined, other patient reasons, or other reasons attributable to the healthcare system) **(G8451)**

OR

Left ventricular ejection fraction (LVEF) ≥ 40% or documentation as normal or mildly depressed left ventricular systolic function **(G8395)**

OR

Left ventricular ejection fraction (LVEF) not performed or documented **(G8396)**

OR

Beta-blocker therapy **not** prescribed **(G8452)**

AND

Left ventricular ejection fraction (LVEF) < 40% or documentation of moderately or severely depressed left ventricular systolic function **(G8923)**

MEASURE #198 (NQF 0079): HEART FAILURE: LEFT VENTRICULAR EJECTION FRACTION (LVEF) ASSESSMENT

DESCRIPTION:

Percentage of patients aged 18 years and older with a diagnosis of heart failure for whom the quantitative or qualitative results of a recent or prior (any time in the past) LVEF assessment is documented within a 12 month period

NUMERATOR:

Patients for whom the quantitative or qualitative results of a recent or prior (any time in the past) LVEF assessment is documented within a 12 month period

Numerator Instructions: The left ventricular systolic dysfunction may be determined by quantitative or qualitative assessment, which may be current or historical. Examples of a quantitative or qualitative assessment may include an echocardiogram: 1) that provides a numerical value of left ventricular systolic function or 2) that uses descriptive terms such as moderately or severely depressed left ventricular systolic function.

Documentation must include documentation in a progress note of the results of an LVEF assessment, regardless of when the evaluation of ejection fraction was performed.

Definitions:

Qualitative Results Correspond to Numeric Equivalents as Follows:

Hyperdynamic: corresponds to LVEF greater than 70%
Normal: corresponds to LVEF 50% to 70% (midpoint 60%)
Mild dysfunction: corresponds to LVEF 40% to 49% (midpoint 45%)
Moderate dysfunction: corresponds to LVEF 30% to 39% (midpoint 35%)
Severe dysfunction: corresponds to LVEF less than 30%

Numerator Options:

Left ventricular ejection fraction (LVEF) < 40% or documentation as normal or mildly depressed left ventricular systolic function **(G8738)**

OR

Left ventricular ejection fraction (LVEF) ≥ 40% or documentation of severely or moderately depressed left ventricular systolic function **(G8739)**

OR

Left ventricular ejection fraction (LVEF) **not** performed or assessed, reason not given **(G8740)**

CORONARY ARTERY DISEASE (CAD) MEASURES GROUP OVERVIEW

2013 PQRS OPTIONS FOR MEASURES GROUPS: REGISTRY ONLY

2013 PQRS MEASURES IN CORONARY ARTERY DISEASE (CAD) MEASURES GROUP:

#6. Coronary Artery Disease (CAD): Antiplatelet Therapy
#197. Coronary Artery Disease (CAD): Lipid Control
#226. Preventive Care and Screening: Tobacco Use: Screening and Cessation Intervention
#242. Coronary Artery Disease (CAD): Symptom Management

INSTRUCTIONS FOR REPORTING: (These instructions apply to registry reporting. Do not report this measures group via claims.)

• It is not necessary to submit the measures group-specific intent G-code for registry-based submissions. However, the measures group specific intent G-code has been created for registry only measure groups for use by registries that utilize claims data.

G8489: I intend to report the Coronary Artery Disease (CAD) Measures Group

• Report the patient sample method:

20 Patient Sample Method: 20 unique patients (a majority of which must be Medicare Part B FFS [fee for service] patients) meeting patient sample criteria for the measures group during the reporting period (January 1 through December 31, 2013 **OR** July 1 through December 31, 2013).

• Patient sample criteria for the CAD Measures Group are patients aged 18 years and older with a specific diagnosis of CAD accompanied by a specific patient encounter:

One of the following diagnosis codes indicating coronary artery disease:

ICD-9-CM: 410.00, 410.01, 410.02, 410.10, 410.11, 410.12, 410.20, 410.21, 410.22, 410.30, 410.31, 410.32, 410.40, 410.41, 410.42, 410.50, 410.51, 410.52, 410.60, 410.61, 410.62, 410.70, 410.71, 410.72, 410.80, 410.81, 410.82, 410.90, 410.91, 410.92, 411.0, 411.1, 411.81, 411.89, 412, 413.0, 413.1, 413.9, 414.00, 414.01, 414.02, 414.03, 414.04, 414.05, 414.06, 414.07, 414.2, 414.3, 414.8, 414.9, V45.81, V45.82

ICD-10-CM [Reference ONLY/Not Reportable]: I20.0, I20.1, I20.8, I20.9, I21.01, I21.02, I21.09, I21.11, I21.19, I21.21, I21.29, I21.3, I21.4, I22.0, I22.1, I22.2, I22.8, I22.9, I24.0, I24.1, I24.8, I24.9, I25.10, I25.110, I25.111, I25.118, I25.119, I25.2, I25.5, I25.6, I25.700, I25.701, I25.708, I25.709, I25.710, I25.711, I25.718, I25.719, I25.720, I25.721, I25.728, I25.729, I25.730, I25.731, I25.738, I25.739, I25.750, I25.751, I25.758, I25.759, I25.760, I25.761, I25.768,

I25.769, I25.790, I25.791, I25.798, I25.799, I25.82, I25.83, I25.89, I25.9, Z95.1, Z95.5, Z98.61

Accompanied by

One of the following patient encounter codes: 99201, 99202, 99203, 99204, 99205, 99212, 99213, 99214, 99215, 99304, 99305, 99306, 99307, 99308, 99309, 99310, 99324, 99325, 99326, 99327, 99328, 99334, 99335, 99336, 99337, 99341, 99342, 99343, 99344, 99345, 99347, 99348, 99349, 99350

• Report a numerator option on **all applicable** measures within the CAD Measures Group for each patient within the eligible professional's patient sample.

• Instructions for qualifying numerator option reporting for each of the measures within the CAD Measures Group are displayed on the next several pages. The following composite G-code has been created for registry only measures groups for use by registries that utilize claims data. This composite G-code may be reported in lieu of the individual quality-data codes for each of the measures within the group, if all quality actions for the patient have been performed for all the measures within the group. However, it is not necessary to submit the following composite G-code for registry-based submissions.

Composite G-code G8498: All quality actions for the applicable measures in the Coronary Artery Disease (CAD) Measures Group have been performed for this patient

• To report satisfactorily for the CAD Measures Group it requires **all applicable** measures for each patient within the eligible professional's patient sample to be reported a minimum of once during the reporting period.

• Measure #242 is represented differently from the corresponding individual measure. Therefore the individual measures are specified and analyzed in a slightly different manner than the same measures contained within the measures group. Use the measure specifications as defined within the measures group for reporting purposes in order to satisfactorily report the measures group.

• Measures groups containing a measure with a 0% performance rate will not be counted as satisfactorily reporting the measures group. The recommended clinical quality action must be performed on at least one patient for each measure within the measures group reported by the eligible professional. Performance exclusion quality-data codes are not counted in the performance denominator. If the eligible professional submits all performance exclusion quality-data codes, the performance rate would be 0/0 and would be considered satisfactorily reporting.

• When using the 20 Patient Sample Method, report all applicable measures for the 20 unique patients seen a majority of which must be Medicare Part B FFS patients for the 12-month or 6-month reporting period.

MEASURE #197 (NQF 0074): CORONARY ARTERY DISEASE (CAD): LIPID CONTROL

DESCRIPTION:

Percentage of patients aged 18 years and older with a diagnosis of coronary artery disease seen within a 12 month period who have a LDL-C result < 100 mg/dL OR patients who have a LDL-C result ≥ 100 mg/dL and have a documented plan of care to achieve LDL-C < 100 mg/dL, including at a minimum the prescription of a statin

NUMERATOR:

Patients who have a LDL-C result < 100 mg/dL OR patients who have a LDL-C result ≥ 100 mg/dL and have a documented plan of care to achieve LDL-C < 100 mg/dL, including at a minimum the prescription of a statin

Numerator Instructions: The first numerator option can be reported for patients who

have a documented LDL-C < 100 mg/dL at any time during the measurement period (if more than one result, report most current) All patients aged 18 years and older with a diagnosis of coronary artery disease must have an LDL-C result in order to satisfy the measure.

Definitions:

Documented plan of care: Includes the prescription of a statin and may also include: documentation of discussion of lifestyle modifications (diet, exercise) or scheduled re-assessment of LDL-C

Prescribed: May include prescription given to the patient for a statin at one or more visits within the measurement period OR patient already taking a statin as documented in current medication list

Numerator Options:

Most current LDL-C < 100 mg/dL **(G8736)**

OR

Most current LDL-C ≥ 100 mg/dL **(G8737)**

AND

Statin therapy prescribed or currently being taken **(4013F)**

AND

Plan of care to achieve lipid control documented **(0556F)**

OR

Most current LDL-C ≥ 100 mg/dL **(G8737)**

AND

Plan of care to achieve lipid control documented **(0556F)**

AND

Documentation of medical reason(s) for statin therapy not prescribed or currently being taken (e.g., allergy, intolerance to statin medication(s), other medical reasons) **(4013F *with 1*P)**

OR

Documentation of patient reason(s) for statin therapy not prescribed or currently being taken (e.g., patient declined, other patient reasons) **(4013F *with* 2P)**

OR

Documentation of system reason(s) for statin therapy not prescribed or currently being taken (e.g., financial reasons, other system reasons) **(4013F *with* 3P)**

OR

Most current LDL-C ≥ 100 mg/dL **(G8737)**

AND

Statin therapy **not** prescribed or currently being taken, reason not otherwise specified **(4013F *with* 8P)**

OR

Most current LDL-C ≥ 100 mg/dL **(G8737)**

AND

Plan of care to achieve lipid control **not** documented **(0556F *with* 8P)**

OR

LDL-C result not present or not within 12 months prior **(G8943)**

ISCHEMIC VASCULAR DISEASE (IVD) MEASURES GROUP OVERVIEW

2013 PQRS OPTIONS FOR MEASURES GROUPS: CLAIMS, REGISTRY

2013 PQRS MEASURES IN ISCHEMIC VASCULAR DISEASE (IVD) MEASURES GROUP:

#201. Ischemic Vascular Disease (IVD): Blood Pressure Management
#204. Ischemic Vascular Disease (IVD): Use of Aspirin or Another Antithrombotic
#226. Preventive Care and Screening: Tobacco Use: Screening and Cessation Intervention
#241. Ischemic Vascular Disease (IVD): Complete Lipid Panel and Low Density Lipoprotein (LDL-C) Control

INSTRUCTIONS FOR REPORTING: (These instructions apply to both Claims and Registry reporting, unless otherwise specified.)

• Indicate your intention to report the IVD Measures Group by submitting the measures group-specific intent G-code at least once during the reporting period when billing a patient claim for the 20 Patient Sample Method. It is not necessary to submit the measures group-specific intent G-code on more than one claim. It is not necessary to submit the measures group-specific intent G-code for registry-based submissions.

G8547: I intend to report the Ischemic Vascular Disease (IVD) Measures Group

• Select patient sample method:

20 Patient Sample Method via claims: 20 unique Medicare Part B FFS (fee for service) patients meeting patient sample criteria for the measures group.

OR

20 Patient Sample Method via registries: 20 unique patients (a majority of which must be Medicare Part B FFS patients) meeting patient sample criteria for the measures group during the reporting period (January 1 through December 31, 2013 **OR** July 1 through December 31, 2013).

• Patient sample criteria for the IVD Measures Group are patients aged 18 years and older with a specific diagnosis of IVD accompanied by a specific patient encounter OR patients aged 18 years and older with a coronary artery bypass graft (CABG) or percutaneous coronary interventions (PCI):

One of the following diagnosis codes indicating ischemic vascular disease

ICD-9-CM: 410.11, 410.21, 410.31, 410.41, 410.51, 410.61, 410.71, 410.81, 410.91, 411.0, 411.1, 411.81, 411.89, 413.0, 413.1, 413.9, 414.00, 414.01, 414.02, 414.03, 414.04, 414.05, 414.06, 414.07, 414.2, 414.8, 414.9, 429.2,

433.00, 433.01, 433.10, 433.11, 433.20, 433.21, 433.30, 433.31, 433.80, 433.81, 433.90, 433.91, 434.00, 434.01, 434.10, 434.11, 434.90, 434.91, 440.1, 440.20, 440.21, 440.22, 440.23, 440.24, 440.29, 440.4, 444.01, 444.09, 444.1, 444.21, 444.22, 444.81, 444.89, 444.9, 445.01, 445.02, 445.81, 445.89

ICD-10-CM [Reference ONLY/Not Reportable]: I20.0, I20.1, I20.8, I20.9, I21.01, I21.02, I21.09, I21.11, I21.19, I21.21, I21.29, I21.3, I21.4, I24.0, I24.1, I24.8, I24.9, I25.10, I25.110, I25.111, I25.118, I25.119, I25.5, I25.6, I25.700, I25.701, I25.708, I25.709, I25.710, I25.711, I25.718, I25.719, I25.720, I25.721, I25.728, I25.729, I25.730, I25.731, I25.738, I25.739, I25.750, I25.751, I25.758, I25.759, I25.760, I25.761, I25.768, I25.769, I25.790, I25.791, I25.798, I25.799, I25.810, I25.811, I25.812, I25.82, I25.89, I25.9, I63.00, I63.011, I63.012, I63.019, I63.02, I63.031, I63.032, I63.039, I63.09, I63.10, I63.111, I63.112, I63.119, I63.12, I63.131, I63.132, I63.139, I63.19, I63.20, I63.211, I63.212, I63.219, I63.22, I63.231, I63.232, I63.239, I63.29, I63.30, I63.311, I63.312, I63.319, I63.321, I63.322, I63.329, I63.331, I63.332, I63.339, I63.341, I63.342, I63.349, I63.39, I63.40, I63.411, I63.412, I63.419, I63.421, I63.422, I63.429, I63.431, I63.432, I63.439, I63.441, I63.442, I63.449, I63.49, I63.50, I63.511, I63.512, I63.519, I63.521, I63.522, I63.529, I63.531, I63.532, I63.539, I63.541, I63.542, I63.549, I63.59, I63.6, I63.8, I63.9, I65.01, I65.02, I65.03, I65.09, I65.1, I65.21, I65.22, I65.23, I65.29, I65.8, I65.9, I66.01, I66.02, I66.03, I66.09, I66.11, I66.12, I66.13, I66.19, I66.21, I66.22, I66.23, I66.29, I66.3, I66.8, I66.9, I70.1, I70.201, I70.202, I70.203, I70.208, I70.209, I70.211, I70.212, I70.213, I70.218, I70.219, I70.221, I70.222, I70.223, I70.228, I70.229, I70.231, I70.232, I70.233, I70.234, I70.235, I70.238, I70.239, I70.241, I70.242, I70.243, I70.244, I70.245, I70.248, I70.249, I70.25, I70.261, I70.262, I70.263, I70.268, I70.269, I70.291, I70.292, I70.293, I70.298, I70.299, I70.92, I74.01, I74.09, I74.10, I74.11, I74.19, I74.2, I74.3, I74.4, I74.5, I74.8, I74.9, I75.011, I75.012, I75.013, I75.019, I75.021, I75.022, I75.023, I75.029, I75.81, I75.89

Accompanied by

One of the following patient encounter codes: 99201, 99202, 99203, 99204, 99205, 99211, 99212, 99213, 99214, 99215, 99217, 99218, 99219, 99220, 99341, 99342, 99343, 99344, 99345, 99347, 99348, 99349, 99350, 99455, 99456, G0402

OR

One of the following coronary artery bypass graft (CABG) or percutaneous coronary interventions (PCI) surgical procedure codes: 33140, 33510, 33511, 33512, 33513, 33514, 33516, 33517, 33518, 33519, 33521, 33522, 33523, 33533, 33534, 33535, 33536 92920, 92924, 92928, 92933, 92937, 92941, 92943

- Measure #201: IVD Blood Pressure Management contains patient demographic criteria specific to the measure. For example, the age criterion is only applicable *to patients 18-75 years* within the sample population.

- Report quality-data codes (QDCs) on **all applicable** measures within the IVD Measures Group for each patient within the eligible professional's patient sample.

• Instructions for quality-data code reporting for each of the measures within the IVD Measures Group are displayed on the next several pages. If all quality actions for the patient have been performed for all the measures within the group, the following composite G-code may be reported in lieu of the individual quality-data codes for each of the measures within the group. It is not necessary to submit the following composite G-code for registry-based submissions.

Composite G-code G8552: All quality actions for the applicable measures in the Ischemic Vascular Disease (IVD) Measures Group have been performed for this patient

• To report satisfactorily the IVD Measures Group requires **all applicable** measures for each patient within the eligible professional's patient sample to be reported a minimum of once during the reporting period.

• Measures groups containing a measure with a 0% performance rate will not be counted as satisfactorily reporting the measures group. The recommended clinical quality action must be performed on at least one patient for each measure within the measures group reported by the eligible professional. Performance exclusion quality-data codes are not counted in the performance denominator. If the eligible professional submits all performance exclusion quality-data codes, the performance rate would be 0/0 and would be considered satisfactorily reporting. If a measure within a measures group is not applicable to a patient, the patient would not be counted in the performance denominator for that measure (e.g., Preventive Care Measures Group - Measure #39: Screening or Therapy for Osteoporosis for Women Aged 65 Years and Older would not be applicable to male patients according to the patient sample criteria). If the measure is not applicable for all patients within the sample, the performance rate would be 0/0 and would be considered satisfactorily reporting.

• When using the 20 Patient Sample Method via claims, report all measures for the 20 unique Medicare Part B FFS patients seen. When using the 20 Patient Sample Method via registries, report all measures for the 20 unique patients seen, a majority of which must be Medicare Part B FFS patients.

• For claims-based submissions, the Carrier/MAC remittance advice notice sent to the practice will show a denial remark code (N365) for the line item on the claim containing **G8547** (and **G8552** if reported) as well as all other line items containing QDCs. N365 indicates that the code is not payable and is used for reporting/informational purposes only. Other services/codes on the claim will not be affected by the addition of a measures group-specific intent G-code or other QDCs. The N365 remark code does NOT indicate whether the QDC is accurate for that claim or for the measure the eligible professional is attempting to report, but does indicate that the QDC was processed and transmitted to the NCH.

MEASURE #201 (NQF 0073): ISCHEMIC VASCULAR DISEASE (IVD): BLOOD PRESSURE MANAGEMENT

DESCRIPTION:

Percentage of patients aged 18 to 75 years with Ischemic Vascular Disease (IVD) who had most recent blood pressure in control (less than 140/90 mmHg)

NUMERATOR:

Patients whose most recent blood pressure < 140/90 mmHg

Numerator Instructions: To describe both systolic and diastolic blood pressure values, **each must be reported separately**. If there are multiple blood pressures on the same date of service, use the lowest systolic and lowest diastolic blood pressure on that date as the representative blood pressure.

NUMERATOR NOTE: The performance period for this measure is 12 months.

Numerator Quality-Data Coding Options for Reporting Satisfactorily: Most Recent Blood Pressure Measurement Performed

Systolic Pressure **(Select one (1) code from this section): G8588:** Most recent systolic blood pressure < 140 mmHg

OR

G8589: Most recent systolic blood pressure ≥ 140 mmHg

AND

Diastolic Pressure **(Select one (1) code from this section): G8590:** Most recent diastolic blood pressure < 90 mmHg

OR

G8591: Most recent diastolic blood pressure ≥ 90 mmHg

OR

Blood Pressure Measurement not Documented, Reason not Given G8592: No documentation of blood pressure measurement, reason not given

MEASURE #204 (NQF 0068): ISCHEMIC VASCULAR DISEASE (IVD): USE ASPIRIN OR ANOTHER ANTITHROMBOTIC

DESCRIPTION:

Percentage of patients aged 18 years and older with Ischemic Vascular Disease (IVD) with documented use of aspirin or another antithrombotic

NUMERATOR:

Patients who are using aspirin or another antithrombotic therapy

Numerator Instructions: Oral antithrombotic therapy consists of aspirin, clopidogrel or combination of aspirin and extended release dipyridamole

NUMERATOR NOTE: The performance period for this measure is 12 months.

Numerator Quality-Data Coding Options for Reporting Satisfactorily: Aspirin or Another Antithrombotic Therapy Used

G8598: Aspirin or another antithrombotic therapy used

OR

Aspirin or Another Antithrombotic Therapy not Used, Reason not Given
G8599: Aspirin or another antithrombotic therapy **not** used, reason not given

MEASURE #241 (NQF 0075): ISCHEMIC VASCULAR DISEASE (IVD): COMPLETE LIPID PANEL AND LOW DENSITY LIPOPROTEIN (LDL-C) CONTROL

DESCRIPTION:

Percentage of patients aged 18 years and older with Ischemic Vascular Disease (IVD) who received at least one lipid profile within 12 months and whose most recent LDL-C level was in control (less than 100 mg/dL)

NUMERATOR:

Patients who received at least one lipid profile (or ALL component tests) with most recent LDL-C < 100 mg/dL

NUMERATOR NOTE:

The performance period for this measure is 12 months from the date of service.

Numerator Quality-Data Coding Options for Reporting Satisfactorily: Lipid Profile Performed and Most Recent LDL-C < 100 mg/dL

*(Two CPT II codes [***G8593 & G8595***] are required on the claim form to submit this numerator option)*

G8593: Lipid panel results documented and reviewed (must include total cholesterol, HDL-C, triglycerides and calculated LDL-C)

Note: If LDL-C could not be calculated due to high triglycerides, count as complete lipid profile.

AND

G8595: Most recent LDL-C < 100 mg/dL

OR

Lipid Profile not Performed, Reason not Given

*(One CPT II code [***G8594***] is required on the claim form to submit this numerator option)* **G8594:** Lipid profile **not** performed, reason not given

OR

Most Recent LDL-C ≥ 100 mg/dL

*(Two CPT II codes [***G8593 & G8597***] are required on the claim form to submit this numerator option)*

G8593: Lipid panel results documented and reviewed (must include total cholesterol, HDL-C, triglycerides and calculated LDL-C)

AND

G8597: Most recent LDL-C ≥ 100 mg/dL

HIV/AIDS MEASURES GROUP OVERVIEW

2013 PQRS OPTIONS FOR MEASURES GROUPS: REGISTRY ONLY

2013 PQRS MEASURES IN HIV/AIDS MEASURES GROUP:

#159. HIV/AIDS: CD4+ Cell Count or CD4+ Percentage
#160. HIV/AIDS: Pneumocystis Jiroveci Pneumonia (PCP) Prophylaxis
#161. HIV/AIDS: Adolescent and Adult Patients with HIV/AIDS Who Are Prescribed Potent Antiretroviral Therapy
#162. HIV/AIDS: HIV RNA Control After Six Months of Potent Antiretroviral Therapy
#205. HIV/AIDS: Sexually Transmitted Disease Screening for Chlamydia and Gonorrhea
#208. HIV/AIDS: Sexually Transmitted Disease Screening for Syphilis

INSTRUCTIONS FOR REPORTING: (These instructions apply to registry reporting. Do not report this measures group via claims.)

• It is not necessary to submit the measures group-specific intent G-code for registry-based submissions. However, the measures group-specific intent G-code has been created for registry only measures groups for use by registries that utilize claims data.

G8491: I intend to report the HIV/AIDS Measures Group

• Report the patient sample method:

20 Patient Sample Method: 20 unique patients (a majority of which must be Medicare Part B FFS [fee for service] patients) meeting patient sample criteria for the measures group during the reporting period (January 1 through December 31, 2013 **OR** July 1 through December 31, 2013).

• Patient sample criteria for the HIV/AIDS Measures Group are patients aged 13 years and older with a specific diagnosis of HIV/AIDS accompanied by a specific patient encounter:

One of the following diagnosis codes indicating HIV/AIDS: ICD-9-CM: 042, V08

ICD-10-CM [Reference ONLY/Not Reportable]: Z21, B20

Accompanied by

One of the following patient encounter codes: 99201, 99202, 99203, 99204, 99205, 99212, 99213, 99214, 99215, G0402

• Report a numerator option on **all** measures within the HIV/AIDS Measures Group for each patient within the eligible professional's patient sample.

• Instructions for qualifying numerator option reporting for each of the measures within the HIV/AIDS Measures Group are displayed on the next several pages. The following composite G-code has been created for registry only measures groups for use by registries that utilize claims data. This composite G-code may be reported in lieu of the individual quality-data codes for each of the measures within the group, if all quality actions for the patient have been performed for all the measures within the group. However, it is not necessary to submit the following composite G-code for registry-based submissions.

Composite G-code G8500: All quality actions for the applicable measures in the HIV/AIDS Measures Group have been performed for this patient

• To report satisfactorily for the HIV/AIDS Measures Group it requires **all** measures for each patient within the eligible professional's patient sample to be reported a minimum of once during the reporting period. Measure #159 will be reported once during the reporting period for measures group purposes.

• Measures #160, #161 and #162 are represented differently from the corresponding individual measures. Therefore the individual measures are specified and analyzed in a slightly different manner than the same measures contained within the measures group. Use the measure specifications as defined within the measures group for reporting purposes in order to satisfactorily report the measures group.

• Measures groups containing a measure with a 0% performance rate will not be counted as satisfactorily reporting the measures group. The recommended clinical quality action must be performed on at least one patient for each measure within the measures group reported by the eligible professional. Performance exclusion quality-data codes are not counted in the performance denominator. If the eligible professional submits all performance exclusion quality-data codes, the performance rate would be 0/0 and would be considered satisfactorily reporting.

• When using the 20 Patient Sample Method, report all applicable measures for the 20 unique patients seen a majority of which must be Medicare Part B FFS patients for the 12-month or 6-month reporting period.

ASTHMA MEASURES GROUP OVERVIEW

2013 PQRS OPTIONS FOR MEASURES GROUPS: CLAIMS, REGISTRY

2013 PQRS MEASURES IN ASTHMA MEASURES GROUP:

#53. Asthma: Pharmacologic Therapy for Persistent Asthma – Ambulatory Care Setting
#64. Asthma: Assessment of Asthma Control – Ambulatory Care Setting
#231. Asthma: Tobacco use: Screening – Ambulatory Care Setting
#232. Asthma: Tobacco Use: Intervention – Ambulatory Care Setting

INSTRUCTIONS FOR REPORTING: (These instructions apply to both Claims and Registry reporting, unless otherwise specified.)

• Indicate your intention to report the Asthma Measures Group by submitting the measures group-specific intent G-code at least once during the reporting period when billing a patient claim for the 20 Patient Sample Method. It is not necessary to submit the measures group-specific intent G-code on more than one claim. It is not necessary to submit the measures group-specific intent G-code for registry-based submissions.

G8645: I intend to report the Asthma Measures Group

• Select patient sample method:

20 Patient Sample Method via claims: 20 unique Medicare Part B FFS (fee for service) patients meeting patient sample criteria for the measures group.

OR

20 Patient Sample Method via registries: 20 unique patients (a majority of which must be Medicare Part B FFS patients) meeting patient sample criteria for the measures group during the reporting period (January 1 through December 31, 2013 **OR** July 1 through December 31, 2013).

• Patient sample criteria for the Asthma Measures Group are patients aged 5 through 50 years with a specific diagnosis of Asthma accompanied by a specific patient encounter:

Diagnosis for asthma

ICD-9-CM: 493.00, 493.01, 493.02, 493.10, 493.11, 493.12, 493.20, 493.21, 493.22, 493.81, 493.82, 493.90, 493.91, 493.92

ICD-10-CM [Reference ONLY/Not Reportable]: J45.20, J45.21, J45.22, J45.30, J45.31, J45.32,

J45.40, J45.41, J45.42, J45.50, J45.51, J45.52, J45.901, J45.902, J45.909, J45.990, J45.991, J45.998

Accompanied by

One of the following patient encounter codes: 99201, 99202, 99203, 99204, 99205, 99212, 99213, 99214, 99215, 99341, 99342, 99343, 99344, 99345, 99347, 99348, 99349, 99350

• Report quality-data codes (QDCs) on **all applicable** measures within the Asthma Measures Group for each patient within the sample.

• Instructions for quality-data code reporting for each of the measures within the Asthma Measures Group are displayed on the next several pages. If all quality actions for the patient have been performed for all the measures within the group, the following composite G-code may be reported in lieu of the individual quality-data codes for each of the measures within the group. It is not necessary to submit the following composite G-code for registry-based submissions.

Composite G-code G8646: All quality actions for the applicable measures in the Asthma Measures Group have been performed for this patient

• To report satisfactorily the Asthma Measures Group requires **all applicable** measures for each patient within the eligible professional's patient sample to be reported a minimum of once during the reporting period.

• Measures groups containing a measure with a 0% performance rate will not be counted as satisfactorily reporting the measures group. The recommended clinical quality action must be performed on at least one patient for each measure within the measures group reported by the eligible professional. Performance exclusion quality-data codes are not counted in the performance denominator. If the eligible professional submits all performance exclusion quality-data codes, the performance rate would be 0/0 and would be considered satisfactorily reporting.

• When using the 20 Patient Sample Method via claims, report all measures for the 20 unique Medicare Part B FFS patients seen. When using the 20 Patient Sample Method via registries, report all measures for the 20 unique patients seen, a majority of which must be Medicare Part B FFS patients.

• For claims-based submissions, the Carrier/MAC remittance advice notice sent to the practice will show a denial remark code (N365) for the line item on the claim containing **G8485** (and **G8494** if reported) as well as all other line items containing QDCs. N365 indicates the code is not payable and is used for reporting/informational purposes only. Other services/codes on the claim will not be affected by the addition of a measures group-specific intent G-code or other QDCs. The N365 remark code does NOT indicate whether the QDC is accurate for that claim or for the measure the eligible professional is attempting to report, but does indicate that the QDC was processed and transmitted to the NCH.

MEASURE #232: ASTHMA: TOBACCO USE: INTERVENTION - AMBULATORY CARE SETTING

DESCRIPTION:

Percentage of patients (or their primary caregiver) aged 5 through 50 years with a diagnosis of asthma who were identified as tobacco users (patients who currently use tobacco AND patients who do not currently use tobacco, but are exposed to second hand smoke in their home environment) who received tobacco cessation intervention at least once during the one-year measurement period

NUMERATOR:

Patients (or their primary caregiver) who received tobacco use cessation intervention

Numerator Instructions: Practitioners providing tobacco cessation interventions to a pediatric patient's primary caregiver are still numerator compliant even if the primary caregiver is not the source of second hand smoke in the home.

Definitions:

Tobacco Users – Tobacco users include patients who currently use tobacco AND patients who do not currently use tobacco, but are exposed to second hand smoke in their home environment. **Tobacco Use Cessation Intervention** – May include brief counseling (3 minutes or less) and/or pharmacotherapy.

NUMERATOR NOTE: For the purpose of this measure, "tobacco user" refers to tobacco smokers and "tobacco non-user" refers to non-smokers (including smokeless tobacco users e.g., chew, snuff).

Numerator Quality-Data Coding Options for Reporting Satisfactorily: Patients who Received Tobacco Use Cessation Intervention

*(Two CPT II codes [***40xxF & 1032F***] are required on the claim form to submit this numerator option)*

CPT II 4000F: Tobacco use cessation intervention, counseling

OR

CPT II 4001F: Tobacco use cessation intervention, pharmacologic therapy

AND

Current Tobacco Smoker OR Current Exposure to Second Hand Smoke

CPT II 1032F: Current tobacco smoker OR currently exposed to second hand smoke

OR

If patient is not eligible for this measure because patient is a non-tobacco user AND has no exposure to second hand smoke, report:

*(One CPT II code [***1033F***] is required on the claim form to submit this numerator option)*

CPT II 1033F: Current tobacco non-smoker AND not currently exposed to second hand smoke

OR

Tobacco Use, not Assessed, Reason Not Given

*(One G-code [***G8751***] is required on the claim form to submit this numerator option)*

G8751: Smoking status and exposure to second hand smoke in the home **not** assessed, reason not given

OR

Tobacco Use Cessation Intervention not Performed, Reason not Otherwise Specified Append a reporting modifier (**8P**) to CPT Category II code **4000F OR 4001F** to report circumstances when the action described in the numerator is not performed and the reason is not otherwise specified.

*(Two CPT II codes [***400xF-8P & 1032F***] are required on the claim form to submit this numerator option)*

4000F *with* 8P: Tobacco use cessation intervention, counseling, **not** performed, reason not otherwise specified

OR

4001F *with* 8P: Tobacco use cessation intervention, pharmacologic therapy, **not** performed, reason not otherwise specified

AND

Current Tobacco Smoker OR Currently Exposed to Second Hand Smoke

CPT II 1032F: Current tobacco smoker OR currently exposed to second hand smoke

CHRONIC OBSTRUCTIVE PULMONARY DISEASE (COPD) MEASURES GROUP OVERVIEW

2013 PQRS OPTIONS FOR MEASURES GROUPS: CLAIMS, REGISTRY

2013 PQRS MEASURES IN COPD MEASURES GROUP:

#51. Chronic Obstructive Pulmonary Disease (COPD): Spirometry Evaluation
#52. Chronic Obstructive Pulmonary Disease (COPD): Bronchodilator Therapy
#110. Preventive Care and Screening: Influenza Immunization
#111. Preventive Care and Screening: Pneumococcal Vaccination for Patients 65 Years and Older
#226. Preventive Care and Screening: Tobacco Use: Screening and Cessation Intervention

INSTRUCTIONS FOR REPORTING: (These instructions apply to both Claims and Registry reporting, unless otherwise specified.)

• Indicate your intention to report the COPD Measures Group by submitting the measures group-specific intent G-code at least once during the reporting period when billing a patient claim for the 20 Patient Sample Method. It is not necessary to submit the measures group-specific intent G-code on more than one claim. It is not necessary to submit the measures group-specific intent G-code for registry-based submissions.

G8898: I intend to report the COPD Measures Group

• elect patient sample method:

20 Patient Sample Method via claims: 20 unique Medicare Part B FFS (fee for service) patients meeting patient sample criteria for the measures group.

OR

20 Patient Sample Method via registries: 20 unique patients (a majority of which must be Medicare Part B FFS patients) meeting patient sample criteria for the measures group during the reporting period (January 1 through December 31, 2013 **OR** July 1 through December 31, 2013).

• Patient sample criteria for the COPD Measures Group are patients aged ≥ 18 years with a specific diagnosis of COPD accompanied by a specific patient encounter:

One of the following diagnosis codes indicating COPD:

ICD-9-CM: 491.0, 491.1, 491.20, 491.21, 491.22, 491.8, 491.9, 492.0, 492.8, 493.20, 493.21, 493.22, 496

ICD-10-CM [Reference ONLY/Not Reportable]: J41.0, J41.1, J41.8, J42, J43.0, J43.1, J43.2, J43.8, J43.9, J44.0, J44.1, J44.9

Accompanied by

One of the following patient encounter codes: 99201, 99202, 99203, 99204, 99205, 99212, 99213, 99214, 99215

• Report quality-data codes (QDCs) on **all applicable** measures within the COPD Measures Group for each patient within the eligible professional's patient sample.

• Measure #111 is only applicable for patients aged 65 years and older.

• Measure #110 need only be reported a minimum of once during the reporting period when the patient's visit included in the patient sample population is between January and March for the 2012-2013 influenza season **OR** between October and December for the 2013-2014 influenza season. When the patient's office visit is between April and September, Measure #110 is not applicable and will not affect the eligible provider's reporting or performance rate. Measure #110 need only be reported on patients 18 years and older.

• Instructions for quality-data code reporting for each of the measures within the COPD Measures Group are displayed on the next several pages. If all quality actions for the patient have been performed for all measures within the group, the following composite G-code may be reported in lieu of the individual quality-data codes for each of the measures within the group. It is not necessary to submit the following composite G-code for registry-based submissions.

Composite G-code G8757: All quality actions for the applicable measures in the COPD Measures Group have been performed for this patient

• To report satisfactorily for the COPD Measures Group it requires **all applicable** measures for each patient within the eligible professional's patient sample to be reported a minimum of once during the reporting period.

• Measures groups containing a measure with a 0% performance rate will not be counted as satisfactorily reporting the measures group. The recommended clinical quality action must be performed on at least one patient for each measure within the measures group reported by the eligible professional. Performance exclusion quality-data codes are not counted in the performance denominator. If the eligible professional submits all performance exclusion quality-data codes, the performance rate would be 0/0 and would be considered satisfactorily reporting. If a measure within a measures group is not applicable to a patient, the patient would not be counted in the performance denominator for that measure (e.g., Preventive Care Measures Group - Measure #39: Screening or Therapy for Osteoporosis for Women Aged 65 Years and Older would not be applicable to male patients according to the patient sample criteria). If the measure is not applicable for all patients within the sample, the performance rate would be 0/0 and would be considered satisfactorily reporting.

• When using the 20 Patient Sample Method via claims, report all measures for the 20 unique Medicare Part B FFS patients seen. When using the 20 Patient

Sample Method via registries, report all measures for the 20 unique patients seen, a majority of which must be Medicare Part B FFS patients.

• For claims-based submissions, the Carrier/MAC remittance advice notice sent to the practice will show a denial remark code (N365) for the line item on the claim containing **G8546** (and **G8550** if reported) as well as all other line items containing QDCs. N365 indicates that the code is not payable and is used for reporting/informational purposes only. Other services/codes on the claim will not be affected by the addition of a measures group-specific intent G-code or other QDCs. The N365 remark code does NOT indicate whether the QDC is accurate for that claim or for the measure the eligible professional is attempting to report, but does indicate that the QDC was processed and transmitted to the NCH.

MEASURE #52 (NQF 0102): CHRONIC OBSTRUCTIVE PULMONARY DISEASE (COPD): BRONCHODILATOR THERAPY

DESCRIPTION:

Percentage of patients aged 18 years and older with a diagnosis of COPD and who have an FEV /FVC less than 60% and have symptoms who were prescribed an inhaled bronchodilator

NUMERATOR:

Patients who were prescribed an inhaled bronchodilator

Definition:

Prescribed – Includes patients who are currently receiving medication(s) that follow the treatment plan recommended at an encounter during the reporting period, even if the prescription for that medication was ordered prior to the encounter.

NUMERATOR NOTE: *The correct combination of numerator code(s) must be reported on the claim form in order to properly report this measure. The "correct combination" of codes may require the submission of multiple numerator codes.*

Numerator Quality-Data Coding Options for Reporting Satisfactorily: Patient Prescribed Inhaled Bronchodilator Therapy

*(One CPT II code [***4025F***] & one G code [***G8924***] are required on the claim form to submit this numerator option)*

CPT II 4025F: Inhaled bronchodilator prescribed

AND

G8924: Spirometry test results demonstrate FEV /FVC < 60% with COPD symptoms (e.g., dyspnea, cough/sputum, wheezing)

OR

Patient not Documented to have Inhaled Bronchodilator Prescribed for Medical, Patient, or System Reasons

*(One CPT II code [***4025F-xP***] & one G code [***G8924***] are required on the claim form to submit this numerator option)*

Append a modifier (**1P, 2P or 3P**) to CPT Category II code **4025F** to report documented circumstances that appropriately exclude patients from the denominator.

4025F *with* 1P: Documentation of medical reason(s) for not prescribing an inhaled bronchodilator **4025F *with* 2P:** Documentation of patient reason(s) for not prescribing an inhaled bronchodilator **4025F *with* 3P:** Documentation of system reason(s) for not prescribing an inhaled bronchodilator

AND

G8924: Spirometry test results demonstrate FEV /FVC < 60% with COPD symptoms (e.g., dyspnea, cough/sputum, wheezing)

OR

If patient is not eligible for this measure because spirometry results demonstrate FEV /FVC ≥ 60% or patient does not have COPD symptoms, report:

Spirometry Results Demonstrate FEV /FVC ≥ 60% or Patient does not have COPD symptoms

*(One G-Code [***G8925 or G8926***] is required on the claim form to submit this numerator option)* **G8925:** Spirometry test results demonstrate FEV /FVC ≥ 60% or patient does not have COPD symptoms

OR

Spirometry Test not Performed or Documented

G8926: Spirometry test **not** performed or documented, reason not given

OR

Patient not Documented to have Inhaled Bronchodilator Prescribed, Reason not Otherwise Specified

*(One CPT II code [***4025F-8P***] & one G-Code [***G8924***] are required on the claim form to submit this numerator option)*

Append a reporting modifier (**8P**) to CPT Category II code **4025F** to report circumstances when the action described in the numerator is not performed and the reason is not otherwise specified. **4025F *with* 8P:** Inhaled bronchodilator **not** prescribed, reason not otherwise specified

AND

G8924: Spirometry test results demonstrate FEV /FVC < 60% with COPD symptoms (e.g., dyspnea, cough/sputum, wheezing)

MEASURE #110 (NQF 0041): PREVENTIVE CARE AND SCREENING: INFLUENZA IMMUNIZATION

DESCRIPTION:

Percentage of patients aged 6 months and older seen for a visit between October 1 and March 31 who received an influenza immunization OR who reported previous receipt of an influenza immunization

NUMERATOR:

Patients who received an influenza immunization OR who reported previous receipt of influenza immunization

Numerator Instructions:

- If reporting this measure between January 1, 2013 and March 31, 2013, G-code **G8482** should be reported when the influenza immunization is ordered or administered to the patient during the months of August, September, October, November, and December of 2012 or January, February, and March of 2013 for the flu season ending March 31, 2013.

- If reporting this measure between October 1, 2013 and December 31, 2013, G-code **G8482** should be reported when the influenza immunization is ordered or administered to the patient during the months of August, September, October, November, and December of 2013 for the flu season ending March 31, 2014.

- Influenza immunizations administered during the month of August or September of a given flu season (either 2012-2013 flu season OR 2013-2014 flu season) can be reported when a visit occurs during the flu season (October 1 - March 31). In these cases, **G8482** should be reported.

Definition:

Previous Receipt - Receipt of the current season's influenza immunization from another provider OR from same provider prior to the visit to which the measure is applied (typically, prior vaccination would include influenza vaccine given since August 1st).

Numerator Quality-Data Coding Options for Reporting Satisfactorily: Influenza Immunization Administered

G8482: Influenza immunization administered or previously received

OR

Influenza Immunization not Administered for Documented Reasons

G8483: Influenza immunization was not ordered or administered for reasons documented by clinician (e.g., patient allergy or other medical reason, patient declined or other patient reasons, or other system reasons)

OR

Influenza Immunization Ordered or Recommended, but not Administered

G0919: Influenza immunization ordered or recommended (to be given at alternate location or alternate provider); vaccine not available at time of visit

OR

Influenza Immunization not Administered, Reason not Given

G8484: Influenza immunization was **not** ordered or administered, reason not given

INFLAMMATORY BOWEL DISEASE (IBD) MEASURES GROUP OVERVIEW

2013 PQRS OPTIONS FOR MEASURES GROUPS: REGISTRY ONLY

2013 PQRS MEASURES IN INFLAMMATORY BOWEL DISEASE (IBD) MEASURES GROUP:

#226. Preventive Care and Screening: Tobacco Use: Screening and Cessation Intervention
#269. Inflammatory Bowel Disease (IBD): Type, Anatomic Location and Activity All Documented
#270. Inflammatory Bowel Disease (IBD): Preventive Care: Corticosteroid Sparing Therapy
#271. Inflammatory Bowel Disease (IBD): Preventive Care: Corticosteroid Related Iatrogenic Injury – Bone Loss Assessment
#272. Inflammatory Bowel Disease (IBD): Preventive Care: Influenza Immunization
#273. Inflammatory Bowel Disease (IBD): Preventive Care: Pneumococcal Immunization
#274. Inflammatory Bowel Disease (IBD): Testing for Latent Tuberculosis (TB) Before Initiating Anti-TNF (Tumor Necrosis Factor) Therapy
#275. Inflammatory Bowel Disease (IBD): Assessment of Hepatitis B Virus (HBV) Status Before Initiating Anti-TNF (Tumor Necrosis Factor) Therapy

INSTRUCTIONS FOR REPORTING: (These instructions apply to registry reporting. Do not report this measures group via claims.)

• It is not necessary to submit the measures group-specific intent G-code for registry-based submissions. However, the measures group-specific intent G-code has been created for registry only measures groups for use by registries that utilize claims data.

G8899: I intend to report the Inflammatory Bowel Disease (IBD) Measures Group

• Report the patient sample method:

20 Patient Sample Method: 20 unique patients (a majority of which must be Medicare Part B FFS [fee for service] patients) meeting patient sample criteria for the measures group during the reporting period (January 1 through December 31, 2013 **OR** July 1 through December 31, 2013).

• Patient sample criteria for the IBD Measures Group are patients aged 18 years and older with a specific diagnosis of IBD accompanied by a specific patient encounter:

One of the following diagnosis codes indicating IBD:

ICD-9-CM: 555.0, 555.1, 555.2, 555.9, 556.0, 556.1, 556.2, 556.3, 556.4, 556.5, 556.6, 556.8, 556.9

ICD-10-CM [Reference ONLY/Not Reportable]: K50.00, K50.011, K50.012, K50.013, K50.014, K50.018, K50.019, K50.10, K50.111, K50.112, K50.113, K50.114, K50.118, K50.119, K50.80, K50.811, K50.812, K50.813, K50.814, K50.818, K50.819, K50.90, K50.911, K50.912, K50.913, K50.914, K50.918, K50.919, K51.00, K51.011, K51.012, K51.013, K51.014, K51.018, K51.019, K51.20, K51.211, K51.212, K51.213, K51.214, K51.218, K51.219, K51.30, K51.311, K51.312, K51.313, K51.314, K51.318, K51.319, K51.40, K51.411, K51.412, K51.413, K51.414, K51.418, K51.419, K51.50, K51.511, K51.512, K51.513, K51.514, K51.518, K51.519, K51.80, K51.811, K51.812, K51.813, K51.814, K51.818, K51.819, K51.90, K51.911, K51.912, K51.913, K51.914, K51.918, K51.919

Accompanied by

One of the following patient encounter codes: 99201, 99202, 99203, 99204, 99205, 99212, 99213, 99214, 99215, 99406, 99407

• Report a numerator option on **all** measures within the IBD Measures Group for each patient within the eligible professional's patient sample.

• Instructions for qualifying numerator option reporting for each of the measures within the IBD Measures Group are displayed on the next several pages. The following composite G-code has been created for registry only measures groups for use by registries that utilize claims data. This composite G-code may be reported in lieu of the individual quality-data codes for each of the measures within the group, if all quality actions for the patient have been performed for all the measures within the group. However, it is not necessary to submit the following composite G-code for registry-based submissions.

Composite G-code G8758: All quality actions for the applicable measures in the Inflammatory Bowel Disease (IBD) Measures Group have been performed for this patient

• To report satisfactorily the IBD Measures Group it requires **all** measures for each patient within the eligible professional's patient sample to be reported a minimum of once during the reporting period.

• Measures groups containing a measure with a 0% performance rate will not be counted as satisfactorily reporting the measures group. The recommended clinical quality action must be performed on at least one patient for each measure within the measures group reported by the eligible professional. Performance exclusion quality-data codes are not counted in the performance denominator. If the eligible professional submits all performance exclusion quality-data codes, the performance rate would be 0/0 and would be considered satisfactorily reporting.

• When using the 20 Patient Sample Method, report all applicable measures for the 20 unique patients seen a majority of which must be Medicare Part B FFS patients for the 12-month or 6-month reporting period.

MEASURE #269: INFLAMMATORY BOWEL DISEASE (IBD): TYPE, ANATOMiC LOCATION AND ACTIVITY ALL DOCUMENTED

DESCRIPTION:

Percentage of patients aged 18 years and older with a diagnosis of inflammatory bowel disease who have documented the disease type, anatomic location and activity, at least once during the reporting year

NUMERATOR:

Patients who were assessed for disease type and anatomic location and activity

Numerator Instructions: Patients are considered to have appropriate documentation of inflammatory bowel disease type, anatomic location, **and** activity if all of the following are documented:

a. Type of inflammatory bowel disease (Crohn's, ulcerative colitis or IBD-unclassified)

b. Anatomic location of disease based on current or historic endoscopic and/or radiologic data (Note: this element does not prescribe frequency of studies).

c. Luminal disease activity (quiescent, mild, moderate, severe) and presence of extraintestinal manifestations

Numerator Options:

Type, anatomic location, and activity all documented **(G0920)**

OR

Documentation of patient reason(s) for not being able to assess (e.g., patient refuses endoscopic and/or radiologic assessment) **(G0921)**

OR

No documentation of disease type, anatomic location and activity, reason not given **(G0922)**

MEASURE #270: INFLAMMATORY BOWEL DISEASE (IBD): PREVENTIVE CARE: CORTICOSTEROID SPARING THERAPY

DESCRIPTION:

Percentage of patients aged 18 years and older with a diagnosis of inflammatory bowel disease who have been managed by corticosteroids greater than or equal to 10 mg/day for 60 or greater consecutive days that have been prescribed corticosteroid sparing therapy in the last reporting year

NUMERATOR:

Patients managed with corticosteroids greater than or equal to 10 mg/day for 60 or greater consecutive days AND prescribed a corticosteroid sparing therapy (e.g., thiopurines, methotrexate, or anti-TNF agents)

Definition:

Corticosteroids - Prednisone equivalents used expressly for the treatment of IBD and not for other indications (including premedication before anti-TNF therapy, non-IBD indications) can be determined using the following: 1 mg of prednisone = 1 mg of prednisolone; 5 mg of cortisone; 4 mg of hydrocortisone; 0.8 mg of triamcinolone; 0.8 mg of methylprednisolone; 0.15 mg of dexamethasone; 0.15 mg of betamethasone.

Numerator Options:

Patient receiving corticosteroids greater than or equal to 10 mg/day for 60 or greater consecutive days **(G8859)**

AND

Corticosteroid sparing therapy prescribed **(4142F)**

OR

Patient not receiving corticosteroids greater than or equal to 10 mg/day for 60 or greater consecutive days **(3750F)**

OR

Patient receiving corticosteroids greater than or equal to 10 mg/day for 60 or greater consecutive days **(G8859)**

AND

Documentation of medical reason(s) for not treating with corticosteroid sparing therapy (e.g., benefits of continuing steroid therapy outweigh the risk of weaning patient off steroids or initiating steroid sparing therapy) **(4142F *with* 1P)**

OR

Patient receiving corticosteroids greater than or equal to 10 mg/day for 60 or greater consecutive days **(G8859)**

AND

Documentation of patient reason(s) for not treating with corticosteroid sparing therapy (e.g., patient refuses to initiate steroid sparing therapy) **(4142F *with* 2P)**

OR

Patient receiving corticosteroids greater than or equal to 10 mg/day for 60 or greater consecutive days **(G8859)**

AND

Corticosteroid sparing therapy **not** prescribed, reason not otherwise specified **(4142F *with* 8P)**

MEASURE #271: INFLAMMATORY BOWEL DISEASE (IBD): PREVENTIVE CARE: CORTICOSTEROID RELATED IATROGENIC INJURY – BONE LOSS ASSESSMENT

DESCRIPTION:

Percentage of patients aged 18 years and older with a diagnosis of inflammatory bowel disease who have received dose of corticosteroids greater than or equal to 10 mg/day for 60 or greater consecutive days and were assessed for risk of bone loss once per the reporting year

NUMERATOR:

Patients who have received dose of corticosteroids greater than or equal to 10 mg/day for 60 or greater consecutive days and who were assessed for risk of bone loss

Definitions:

Corticosteroids - Prednisone equivalents used expressly for the treatment of IBD and not for other indications (including premedication before anti-TNF therapy, non-IBD indications) can be determined using the following: 1 mg of prednisone = 1 mg of prednisolone; 5 mg of cortisone; 4 mg of hydrocortisone; 0.8 mg of triamcinolone; 0.8 mg of methylprednisolone; 0.15 mg of dexamethasone; 0.15 mg of betamethasone.

Assessed - Documentation that an assessment for risk of bone loss has been performed or ordered. This includes, but is not limited to, review of systems and medication history, and ordering of Central Dual-energy X-Ray Absorptiometry (DXA) scan.

Numerator Options:

Patients who have received dose of corticosteroids greater than or equal to 10 mg/day for 60 or greater consecutive days **(G8860)**

AND

Central Dual-energy X-Ray Absorptiometry (DXA) ordered or documented, review of systems and medication history or pharmacologic therapy (other than minerals/vitamins) for osteoporosis prescribed **(G8861)**

OR

Patients not receiving corticosteroids greater than or equal to 10 mg/day for 60 or greater consecutive days **(G8862)**

OR

Patients who have received dose of corticosteroids greater than or equal to 10 mg/day for 60 or greater consecutive days **(G8860)**

AND

Patients **not** assessed for risk of bone loss, reason not given **(G8863)**

MEASURE #273: INFLAMMATORY BOWEL DISEASE (IBD): PREVENTIVE CARE: PNEUMOCOCCAL IMMUNIZATION

DESCRIPTION:

Percentage of patients aged 18 years and older with a diagnosis of inflammatory bowel disease that had pneumococcal vaccination administered or previously received

NUMERATOR:

Patients for whom pneumococcal vaccine administered or previously received

Numerator Options:

Pneumococcal vaccine administered or previously received **(G8864)**

OR

Documentation of medical reason(s) for not administering or previously receiving pneumococcal vaccine (e.g., patient allergic reaction, potential adverse drug reaction) **(G8865)**

OR

Documentation of patient reason(s) for not administering or previously receiving pneumococcal vaccine (e.g., patient refusal) **(G8866)**

OR

Pneumococcal vaccine **not** administered or previously received, reason not given **(G8867)**

MEASURE #275: INFLAMMATORY BOWEL DISEASE (IBD): ASSESSMENT OF HEPATITIS B VIRUS (HBV) STATUS BEFORE INITIATING ANTI-TNF (TUMOR NECROSIS FACTOR) THERAPY

DESCRIPTION:

Percentage of patients aged 18 years and older with a diagnosis of inflammatory bowel disease (IBD) who had Hepatitis B Virus (HBV) status assessed and results interpreted within one year prior to receiving a first course of anti-TNF (tumor necrosis factor) therapy

NUMERATOR:

Patients who had HBV status assessed and results interpreted within one year prior to receiving a first course of anti-TNF therapy

Numerator Instructions: HBV status must be assessed by one of the following: HBsAg, HBsAg neutralization, HBcAb total, HBcAb IgM, HBsAb

Definition:

First Course of anti-TNF therapy: the first **(ever)** course of anti-TNF therapy

Numerator Options:

Hepatitis B Virus (HBV) status assessed and results interpreted within one year prior to receiving a first course of anti-TNF (tumor necrosis factor) therapy **(3517F)**

OR

Patient has documented immunity to hepatitis B and is receiving a first course of anti-TNF therapy **(G8869)**

OR

Hepatitis B vaccine injection administered or previously received and is receiving a first course of anti-TNF therapy **(G8870)**

OR

Patient not receiving a first course of anti-TNF therapy **(G8871)**

OR

Documentation of medical reason(s) for not assessing Hepatitis B Virus (HBV) (eg, potential drug interaction, potential for allergic reaction) status within one year prior to receiving first course of anti-TNF therapy **(3517F *with* 1P)**

OR

Documentation of patient reason(s) for not assessing Hepatitis B Virus (HBV) status (eg, patient declined) within one year prior to receiving first course of anti-TNF therapy **(3517F *with* 2P)**

OR

Hepatitis B Virus (HBV) status **not** assessed and results interpreted within one year prior to receiving a first course of anti-TNF (tumor necrosis factor) therapy, reason not otherwise specified **(3517F *with* 8P)**

SLEEP APNEA MEASURES GROUP OVERVIEW

2013 PQRS OPTIONS FOR MEASURES GROUP: REGISTRY ONLY

2013 PQRS MEASURES IN SLEEP APNEA MEASURES GROUP:

#276. Sleep Apnea: Assessment of Sleep Symptoms
#277. Sleep Apnea: Severity Assessment at Initial Diagnosis
#278. Sleep Apnea: Positive Airway Pressure Therapy Prescribed
#279. Sleep Apnea: Assessment of Adherence to Positive Airway Pressure Therapy

INSTRUCTIONS FOR REPORTING: (These instructions apply to registry reporting. Do not report this measures group via claims.)

• It is not necessary to submit the measures group-specific intent G-code for registry-based submissions. However, the measures group-specific intent G-code has been created for registry only measures groups for use by registries that utilize claims data.

G8900: I intend to report the Sleep Apnea Measures Group

• Report the patient sample method:

20 Patient Sample Method: 20 unique patients (a majority of which must be Medicare Part B FFS [fee for service] patients) meeting patient sample criteria for the measures group during the reporting period (January 1 through December 31, 2013 **OR** July 1 through December 31, 2013).

• Patient sample criteria for the Sleep Apnea Measures Group are patients aged 18 years and older with a specific diagnosis of Sleep Apnea accompanied by a specific patient encounter:

One of the following diagnosis codes indicating Sleep Apnea: ICD-9-CM: 327.23, 780.51, 780.53, 780.57

ICD-10-CM [Reference ONLY/Not Reportable]: G47.30, G47.33

Accompanied by

One of the following patient encounter codes: 99201, 99202, 99203, 99204, 99205, 99212, 99213, 99214, 99215

• Report a numerator option on **all** measures within the Sleep Apnea Measures Group for each patient within the eligible professional's patient sample.

• Instructions for qualifying numerator option reporting for each of the measures within the Sleep Apnea Measures Group are displayed on the next several pages. The following composite G-code has been created for registry only measures groups for use by registries that utilize claims data. This composite G-code may be reported in lieu of the individual quality-data codes for each of the measures within the group, if all quality actions for the patient have been performed for all the measures within the group. However, it is not necessary to submit the following composite G-code for registry-based submissions.

Composite G-code G8759: All quality actions for the applicable measures in the Sleep Apnea Measures Group have been performed for this patient.

• To report satisfactorily the Sleep Apnea Measures Group it requires **all** measures for each patient within the eligible professional's patient sample to be reported a minimum of once during the reporting period. In measures group reporting, measures that are based on patient visits need only be reported a minimum of once per reporting period – they do not need to be reported each visit.

• Measures groups containing a measure with a 0% performance rate will not be counted as satisfactorily reporting the measures group. The recommended clinical quality action must be performed on at least one patient for each measure within the measures group reported by the eligible professional. Performance exclusion quality-data codes are not counted in the performance denominator. If the eligible professional submits all performance exclusion quality-data codes, the performance rate would be 0/0 and would be considered satisfactorily reporting.

• When using the 20 Patient Sample Method, report all applicable measures for the 20 unique patients seen a majority of which must be Medicare Part B FFS patients for the 12-month or 6-month reporting period.

MEASURE #277: SLEEP APNEA: SEVERITY ASSESSMENT AT INITIAL DIAGNOSIS

DESCRIPTION:

Percentage of patients aged 18 years and older with a diagnosis of obstructive sleep apnea who had an apnea hypopnea index (AHI) or a respiratory disturbance index (RDI) measured at the time of initial diagnosis

NUMERATOR:

Patients who had an apnea hypopnea index (AHI) or a respiratory disturbance index (RDI) measured at the time of initial diagnosis

Definitions:

Apnea-Hypopnea Index (AHI) for Polysomnography performed in a sleep lab is defined as (Total Apneas + Hypopneas per hour of sleep); Apnea-Hypopnea Index (AHI) for a home sleep study is defined as (Total Apneas + Hypopneas per hour of monitoring)

Respiratory Disturbance Index (RDI) is defined as (Total Apneas + Hypopneas + Respiratory-Effort-Related-Arousals per hour of sleep)

Numerator Options:

Apnea hypopnea index (AHI) or respiratory disturbance index (RDI) measured at the time of initial diagnosis **(G8842)**

OR

Documentation of reason(s) for not measuring an apnea hypopnea index (AHI) or a respiratory disturbance index (RDI) at the time of initial diagnosis (e.g., abnormal anatomy, patient declined, financial, insurance coverage) **(G8843)**

OR

Apnea hypopnea index (AHI) or respiratory disturbance index (RDI) **not** measured at the time of initial diagnosis, reason not given **(G8844)**

MEASURE #278: SLEEP APNEA: POSITIVE AIRWAY PRESSURE THERAPY PRESCRIBED

DESCRIPTION:

Percentage of patients aged 18 years and older with a diagnosis of moderate or severe obstructive sleep apnea who were prescribed positive airway pressure therapy

NUMERATOR:

Patients who were prescribed positive airway pressure therapy

Definition: Moderate or severe sleep apnea is defined as apnea hypopnea index (AHI) or a respiratory disturbance index (RDI) greater than or equal to 15 episodes per hour of sleep

Numerator Options:

Positive airway pressure therapy prescribed **(G8845)**

AND

Moderate or severe obstructive sleep apnea (apnea hypopnea index (AHI) or respiratory disturbance index (RDI) of 15 or greater) **(G8846)**

OR

Mild obstructive sleep apnea (apnea hypopnea index (AHI) or respiratory disturbance index (RDI) of less than 15) **(G8848)**

OR

Documentation of reason(s) for not prescribing positive airway pressure therapy (e.g., patient unable to tolerate, alternative therapies used, patient declined, financial, insurance coverage) **(G8849)**

AND

Moderate or severe obstructive sleep apnea (apnea hypopnea index (AHI) or respiratory disturbance index (RDI) of 15 or greater) **(G8846)**

OR

Positive airway pressure therapy **not** prescribed, reason not given **(G8850)**

AND

Moderate or severe obstructive sleep apnea (apnea hypopnea index (AHI) or respiratory disturbance index (RDI) of 15 or greater) **(G8846)**

MEASURE #279: SLEEP APNEA: ASSESSMENT OF ADHERENCE TO POSITIVE AIRWAY PRESSURE THERAPY

DESCRIPTION:

Percentage of visits for patients aged 18 years and older with a diagnosis of obstructive sleep apnea who were prescribed positive airway pressure therapy who had documentation that adherence to positive airway pressure therapy was objectively measured

NUMERATOR:

Patient visits with documentation that adherence to positive airway pressure therapy was objectively measured

Definition: Objectively measured is defined as: positive airway pressure machine-generated measurement of hours of use.

Numerator Options:

Objective measurement of adherence to positive airway pressure therapy, documented **(G8851) AND**

Positive airway pressure therapy was prescribed **(G8852)**

OR

Positive airway pressure therapy not prescribed **(G8853)**

OR

Documentation of reason(s) for not objectively measuring adherence to positive airway pressure therapy (e.g., patient didn't bring data from continuous positive airway pressure [CPAP], therapy not yet initiated, not available on machine) **(G8854)**

AND

Positive airway pressure therapy was prescribed **(G8852)**

OR

Objective measurement of adherence to positive airway pressure therapy **not** performed, reason not given **(G8855)**

AND

Positive airway pressure therapy was prescribed **(G8852)**

DEMENTIA MEASURES GROUP OVERVIEW

2013 PQRS OPTIONS FOR MEASURES GROUPS: CLAIMS, REGISTRY

2013 PQRS MEASURES IN DEMENTIA MEASURES GROUP:

#280. Dementia: Staging of Dementia
#281. Dementia: Cognitive Assessment
#282. Dementia: Functional Status Assessment
#283. Dementia: Neuropsychiatric Symptom Assessment
#284. Dementia: Management of Neuropsychiatric Symptoms
#285. Dementia: Screening for Depressive Symptoms
#286. Dementia: Counseling Regarding Safety Concerns
#287. Dementia: Counseling Regarding Risks of Driving

#288. Dementia: Caregiver Education and Support

INSTRUCTIONS FOR REPORTING: (These instructions apply to both Claims and Registry reporting, unless otherwise specified.)

• Indicate your intention to report the Dementia Measures Group by submitting the measures group-specific intent G-code at least once during the reporting period when billing a patient claim for the 20 Patient Sample Method. It is not necessary to submit the measures group-specific intent G-code on more than one claim. It is not necessary to submit the measures group-specific intent G-code for registry-based submissions.

G8902: I intend to report the Dementia Measures Group

• Select patient sample method:

20 Patient Sample Method via claims: 20 unique Medicare Part B FFS (fee for service) patients meeting patient sample criteria for the measures group.

OR

20 Patient Sample Method via registries: 20 unique patients (a majority of which must be Medicare Part B FFS patients) meeting patient sample criteria for the measures group during the reporting period (January 1 through December 31, 2013 **OR** July 1 through December 31, 2013).

• Patient sample criteria for the Dementia Measures Group are all patients regardless of age, with a specific diagnosis of dementia accompanied by a specific patient encounter:

One of the following diagnosis codes indicating Dementia:

ICD-9-CM: 094.1, 290.0, 290.10, 290.11, 290.12, 290.13, 290.20, 290.21, 290.3, 290.40, 290.41, 290.42, 290.43, 290.8, 290.9, 294.10, 294.11, 294.20, 294.21, 294.8, 331.0, 331.11, 331.19, 331.82

ICD-10-CM [Reference ONLY/Not Reportable]: A52.17, F01.50, F01.51, F02.80, F02.81, F03.90, F03.91, F05, F06.0, F06.8, G30.0, G30.1, G30.8, G30.9, G31.01, G31.09, G31.83

Accompanied by

One of the following patient encounter codes: 90791, 90792, 90832, 90834, 90837, 96116, 96118, 96119, 96120, 96150, 96151, 96152, 96154, 97003, 97004, 99201, 99202, 99203, 99204, 99205, 99212, 99213, 99214, 99215, 99304, 99305, 99306, 99307, 99308, 99309, 99310, 99324, 99325, 99326, 99327, 99328, 99334, 99335, 99336, 99337, 99341, 99342, 99343, 99344, 99345, 99347, 99348, 99349, 99350

• Report quality-data codes (QDCs) on **all** measures within the Dementia Measures Group for each patient within the eligible professional's patient sample.

• Instructions for quality-data code reporting for each of the measures within the Dementia Measures Group are displayed on the next several pages. If all quality actions for the patient have been performed for all the measures within the group, the following composite G-code may be reported in lieu of the individual quality-data codes for each of the measures within the group. It is not necessary to submit the following composite G-code for registry-based submissions.

Composite G-code G8761: All quality actions for the applicable measures in the Dementia Measures Group have been performed for this patient

• To report satisfactorily the Dementia Measures Group it requires **all** measures for each patient within the eligible professional's patient sample to be reported a minimum of once during the reporting period.

• Measures groups containing a measure with a 0% performance rate will not be counted as satisfactorily reporting the measures group. The recommended clinical quality action must be performed on at least one patient for each measure within the measures group reported by the eligible professional. Performance exclusion quality-data codes are not counted in the performance denominator. If the eligible professional submits all performance exclusion quality-data codes, the performance rate would be 0/0 and would be considered satisfactorily reporting.

• When using the 20 Patient Sample Method via claims, report all measures for the 20 unique Medicare Part B FFS patients seen. When using the 20 Patient Sample Method via registries, report all measures for the 20 unique patients seen, a majority of which must be Medicare Part B FFS patients.

• For claims-based submissions, the Carrier/MAC remittance advice notice sent to the practice will show a denial remark code (N365) for the line item on the claim containing **G8902** (and **G8761** if reported) as well as all other line items containing QDCs. N365 indicates the code is not payable and is used for reporting/informational purposes only. Other services/codes on the claim will not be affected by the addition of a measures group-specific intent G-code or other QDCs. The N365 remark code does NOT indicate whether the QDC is accurate for that claim or for the measure the eligible professional is attempting to report, but does indicate that the QDC was processed and transmitted to the NCH.

MEASURE #284: DEMENTIA: MANAGEMENT OF NEUROPSYCHIATRIC SYMPTOMS

DESCRIPTION:

Percentage of patients, regardless of age, with a diagnosis of dementia who have one or more neuropsychiatric symptoms who received or were recommended to receive an intervention for neuropsychiatric symptoms within a 12 month period

NUMERATOR:

Patients who received or were recommended to receive an intervention for neuropsychiatric symptoms within a 12 month period

Numerator Quality-Data Coding Options for Reporting Satisfactorily:

Neuropsychiatric Intervention Ordered or Received, if Neuropsychiatric Symptoms Present *(One G-code [***G8947***] & one CPT II code [***452xF***] are required on the claim form to submit this numerator option)*

G8947: One or more neuropsychiatric symptoms **AND**

CPT II 4525F: Neuropsychiatric intervention ordered

OR

CPT II 4526F: Neuropsychiatric intervention received

OR

G8948: No neuropsychiatric symptoms

OR

Neuropsychiatric Symptoms Present and Neuropsychiatric Intervention not Ordered or Received, Reason not Otherwise Specified

*(One G-code [***G8947***] & one CPT II code [***452xF-8P***] are required on the claim form to submit this numerator option)*

Append a modifier (**8P**) to CPT Category II code **4025F** or **4026F** to report documented circumstances that appropriately exclude patients from the denominator.

G8947: One or more neuropsychiatric symptoms

AND

4525F ***with*** **8P:** Neuropsychiatric Intervention **not** ordered, reason not otherwise specified

OR

4526F ***with*** **8P:** Neuropsychiatric Intervention **not** received, reason not otherwise specified

PARKINSON'S DISEASE MEASURES GROUP OVERVIEW

2013 PQRS OPTIONS FOR MEASURES GROUPS: REGISTRY ONLY

2013 PQRS MEASURES IN PARKINSON'S DISEASE MEASURES GROUP:

#289. Parkinson's Disease: Annual Parkinson's Disease Diagnosis Review
#290. Parkinson's Disease: Psychiatric Disorders or Disturbances Assessment
#291. Parkinson's Disease: Cognitive Impairment or Dysfunction Assessment
#292. Parkinson's Disease: Querying about Sleep Disturbances
#293. Parkinson's Disease: Rehabilitative Therapy Options
#294. Parkinson's Disease: Parkinson's Disease Medical and Surgical Treatment Options Reviewed

INSTRUCTIONS FOR REPORTING: (These instructions apply to registry reporting. Do not report this measures group via claims.)

• It is not necessary to submit the measures group-specific intent G-code for registry-based submissions. However, the measures group-specific intent G-code has been created for registry only measures groups for use by registries that utilize claims data.

G8903: I intend to report the Parkinson's Disease Measures Group

• Report the patient sample method:

20 Patient Sample Method: 20 unique patients (a majority of which must be Medicare Part B FFS [fee for service] patients) meeting patient sample criteria for the measures group during the reporting period (January 1 through December 31, 2013 **OR** July 1 through December 31, 2013).

• Patient sample criteria for the Parkinson's Disease Measures Group are patients aged 18 years and older with a specific diagnosis of Parkinson's Disease accompanied by a specific patient encounter:

The following diagnosis code indicating Parkinson's disease: ICD-9-CM: 332.0

ICD-10-CM [Reference ONLY/Not Reportable]: G20

Accompanied by

One of the following patient encounter codes: 99201, 99202, 99203, 99204, 99205, 99212, 99213, 99214, 99215, 99304, 99305, 99306, 99307, 99308, 99309, 99310

• Report a numerator option on **all** measures within the Parkinson's Disease Measures Group for each patient within the eligible professional's patient sample.

• Instructions for qualifying numerator option reporting for each of the measures within the Parkinson's Disease Measures Group are displayed on the next several pages. The following composite G-code has been created for registry only measures groups for use by registries that utilize claims data. This composite G-code may be reported in lieu of the individual quality-data codes for each of the measures within the group, if all quality actions for the patient have been performed for all the measures within the group. However, it is not necessary to submit the following composite G-code for registry-based submissions.

Composite G-code G8762: All quality actions for the applicable measures in the Parkinson's Disease Measures Group have been performed for this patient

• To report satisfactorily the Parkinson's Disease Measures Group it requires **all** measures for each patient within the eligible professional's patient sample to be reported a minimum of once during the reporting period.

• Measures groups containing a measure with a 0% performance rate will not be counted as satisfactorily reporting the measures group. The recommended clinical quality action must be performed on at least one patient for each measure within the measures group reported by the eligible professional. Performance exclusion quality-data codes are not counted in the performance denominator. If the eligible professional submits all performance exclusion quality-data codes, the performance rate would be 0/0 and would be considered satisfactorily reporting.

• When using the 20 Patient Sample Method, report all applicable measures for the 20 unique patients seen a majority of which must be Medicare Part B FFS patients for the 12-month or 6-month reporting period.

HYPERTENSION MEASURES GROUP OVERVIEW

2013 PQRS OPTIONS FOR MEASURES GROUPS: REGISTRY ONLY

2013 PQRS MEASURES IN HYPERTENSION MEASURES GROUP:

#295. Hypertension: Appropriate Use of Aspirin or Other Antithrombotic Therapy
#296. Hypertension: Complete Lipid Profile
#297. Hypertension: Urine Protein Test
#298. Hypertension: Annual Serum Creatinine Test
#299. Hypertension: Diabetes Mellitus Screening Test
#300. Hypertension: Blood Pressure Control
#301. Hypertension: Low Density Lipoprotein (LDL-C) Control
#302. Hypertension: Dietary and Physical Activity Modifications Appropriately Prescribed

INSTRUCTIONS FOR REPORTING: (These instructions apply to registry reporting. Do not report this measures group via claims.)

• It is not necessary to submit the measures group-specific intent G-code for registry-based submissions. However, the measures group-specific intent G-code has been created for registry only measures groups for use by registries that utilize claims data.

G8904: I intend to report the Hypertension (HTN) Measures Group

• Report the patient sample method:

20 Patient Sample Method: 20 unique patients (a majority of which must be Medicare Part B FFS [fee for service] patients) meeting patient sample criteria for the measures group during the reporting period (January 1 through December 31, 2013 **OR** July 1 through December 31, 2013).

• Patient sample criteria for the Hypertension Measures Group are patients aged 18 through 90 years with a specific diagnosis of hypertension, and without a diagnosis of stage 5 chronic kidney disease (GFR of < 15ml/min per 1.72 m2 or end-stage kidney disease), accompanied by a specific patient encounter:

One of the following diagnosis codes indicating hypertension:

ICD-9-CM: 401.0, 401.1, 401.9, 402.00, 402.01, 402.10, 402.11, 402.90, 402.91, 403.00, 403.10, 403.90, 404.00, 404.01, 404.10, 404.11, 404.90, 404.91

ICD-10-CM [Reference ONLY/Not Reportable]: I10, I11.0, I11.9, I12.9, I13.0, I13.10

Accompanied by

One of the following patient encounter codes: 99201, 99202, 99203, 99204, 99205, 99212, 99213, 99214, 99215, 99304, 99305, 99306, 99307, 99308, 99309, 99310, 99324, 99325, 99326, 99327, 99328, 99334, 99335, 99336, 99337, 99341, 99342, 99343, 99344, 99345, 99347, 99348, 99349, 99350, G0438, G0439

AND NOT

Diagnosis for stage 5 chronic kidney disease:

ICD-9-CM: 403.01, 403.11, 403.91, 404.02, 404.03, 404.12, 404.13, 404.92, 404.93, 585.5, 585.6

ICD-10-CM [Reference ONLY/Not Reportable]: I12.0, I13.11, I13.2, N18.5, N18.6

• Report a numerator option on **all applicable** measures within the Hypertension Measures Group for each patient within the eligible professional's patient sample.

• Applicable measures contain patient demographic criteria specific to the measure. For example, Hypertension: Appropriate Use of Aspirin or Other Antithrombotic Therapy criteria is applicable *only to patients 30-90 years* within the sample population, while all other measures within this group apply to *all* patients 18-90 years. Reporting measure(s) from the group that are inapplicable to an individual patient will not affect the eligible provider's reporting or performance rate.

• Instructions for qualifying numerator option reporting for each of the measures within the Hypertension Measures Group are displayed on the next several pages. The following composite G-code has been created for registry only measures groups for use by registries that utilize claims data. This composite G-code may be reported in lieu of the individual quality-data codes for each of the measures within the group, if all quality actions for the patient have been performed for all the measures within the group. However, it is not necessary to submit the following composite G-code for registry-based submissions.

Composite G-code G8763: All quality actions for the applicable measures in the Hypertension (HTN) Measures Group have been performed for this patient

• To report satisfactorily the Hypertension Measures Group it requires **all** measures for each patient within the eligible professional's patient sample to be reported a minimum of once during the reporting period.

• Measures groups containing a measure with a 0% performance rate will not be counted as satisfactorily reporting the measures group. The recommended clinical quality action must be performed on at least one patient for each measure within the measures group reported by the eligible professional. Performance exclusion quality-data codes are not counted in the performance denominator. If the eligible professional submits all performance exclusion quality-data codes, the performance rate would be 0/0 and would be considered satisfactorily reporting.

• When using the 20 Patient Sample Method, report all applicable measures for the 20 unique patients seen a majority of which must be Medicare Part B FFS patients for the 12-month or 6-month reporting period.

MEASURE #297: HYPERTENSION: URINE PROTEIN TEST

DESCRIPTION:

Percentage of patients aged 18 through 90 years old with a diagnosis of hypertension who either have chronic kidney disease diagnosis documented or had a urine protein test done within **36 months**

NUMERATOR:

Patients who either have chronic kidney disease diagnosis documented OR had a urine protein test done within **36 months**

Numerator Instructions: This measure is looking for a urine protein screening test or evidence of existing chronic kidney disease. A urine protein test consists of tests for albuminuria, microalbuminuria, or proteinuria. Patients for whom the goals of care are predominantly palliative or for whom treatment of hypertension with standard treatment goals is not clinically appropriate should be excluded.

Definitions:

Treatment of hypertension with standard treatment goals is not clinically appropriate - For some patients, treatment of hypertension with standard goals may not be relevant, as might be the case for a patient with severe Alzheimer's disease.

*NUMERATOR NOTE: The performance period for this measure is **36 months**.*

Numerator Options:

Urine Protein test result documented and reviewed **(G8770)**

OR

Documentation of diagnosis of chronic kidney disease **(G8771)**

OR

Documentation of medical reason(s) for not performing urine protein test (e.g., patients with palliative goals or for whom treatment of hypertension with standard treatment goals is not clinically appropriate) **(G8772)**

OR

Urine protein test was **not** performed, reason not given **(G8773)**

MEASURE #298: HYPERTENSION: ANNUAL SERUM CREATININE TEST

DESCRIPTION:

Percentage of patients aged 18 through 90 years old with a diagnosis of hypertension who had a serum creatinine test done within **12 months**

NUMERATOR:

Patients who had most recent serum creatinine test done within **12 months**

Numerator Instructions: Patients for whom the goals of care are predominantly palliative or for whom treatment of hypertension with standard treatment goals is not clinically appropriate should be excluded.

Definitions:

Treatment of hypertension with standard treatment goals is not clinically appropriate - For some patients, treatment of hypertension with standard goals may not be relevant, as might be the case for a patient with severe Alzheimer's disease.

*NUMERATOR NOTE: The performance period for this measure is **12 months**.*

Numerator Options:

Serum creatinine test result documented and reviewed **(G8774)**

OR

Documentation of medical reason(s) for not performing serum creatinine test (e.g., patients with palliative goals or for whom treatment of hypertension with standard treatment goals is not clinically appropriate) **(G8775)**

OR

Serum creatinine test **not** performed, reason not given **(G8776)**

MEASURE #299: HYPERTENSION: DIABETES MELLITUS SCREENING TEST

DESCRIPTION:

Percentage of patients aged 18 through 90 years old with a diagnosis of hypertension who had a diabetes screening test within **36 months**

NUMERATOR:

Patients who had a diabetes screening test done within **36 months**

Numerator Instructions: Diabetes screening test consists of either a fasting glucose measurement, glycosylated hemoglobin test, or a two hour glucose tolerance test (three specimens). Patients for whom the goals of care are predominantly palliative or for whom treatment of hypertension with standard treatment goals is not clinically appropriate should be excluded.

Definitions:

Treatment of hypertension with standard treatment goals is not clinically appropriate - For some patients, treatment of hypertension with standard goals may not be relevant, as might be the case for a patient with severe Alzheimer's disease.

NUMERATOR NOTE: The performance period for this measure is ***36 months****.*

Numerator Options:

Diabetes screening test performed **(G8777)**

OR

Documentation of medical reason(s) for not performing diabetes screening test (e.g., patients with palliative goals or for whom treatment of hypertension with standard treatment goals is not clinically appropriate) **(G8778)**

OR

Diabetes screening test **not** performed, reason not given **(G8779)**

MEASURE #300: HYPERTENSION: BLOOD PRESSURE CONTROL

DESCRIPTION:

Percentage of patients aged 18 through 90 years old with a diagnosis of hypertension who had most recent blood pressure level under control (at goal)

NUMERATOR:

Patients who had most recent blood pressure under control

Numerator Instructions: Patients are considered to have most recent blood pressure under control if any of the following are documented:

- < 130/80 mmHg for those with chronic kidney disease OR diabetes
- < 140/90 mmHg for those without conditions listed above

If there are multiple blood pressures on the same date of service, use the lowest systolic and lowest diastolic blood pressure on that date as the representative blood pressure. To be "under control", both systolic and diastolic blood pressures must be below the target values (e.g., for a diabetes patient, systolic BP =136 mmHg and diastolic BP =70 mmHg is not "under control").

Patients for whom the goals of care are predominantly palliative or for whom treatment of hypertension with standard treatment goals is not clinically appropriate should be excluded.

Definitions:

Treatment of hypertension with standard treatment goals is not clinically appropriate - For some patients, treatment of hypertension with standard goals may not be relevant, as might be the case for a patient with severe Alzheimer's disease.

NUMERATOR NOTE: *The performance period for this measure is* ***12 months****.*

Numerator Options:

Most recent blood pressure under control **(G8886)**

OR

Documentation of medical reason(s) for most recent blood pressure **not** being under control (e.g., patients with palliative goals or for whom treatment of hypertension with standard treatment goals is not clinically appropriate) **(G8887)**

OR

Most recent blood pressure **not** under control, results documented and reviewed **(G8888)**

OR

No documentation of blood pressure measurement, reason not given **(G8889)**

MEASURE #301: HYPERTENSION: LOW DENSITY LIPOPROTEIN (LDL-C) CONTROL

DESCRIPTION:

Percentage of patients aged 18 through 90 years old with a diagnosis of hypertension who had most recent LDL cholesterol level under control (at goal)

NUMERATOR:

Patients who had most recent LDL-C level under control during the **60-month** period

Numerator Instructions: Patients are considered to have most recent LDL-C level under control if any of the following are documented:

• < 100 mg/dL for those with coronary heart disease, OR stroke or transient ischemic attack, OR peripheral artery disease, OR diabetes

•< 130 mg/dL for those without conditions listed above, but with one or more additional risk factors for CHD (Low HDL (< 40 mg/dL) or on HDL-raising medication, risk age (men ≥ 45, women ≥ 55), family history of premature CHD, smoking); HDL cholesterol ≥ 60 acts as a negative risk factor

• < 160 mg/dL for those without conditions listed above, **and without additional** risk factors for CHD (Low HDL (< 40 mg/dL) or on HDL-raising medication, risk age (men ≥ 45, women ≥ 55), family history of premature CHD, smoking); HDL cholesterol ≥ 60 acts as a negative risk factor

Patients for whom the goals of care are predominantly palliative or for whom treatment of hypertension with standard treatment goals is not clinically appropriate should be excluded.

Definitions:

Treatment of hypertension with standard treatment goals is not clinically appropriate - For some patients, treatment of hypertension with standard goals may not be relevant, as might be the case for a patient with severe Alzheimer's disease.

*NUMERATOR NOTE: The performance period for this measure is **60 months**.*

Numerator Options:

Most recent LDL-C under control, results documented and reviewed **(G8890)**

OR

Documentation of medical reason(s) for most recent LDL-C not under control (e.g., patients with palliative goals or for whom treatment of hypertension with standard treatment goals is not clinically appropriate) **(G8891)**

OR

Documentation of medical reason(s) for not performing LDL-C test (e.g., patients with palliative goals or for whom treatment of hypertension with standard treatment goals is not clinically appropriate) **(G8892)**

OR

Most recent LDL-C **not** under control, results documented and reviewed **(G8893)**

OR

LDL-C **not** performed, reason not given **(G8894)**

MEASURE #302: HYPERTENSION: DIETARY AND PHYSICAL ACTIVITY MODIFICATIONS APPROPRIATELY PRESCRIBED

DESCRIPTION:

Percentage of patients aged 18 through 90 years old with a diagnosis of hypertension who received dietary and physical activity counseling at least once within **12 months**

NUMERATOR:

Patients who received dietary and physical activity counseling at least once within **12 months**

Numerator Instructions: Patients for whom the goals of care are predominantly palliative or for whom treatment of hypertension with standard treatment goals is not clinically appropriate should be excluded.

Definitions:

Treatment of hypertension with standard treatment goals is not clinically appropriate - For some patients, treatment of hypertension with standard goals may not be relevant, as might be the case for a patient with severe Alzheimer's disease.

Counseling – May include documentation of prescribing any of the following dietary modifications: dietary saturated fat and cholesterol restriction, calorie restriction as part of weight reduction program for overweight/obese patients, DASH eating plan, dietary sodium restriction, increased fruits, vegetables and/or soluble fiber; and documentation of activity status for active patients or discussion of increase exercise or physical activity for inactive patients.

NUMERATOR NOTE: *The performance period for this measure is* ***12 months****.*

Numerator Options:

Counseling for Diet and Physical Activity Performed **(G8780)**

OR

Documentation of medical reason(s) for patient not receiving counseling for diet and physical activity (e.g., patients with palliative goals or for whom treatment of hypertension with standard treatment goals is not clinically appropriate) **(G8781)**

OR

Documentation of patient reason(s) for patient not receiving counseling for diet and physical activity (e.g., patient is not willing to discuss diet or exercise interventions to help control blood pressure, or the patient said he/she refused to make these changes) **(G8949)**

OR

Counseling for Diet and Physical Activity **not** performed, reason not given **(G8782)**

CARDIOVASCULAR PREVENTION MEASURES GROUP OVERVIEW

2013 PQRS OPTIONS FOR MEASURES GROUPS: CLAIMS, REGISTRY

2013 PQRS MEASURES IN CARDIOVASCULAR PREVENTION MEASURES GROUP:

#2.Diabetes Mellitus: Low Density Lipoprotein (LDL-C) Control
#204. Ischemic Vascular Disease (IVD): Use of Aspirin or Another Antithrombotic
#226. Preventive Care: Tobacco Use: Screening and Cessation Intervention
#236. Hypertension (HTN): Controlling High Blood Pressure
#241. Ischemic Vascular Disease (IVD): Complete Lipid Panel and Low Density Lipoprotein (LDL-C) Control
#317. Preventive Care and Screening: Screening for High Blood Pressure and Follow-Up Documented

INSTRUCTIONS FOR REPORTING: (These instructions apply to both Claims and Registry reporting, unless otherwise specified.)

• Indicate your intention to report the Cardiovascular Preventive Measures Group by submitting the measures group-specific intent G-code at least once during the reporting period when billing a patient claim for the 20 Patient Sample Method. It is not necessary to submit the measures group-specific intent G-code on more than one claim. It is not necessary to submit the measures group-specific intent G-code for registry-based submissions.

G8905: I intend to report the Cardiovascular Prevention Measures Group

• Select patient sample method:

20 Patient Sample Method via claims: 20 unique Medicare Part B FFS (fee for service) patients meeting patient sample criteria for the measures group.

OR

20 Patient Sample Method via registries: 20 unique patients (a majority of which must be Medicare Part B FFS patients) meeting patient sample criteria for the measures group during the reporting period (January 1 through December 31, 2013 **OR** July 1 through December 31, 2013).

• Patient sample criteria for the Cardiovascular Prevention Measures Group are patients aged ≥ 18 and older with a specific diagnosis of Diabetes Mellitus or Ischemic Vascular Disease and accompanied by a specific patient encounter:

One of the following diagnosis codes indicating diabetes mellitus:

ICD-9-CM: 250.00, 250.01, 250.02, 250.03, 250.10, 250.11, 250.12, 250.13, 250.20, 250.21, 250.22, 250.23, 250.30, 250.31, 250.32, 250.33, 250.40, 250.41, 250.42, 250.43, 250.50, 250.51, 250.52, 250.53, 250.60, 250.61, 250.62, 250.63, 250.70, 250.71, 250.72, 250.73, 250.80, 250.81, 250.82, 250.83, 250.90, 250.91, 250.92, 250.93, 357.2, 362.01, 362.02, 362.03, 362.04, 362.05, 362.06, 362.07, 366.41, 648.00, 648.01, 648.02, 648.03, 648.04

ICD-10-CM [Reference ONLY/Not Reportable]: E10.10, E10.11, E10.21, E10.22, E10.29, E10.311, E10.319, E10.321, E10.329, E10.331, E10.339, E10.341, E10.349, E10.351, E10.359, E10.36, E10.39, E10.40, E10.41, E10.42, E10.43, E10.44, E10.49, E10.51, E10.52, E10.59, E10.610, E10.618, E10.620, E10.621, E10.622, E10.628, E10.630, E10.638, E10.641, E10.649, E10.65, E10.69,E10.8, E10.9, E11.00, E11.01, E11.21, E11.22, E11.29, E11.311, E11.319, E11.321, E11.329, E11.331, E11.339, E11.341, E11.349, E11.351, E11.359, E11.36, E11.39, E11.40, E11.41, E11.42, E11.43, E11.44, E11.49, E11.51, E11.52, E11.59, E11.610, E11.618, E11.620, E11.621, E11.622, E11.628, E11.630, E11.638, E11.641, E11.649, E11.65, E11.69, E11.8, E11.9, O24.011, O24.012, O24.013, O24.019, O24.02, O24.03, O24.111, O24.112, O24.113, O24.119, O24.12, O24.13

AND/OR

One of the following diagnosis codes indicating ischemic vascular disease:

ICD-9-CM: 410.11, 410.21, 410.31, 410.41, 410.51, 410.61, 410.71, 410.81, 410.91, 411.0, 411.1, 411.81, 411.89, 413.0, 413.1, 413.9, 414.00, 414.01, 414.02, 414.03, 414.04, 414.05, 414.06, 414.07, 414.2, 414.8, 414.9, 429.2, 433.00, 433.01, 433.10, 433.11, 433.20, 433.21, 433.30, 433.31, 433.80, 433.81, 433.90, 433.91, 434.00, 434.01, 434.10, 434.11, 434.90, 434.91, 444.01, 444.09, 440.1, 440.20, 440.21, 440.22, 440.23, 440.24, 440.29, 440.4, 444.1, 444.21, 444.22, 444.81, 444.89, 444.9, 445.01, 445.02, 445.81, 445.89

ICD-10-CM [Reference ONLY/Not Reportable]: I20.0, I20.1, I20.8, I20.9, I21.01, I21.02, I21.09, I21.11, I21.19, I21.21, I21.29, I21.3, I21.4, I24.0, I24.1, I24.8, I24.9, I25.10, I25.110, I25.111, I25.118, I25.119, I25.5, I25.6, I25.700, I25.701, I25.708, I25.709, I25.710, I25.711, I25.718, I25.719, I25.720, I25.721, I25.728, I25.729, I25.730, I25.731, I25.738, I25.739, I25.750, I25.751, I25.758,

I25.759, I25.760, I25.761, I25.768, I25.769, I25.790, I25.791, I25.798, I25.799, I25.810, I25.811, I25.812, I25.82, I25.89, I25.9, I63.00, I63.011, I63.012, I63.019, I63.02, I63.031, I63.032, I63.039, I63.09, I63.10, I63.111, I63.112, I63.119, I63.12, I63.131, I63.132, I63.139, I63.19, I63.20, I63.211, I63.212, I63.219, I63.22, I63.231, I63.232, I63.239, I63.29, I63.30, I63.311, I63.312, I63.319, I63.321, I63.322, I63.329, I63.331, I63.332, I63.339, I63.341, I63.342, I63.349, I63.39, I63.40, I63.411, I63.412, I63.419, I63.421, I63.422, I63.429, I63.431, I63.432, I63.439, I63.441, I63.442, I63.449, I63.49, I63.50, I63.511, I63.512, I63.519, I63.521, I63.522, I63.529, I63.531, I63.532, I63.539, I63.541, I63.542, I63.549, I63.59, I63.6, I63.8, I63.9, I65.01, I65.02, I65.03, I65.09, I65.1, I65.21, I65.22, I65.23, I65.29, I65.8, I65.9, I66.01, I66.02, I66.03, I66.09, I66.11, I66.12, I66.13, I66.19, I66.21, I66.22, I66.23, I66.29, I66.3, I66.8, I66.9, I70.1, I70.201, I70.202, I70.203, I70.208, I70.209, I70.211, I70.212, I70.213, I70.218, I70.219, I70.221, I70.222, I70.223, I70.228, I70.229, I70.231, I70.232, I70.233, I70.234, I70.235, I70.238, I70.239, I70.241, I70.242, I70.243, I70.244, I70.245, I70.248, I70.249, I70.25, I70.261, I70.262, I70.263, I70.268, I70.269, I70.291, I70.292, I70.293, I70.298, I70.299, I70.92, I74.0, I74.10, I74.11, I74.19, I74.2, I74.3, I74.4, I74.5, I74.8, I74.9, I75.011, I75.012, I75.013, I75.019, I75.021, I75.022, I75.023, I75.029, I75.81, I75.89

Accompanied by

One of the following patient encounter codes: 99201, 99202, 99203, 99204, 99205, 99212, 99213, 99214, 99215

• Report quality-data codes (QDCs) on **all applicable** measures within the Cardiovascular Prevention Measures Group for each patient within the sample.

• Applicable measures contain patient demographic criteria specific to the measure. For example, Diabetes Mellitus criteria is applicable *only to patients 18-75 years* within the sample population, while the Tobacco Use: Screening and Cessation Intervention measure within this group applies to *all* patients ≥ 18 years and older. Reporting measure(s) from the group that are inapplicable to an individual patient will not affect the eligible provider's reporting or performance rate.

• Only patients with IVD or DM are included in this measures group.

• For patients with DM diagnosis, only need to report for those aged 18 – 75 years.

• If patient also has a diagnosis of HTN measure #236 should be reported.

ICD-9-CM: 401.0, 401.1, 401.9, 402.00, 402.01, 402.10, 402.11, 402.90, 402.91, 403.00, 403.01, 403.10, 403.11, 403.90, 403.91, 404.00, 404.01, 404.02, 404.03, 404.10, 404.11, 404.12, 404.13, 404.90, 404.91, 404.92, 404.93, 405.01, 405.09, 405.10, 405.19, 405.91, 405.99

ICD-10-CM [Reference ONLY/Not Reportable]: I10, I11.0, I11.9, I12.0, I12.9, I13.0, I13.10, I13.11, I13.2, I15.0, I15.1, I15.2, I15.8, I15.9

• If a patient does not have a diagnosis of HTN, measure #317 should be reported.

• The table below illustrates the applicable measures to report based on the denominator criteria the patient meets.

Diagnosis	Has HTN Diagnosis – Report these measures	Does not have HTN Diagnosis – Report these measures
DM only	2*, 226, 236	2*, 226, 317
IVD Only	204, 226, 236, 241	204, 226, 241, 317
DM & IVD	2*, 204, 226, 236, 241	2*, 204, 226, 241, 317

***Only report for patients aged 18-75 years**

• Instructions for quality-data code reporting for each of the measures within the Cardiovascular Prevention Measures Group are displayed on the next several pages. If all quality actions for the patient have been performed for all the measures within the group, the following composite G-code may be reported in lieu of the individual quality-data codes for each of the measures within the group. It is not necessary to submit the following composite G-code for registry-based submissions.

Composite G-code G8764: All quality actions for the applicable measures in the Cardiovascular Prevention Measures Group have been performed for this patient

• To report satisfactorily the Cardiovascular Prevention Measures Group requires **all applicable** measures for each patient within the eligible professional's patient sample to be reported a minimum of once during the reporting period.

• Measures groups containing a measure with a 0% performance rate will not be counted as satisfactorily reporting the measures group. The recommended clinical quality action must be performed on at least one patient for each measure within the measures group reported by the eligible professional. Performance exclusion quality-data codes are not counted in the performance denominator. If the eligible professional submits all performance exclusion quality-data codes, the performance rate would be 0/0 and would be considered satisfactorily reporting. If a measure within a measures group is not applicable to a patient, the patient would not be counted in the performance denominator for that measure (e.g., Preventive Care Measures Group - Measure #39: Screening or Therapy for Osteoporosis for Women Aged 65 Years and Older would not be applicable to male patients according to the patient sample criteria). If the measure is not applicable for all patients within the sample, the performance rate would be 0/0 and would be considered satisfactorily reporting.

• When using the 20 Patient Sample Method via claims, report all measures for the 20 unique Medicare Part B FFS patients seen. When using the 20 Patient

Sample Method via registries, report all measures for the 20 unique patients seen, a majority of which must be Medicare Part B FFS patients.

• For claims-based submissions, the Carrier/MAC remittance advice notice sent to the practice will show a denial remark code (N365) for the line item on the claim containing **G8485** (and **G8494** if reported) as well as all other line items containing QDCs. N365 indicates the code is not payable and is used for reporting/informational purposes only. Other services/codes on the claim will not be affected by the addition of a measures group-specific intent G-code or other QDCs. The N365 remark code does NOT indicate whether the QDC is accurate for that claim or for the measure the eligible professional is attempting to report, but does indicate that the QDC was processed and transmitted to the NCH.

MEASURE #204 (NQF 0068): ISCHEMIC VASCULAR DISEASE (IVD): USE OF ASPIRIN OR ANOTHER ANTITHROMBOTIC

DESCRIPTION:

Percentage of patients aged 18 years and older with Ischemic Vascular Disease (IVD) with documented use of aspirin or another antithrombotic

NUMERATOR:

Patients who are using aspirin or another antithrombotic therapy

Numerator Instructions: Oral antithrombotic therapy consists of aspirin, clopidogrel or combination of aspirin and extended release dipyridamole.

NUMERATOR NOTE: The performance period for this measure is 12 months from the date of service

Numerator Quality-Data Coding Options for Reporting Satisfactorily: Aspirin or Another Antithrombotic Therapy Used

G8598: Aspirin or another antithrombotic therapy used

OR

Aspirin or Another Antithrombotic Therapy not Used, Reason not Given
G8599: Aspirin or another antithrombotic therapy **not** used, reason not given

MEASURE #236 (NQF 0018): HYPERTENSION (HTN): CONTROLLING HIGH BLOOD PRESSURE

DESCRIPTION:

Percentage of patients aged 18 through 85 years who had a diagnosis of hypertension (HTN) and whose blood pressure (BP) was adequately controlled (< 140/90 mmHg)

NUMERATOR:

Patients whose most recent blood pressure < 140/90 mmHg

Numerator Instructions: To describe both systolic and diastolic blood pressure values, **each must be reported separately**. If there are multiple blood pressures on the same date of service, use the lowest systolic and lowest diastolic blood pressure on that date as the representative blood pressure.

Numerator Quality-Data Coding Options for Reporting Satisfactorily: Most Recent Blood Pressure Measurement Performed

Systolic pressure **(Select one (1) code from this section): G8752:** Most recent systolic blood pressure < 140 mmHg

OR

G8753: Most recent systolic blood pressure ≥ 140 mmHg

AND

Diastolic pressure **(Select one (1) code from this section): G8754:** Most recent diastolic blood pressure < 90 mmHg

OR

G8755: Most recent diastolic blood pressure ≥ 90 mmHg

OR

Blood Pressure Measurement not Documented, Reason not Given G8756: No documentation of blood pressure measurement, reason not given

MEASURE #241 (NQF 0075): ISCHEMIC VASCULAR DISEASE (IVD): COMPLETE LIPID PANEL AND LOW DENSITY LIPOPROTEIN (LDL-C) CONTROL

DESCRIPTION:

Percentage of patients aged 18 years and older with Ischemic Vascular Disease (IVD) who received at least one lipid profile within 12 months and whose most recent LDL-C level was in control (less than 100 mg/dL)

NUMERATOR:

Patients who received at least one lipid profile (or ALL component tests) with most recent LDL-C < 100 mg/dL

NUMERATOR NOTE: *The performance period for this measure is 12 months from the date of service.*

Numerator Quality-Data Coding Options for Reporting Satisfactorily: Lipid Profile Performed and Most Recent LDL-C < 100 mg/dL

G8593: Lipid panel results documented and reviewed (must include total cholesterol, HDL-C, triglycerides and calculated LDL-C)

Note: If LDL-C could not be calculated due to high triglycerides, count as complete lipid profile.

AND

G8595: Most recent LDL-C < 100 mg/dL

OR

Lipid Profile not Performed, Reason not Given G8594: Lipid profile **not** performed, reason not given

OR

Most Recent LDL-C ≥ 100 mg/dL

G8593: Lipid panel results documented and reviewed (must include total cholesterol, HDL-C, triglycerides and calculated LDL-C)

AND

G8597: Most recent LDL-C ≥ 100 mg/dL

MEASURE #317: PREVENTIVE CARE AND SCREENING: SCREENING FOR HIGH BLOOD PRESSURE AND FOLLOW-UP DOCUMENTED

DESCRIPTION:

Percentage of patients aged 18 years and older seen during the reporting period who were screened for high blood pressure (BP) AND a recommended follow-up plan is documented based on the current blood pressure reading as indicated

NUMERATOR:

Patients who were screened for high blood pressure **and a recommended follow-up plan is documented as indicated if the blood pressure is pre-hypertensive or hypertensive**

Numerator Note: *Although recommended screening interval for a normal BP reading is every 2 years, to meet the intent of this measure, a BP screening must be performed once per measurement period. The intent of this measure is to screen patients for high blood pressure and provide recommended follow-up as indicated.*

Definitions:

BP Classification: BP is defined by four BP reading classifications as listed in the "Recommended Blood Pressure Follow-Up" table below including Normal, Pre-Hypertensive, First Hypertensive, and Second Hypertensive Readings

Recommended BP Follow-Up: The current *Report of the Joint National Committee on the Prevention, Detection, Evaluation, and Treatment of High Blood Pressure* (JNC) recommends BP screening intervals, lifestyle modifications and interventions based on BP Classification of the current BP reading as listed in the "Recommended BP Follow-Up" table below

Lifestyle Modifications: The current JNC report outlines lifestyle modifications which must include one or more of the following as indicated: Weight Reduction, DASH Eating Plan, Dietary Sodium Restriction, Increased Physical Activity, or Moderation in Alcohol Consumption

Second Hypertensive Reading: Requires both a BP reading of Systolic BP ≥ 140 mmHg OR Diastolic BP ≥ 90 mmHg during the current encounter AND a most recent BP reading within the last 12 months Systolic BP ≥ 140 mmHg OR Diastolic BP ≥ 90 mmHg

Second Hypertensive Reading Interventions: The current JNC report outlines interventions based on BP Readings shown in the "Recommended BP Follow-up" table and must include one or more of the following as indicated: Anti-Hypertensive Pharmacologic Therapy, Laboratory Tests, or Electrocardiogram (ECG)

Recommended Blood Pressure Follow-Up Table

BP Classification	**Systolic BP mmHg**	**Diastolic BP mmHg**	**Recommended Follow-Up** ***(must include all indicated actions for each BP classification)***
Normal BP Reading	< 120	AND < 80	• No Follow-Up required

Pre-Hypertensiv e BP Reading	≥ 120 AND ≤ 139	OR ≥ 80 AND ≤ 89	• Rescreen BP within a minimum of 1 year *AND* Recommend Lifestyle Modifications OR • Referral to Alternative / Primary Care Provider
First Hypertensive BP Reading	≥ 140	OR ≥ 90	• Rescreen BP within a minimum of ≥ 1 day and ≤ 4 weeks *AND* Recommend Lifestyle Modifications OR • Referral to Alternative / Primary Care Provider
Second Hypertensive BP Reading	≥ 140	OR ≥ 90	• Recommend Lifestyle Modifications *AND* one or more of the Second Hypertensive Reading Interventions (see definitions) OR • Referral to Alternative / Primary Care Provider

Not Eligible – A patient is **not** eligible if one or more of the following reasons exist:

- Patient has an active diagnosis of hypertension
- Patient refuses BP measurement
- Patient is in an urgent or emergent situation where time is of the essence and to delay treatment would jeopardize the patient's health status. This may include but is not limited to severely elevated BP when immediate medical treatment is indicated

Numerator Quality-Data Coding Options for Reporting Satisfactorily: Normal Blood Pressure Reading Documented, Follow-Up not Required
G8783: Normal blood pressure reading documented, follow-up not required

OR

Pre-Hypertensive or Hypertensive Blood Pressure Reading Documented, Indicated Follow-Up Documented

G8950: Pre-hypertensive or Hypertensive blood pressure reading documented, indicated follow-up documented

OR

Blood Pressure Reading not Documented, Patient not Eligible/not Appropriate G8784: Blood pressure reading not documented, patient not eligible/not appropriate

OR

Pre-Hypertensive or Hypertensive Blood Pressure Reading Documented, Indicated Follow-Up not Documented, Patient not Eligible/not Appropriate

G8951: Pre-Hypertensive or Hypertensive blood pressure reading documented, indicated follow-up not documented, patient not eligible/not appropriate

OR

Blood Pressure Reading not Documented, Reason not Given

G8785: Blood pressure reading **not** documented, reason not given

OR

Pre-Hypertensive or Hypertensive Blood Pressure Reading Documented, Indicated Follow-Up not Documented, Reason not Given

G8952: Pre-Hypertensive or Hypertensive blood pressure reading documented, indicated follow-up **not** documented, reason not given

CATARACTS MEASURES GROUP OVERVIEW

2013 PQRS OPTIONS FOR MEASURES GROUPS: REGISTRY ONLY

2013 PQRS MEASURES IN CATARACTS MEASURES GROUP:

#191. Cataracts: 20/40 or Better Visual Acuity within 90 Days Following Cataract Surgery
#192. Cataracts: Complications within 30 Days Following Cataract Surgery Requiring Additional Surgical Procedures
#303. Cataracts: Improvement in Patient's Visual Function within 90 Days Following Cataract Surgery
#304. Cataracts: Patient Satisfaction within 90 Days Following Cataract Surgery

INSTRUCTIONS FOR REPORTING: (These instructions apply to registry reporting. Do not report this measures group via claims.)

• It is not necessary to submit the measures group-specific intent G-code for registry-based submissions. However, the measures group-specific intent G-code has been created for registry only measures groups for use by registries that utilize claims data.

G8906: I intend to report the Cataracts Measures Group

• Report the patient sample method:

20 Patient Sample Method: 20 unique procedures (patients – a majority of which must be Medicare Part B FFS [fee for service] patients) meeting patient sample criteria for the measures group during the reporting period (January 1 through December 31, 2013 **OR** July 1 through December 31, 2013).

• Patient sample criteria for the Cataracts Measures Group are patients aged 18 years and older that have a specific procedure for cataract surgery performed:

One of the following procedure codes indicating cataract surgery: 66840, 66850, 66852, 66920, 66930, 66940, 66983, 66984

WITHOUT

Modifier 56 (preoperative management only)

• For purposes of satisfactory reporting **all** measures contained within the Cataracts Measures Group, include only procedures performed through September 30 of the reporting period. Procedures performed October 1 through December 31 of the reporting period are not included.

• Measures #191 and #192 need only be reported when the patient also has a diagnosis of uncomplicated cataract. Refer to the measure specification on the following pages for specific codes indicating a diagnosis of uncomplicated cataract for each of these two measures. Measures #303 and #304 need **not** be reported when the cataract surgery includes a modifier 55 (post-operative management only).

• Report a numerator option on **all applicable** measures within the Cataracts Measures Group for each procedure (patient) within the eligible professional's patient sample.

• Instructions for qualifying numerator option reporting for each of the measures within the Cataracts Measures Group are displayed on the next several pages. The following composite G-code has been created for registry only measures groups for use by registries that utilize claims data. This composite G-code may be reported in lieu of the individual quality-data codes for each of the measures within the group, if all quality actions for the patient have been performed for all the measures within the group. However, it is not necessary to submit the following composite G-code for registry-based submissions.

Composite G-code G8765: All quality actions for the applicable measures in the Cataracts Measures Group have been performed for this patient

• To report satisfactorily the Cataracts Measures Group it requires **all applicable** measures for each patient within the eligible professional's patient sample to be reported each time a cataract surgery is performed during the reporting period.

• Measures groups containing a measure with a 0% performance rate will not be counted as satisfactorily reporting the measures group. The recommended clinical quality action must be performed on at least one patient for each measure within the measures group reported by the eligible professional. Performance exclusion quality-data codes are not counted in the performance denominator. If the eligible professional submits all performance exclusion quality-data codes, the performance rate would be 0/0 and would be considered satisfactorily reporting. If a measure within a measures group is not applicable to a patient, the patient would not be counted in the performance denominator for that measure (e.g., Preventive Care Measures Group - Measure #39: Screening or Therapy for Osteoporosis for Women Aged 65 Years and Older would not be applicable to male patients according to the patient sample criteria). If the measure is not applicable for all patients within the sample, the performance rate would be 0/0 and would be considered satisfactorily reporting. When a lower rate indicates better performance, such as Measure #192, a 0% performance rate will be counted as satisfactorily reporting (100% performance rate would not be considered satisfactorily reporting).

• When using the 20 Patient Sample Method, report all applicable measures for the 20 unique procedures performed (patients seen) a majority of which must be Medicare Part B FFS procedures (patients) for the 12-month or 6-month reporting period.

ONCOLOGY MEASURES GROUP OVERVIEW

2013 PQRS OPTIONS FOR MEASURES GROUPS: REGISTRY ONLY

2013 PQRS MEASURES IN ONCOLOGY MEASURES GROUP:

#71. Breast Cancer: Hormonal Therapy for Stage IC - IIIC Estrogen Receptor/Progesterone Receptor (ER/PR) Positive Breast Cancer
#72. Colon Cancer: Chemotherapy for AJCC Stage III Colon Cancer Patients
#110. Preventive Care and Screening: Influenza Immunization
#130. Documentation of Current Medications in the Medical Record
#143. Oncology: Medical and Radiation – Pain Intensity Quantified
#144. Oncology: Medical and Radiation – Plan of Care for Pain
#194. Oncology: Cancer Stage Documented
#226. Preventive Care and Screening: Tobacco Use: Screening and Cessation Intervention

INSTRUCTIONS FOR REPORTING: (These instructions apply to registry reporting. Do not report this measures group via claims.)

• It is not necessary to submit the measures group-specific intent G-code for registry-based submissions. However, the measures group-specific intent G-code has been created for registry only measures groups for use by registries that utilize claims data.

G8977: I intend to report the Oncology Measures Group

• Report the patient sample method:

20 Patient Sample Method: 20 unique procedures (patients – a majority of which must be Medicare Part B FFS [fee for service] patients) meeting patient sample criteria for the measures group during the reporting period (January 1 through December 31, 2013 **OR** July 1 through December 31, 2013).

• Patient sample criteria for the Oncology Measures Group are patients aged 18 years and older with a specific diagnosis of cancer, accompanied by a specific patient encounter:

One of the following diagnosis codes indicating cancer

ICD-9-CM: 140.0, 140.1, 140.3, 140.4, 140.5, 140.6, 140.8, 140.9, 141.0, 141.1, 141.2, 141.3, 141.4, 141.5, 141.6, 141.8, 141.9, 142.0, 142.1, 142.2, 142.8, 142.9, 143.0, 143.1, 143.8, 143.9, 144.0, 144.1, 144.8, 144.9, 145.0, 145.1, 145.2, 145.3, 145.4, 145.5, 145.6, 145.8, 145.9, 146.0, 146.1, 146.2, 146.3, 146.4, 146.5, 146.6, 146.7, 146.8, 146.9, 147.0, 147.1, 147.2, 147.3, 147.8, 147.9, 148.0, 148.1, 148.2, 148.3, 148.8, 148.9, 149.0, 149.1, 149.8, 149.9, 150.0, 150.1, 150.2, 150.3, 150.4, 150.5, 150.8, 150.9, 151.0, 151.1, 151.2, 151.3, 151.4, 151.5, 151.6, 151.8, 151.9, 152.0, 152.1, 152.2, 152.3, 152.8, 152.9, 153.0, 153.1, 153.2, 153.3, 153.4, 153.5, 153.6, 153.7, 153.8, 153.9, 154.0, 154.1, 154.2, 154.3, 154.8, 155.0, 155.1, 155.2, 156.0, 156.1,

156.2, 156.8, 156.9, 157.0, 157.1, 157.2, 157.3, 157.4, 157.8, 157.9, 158.0, 158.8, 158.9, 159.0, 159.1, 159.8, 159.9, 160.0, 160.1, 160.2, 160.3, 160.4, 160.5, 160.8, 160.9, 161.0, 161.1, 161.2, 161.3, 161.8, 161.9, 162.0, 162.2, 162.3, 162.4, 162.5, 162.8, 162.9, 163.0, 163.1, 163.8, 163.9, 164.0, 164.1, 164.2, 164.3, 164.8, 164.9, 165.0, 165.8, 165.9, 170.0, 170.1, 170.2, 170.3, 170.4, 170.5, 170.6, 170.7, 170.8, 170.9, 171.0, 171.2, 171.3, 171.4, 171.5, 171.6, 171.7, 171.8, 171.9, 172.0, 172.1, 172.2, 172.3, 172.4, 172.5, 172.6, 172.7, 172.8, 172.9, 173.00, 173.01, 173.02, 173.09, 173.10, 173.11, 173.12, 173.19, 173.20, 173.21, 173.22, 173.29, 173.30, 173.31, 173.32, 173.39, 173.40, 173.41, 173.42, 173.49, 173.50, 173.51, 173.52, 173.59, 173.60, 173.61, 173.62, 173.69, 173.70, 173.71, 173.72, 173.79, 173.80, 173.81, 173.82, 173.89, 173.90, 173.91, 173.92, 173.99, 174.0, 174.1, 174.2, 174.3, 174.4, 174.5, 174.6, 174.8, 174.9, 175.0, 175.9, 176.0, 176.1, 176.2, 176.3, 176.4, 176.5, 176.8, 176.9, 179, 180.0, 180.1, 180.8, 180.9, 181, 182.0, 182.1, 182.8, 183.0, 183.2, 183.3, 183.4, 183.5, 183.8, 183.9, 184.0, 184.1, 184.2, 184.3, 184.4, 184.8, 184.9, 185, 186.0, 186.9, 187.1, 187.2, 187.3, 187.4, 187.5, 187.6, 187.7, 187.8, 187.9, 188.0, 188.1, 188.2, 188.3, 188.4, 188.5, 188.6, 188.7, 188.8, 188.9, 189.0, 189.1, 189.2, 189.3, 189.4, 189.8, 189.9, 190.0, 190.1, 190.2, 190.3, 190.4, 190.5, 190.6, 190.7, 190.8, 190.9, 191.0, 191.1, 191.2, 191.3, 191.4, 191.5, 191.6, 191.7, 191.8, 191.9, 192.0, 192.1, 192.2, 192.3, 192.8, 192.9, 193, 194.0, 194.1, 194.3, 194.4, 194.5, 194.6, 194.8, 194.9, 195.0, 195.1, 195.2, 195.3, 195.4, 195.5, 195.8, 196.0, 196.1, 196.2, 196.3, 196.5, 196.6, 196.8, 196.9, 197.0, 197.1, 197.2, 197.3, 197.4, 197.5, 197.6, 197.7, 197.8, 198.0, 198.1, 198.2, 198.3, 198.4, 198.5, 198.6, 198.7, 198.81, 198.82, 198.89, 199.0, 199.1, 199.2, 200.00, 200.01, 200.02, 200.03, 200.04, 200.05, 200.06, 200.07, 200.08, 200.10, 200.11, 200.12, 200.13, 200.14, 200.15, 200.16, 200.17, 200.18, 200.20, 200.21, 200.22, 200.23, 200.24, 200.25, 200.26, 200.27, 200.28, 200.30, 200.31, 200.32, 200.33, 200.34, 200.35, 200.36, 200.37, 200.38, 200.40, 200.41, 200.42, 200.43, 200.44, 200.45, 200.46, 200.47, 200.48, 200.50, 200.51, 200.52, 200.53, 200.54, 200.55, 200.56, 200.57, 200.58, 200.60, 200.61, 200.62, 200.63, 200.64, 200.65, 200.66, 200.67, 200.68, 200.70, 200.71, 200.72, 200.73, 200.74, 200.75, 200.76, 200.77, 200.78, 200.80, 200.81, 200.82, 200.83, 200.84, 200.85, 200.86, 200.87, 200.88, 201.00, 201.01, 201.02, 201.03, 201.04, 201.05, 201.06, 201.07, 201.08, 201.10, 201.11, 201.12, 201.13, 201.14, 201.15, 201.16, 201.17, 201.18, 201.20, 201.21, 201.22, 201.23, 201.24, 201.25, 201.26, 201.27, 201.28, 201.40, 201.41, 201.42, 201.43, 201.44, 201.45, 201.46, 201.47, 201.48, 201.50, 201.51, 201.52, 201.53, 201.54, 201.55, 201.56, 201.57, 201.58, 201.60, 201.61, 201.62, 201.63, 201.64, 201.65, 201.66, 201.67, 201.68, 201.70, 201.71, 201.72, 201.73, 201.74, 201.75, 201.76, 201.77, 201.78, 201.90, 201.91, 201.92, 201.93, 201.94, 201.95, 201.96, 201.97, 201.98, 202.00, 202.01, 202.02, 202.03, 202.04, 202.05, 202.06, 202.07, 202.08, 202.10, 202.11, 202.12, 202.13, 202.14, 202.15, 202.16, 202.17, 202.18, 202.20, 202.21, 202.22, 202.23, 202.24, 202.25, 202.26, 202.27, 202.28, 202.30, 202.31, 202.32, 202.33, 202.34, 202.35, 202.36, 202.37, 202.38, 202.40, 202.41, 202.42, 202.43, 202.44, 202.45, 202.46, 202.47, 202.48, 202.50, 202.51, 202.52, 202.53, 202.54, 202.55, 202.56, 202.57, 202.58, 202.60, 202.61, 202.62, 202.63, 202.64, 202.65, 202.66, 202.67, 202.68, 202.70, 202.71, 202.72, 202.73, 202.74, 202.75, 202.76, 202.77, 202.78, 202.80, 202.81, 202.82, 202.83, 202.84, 202.85, 202.86, 202.87, 202.88, 202.90, 202.91, 202.92, 202.93, 202.94, 202.95, 202.96, 202.97, 202.98, 203.00, 203.01, 203.02, 203.10, 203.11, 203.12, 203.80, 203.81, 203.82, 204.00, 204.01, 204.02, 204.10, 204.11, 204.12, 204.20, 204.21, 204.22, 204.80, 204.81, 204.82, 204.90, 204.91,

204.92, 205.00, 205.01, 205.02, 205.10, 205.11, 205.12, 205.20, 205.21, 205.22, 205.30, 205.31, 205.32, 205.80, 205.81, 205.82, 205.90, 205.91, 205.92, 206.00, 206.01, 206.02, 206.10, 206.11, 206.12, 206.20, 206.21, 206.22, 206.80, 206.81, 206.82, 206.90, 206.91, 206.92, 207.00, 207.01, 207.02, 207.10, 207.11, 207.12, 207.20, 207.21, 207.22, 207.80, 207.81, 207.82, 208.00, 208.01, 208.02, 208.10, 208.11, 208.12, 208.20, 208.21, 208.22, 208.80, 208.81, 208.82, 208.90, 208.91, 208.92, 209.00, 209.01, 209.02, 209.03, 209.10, 209.11, 209.12, 209.13, 209.14, 209.15, 209.16, 209.17, 209.20, 209.21, 209.22, 209.23, 209.24, 209.25, 209.26, 209.27, 209.29, 209.30, 209.31, 209.32, 209.33, 209.34, 209.35, 209.36, 209.70, 209.71, 209.72, 209.73, 209.74, 209.75, 209.79, 235.0, 235.1, 235.2, 235.3, 235.4, 235.5, 235.6, 235.7, 235.8, 235.9, 236.0, 236.1, 236.2, 236.3, 236.4, 236.5, 236.6, 236.7, 236.90, 236.91, 236.99, 237.0, 237.1, 237.2, 237.3, 237.4, 237.5, 237.6, 237.70, 237.71, 237.72, 237.73, 238.79, 237.79, 237.9, 238.0, 238.1, 238.2, 238.3, 238.4, 238.5, 238.6, 238.71, 238.72, 238.73, 238.74, 238.75, 238.76, 238.77, 238.8, 238.9, 239.0, 239.1, 239.2, 239.3, 239.4, 239.5, 239.6, 239.7, 239.81, 239.89, 239.9

ICD-10-CM [Reference ONLY/Not Reportable]: C00.0, C00.1, C00.2, C00.3, C00.4, C00.5, C00.6, C00.8, C00.9, C01, C02.0, C02.1, C02.2, C02.3, C02.4, C02.8, C02.9, C03.0, C03.1, C03.9, C04.0, C04.1, C04.8, C04.9, C05.0, C05.1, C05.2, C05.8, C05.9, C06.0, C06.1, C06.2, C06.80, C06.89, C06.9, C07, C08.0, C08.1, C08.9, C09.0, C09.1, C09.8, C09.9, C10.0, C10.1, C10.2, C10.3, C10.4, C10.8, C10.9, C11.0, C11.1, C11.2, C11.3, C11.8, C11.9, C12, C13.0, C13.1, C13.2, C13.8, C13.9, C14.0, C14.2, C14.8, C15.3, C15.4, C15.5, C15.8, C15.9, C16.0, C16.1, C16.2, C16.3, C16.4, C16.5, C16.6, C16.8, C16.9, C17.0, C17.1, C17.2, C17.3, C17.8, C17.9, C18.0, C18.1, C18.2, C18.3, C18.4, C18.5, C18.6, C18.7, C18.8, C18.9, C19, C20, C21.0, C21.1, C21.2, C21.8, C22.0, C22.1, C22.2, C22.3, C22.4, C22.7, C22.8, C22.9, C23, C24.0, C24.1, C24.8, C24.9, C25.0, C25.1, C25.2, C25.3, C25.4, C25.7, C25.8, C25.9,C26.0, C26.1, C26.9, C30.0, C30.1, C31.0, C31.1, C31.2, C31.3, C31.8, C31.9, C32.0, C32.1, C32.2, C32.3, C32.8, C32.9, C33, C34.00, C34.01, C34.02, C34.10, C34.11, C34.12, C34.2, C34.30, C34.31, C34.32, C34.80, C34.81, C34.82, C34.90, C34.91, C34.92, C37, C38.0, C38.1, C38.2, C38.3, C38.4, C38.8, C39.0, C39.9, C40.00, C40.01, C40.02, C40.10, C40.11, C40.12, C40.20, C40.21, C40.22, C40.30, C40.31, C40.32, C40.80, C40.81, C40.82, C40.90, C40.91, C40.92, C41.0, C41.1, C41.2, C41.3, C41.4, C41.9, C43.0, C43.10, C43.31, C43.39, C43.4, C43.51, C43.52, C43.59, C43.60, C43.61, C43.62, C43.11, C43.70, C43.71, C43.72, C43.8, C43.12, C43.9, C43.20, C43.21, C43.22, C43.30, C44.00, C44.01, C44.02, C44.09, C44.101, C44.102, C44.109, C44.111, C44.112, C44.119, C44.121, C44.122, C44.129, C44.191, C44.192, C44.199, C44.201, C44.202, C44.209, C44.211, C44.212, C44.219, C44.221, C44.222, C44.229, C44.291, C44.292, C44.299, C44.300, C44.301, C44.309, C44.310, C44.311, C44.319, C44.320, C44.321, C44.329, C44.390, C44.391, C44.399, C44.40, C44.41, C44.42, C44.49, C44.500, C44.501, C44.509, C44.510, C44.511, C44.519, C44.520, C44.521, C44.529, C44.590, C44.591, C44.599, C44.601, C44.602, C44.609, C44.611, C44.612, C44.619, C44.621, C44.622, C44.629, C44.691, C44.692, C44.699, C44.701, C44.702, C44.709, C44.711, C44.712, C44.719, C44.721, C44.722, C44.729, C44.791, C44.792, C44.799, C44.80, C44.81, C44.82,C44.89, C44.90, C44.91, C44.92, C44.99, C45.0, C45.1, C45.2, C45.7, C45.9, C46.0, C46.1, C46.2, C46.3, C46.4, C46.50, C46.51, C46.52, C46.7, C46.9, C47.0, C47.10, C47.11, C44.30, C47.12, C47.20, C47.21, C47.22, C47.3, C47.4, C47.5, C47.6, C47.8, C47.9, C48.0, C48.1, C48.2, C48.8, C49.0, C49.10, C49.11, C49.12, C49.20, C49.21, C49.22, C49.3, C49.4,

C49.5, C49.6, C49.8, C49.9, C4A.0, C4A.10, C4A.11, C4A.12, C4A.20, C4A.21, C4A.22, C4A.30, C4A.31, C4A.39, C4A.4, C4A.51, C4A.52, C4A.59, C4A.60, C4A.61, C4A.62, C4A.70, C4A.71, C4A.72, C4A.8, C4A.9, C50.011, C50.012, C50.019, C50.021, C50.022, C50.029, C50.111, C50.112, C50.119, C50.121, C50.122, C50.129, C50.211, C50.212, C50.219, C50.221, C50.222, C50.229, C50.311, C50.312, C50.319, C50.321, C50.322, C50.329, C50.411, C50.412, C50.419, C50.421, C50.422, C50.429, C50.511, C50.512, C50.519, C50.521, C50.522, C50.529, C50.611, C50.612, C50.619, C50.621, C50.622, C50.629, C50.811, C50.812, C50.819, C50.821, C50.822, C50.829, C50.911, C50.912, C50.919, C50.921, C50.922, C50.929, C51.0, C51.1, C51.2, C51.8, C51.9, C52, C53.0, C53.1, C53.8, C53.9, C54.0, C54.1, C54.2, C54.3, C54.8, C54.9, C55, C56.1, C56.2, C56.9, C57.00, C57.01, C57.02, C57.10, C57.11, C57.12, C57.20, C57.21, C57.22, C57.3, C57.4, C57.7, C57.8, C57.9, C58, C60.0, C60.1, C60.2, C60.8, C60.9, C61, C62.00, C62.01, C62.02, C62.10, C62.11, C62.12, C62.90, C62.91, C62.92, C63.00, C63.01, C63.02, C63.10, C63.11, C63.12, C63.2, C63.7, C63.8, C63.9, C64.1, C64.2, C64.9, C65.1, C65.2, C65.9, C66.1, C66.2, C66.9, C67.0, C67.1, C67.2, C67.3, C67.4, C67.5, C67.6, C67.7, C67.8, C67.9, C68.0, C68.1, C68.8, C68.9, C69.00, C69.01, C69.02, C69.10, C69.11, C69.12, C69.20, C69.21, C69.22, C69.30, C69.31, C69.32, C69.40, C69.41, C69.42, C69.50, C69.51, C69.52, C69.60, C69.61, C69.62, C69.80, C69.81, C69.82, C69.90, C69.91, C69.92, C70.0, C70.1, C70.9, C71.0, C71.1, C71.2, C71.3, C71.4, C71.5, C71.6, C71.7, C71.8, C71.9, C72.0, C72.1, C72.20, C72.21, C72.22, C72.30, C72.31, C72.32, C72.40, C72.41, C72.42, C72.50, C72.59, C72.9, C73, C74.00, C74.01, C74.02, C74.10, C74.11, C74.12, C74.90, C74.91, C74.92, C75.0, C75.1, C75.2, C75.3, C75.4, C75.5, C75.8, C75.9, C76.0, C76.1, C76.2, C76.3, C76.40, C76.41, C76.42, C76.50, C76.51, C76.52, C76.8, C77.0, C77.1, C77.2, C77.3, C77.4, C77.5, C77.8, C77.9, C78.00, C78.01, C78.02, C78.1, C78.2, C78.30, C78.39, C78.4, C78.5, C78.6, C78.7, C78.80, C78.89, C79.00, C79.01, C79.02, C79.10, C79.11, C79.19, C79.2, C79.31, C79.32, C79.40, C79.49, C79.51, C79.52, C79.60, C79.61, C79.62, C79.70, C79.71, C79.72, C79.81, C79.82, C79.89, C79.9, C7A.00, C7A.010, C7A.011, C7A.012, C7A.019, C7A.020, C7A.021, C7A.022, C7A.023, C7A.024, C7A.025, C7A.026, C7A.029, C7A.090, C7A.091, C7A.092, C7A.093, C7A.094, C7A.095, C7A.096, C7A.098, C7A.1, C7A.8, C7B.00, C7B.01, C7B.02, C7B.03, C7B.04, C7B.09, C7B.1, C7B.8, C80.0, C80.1, C80.2, C81.00, C81.01, C81.02, C81.03, C81.04, C81.05, C81.06, C81.07, C81.08, C81.09, C81.10, C81.11, C81.12, C81.13, C81.14, C81.15, C81.16, C81.17, C81.18, C81.19, C81.20, C81.21, C81.22, C81.23, C81.24, C81.25, C81.26, C81.27, C81.28, C81.29, C81.30, C81.31, C81.32, C81.33, C81.34, C81.35, C81.36, C81.37, C81.38, C81.39, C81.40, C81.41, C81.42, C81.43, C81.44, C81.45, C81.46, C81.47, C81.48, C81.49, C81.70, C81.71, C81.72, C81.73, C81.74, C81.75, C81.76, C81.77, C81.78, C81.79, C81.90, C81.91, C81.92, C81.93, C81.94, C81.95, C81.96, C81.97, C81.98, C81.99, C82.00, C82.01, C82.02, C82.03, C82.04, C82.05, C82.06, C82.07, C82.08, C82.09, C82.10, C82.11, C82.12, C82.13, C82.14, C82.15, C82.16, C82.17, C82.18, C82.19, C82.20, C82.21, C82.22, C82.23, C82.24, C82.25, C82.26, C82.27, C82.28, C82.29, C82.30, C82.31, C82.32, C82.33, C82.34, C82.35, C82.36, C82.37, C82.38, C82.39, C82.40, C82.41, C82.42, C82.43, C82.44, C82.45, C82.46, C82.47, C82.48, C82.49, C82.50, C82.51, C82.52, C82.53, C82.54, C82.55, C82.56, C82.57, C82.58, C82.59, C82.60, C82.61, C82.62, C82.63, C82.64, C82.65, C82.66, C82.67, C82.68, C82.69, C82.80, C82.81, C82.82, C82.83, C82.84, C82.85, C82.86, C82.87, C82.88, C82.89, C82.90, C82.91, C82.92, C82.93, C82.94, C82.95, C82.96, C82.97, C82.98, C82.99, C83.00, C83.01, C83.02, C83.03, C83.04, C83.05, C83.06, C83.07,

C83.08, C83.09, C83.10, C83.11, C83.12, C83.13, C83.14, C83.15, C83.16, C83.17, C83.18, C83.19, C83.30, C83.31, C83.32, C83.33, C83.34, C83.35, C83.36, C83.37, C83.38, C83.39, C83.50, C83.51, C83.52, C83.53, C83.54, C83.55, C83.56, C83.57, C83.58, C83.59, C83.70, C83.71, C83.72, C83.73, C83.74, C83.75, C83.76, C83.77, C83.78, C83.79, C83.80, C83.81, C83.82, C83.83, C83.84, C83.85, C83.86, C83.87, C83.88, C83.89, C83.90, C83.91, C83.92, C83.93, C83.94, C83.95, C83.96, C83.97, C83.98, C83.99, C84.00, C84.01, C84.02, C84.03, C84.04, C84.05, C84.06, C84.07, C84.08, C84.09, C84.10, C84.11, C84.12, C84.13, C84.14, C84.15, C84.16, C84.17, C84.18, C84.19, C84.40, C84.41, C84.42, C84.43, C84.44, C84.45, C84.46, C84.47, C84.48, C84.49, C84.60, C84.61, C84.62, C84.63, C84.64, C84.65, C84.66, C84.67, C84.68, C84.69, C84.70, C84.71, C84.72, C84.73, C84.74, C84.75, C84.76, C84.77, C84.78, C84.79, C84.90, C84.91, C84.92, C84.93, C84.94, C84.95, C84.96, C84.97, C84.98, C84.99, C84.A0, C84.A1, C84.A2, C84.A3, C84.A4, C84.A5, C84.A6, C84.A7, C84.A8, C84.A9, C84.Z0, C84.Z1, C84.Z2, C84.Z3, C84.Z4, C84.Z5, C84.Z6, C84.Z7, C84.Z8, C84.Z9, C85.10, C85.11, C85.12, C85.13, C85.14, C85.15, C85.16, C85.17, C85.18, C85.19, C85.20, C85.21, C85.22, C85.23, C85.24, C85.25, C85.26, C85.27, C85.28, C85.29, C85.80, C85.81, C85.82, C85.83, C85.84, C85.85, C85.86, C85.87, C85.88, C85.89, C85.90, C85.91, C85.92, C85.93, C85.94, C85.95, C85.96, C85.97, C85.98, C85.99, C86.0, C86.1, C86.2, C86.3, C86.4, C86.5, C86.6, C88.0, C88.2, C88.3, C88.4, C88.8, C88.9, C90.00, C90.01, C90.02, C90.10, C90.11, C90.12, C90.20, C90.21, C90.22, C90.30, C90.31, C90.32, C91.00, C91.01, C91.02, C91.10, C91.11, C91.12, C91.30, C91.31, C91.32, C91.40, C91.41, C91.42, C91.50, C91.51, C91.52, C91.60, C91.61, C91.62, C91.90, C91.91, C91.92, C91.A0, C91.A1, C91.A2, C91.Z0, C91.Z1, C91.Z2, C92.00, C92.01, C92.02, C92.10, C92.11, C92.12, C92.20, C92.21, C92.22, C92.30, C92.31, C92.32, C92.40, C92.41, C92.42, C92.50, C92.51, C92.52, C92.60, C92.61, C92.62, C92.90, C92.91, C92.92, C92.A0, C92.A1, C92.A2, C92.Z0, C92.Z1, C92.Z2, C93.00, C93.01, C93.02, C93.10, C93.11, C93.12, C93.30, C93.31, C93.32, C93.90, C93.91, C93.92, C93.Z0, C93.Z1, C93.Z2, C94.00, C94.01, C94.02, C94.20, C94.21, C94.22, C94.30, C94.31, C94.32, C94.40, C94.41, C94.42, C94.6, C94.80, C94.81, C94.82, C95.00, C95.01, C95.02, C95.10, C95.11, C95.12, C95.90, C95.91, C95.92, C96.0, C96.2, C96.4, C96.5,C96.6, C96.9, C96.A, C96.Z, D37.01, D37.02, D37.030, D37.031, D37.032, D37.039, D37.04, D37.05, D37.09, D37.1, D37.2, D37.3, D37.4, D37.5, D37.6, D37.8, D37.9, D38.0, D38.1, D38.2, D38.3, D38.4, D38.5, D38.6, D39.0, D39.10, D39.11, D39.12, D39.2, D39.8, D39.9, D40.0, D40.10, D40.11, D40.12, D40.8, D40.9, D41.00, D41.01, D41.02, D41.10, D41.11, D41.12, D41.20, D41.21, D41.22, D41.3, D41.4, D41.8, D41.9, D42.0, D42.1, D42.9, D43.0, D43.1, D43.2, D43.3, D43.4, D43.8, D43.9, D44.0, D44.10, D44.11, D44.12, D44.2, D44.3, D44.4, D44.5, D44.6, D44.7, D44.8, D44.9, D45, D46.0, D46.1, D46.20, D46.21, D46.22, D46.4, D46.9, D46.A, D46.B, D46.C, D46.Z, D47.0, D47.1, D47.2, D47.3, D47.4, D47.9, D47.Z1, D47.Z9, D48.0, D48.1, D48.2, D48.3, D48.4, D48.5, D48.60, D48.61, D48.62, D48.7, D48.9, D49.0, D49.1, D49.2, D49.3, D49.4, D49.5, D49.6, D49.7, D49.81, D49.89, D49.9, Q85.00, Q85.01, Q85.02, Q85.03, Q85.09

Accompanied by

One of the following patient encounter codes: 77427, 77431, 77432, 77435, 77470

OR

One of the following patient encounter codes: 99201, 99202, 99203, 99204, 99205, 99212, 99213, 99214, 99215

AND

One of the following patient encounter codes – Procedure codes: 51720, 96401, 96402, 96405, 96406, 96409, 96411, 96413, 96415, 96416, 96417, 96420, 96422, 96423, 96425, 96440, 96446, 96450, 96521, 96522, 96523, 96542, 96549

• Measure #71 only needs to be reported when the patient is female and has the following diagnosis code indicating breast cancer:

ICD-9-CM: 174.0, 174.1, 174.2, 174.3, 174.4, 174.5, 174.6, 174.8, 174.9

ICD-10-CM [Reference ONLY/Not Reportable]: C50.011, C50.012, C50.019, C50.111, C50.112, C50.119, C50.211, C50.212, C50.219, C50.311, C50.312, C50.319, C50.411, C50.412, C50.419, C50.511, C50.512, C50.519, C50.611, C50.612, C50.619, C50.811, C50.812, C50.819, C50.911, C50.912, C50.919

• Measure #72 only needs to be reported when the patient is 18 through 80 years old and has the following diagnosis code indicating colon cancer:

ICD-9-CM: 153.0, 153.1, 153.2, 153.3, 153.4, 153.6, 153.7, 153.8, 153.9

ICD-10-CM [Reference ONLY/Not Reportable]: C18.0, C18.2, C18.3, C18.4, C18.5, C18.6, C18.7, C18.8, C18.9

• Measure #144 only needs to be reported when patients are identified in Measure #143 with pain present (1125F).

• Report a numerator option on **all applicable** measures within the Oncology Measures Group for each patient within the eligible professional's patient sample.

• Instructions for qualifying numerator option reporting for each of the measures within the Oncology Measures Group are displayed on the next several pages. The following composite G-code has been created for registry only measures groups for use by registries that utilize claims data. This composite G-code may be reported in lieu of the individual quality-data codes for each of the measures within the group, if all quality actions for the patient have been performed for all the measures within the group. However, it is not necessary to submit the following composite G-code for registry-based submissions.

Composite G-code G8953: All quality actions for the applicable measures in the Oncology Measures Group have been performed for this patient

• To report satisfactorily the Oncology Measures Group requires **all applicable** measures for each patient within the eligible professional's patient sample to be reported a minimum of once during the reporting period.

• Measure #110 need only be reported a minimum of once during the reporting period when the patient's visit included in the patient sample population is between January and March for the 2012-2013 influenza season **OR** between October and December for the 2013-2014 influenza season. When the patient's office visit is between April and September, Measure #110 is not applicable and will not affect the eligible provider's reporting or performance rate. Measure #110 need only be reported on patients 18 years and older.

• Measures groups containing a measure with a 0% performance rate will not be counted as satisfactorily reporting the measures group. The recommended clinical quality action must be performed on at least one patient for each measure within the measures group reported by the eligible professional. Performance exclusion quality-data codes are not counted in the performance denominator. If the eligible professional submits all performance exclusion quality-data codes, the performance rate would be 0/0 and would be considered satisfactorily reporting. If a measure within a measures group is not applicable to a patient, the patient would not be counted in the performance denominator for that measure (e.g., Oncology Measures Group - Measure #71: Breast Cancer: Hormonal Therapy for Stage IC-IIIC Estrogen Receptor/Progesterone Receptor (ER/PR) Positive Breast Cancer would not be applicable to male patients according to the patient sample criteria). If the measure is not applicable for all patients within the sample, the performance rate would be 0/0 and would be considered satisfactorily reporting.

• When using the 20 Patient Sample Method, report all applicable measures for the 20 unique procedures performed (patients seen) a majority of which must be Medicare Part B FFS procedures (patients) for the 12-month or 6-month reporting period.

MEASURE #72 (NQF 0385): COLON CANCER: CHEMOTHERAPY FOR AJCC STAGE III COLON CANCER PATIENTS

DESCRIPTION:

Percentage of patients aged 18 through 80 years with AJCC Stage III colon cancer who are referred for adjuvant chemotherapy, prescribed adjuvant chemotherapy, or have previously received adjuvant chemotherapy within the 12-month reporting period

NUMERATOR:

Patients who are referred for adjuvant chemotherapy, prescribed adjuvant chemotherapy, or who have previously received adjuvant chemotherapy within the 12-month reporting period

Definitions:

Adjuvant Chemotherapy – According to current NCCN guidelines, the following therapies are recommended: 5-FU/LV/oxaliplatin (mFOLFOX6) as the standard of care (category 1); bolus 5-FU/LV/oxaliplatin (FLOX, category 1); capecitabine/oxaliplatin (CapeOx, category 1); or single agent capecitabine (category 2A) or 5-FU/LV (category 2A) in patients felt to be inappropriate for oxaliplatin therapy (NCCN). See clinical recommendation statement for cases where leucovorin is not available.

Prescribed – May include prescription ordered for the patient for adjuvant chemotherapy at one or more visits in the 12-month period OR patient already receiving adjuvant chemotherapy as documented in the current medication list.

NUMERATOR NOTE: *The correct combination of numerator code(s) must be reported on the claim form in order to properly report this measure. The "correct combination" of codes may require the submission of multiple numerator codes.*

Numerator Quality-Data Coding Options for Reporting Satisfactorily: Adjuvant Chemotherapy Referred, Prescribed or Previously Received

*(One G-Code [**G8927**] and one CPT II code [**3388F**] are required on the claim form to submit this numerator option)*

G8927: Adjuvant chemotherapy referred, prescribed or previously received for AJCC Stage III colon cancer

AND

CPT II 3388F: AJCC Colon Cancer Stage III, documented

OR

Adjuvant Chemotherapy not Referred, Prescribed or Previously Received for Documented Reasons

*(One G-code [**G8928**] and one CPT II code [**3388F**] are required on the claim form to submit this numerator option)*

G8928: Adjuvant chemotherapy **not** prescribed or previously received, reason specified **AND**

CPT II 3388F: AJCC Colon Cancer Stage III, documented

OR

If patient is not eligible for this measure because patient is not stage III colon cancer, report:

Patient not Stage III Colon Cancer

*(One CPT II code [**33xxF**] is required on the claim form to submit this numerator option)* **CPT II 3382F:** AJCC Colon Cancer Stage 0, documented

OR

CPT II 3384F: AJCC Colon Cancer Stage I, documented

OR

CPT II 3386F: AJCC Colon Cancer Stage II, documented

OR

CPT II 3390F: AJCC Colon Cancer Stage IV, documented

OR

If patient is not eligible for this measure because cancer stage is not documented, report: Cancer Stage not Documented

*(One CPT II code [***3382F-8P***] is required on the claim form to submit this category)*

Append a reporting modifier (**8P**) to CPT Category II code **3382F** to report circumstances when the patient is not eligible for the measure.

3382F ***with*** **8P: No** documentation of cancer stage

OR

Adjuvant Chemotherapy not Referred, Prescribed or Previously Received, Reason not Given *(One G-code [***G8929***] and one CPT II code [***3388F***] are required on the claim form to submit this numerator option)*

G8929: Adjuvant chemotherapy **not** prescribed or previously received, reason not given **AND**

CPT II 3388F: AJCC Colon Cancer Stage III, documented

MEASURE #110 (NQF 0041): PREVENTIVE CARE AND SCREENING: INFLUENZA IMMUNIZATION

DESCRIPTION:

Percentage of patients aged 6 months and older seen for a visit between October 1 and March 31 who received an influenza immunization OR who reported previous receipt of an influenza immunization

NUMERATOR:

Patients who received an influenza immunization OR who reported previous receipt of influenza immunization

Numerator Instructions:

• If reporting this measure between January 1, 2013 and March 31, 2013, G-code **G8482** should be reported when the influenza immunization is ordered or administered to the patient during the months of August, September, October, November, and December of 2012 or January, February, and March of 2013 for the flu season ending March 31, 2013.

• If reporting this measure between October 1, 2013 and December 31, 2013, G-code **G8482** should be reported when the influenza immunization is ordered or administered to the patient during the months of August, September, October, November, and December of 2013 for the flu season ending March 31, 2014.

• Influenza immunizations administered during the month of August or September of a given flu season (either 2012-2013 flu season OR 2013-2014 flu season) can be reported when a visit occurs during the flu season (October 1 - March 31). In these cases, **G8482** should be reported.

Definition:

Previous Receipt - Receipt of the current season's influenza immunization from another provider OR from same provider prior to the visit to which the measure is applied (typically, prior vaccination would include influenza vaccine given since August 1st).

Numerator Quality-Data Coding Options for Reporting Satisfactorily: Influenza Immunization Administered

G8482: Influenza immunization administered or previously received

OR

Influenza Immunization not Administered for Documented Reasons

G8483: Influenza immunization was not ordered or administered for reasons documented by clinician (e.g., patient allergy or other medical reason, patient declined or other patient reasons, or other system reasons)

OR

Influenza Immunization Ordered or Recommended, but not Administered

G0919: Influenza immunization ordered or recommended (to be given at alternate location or alternate provider); vaccine not available at time of visit

OR

Influenza Immunization not Administered, Reason not Given

G8484: Influenza immunization was **not** ordered or administered, reason not given

MEASURE #130 (NQF 0419): DOCUMENTATION OF CURRENT MEDICATIONS IN THE MEDICAL RECORD

DESCRIPTION:

Percentage of specified visits for patients aged 18 years and older for which the eligible professional attests to documenting a list of current medications to the best of his/her knowledge and ability. This list ***must*** include ALL prescriptions, over-the-counters, herbals, and vitamin/mineral/dietary (nutritional) supplements AND ***must*** contain the medications' name, dosage, frequency and route of administration

NUMERATOR:

Eligible professional attests to documenting a list of current medications to the best of his/her knowledge and ability. This list ***must*** include ALL prescriptions, over-the counters, herbals, and vitamin/mineral/dietary (nutritional) supplements AND ***must*** contain the medications' name, dosages, frequency and route of administration

Definitions:

Current Medications – Medications the patient is presently taking including all prescriptions, over-the-counters, herbals and vitamin/mineral/dietary (nutritional) supplements with each medication's name, dosage, frequency and administered route.

Not Eligible – A patient is **not** eligible if the following reason exists:

• Patient is in an urgent or emergent medical situation where time is of the essence and to delay treatment would jeopardize the patient's health status.

*NUMERATOR NOTE: By reporting **G8427**, the eligible professional is attesting the documented medication information is current, accurate and complete to the best of his/her knowledge and ability at the time of the patient encounter. This code should also be reported if the eligible professional documented the patient is not currently taking any medications. Eligible professionals reporting this measure may document medication information received from the patient, authorized representative(s), caregiver(s) or other available healthcare resources.*

Numerator Quality-Data Coding Options for Reporting Satisfactorily: Current Medications Documented

G8427: Eligible professional attests to documenting the patient's current medications to the best of his/her knowledge and ability

OR

Current Medications not Documented, Patient not Eligible

G8430: Eligible professional attests the patient is not eligible for medication documentation

OR

Current Medications with Name, Dosage, Frequency, Route not Documented, Reason not Given

G8428: Current medications **not** documented by the eligible professional, reason not given

MEASURE #143 (NQF 0384): ONCOLOGY: MEDICAL AND RADIATION – PAIN INTENSITY QUANTIFIED

DESCRIPTION:

Percentage of patient visits, regardless of patient age, with a diagnosis of cancer currently receiving chemotherapy or radiation therapy in which pain intensity is quantified

NUMERATOR:

Patient visits in which pain intensity is quantified

Numerator Instructions: Pain intensity should be quantified using a standard instrument, such as a 0-10 numeric rating scale, a categorical scale, or the pictorial scale.

Numerator Options:

Pain severity quantified; pain present **(1125F)**

OR

Pain severity quantified; no pain present **(1126F)**

OR

Pain severity **not** documented, reason not otherwise specified **(1125F with 8P)**

This page intentionally left blank

INDEX

A

B

C

D

E

F

G

H

I

J

K

L

M

N

O

P

Q

R

S

T

U

V

W

X

Y

Z